Isolation, Characterization, and Utilization of T Lymphocyte Clones

Contributors

M. E. Andrew
Barbara A. Araneo
Esther Arman
Yoshihiro Asano
Thomas M. Aune
Fritz H. Bach
Barbara N. Beck
T. J. Braciale
V. L. Braciale
Jennifer Bruce
K. Theodor Brunner
Hartwig Bunzendahl
Harvey Cantor
Jean-Charles Cerottini
Chuan Chen
Robert W. Chesnut
Jacques M. Chiller
Maurizio Cianfriglia
Andreas Conzelmann
Patricia Corthesy
Elaine C. DeFreitas
Helen Derry
Michel Dy
Klaus Eichmann
John M. Ely
C. Garrison Fathman
Anthony S. Fauci
Frank W. Fitch
Varda Friedman
Igal Gery
Steven Gillis
Andrew L. Glasebrook
Jörg Goronzy
Marie-Lise Gougeon
Sam D. Graham, Jr.
Howard M. Grey
Elizabeth A. Grimm
Ute Hamann
Günter Hämmerling
Karen S. Hathcock
Hans Hengartner
Richard J. Hodes
Leroy E. Hood
Suzanna J. Horvath
Lothar Hültner
A. J. Infante
Peter Isakson
Jun Iwaki
Judith P. Johnson
Judith A. Kapp
John W. Kappler
Ursula Kees
Anne Kelso
Masao Kimoto
Ellen Kraig
Peter H. Krammer
Mitchell Kronenberg
Rudolf C. Kuppers
Lise Leclercq
H. James Leibson
Marie-Luise Lohmann-Matthes
Peter Lonai
H. Robson MacDonald
Bernard Malissen
Fabrizio Marcucci
Philippa Marrack
Claude Mawas
Inga Melchers
Andrea Michnay
R. G. Miller
N. A. Mitchison
S. B. Mizel
Diane Mochizuki
Katherine Molnar-Kimber
Jean-Louis Moreau
Markus Nabholz
Makoto Nonaka
Carl W. Pierce
Michael B. Prystowsky
Ellen Puré
Joseph Puri
Neal Roehm
Steven A. Rosenberg
Huub F. C. Savelkoul
Anneliese Schimpl
Ronald H. Schwartz
Miriam Segall
Rafick P. Sekaly
Linda A. Sherman
Minoru Shigeta
Markus M. Simon
Alfred Singer
Barry J. Skidmore
Gerard Somme
Craig M. Sorensen
Jonathan Sprent
Benjamin Sredni
Fritz Staber
Tomio Tada
Michael J. Taussig
Jacques Thèze
Ellen S. Vitetta
David Volkman
Michael Waller
James Watson
Susan R. Webb
Siew-Lin Wee
Dale Wegmann
Arthur Weiss
Cornelia Weyand
Darcy B. Wilson
Gabriele Zahn
Rudolf H. Zubler

Isolation, Characterization, and Utilization of T Lymphocyte Clones

Edited by

C. GARRISON FATHMAN
Division of Immunology
Department of Medicine
Stanford University
Stanford, California

FRANK W. FITCH
Department of Pathology and
Committee on Immunology
University of Chicago
Chicago, Illinois

1982

ACADEMIC PRESS
A Subsidiary of Harcourt Brace Jovanovich, Publishers
New York London
Paris San Diego San Francisco São Paulo Sydney Tokyo Toronto

ACADEMIC PRESS, INC.
111 Fifth Avenue, New York, New York 10003

United Kingdom Edition published by
ACADEMIC PRESS, INC. (LONDON) LTD.
24/28 Oval Road, London NW1 7DX

LIBRARY OF CONGRESS CATALOG CARD NUMBER: 82-72508

ISBN 0-12-249920-4

PRINTED IN THE UNITED STATES OF AMERICA

82 83 84 85 9 8 7 6 5 4 3 2 1

Contents

CONTRIBUTORS xxi

PREFACE xxvii

1 Introduction and Historical Overview

Frank W. Fitch and Jean-Charles Cerottini

Text 1
References 7

2 Differentiation within the Immune System: The Importance of Cloning

N. A. Mitchison

I. Comparison with the Nervous System 11
II. Cloning Methods 13
III. Questions of the Day 14
References 16

I. IL-1 (Lymphocyte Activating Factor) and IL-2 (T Cell Growth Factor)

3 Biochemical Characterization of Interleukin-2 (T Cell Growth Factor)

Steven Gillis, James Watson, and Diane Mochizuki

I. IL-2 Microassay 24
II. Purification of Human and Murine IL-2 24

III. Temperature, Chemical, and Enzymatic Treatments of IL-2 26
IV. Improved Cellular Sources for IL-2 Production and Characterization 26
V. Polyacrylamide Gel Electrophoresis of IL-2 30
VI. Molecular Prospects for the Future 36
VII. Conclusions 38
References 38

4 Production and Assay of Interleukin-1 (IL-1)

Igal Gery

I. Production of IL-1 42
II. IL-1 Assay 49
III. Conclusions 52
References 53

5 Production and Properties of Human IL-2

Elizabeth A. Grimm and Steven A. Rosenberg

I. Introduction 57
II. Culture Conditions for Generation of Human IL-2 58
III. Testing of Culture Supernatant for IL-2 Content 63
IV. Removal of PHA from IL-2-Containing Culture Supernatants 66
V. Long-Term Growth of Cytotoxic T Lymphocytes in IL-2 69
VI. Use of IL-2-Containing Preparations for Activation of Cytolytic Lymphocytes: IL-2 Providing the Proliferative Stimulus Necessary for Allogeneic IVS 77
VII. Conclusions 79
References 79

6 Signal Requirement for T Lymphocyte Activation

Jacques M. Chiller, Elaine C. DeFreitas, Robert W. Chesnut, Howard M. Grey, and Barry J. Skidmore

I. T Lymphocyte Propagation 83
II. T Lymphocyte Activation 86
References 89

II. T Cell Hybridomas and Their Products

7 An Overview

Tomio Tada and Makoto Nonaka

I. A Catalog 97
II. Problems 99
III. Lessons 101
IV. Conclusions 105
References 105

8 Factors, Receptors, and Their Ligands: Studies with *H-2* Restricted Helper Hybridoma Clones

Peter Lonai, Esther Arman, Huub F. C. Savelkoul, Varda Friedman, Joseph Puri, and Günter Hämmerling

I. Ia-Associated Antigen Complex 109
II. Isolation of T Hybridomas 111
III. Characterization of the Hybridoma Clones 111
IV. Analysis of the Altered Self-Dual Recognition Problem 112
V. Isolation of Helper Factors 116
References 116

9 Properties of Antigen-Specific *H-2* Restricted T Cell Hybridomas

Philippa Marrack, Sam D. Graham, Jr., H. James Leibson, Neal Roehm, Dale Wegmann, and John W. Kappler

I. Factor Production by T Cell Hybridomas 120
II. Use of T Cell Hybridomas to Examine Properties of the T Cell Receptor 122
III. T Cell Hybridomas Do Not Express Unexpected H-2 Specificites 123
IV. Karyotypic Analysis of T Cell Hybridomas 124
References 126

10 Studies on an Antigen-Specific Suppressor Factor Produced by a T Hybrid Line

Michael J. Taussig

I. Derivation and Specificity of the A1 Supressor Line 128
II. B Cells as the Targets for A1 Factor 129
III. Genetic Control of Suppression 130
IV. Interaction between Suppressor Factor and Monoclonal Antibodies in Regulation of the Immune Response 132
V. Conclusion 134
References 135

11 Characterization of Antigen-Specific Suppressor Factors from T Cell Hybridomas

Judith A. Kapp and Barbara A. Araneo

I. Experimental Systems Used to Identify Suppressor T Cells and Their Products 138
II. Characterization of GAT- and GT-Specific TsF 140
III. Comparison of GAT-TsF and GT-TsF to Other Suppressor T Cell Factors 144
References 145

12 Suppression of Antibody Responses by a T Cell Hybridoma-Derived Haplotype-Specific Suppressor Factor

Craig M. Sorensen and Carl W. Pierce

I. Properties of TsF-H 150
II. Mechanism of Action of TsF-H 152
III. Conclusions 153
References 155

13 Soluble Immune Response Suppressor (SIRS) Derived from T Cell Hybridomas

Thomas M. Aune and Carl W. Pierce

I. Characteristics of SIRS 158
II. Speculations 161
References 161

III. The Somatic Cell Genetic Analysis of Cytolytic T Lymphocyte Functions

14 An Overview

Markus Nabholz

I. CTL Lines 166
II. Mutants 170
III. Somatic Cell Hybrids 173
IV. Outlook 176
References 179

15 Karyotype Evolution of Cytolytic T Cell Lines

Judith P. Johnson, Maurizio Cianfriglia, Andrew L. Glasebrook, and Markus Nabholz

I. Karyotype Analysis of Functional T Cell Lines 183
II. Discussion 189
References 190

16 Growth Regulation of Cytolytic T Cell Lines by Interleukin-2

Rafick P. Sekaly, H. Robson MacDonald, and Markus Nabholz

I. Mechanisms of Action of Growth Factors 194
II. Mechanisms of Action of TCGF on a Cloned CTL Line 196
References 202

17 Correlation between Cytolytic Activity, Growth Factor Dependence, and Lectin Resistance in Cytolytic T Cell Hybrids

Andreas Conzelmann, Patricia Corthesy, and Markus Nabholz

I. Introduction 205
II. Origin of CTL Hybrids 206
III. CTL Activity, VV Resistance, and CS Dependence of Hybrids 206

IV. Selection of CS^- Variants from Cloned CS^+ Cytolytic Hybrids 210
V. Conclusions 213
References 214

IV. Clonal Analysis by Limiting Dilution

18 An Overview

R. G. Miller

I. Theory of Limiting Dilution 220
II. Experimental Conditions Required for Limiting Dilution Analysis of CTL-P Frequencies 224
III. The CTL-P Frequency Problem 228
References 230

19 Clonal Analysis of Helper and Cytolytic T Cells: Multiple, Independently Regulated Precursor Sets at Frequencies Suggesting a Limited Repertoire

Klaus Eichmann, Jörg Goronzy, Ute Hamann, Peter H. Krammer, Rudolf C. Kuppers, Inga Melchers, Markus M. Simon, and Gabriele Zahn

I. The Assay 234
II. Multiple Populations of T Precursor Cells 236
III. Independent Regulation of Each Precursor Population 238
IV. Lyt-Phenotypic Differences between T Precursor Populations 241
V. Conclusions 241
References 243

20 Frequency, Regulation, and H-2 Epitope Specificity of Alloreactive and *H-2* Restricted CTL Clones

Günter J. Hämmerling, Cornelia Weyand, and Jörg Goronzy

I. Topographic Arrangement of Alloantigenic Determinants on the $H\text{-}2K^k$ Molecule 245

II. Distinct CTL Subpopulations with Different Precursor Frequencies Detected by Limiting Dilution Analysis 246
III. Target Inhibition by mc Anti-H-2 of CTL Clones Generated in the Limiting Dilution System 247
IV. Target Inhibition of $H\text{-}2K^k$-Restricted, TNP-Specific CTL Clones 248
Conclusions 249
References 251

21 Production of Lymphokines by Murine T Cells Grown in Limiting Dilution and Long-Term Cultures

Peter H. Krammer, Michel Dy, Lothar Hültner, Peter Isakson, Ursula Kees, Marie-Luise Lohmann-Matthes, Fabrizio Marcucci, Andrea Michnay, Ellen Puré, Anneliese Schimpl, Fritz Staber, Ellen S. Vitetta, and Michael Waller

I. Introduction 253
II. Analysis of Lymphokine Release in Limiting Dilution Microcultures 254
III. Analysis of Lymphokine Production from Long-Term T Cell Clones and Lines 258
IV. Conclusions 261
References 261

V. Murine T Cell Clones Reactive with Alloantigens

22 An Overview

Andrew L. Glasebrook and Frank W. Fitch

I Conditions for Deriving T Cell Clones 266
II. Cytolytic T Cell Clones 269
III. Noncytolytic T Cell Clones 273
IV. Factors Produced by Alloreactive T Cell Clones 276
V. Conclusions 278
References 280

23 Cloned Continuous Lines of *H-2*-Restricted Influenza Virus-Specific CTL: Probes of T Lymphocyte Specificity and Heterogeneity

T. J. Braciale, V. L. Braciale, and M. E. Andrew

I. Properties of Influenza-Specific CTL Clones 286
II. Conclusions 293
References 294

24 Cytolytic T Lymphocyte Clones Recognizing Murine Sarcoma Virus-Induced Tumor Antigens

K. Theodor Brunner, Arthur Weiss, H. Robson MacDonald, and Jean-Charles Cerottini

I. Optimal Microculture Conditions for the Generation of MoLV-Specific CTL Clones 298
II. Frequency Determination of MoLV-Specific CTL Precursors 300
III. Isolation and Maintenance of MoLV-Specific CTL Clones 301
IV. Specificity of MoLV-Specific CTL Clones 302
V. Surface Phenotype of MoLV-Specific CTL Clones 309
VI. Conclusions 309
References 310

25 The Specificity Repertoire of Cytolytic T Lymphocytes

Linda A. Sherman

I. Analysis of Receptor Specificity 314
II. CTL Receptor Repertoire of the B10.D2 Anti-H-$2K^b$ Response 315
III. Specificity Repertoire of the bm11 Anti-H-$2K^b$ Response 317
IV. The C57BL/6 Anti-bm11 CTL Response: A Model for Determinant Recognition 319
V. The Influence of MHC on Receptor Repertoire 320
References 322

26 Alloreactive T Cell Clones Which Recognize Hybrid Determinants

Barbara N. Beck and C. Garrison Fathman

Text 325
References 328

27 Anti-H-2 Reactivity of Mls-Specific T Cell Clones

Susan R. Webb, Jennifer Bruce, Katherine Molnar-Kimber, Darcy B. Wilson, and J. Sprent

I. H-2 Specificity of Uncloned Mls-Reactive T Cell Lines 332
II. Anti-H-2 and Anti-Mls Reactivity of T Cell Clones 334
III. Characteristics of Cloned Mls-Reactive T Cell Lines 336
IV. Conclusions 336
References 338

28 Lymphokine Production by Cytolytic and Noncytolytic Alloreactive T Cell Clones

Andrew L. Glasebrook, Anne Kelso, Rudolf H. Zubler, John M. Ely, Michael B. Prystowsky, and Frank W. Fitch

I. Analysis of Lymphokine Production by a Noncytolytic T Cell Clone and Its Variant upon Alloantigenic Stimulation 342
II. Analysis of Lymphokine Production by Noncytolytic and Cytolytic Alloreactive T Cell Clones after Stimulation with Mitogen 345
III. Biological Separation of Lymphokine Activities Using Different T Cell Clones 348
IV. Heterogeneity of Cell Clones Producing Lymphokines 350
V. Conclusions 352
References 353

VI. Murine T Cell Clones Reactive with Soluble Antigens

29 An Overview

C. Garrison Fathman

Text 357
References 364

30 An Analysis of T Cell Antigen Recognition Utilizing T Cell Clones

A. J. Infante, M. Kimoto, and C. G. Fathman

I. Experimental Design 368
II. T Cell Antigen Specificity 368
III. Conformational Requirements of T Cell Antigen Recognition 369
IV. Antigen-Presenting Cell Function 370
V. *Ia* Restriction and *Ir* Gene Function 371
VI. Conclusions 373
References 373

31 Alloreactivity of Antigen-Specific T Cell Clones

Ronald H. Schwartz and Benjamin Sredni

Text 375
References 382

32 Mechanism of B Cell Activation by Monoclonal T Helper Cell Populations

Richard J. Hodes, Yoshihiro Asano, Minoru Shigeta, Karen S. Hathcock, Masao Kimoto, C. Garrison Fathman, and Alfred Singer

I. KLH-Specific Cloned T Cells Provide *H-2* Restricted Help for Antibody Responses to TNP-KLH 386
II. Cloned T_h Cells Can Be *H-2* Restricted in Their Recognition of Accessory Cells but Not B Cells 388
III. After Specific Activation T Cell Clones Can Provide Antigen-Nonspecific Helper Activity 389
IV. Cloned T_h Cell Supernatant Mediates Antigen-Nonspecific Help 389

V. Cloned T_h Cells Can Function through a Pathway Requiring Lyb-5$^+$ B Cells 390
VI. The Same Cloned T_h Cells Function through Pathways Which Are either Restricted or Unrestricted for T_h Cell Recognition of B Cell MHC Determinants 391
VII. The Same Cloned T_h Cells Function through Pathways Which Activate Different B Cell Subpopulations 393
VIII. Conclusions 394
References 395

33 T Cell Lines and T Cell Clones Bearing Cross-Reactive Idiotype

Jacques Thèze, Masao Kimoto, Marie-Lise Gougeon, Jean-Louis Moreau, Gerard Somme, Lise Leclercq, and C. Garrison Fathman

I. Functional Characterization of the Helper Activity of Cell Line L.14 398
II. L.14 Cells Expressing Idiotypic-Like Determinants 400
III. Effect of Anti-Idiotypic Serum B658 on the Activity of Clone C.14.14 401
IV. Conclusions 402
References 403

34 Specific Regulation of Immune Responses by Products of T Cell Clones

Harvey Cantor

Text 405
References 408

VII. Human T Cell Clones

35 Cloning of T Lymphocytes in Man

Fritz H. Bach, Hartwig Bunzendahl, Siew-Lin Wee, Jun Iwaki, and Miriam Segall

I. PLT-Reactive Clones 414
II. Cytotoxic (CTL) Clones 417

III. Conclusions 422
References 423

36 Human T Cell Clones: Function, Specificity, and Cell Surface Markers

Bernard Malissen and Claude Mawas

I. T Cell Clones Obtained Following Sensitization *in Vitro* 426
II. T Cell Clones following *in Vivo* Immunization 430
III. Surface Markers of Human T Cell Clones: Monoclonal Antibodies (mAB) Interacting with the Cytolytic Function 433
IV. Conclusions 435
References 435

37 Human T Cell Clones Reactive with Soluble Antigens: Methodology, Specificity, and MHC Restriction

Benjamin Sredni, David Volkman, Ronald H. Schwartz, and Anthony S. Fauci

I. Antigen Specificity of Soft Agar Colonies of Human T Cells 440
II. Genetic Requirements for Antigen Stimulation 442
References 445

VIII. Future Perspectives in the Utilization of T Cell Clones

38 Potential Use of Expanded T Lymphoid Cells and T Cell Clones for the Immunotherapy of Cancer

Steven A. Rosenberg

I. Traffic *in Vivo* of Cells Grown in T Cell Growth Factor 453
II. Effect *in Vivo* of Adoptively Transferred Cells Expanded in T Cell Growth Factor 456

III. Isolation of T Lymphocyte Clones Specifically Reactive with Tumor 459
IV. The Lysis of Fresh Syngeneic or Autologous Tumor Cells by Lymphoid Cells Expanded in T Cell Growth Factor 463
V. Conclusions 465
References 465

39 Cloned T Cells as a Tool for Molecular Geneticists: Approaches to Cloning Genes Which Encode T Cell Antigen Receptors

Mitchell Kronenberg, Ellen Kraig, Suzanna J. Horvath, and Leroy E. Hood

I. Immunoglobulin Expression in Cloned T Cells 468
II. Cloning Nonimmunoglobulin Genes from T Cells 480
III. Conclusions 486
References 487

IX. Appendix

I. Factors which Influence the Growth of T Lymphocyte Clones 495

A. Assay for Interleukin-1 (IL-1) 495
Igal Gery

B. T Cell Lymphoma Model for the Analysis of Interleukin-1 (IL-1) 497
Steven Gillis and S. B. Mizel

C. Preparation of TCGF from Rat Spleen Cells 498
Klaus Eichmann

D. Preparation of TCGF from a T Cell Tumor (EL-4) 499
Chuan Chen and Ronald H. Schwartz

E. Production of Human TCGF 499
Elizabeth A. Grimm and Steven A. Rosenberg

F. Preparation of TCGF from Human Spleen Cells 500
Fritz H. Bach

G. IL-2 Microassay 501
Steven Gillis

H. Purification and Characterization of IL-2 503
Steven Gillis, James Watson, and Diane Mochizuki

II. Cell Fusion as a Technique for Generation of T Cell Clones 507

A. Production of Antigen-Specific, *H-2* Restricted T Cell Hybridomas 508
Philippa Marrack

III. Clonal Analysis by Limiting Dilution 510

A. Measurement and Calculation of CTL-P Frequencies 510
Helen Derry and R. G. Miller

B. Limit Dilution Analysis of Functional T Cell Precursors 515
Klaus Eichmann

C. Limit Dilution Analysis of T Cells Releasing Lymphokines 516
Peter Krammer

IV. Murine T Cell Clones Reactive with Alloantigens 519
519

A. Clones of Noncytolytic Alloreactive Murine T Cells 519
C. G. Fathman and Hans Hengartner

B. Cloning of Alloreactive Murine T Cells 522
A. L. Glasebrook and Frank W. Fitch

C. Isolation of Virus-Specific CTL Clones 524
T. J. Braciale and V. L. Braciale

V. Murine T Cell Clones Reactive with Soluble Antigens 525

A. Immunization and Long-Term Culture of Murine Immune Lymph Node Cells 525
M. Kimoto and C. G. Fathman

B. Cloning of Soluble Antigen-Reactive Murine T Inducer (T_h) Cells 527
M. Kimoto and C. G. Fathman

C. Soft Agar Technique for Obtaining Antigen-Specific T Cell Clones 528
Chuan Chen and Ronald H. Schwartz

VI. Human T Cell Clones Reactive with Alloantigens and Soluble Antigens 529

A. Cloning of Alloreactive Human T Cells 530
Fritz H. Bach

B. Cloning and Expansion of Human Alloreactive T Lymphocytes 533
Bernard Mallissen and Claude Mawas

C. Establishment of Colonies of Antigen-Reactive Human T Cells 535
Benjamin Sredni

INDEX 539

Contributors

Numbers in parentheses indicate the pages on which the authors' contributions begin.

M. E. Andrew (285), Department of Pathology, Washington University School of Medicine, St. Louis, Missouri 63110

Barbara A. Araneo (137), Department of Pathology and Laboratory Medicine, The Jewish Hospital of St. Louis, and Department of Pathology, Washington University School of Medicine, St. Louis, Missouri 63110

Esther Arman (109), Department of Chemical Immunology, The Weizmann Institute of Science, Rehovot, Israel

Yoshihiro Asano (385), Immunology Branch, National Cancer Institute, National Institutes of Health, Bethesda, Maryland 20014

Thomas M. Aune (157), Department of Pathology and Laboratory Medicine, The Jewish Hospital of St. Louis, and Department of Pathology, Washington University School of Medicine, St. Louis, Missouri 63110

Fritz H. Bach (413, 500, 530), Immunobiology Research Center, University of Minnesota, Minneapolis, Minnesota 55455

Barbara N. Beck (325), Department of Immunology, Mayo Clinic, Rochester, Minnesota 55901

T. J. Braciale (285, 524), Department of Pathology, Washington University School of Medicine, St. Louis, Missouri 63110

V. L. Braciale (285, 524), Department of Pathology, Washington University School of Medicine, St. Louis, Missouri 63110

Jennifer Bruce (331), Division of Research Immunology, Department of Pathology and Laboratory Medicine, University of Pennsylvania School of Medicine, Philadelphia, Pennsylvania 19104

K. Theodor Brunner (297), Department of Immunology, Swiss Institute for Experimental Cancer Research, Epalinges S./Lausanne, Switzerland

Hartwig Bunzendahl (413), Immunobiology Research Center, University of Minnesota, Minneapolis, Minnesota 55455

Harvey Cantor (405), Department of Pathology, Harvard Medical School, Boston, Massachusetts 02115

Jean-Charles Cerottini (1, 297), Ludwig Institute for Cancer Research, Epalinges S./ Lausanne, Switzerland

Chuan Chen (499, 528), Laboratory of Immunology, National Institute of Allergy and Infectious Diseases, National Institutes of Health, Bethesda, Maryland 20205

Robert W. Chesnut (83), Department of Medicine, National Jewish Hospital and Research Center, Denver, Colorado 80206

Jacques M. Chiller (83), Department of Immunopathology, Scripps Clinic and Research Foundation, La Jolla, California 92037

Maurizio Cianfriglia[1] (183), Genetics Unit, Swiss Institute for Experimental Cancer Research, Epalinges S./Lausanne, Switzerland

Andreas Conzelmann (205), Genetics Unit, Swiss Institute for Experimental Cancer Research, Epalinges S./Lausanne, Switzerland

Patricia Corthesy (205), Genetics Unit, Swiss Institute for Experimental Cancer Research, Epalinges S./Lausanne, Switzerland

Elaine C. DeFreitas (83), The Wistar Institute, Philadelphia, Pennsylvania 19085

Helen Derry (510), Ontario Cancer Institute, Toronto, Ontario, Canada

Michel Dy (253), INSERM U25, CNRS 122, Hôpital Necker, 75730 Paris Cedex 15, France

Klaus Eichmann[2] (233, 498, 515), Institute for Immunology and Genetics, German Cancer Research Center, D-6900 Heidelberg, Federal Republic of Germany

John M. Ely (341), Department of Pathology and Committee on Immunology, University of Chicago, Chicago, Illinois 60637

C. Garrison Fathman (325, 357, 367, 385, 397, 519, 525, 527), Division of Immunology, Department of Medicine, Stanford University, Stanford, California 94305

Anthony S. Fauci (439), Laboratory of Immunology and Laboratory of Immunoregulation, National Institute of Allergy and Infectious Diseases, National Institutes of Health, Bethesda, Maryland 20205

Frank W. Fitch (1, 265, 341, 522), Department of Pathology and Committee on Immunology, University of Chicago, Chicago, Illinois 60637

Varda Friedman (109), Department of Chemical Immunology, The Weizmann Institute of Science, Rehovot, Israel

Igal Gery (41, 495), Laboratory of Vision Research, National Eye Institute, National Institutes of Health, Bethesda, Maryland 20205

Steven Gillis (21 497, 501, 503), Basic Immunology Program, Fred Hutchinson Cancer Research Center, Seattle, Washington 98104

Andrew L. Glasebrook (183, 265, 341, 522), Department of Immunology, Swiss Institute for Experimental Cancer Research, Epalinges S./Lausanne, Switzerland

Jörg Goronzy (233, 245), Institute for Immunology and Genetics, German Cancer Research Center, D-6900 Heidelberg, Federal Republic of Germany

Marie-Lise Gougeon (397), Department of Immunology, Pasteur Institute, Paris, France

Sam D. Graham, Jr. (119), Department of Medicine, National Jewish Hospital, Denver, Colorado 80206, and Department of Surgery, Duke University, Durham, North Carolina 27706

Howard M. Grey (83), Department of Medicine, National Jewish Hospital and Research Center, Denver, Colorado 80206

[1]Present address: Department of Immunology, SCLAVO Research Centre, Siena 53100, Italy
[2]Present address: Max-Planck-Institute for Immunobiology, Freiburg, Federal Republic of Germany

Elizabeth A. Grimm (57, 499), Surgery Branch, Division of Cancer Treatment, National Cancer Institute, National Institutes of Health, Bethesda, Maryland 20205

Ute Hamann (233), Institute for Immunology and Genetics, German Cancer Research Center, Heidelberg, Federal Republic of Germany

Günter Hämmerling (109, 245), Institute for Immunology and Genetics, German Cancer Research Center, D-6900 Heidelberg, Federal Republic of Germany

Karen S. Hathcock (385), Immunology Branch, National Cancer Institute, National Institutes of Health, Bethesda, Maryland 20205

Hans Hengartner (519), Department for Experimental Pathology, University Hospital, 8091 Zurich, Switzerland

Richard J. Hodes (385), Immunology Branch, National Cancer Institute, National Institutes of Health, Bethesda, Maryland 20205

Leroy E. Hood (467), Biology Division, California Institute of Technology, Pasadena, California 91125

Suzanna J. Horvath (467), Biology Division, California Institute of Technology, Pasadena, California 91125

Lothar Hültner (253), Division of Experimental Hematology, Society of Radiation and Environmental Research, D-8000 Munich 2, Federal Republic of Germany

A. J. Infante (367), Division of Immunology, Department of Medicine, Stanford University, Stanford, California 94305

Peter Isakson (253), Department of Microbiology, University of Texas Health Science Center, Dallas, Texas 75235

Jun Iwaki (413), Immunobiology Research Center, University of Minnesota, Minneapolis, Minnesota, 55812

Judith P. Johnson (183), Institute for Immunology, University of Munich, 8000 Munich 2, Federal Republic of Germany

Judith A. Kapp (137), Departments of Pathology, and Microbiology and Immunology, Washington University School of Medicine, St. Louis, Missouri 63110

John W. Kappler (119), Department of Medicine, National Jewish Hospital and Research Center, and Departments of Microbiology and Medicine, University of Colorado Health Sciences Center, Denver, Colorado 80206

Ursula Kees (253), Institute for Immunology and Genetics, German Cancer Research Center, D-6900 Heidelberg, Federal Republic of Germany

Anne Kelso (341), Department of Immunology, Swiss Institute for Experimental Cancer Research, Epalinges S./Lausanne, Switzerland

Masao Kimoto (367, 385, 397, 525, 527), Department of Internal Medicine, Osaka University, Osaka, Japan

Ellen Kraig (467), Biology Division, California Institute of Technology, Pasadena, California 91125

Peter H. Krammer (233, 253, 516), Institute for Immunology and Genetics, German Cancer Research Center, D-6900 Heidelberg, Federal Republic of Germany

Mitchell Kronenberg (467), Biology Division, California Institute of Technology, Pasadena, California 91125

Rudolf C. Kuppers (233), Institute for Immunology and Genetics, German Cancer Research Center, D-6900 Heidelberg, Federal Republic of Germany

Lise Leclercq (397), Department of Immunology, Pasteur Institute, Paris, France

H. James Leibson (119), Department of Medicine, National Jewish Hospital and Research Center, Denver, Colorado 80206

Marie-Luise Lohmann-Matthes (253), Max-Planck-Institute for Immunobiology, Freiburg, Federal Republic of Germany

Peter Lonai (109), Department of Chemical Immunology, The Weizmann Institute of Science, Rehovot, Israel

H. Robson MacDonald (193, 297), Ludwig Institute for Cancer Research, Epalinges S./ Lausanne, Switzerland

Bernard Malissen (425 533), Centre d'Immunologie, INSERM-CNRS de Marseille-Luminy, Marseille, France

Fabrizio Marcucci (253), Institute for Virology, German Cancer Research Center, D-6900 Heidelberg, Federal Republic of Germany

Philippa Marrack (119, 508), Department of Medicine, National Jewish Hospital and Research Center, Denver, Colorado 80206, and Departments of Biochemistry, Biophysics, and Medicine, University of Colorado Health Sciences Center, Denver, Colorado 80220

Claude Mawas (425, 533), Centre d'Immunologie, INSERM-CNRS de Marseille-Luminy, Marseille, France

Inga Melchers (233), Institute for Immunology and Genetics, German Cancer Research Center, D-6900 Heidelberg, Federal Republic of Germany

Andrea Michnay (253), Institute for Immunology and Genetics, German Cancer Research Center, D-6900 Heidelberg, Federal Republic of Germany

R. G. Miller (219, 510), Ontario Cancer Institute and The University of Toronto, Toronto, Ontario M4X 1K9, Canada

N. A. Mitchison (11), Imperial Cancer Research Fund Tumour Immunology Unit, Department of Zoology, University College London, London, England

S. B. Mizel (497), Departments of Microbiology, Cell Biology, Biochemistry, and Biophysics, College of Science, Pennsylvania State University, University Park, Pennsylvania 16802

Diane Mochizuki (21, 503), Basic Immunology Program, Fred Hutchinson Cancer Research Center, Seattle, Washington 98104

Katherine Molnar-Kimber (331), Institute for Cancer Research, Philadelphia, Pennsylvania 19111

Jean-Louis Moreau (397), Department of Immunology, Pasteur Institute, Paris, France

Markus Nabholz (165, 183, 193, 205), Genetics Unit, Swiss Institute for Experimental Cancer Research, Epalinges S./Lausanne, Switzerland

Makoto Nonaka (95), Department of Immunology, Faculty of Medicine, University of Tokyo, Tokyo, Japan

Carl W. Pierce (149, 157), Department of Pathology and Laboratory Medicine, The Jewish Hospital of St. Louis, and Departments of Pathology, and Microbiology and Immunology, Washington University School of Medicine, St. Louis, Missouri 63110

Michael B. Prystowsky (341), Department of Pathology and Committee on Immunology, University of Chicago, Chicago, Illinois 60637

Ellen Puré (253), Department of Microbiology, University of Texas Health Science Center, Dallas, Texas 75235

Joseph Puri (109), Department of Chemical Immunology, The Weizmann Institute of Science, Rehovot, Israel

Neal Roehm (119), Department of Medicine, National Jewish Hospital and Research Center, Denver, Colorado 80206

Steven A. Rosenberg (57, 451, 499), Surgery Branch, Division of Cancer Treatment, National Cancer Institute, National Institutes of Health, Besthesda, Maryland 20205

Huub F. C. Savelkoul (109), Department of Chemical Immunology, The Weizmann Institute of Science, Rehovot, Israel

Anneliese Schimpl (253), Institute for Virology and Immunobiology, Wurzburg, Federal Republic of Germany

Ronald H. Schwartz (375, 439, 499, 528), Laboratory of Immunology, National Institute of Allergy and Infectious Diseases, National Institutes of Health, Bethesda, Maryland 20205

Miriam Segall (413), Immunobiology Research Center, University of Minnesota, Minneapolis, Minnesota 55455

Rafick P. Sekaly (193), Ludwig Institute for Cancer Research, Epalinges S./Lausanne, Switzerland

Linda A. Sherman (313), Department of Immunopathology, Scripps Clinic and Research Foundation, La Jolla, California 92037

Minoru Shigeta (385), Department of Internal Medicine, Osaka University, Osaka, Japan

Markus M. Simon (233), Institute for Immunology and Genetics, German Cancer Research Center, D-6900 Heidelberg, Federal Republic of Germany

Alfred Singer (385), Immunology Branch, National Cancer Institute, National Institutes of Health, Bethesda, Maryland 20205

Barry J. Skidmore (83), Department of Immunopathology, Scripps Clinic and Research Foundation, La Jolla, California 92037

Gerard Somme (397), Department of Immunology, Pasteur Institute, Paris, France

Craig M. Sorensen (149), Department of Pathology and Laboratory Medicine, The Jewish Hospital of St. Louis, and Department of Pathology, Washington University School of Medicine, St. Louis, Missouri 63110

Jonathan Sprent (331), Division of Research Immunology, Department of Pathology, University of Pennsylvania School of Medicine, and The Wistar Institute, Philadelphia, Pennsylvania 19104

Benjamin Sredni[3] (375, 439, 535), Laboratory of Immunology, National Institute of Allergy and Infectious Diseases, National Institutes of Health, Bethesda, Maryland 20205

Fritz Staber[4] (253), Institute for Hematology, Munich, Federal Republic of Germany

Tomio Tada (95), Department of Immunology, Faculty of Medicine, University of Tokyo, Tokyo, Japan

Michael J. Taussig (127), Department of Immunology, Agricultural Research Council, Institute of Animal Physiology, Babraham, Cambridge, United Kingdom

Jacques Thèze (397), Department of Immunology, Pasteur Institute, Paris, France

[3]Present address: Department of Life Sciences, Bar-Ilan University, Ramat-Gan 52100, Israel

[4]Present address: Labor Struppe e Staber, Ardingganstrasse 21, 8 München 83, Federal Republic of Germany

Ellen S. Vitetta (253), Department of Microbiology, University of Texas Health Science Center, Dallas, Texas 75235

David Volkman (439), Laboratory of Immunology and Laboratory of Immunoregulation, National Institute of Allergy and Infectious Diseases, National Institutes of Health, Bethesda, Maryland 20205

Michael Waller (253), Institute for Immunology and Genetics, German Cancer Research Center, D-6900 Heidelberg, Federal Republic of Germany

James Watson (21, 503), Department of Pathology, University of Auckland, Auckland, New Zealand

Susan R. Webb (331), Division of Research Immunology, Department of Pathology and Laboratory Medicine, University of Pennsylvania School of Medicine, Philadelphia, Pennsylvania 19104

Siew-Lin Wee (413), Immunobiology Research Center, University of Minnesota, Minneapolis, Minnesota 55455

Dale Wegmann (119), Department of Medicine, National Jewish Hospital and Research Center, Denver, Colorado, 80206, and Department of Microbiology, University of Colorado Health Sciences Center, Denver, Colorado 80220

Arthur Weiss (297), Department of Medicine, University of California at San Francisco, San Francisco, California 94102

Cornelia Weyand (245), Institute for Immunology and Genetics, German Cancer Research Center, D-6900 Heidelberg, Federal Republic of Germany

Darcy B. Wilson (331), Division of Research Immunology, Department of Pathology and Laboratory Medicine, University of Pennsylvania School of Medicine, Philadelphia, Pennsylvania 19104

Gabriele Zahn (233), Institute for Immunology and Genetics, German Cancer Research Center, D-6900 Heidelberg, Federal Republic of Germany

Rudolf H. Zubler (341), Department of Immunology, Swiss Institute for Experimental Cancer Research, Epalinges S./Lausanne, Switzerland

Preface

The complexity of cellular interactions which regulate an immune response may never be entirely understood. Efforts to reconstruct *in vitro* the immune responses that occur *in vivo* are subject to a variety of misconceptions at best. In an attempt to more readily understand cellular interactions, great effort has been devoted to the isolation of clones of immunocompetent cells which will allow one to study interactions between cells in a strict reductionist mode. Until recently, such approaches have been dominated by analyses of clones of "immunocompetent" neoplastic cells, particularly myelomas and lymphomas. Such neoplastic cells comprise relatively uniform cell populations, and many important contributions to an understanding of the immune system have resulted from studies of these cloned cell populations. Unfortunately, relatively few different kinds of functional lymphoid tumor cells exist, and the availability of cell lines depends on the chance occurrence of tumors. The limited variety of cell types which have become transformed has meant that there has been only a narrow "window of observations."

Recently, utilizing techniques of somatic cell fusion, it has been possible to create "hybridomas" which maintain many of the immunologically relevant properties of the normal parent cell. Valuable information has been obtained thanks to this technological breakthrough, but the usefulness of such hybridomas in model systems of immune responses in *in vitro* and *in vivo* has been limited because of their neoplastic nature. An alternative approach for obtaining large numbers of identical cells has been the isolation of clones of immunocompetent cells which maintain normal function. Such cells have been used to reconstruct models of normal immune responses *in vitro*.

The most remarkable aspect of our initial conversations when we met 4 years ago was the realization that we both believed that our techniques of cell culture would ultimately allow the type of reconstitution of normal immunological circuitry *in vitro* and *in vivo* that would allow us to dissect the cellular parameters involved in a normal immune response. Over the past 4 years, the number of laboratories working on the isolation and characterization of clones of immunoncompetent T cells has increased greatly. This volume is addressed to the many workers who are currently contemplating joining or have recently joined the field of cloning of immunocompetent T cells. The questions to be addressed are legion and the results will have striking implications not only for the understanding of normal immunoregulation, but also for possible immunotherapeutic intervention. The insights gained from studies *in vitro* are now being applied in attempts to modulate immune responses *in vivo;* these approaches are essential to verify that the interpretations based on observation in culture actually do have relevance in animals.

We asked the contributors not to dwell on previously published data but to attempt to make this book an up-to-date, state-of-the-art treatise. We issue it as an invitation to young scientists interested in plunging into a new ''sea'' of basic research with potential clinical applications—come on in, the water is fine!

Clearly, this volume is a joint effort. The cooperation and prompt responses of the contributors eased our task. We wish to acknowledge our gratitude to Frances Mills for her invaluable secretarial help in preparing the final manuscripts. We appreciate the support and understanding of our families during the preparation of this book.

C. Garrison Fathman
Frank W. Fitch

Isolation, Characterization, and Utilization of T Lymphocyte Clones

1

Introduction and Historical Overview

Frank W. Fitch/Jean-Charles Cerottini

Text 1
References 7

Less than 25 years ago, the function of lymphocytes still was unknown. Trowell (1958) concluded his review on "The Lymphocyte" as follows: "The small lymphocyte seems a poor sort of cell, characterized by mostly negative attributes: small in size, with especially little cytoplasm, unable to multiply, dying on the least provocation, surviving *in vitro* for only a few days, living *in vivo* for perhaps a few weeks. . . . It must be regretfully concluded, however, that the office of this Cinderella cell is still uncertain. There is, in fact, little to add to the statement of Rich (1936) that 'The complete ignorance of the function of this cell is one of the most humiliating and disgraceful gaps in all medical knowledge'." This rather gloomy view of the state of knowledge about lymphocytes was substantiated by immunological publications of the time. In the year that Trowell published his review, 137 papers were published in the *Journal of Immunology*. The word "lymphocyte" was not even listed in the index. Two papers described experiments involving transfer of lymph node cells, but none of the 137 papers were concerned directly with lymphocyte functions.

Perceptions regarding lymphocytes have changed dramatically during the ensuing quarter century. Multiple, functionally distinct lymphocyte subsets have been recognized. In current paradigms, lymphocytes have been assigned central and dominant roles in immune responses. However, the heterogeneity of cell populations found in lymphoid organs has complicated efforts to understand the molecular and cellular mechanisms by which lymphocytes participate in immune responses. Monoclonal myelomas and more recently B lymphocyte hybridomas have made possible the research that has led to the description of the detailed structure of immunoglobulin molecules and to an understanding of the organization of the multiple gene segments which specify immunoglobulin structure.

Only recently has it been possible to obtain monoclonal T lymphocytes which retain their function *in vitro*. As will be reviewed in this treatise, clones of

ISOLATION, CHARACTERIZATION, AND
UTILIZATION OF T LYMPHOCYTE CLONES

ISBN 0-12-249920-4

different types of T lymphocytes now can be grown indefinitely in culture. These cloned cells already have proved to be useful for defining in some detail the antigenic requirements for stimulation of T lymphocytes and for characterizing the molecular products of T cells which influence the functions of B and T lymphocytes as well as other cells. The cloned cells also have provided insights about the repertoire of antigen recognition by cytolytic T lymphocytes (CTL). T lymphocyte clones are certain to contribute to better understanding of regulatory functions that control immune responses. These cloned cells and their products are likely to be useful therapeutically in clinical situations.

The remarkable progress in the understanding of lymphocyte functions can be traced to a relatively few key technical developments which were made in the course of research seeking answers to questions related only vaguely, if at all, to the role of lymphocytes in immune responses. Most of the publications describing these developments have been written to conform to the generally accepted style of "normal science" (Kuhn, 1970). The illusion usually was maintained that the discoveries were made in the course of a a logical, rational approach to a problem. In fact, serendipity has played a major role in nearly all of these developments. Many of them transformed the concepts then in existence and led to the elaboration of new paradigms. It seems useful to recount how some of the advances that have contributed to the almost invisible immunological revolution really came about, since it is likely that chance observations made with T cell clones will be the basis for some of the next series of revolutions in our understanding of lymphocyte functions.

The fact that circulating lymphocytes can be stimulated to divide was made accidentally during the year after Trowell's review article was published (Nowell, 1977 and personal communication). Peter Nowell in Philadelphia had been studying chromosome abnormalities in human patients with leukemia. It was much easier to identify the dividing cells, presumed to be the malignant leukemic cells, if erythrocytes were removed from the blood before cultures were prepared. He chose to use a culture method developed several years earlier (Osgood and Krippaehne, 1955) which employed phytohemagglutinin (PHA) obtained from red kidney beans to clump and rapidly sediment erythrocytes. The remaining leukocyte-rich plasma was then cultured for several days. One day, blood was obtained from a patient before it was realized that his leukemia was in remission and that he did not have leukemic cells in his bloodstream at that particular time. Since cultures had already been prepared, they were examined. Quite unexpectedly, numerous dividing cells were found. The mitogenic effect of PHA for circulating lymphocytes from normal individuals was demonstrated in short order (Nowell, 1960), and other lymphocyte mitogens were soon identified. These and other related observations quickly laid to rest the erroneous notion that circulating lymphocytes were unable to divide.

At least some of the early uncertainties about the function of lymphocytes can be blamed on problems in determining cell lineages. A great deal of evidence, much of it circumstantial, had linked lymphoid tissues with immune responses. For many years, however, there was considerable controversy about which of the several cell types found in lymph nodes was most important. Immunohistochemical techniques (Coons *et al.,* 1955) finally demonstrated conclusively that antibodies were produced by plasma cells, but the developmental pathway of these cells was not generally agreed upon. Incidentally, the story of the origins of immunofluorescence also is interesting (Coons, 1961).

The relatively high frequency of dividing cells in lymph nodes made it clear that lymphocytes were produced in large numbers in normal animals. Evidence for the magnitude of lymphocyte production was obtained by collecting cells from the thoracic duct of rabbits (Sanders *et al.,* 1940); the daily output of lymphocyte was found to be five times the number of cells present in the bloodstream. James Gowans, a student of Lord Florey, followed up these observations using a technique for cannulation of the thoracic duct which permitted collection of the lymph from unanesthetized animals for periods of several days (Bollman *et al.,* 1948). This procedure had been developed to study the physiology of digestion. Gowans found that drainage of thoracic duct lymph for several days was associated with a progressive decrease in daily output of lymphocytes in the lymph and a concomitant depletion of lymphocytes from the lymph nodes and spleen. Reinfusion of the lymphocytes into the bloodstream prevented both effects (Gowans, 1957). These observations suggested that lymphocytes passed from the bloodstream into the lymph and then back to the bloodstream. This conclusion was confirmed by the recovery of isotope-labeled lymphocytes in the thoracic duct lymph after intravenous infusion of labeled cells (Gowans, 1959).

Extension of these studies indicated that lymphocytes were involved in immune responses. Immunological reactivity of rats was impaired markedly by prolonged thoracic duct drainage, and reactivity could be restored by intravenous infusion of syngeneic thoracic duct lymphocytes (Gowans *et al.,* 1962). Ultimately, it was shown that immunological memory could be conferred passively by small thoracic duct lymphocytes from immunized syngeneic donors (Gowans and Uhr, 1966).

Additional evidence for the involvement of lymphocytes in immune responses came in the course of studies concerned with the pathogenesis of leukemia in mice. Thymectomy had been shown to reduce markedly the incidence of lymphocytic leukemias in mice which would otherwise develop the disease spontaneously (McEndy *et al.,* 1944). Since newborn mice were more susceptible to the leukemia virus than adult mice, thymectomy was performed soon after birth to determine whether virus could multiply outside the thymus. More than 50% of mice thymectomized at 1 day of age died between 2 and 4 months later, although none of them developed leukemia (Miller, 1961a). Low numbers of circulating lymphocytes were found in mice thymectomized at birth, germinal centers were absent from lymph nodes and spleens, and only a few plasma cells were seen. Skin allograft survival in such animals was prolonged greatly (Miller, 1961b).

These findings were confirmed in short order in other species (Jankovic *et al.*, 1962; Archer *et al.*, 1962), but the immunological deficit in neonatally thymectomized animals proved to be somewhat complex. While cell-mediated responses were severely impaired, antibody responses to many antigens were apparently normal while the response to others was impaired (reviewed in Miller and Osoba, 1967). Ultimately, it was shown that there were two distinct developmental pathways for lymphocytes. Lymphocytes maturing in the thymus participated directly in cell-mediated responses and indirectly in the regulation of cell-mediated and humoral immune responses. Lymphocytes which produced antibody did not require the thymus for their maturation (Mitchell and Miller, 1968).

Actually, the importance of nonthymic lymphocytes in antibody formation had been demonstrated several years before the role of the thymus was appreciated. However, this observation escaped the immediate attention of most immunologists, probably because it was published in an obscure (at least for immunologists) journal, *Poultry Science*. Bruce Glick and his colleagues had removed various organs, including the bursa of Fabricius, from newly hatched chicks in the course of studies evaluating endocrine influences on the growth of chickens. The bursectomized chicks appeared to develop normally and were set aside. Some months later, they were included in a group of chickens inoculated with a bacterial vaccine to obtain a pool of antiserum. Surprisingly, the bursectomized birds produced practically no antibody. Glick pursued this unexpected finding and confirmed that bursectomy soon after hatching resulted in impaired antibody formation but did not affect cell-mediated responses (Glick *et al.*, 1956).

Although indistinguishable morphologically using conventional microscopic techniques, convenient cell surface markers can distinguish between these two major types of lymphocytes. Surface immunoglobulin serves to identify B lymphocytes. The Thy-1 antigen is a useful indicator for murine T lymphocytes. This antigen was discovered unexpectedly during attempts to develop antibody to leukemic cells. Arnold Reif (Reif and Allen, 1963) immunized C3H mice with leukemic cells from histocompatible AKR mice. The resulting antiserum reacted with thymocytes from AKR mice long before leukemia developed. Puzzled by this finding, he did reciprocal immunizations and found that antisera raised in AKR mice by immunization with C3H thymocytes reacted with thymus cells from 16 different mouse strains tested (Reif and Allen, 1964). Subsequent studies confirmed that this antigen provided a convenient marker for lymphocytes that had matured in the thymic environment, although it also was recognized that the antigen was also found in brain, skin, and some other tissues.

The Lyt-1,2,3 antigens, useful for defining functional subsets of T lymphocytes, also were recognized during the course of studies attempting to define tumor antigens. Cytolytic antibodies reactive with lymphocyte antigens were found in alloantisera raised by immunizing mice with tumors bearing Gross and mammary leukemia antigens. Some of these anti-lymphocyte antibodies remained after the antisera were absorbed thoroughly with mammary tumor tissue (Stück *et al.*, 1964). The allelic nature of these antigens and their expression by only a portion of lymphocytes was shown rather quickly (Boyse *et al.*, 1968). However, more that a decade elapsed before the differential expression of these antigens on functionally distinct subsets of T lymphocytes was fully documented (Shiku *et al.*, 1975; Cantor and Boyse, 1975a,b).

Tissue culture techniques have permitted the study of immune responses by selected populations of cells under conditions which can be controlled to a greater extent than is possible in intact animals. Several of these methods have been developed almost accidentally. The mixed leukocyte culture (MLC), which is used widely to study alloimmune responses, came about because of chance observations during the course of studies on the apparent differential susceptibility of leukemic and normal lymphocytes to the toxic effect of heterologous sera (Schrek and Donnelly, 1961). Enlarged lymphocytes, some of which were dividing, were noted in a culture prepared with a mixture of bloods from two patients with hemochromatosis; these changes were not seen in cultures prepared with blood from 18 individual patients. Other investigators (Bain *et al.*, 1964; Bach and Hirschhorn, 1964) extended these findings and showed that the response was based on the reaction of lymphocytes toward alloantigens. Since the response in MLC appeared to be similar to a primary allograft response *in vivo,* it seemed reasonable to expect that cytotoxic effector cells should be produced. Indeed, this proved to be the case (Häyry and Defendi, 1970; Hodes and Svedmyr, 1970).

The most recent technical advance that was essential for cloning of T lymphocytes involved the serendipitous rediscovery of T cell growth factor. It had been found as early as 1965 that medium obtained from lymphocytes stimulated in mixed leukocyte culture caused other lymphocytes to proliferate (Kasakura and Lowenstein, 1965; Gordon and MacLean, 1965), but the significance of this observation was not appreciated at that time, and cells were grown only for very short periods. Several years later, Robert Gallo and his colleagues at the National Cancer Institute were attempting to grow large numbers of human granulopoietic cells for biochemical and virological studies (R. Gallo, personal communication). Although most sources of colony stimulating factor (CSF) promoted growth of these cells in soft agar, long-term growth in suspension culture was not possible because of "terminal differentiation." A few batches of conditioned medium (CM) from human embryo cells promoted long-term growth of granulopoietic cells, but this source of CM proved to be unreliable. He and his colleagues sought other sources of CM. For several years, they had used PHA-stimulated human lymphocytes for biochemical studies. Conditioned Media from these cells had been evaluated for growth promoting properties in the early

1970s. Gallo and his co-workers showed that this CM did have conventional CSF activity, although granulopoietic cells failed to grow in long-term cultures because of terminal differentiation. They also observed extended growth of lymphoblasts. It was assumed that these were B lymphocytes which had been transformed as the result of infection with Epstein–Barr (EB) virus.

A few years later, they again observed this phenomenon when they attempted again, in their frustration, to use CM from PHA-stimulated lymphocytes for the long-term growth of granulopoietic cells. This time, however, they examined the lymphoblasts for the presence of EB virus, and the cells were found to be negative. Further study demonstrated that they were mature T lymphocytes, and the active agent in the CM was characterized as T cell growth factor (Morgan *et al.*, 1976; Ruscetti and Gallo, 1981).

With the discovery of T cell growth factor, the stage was set for cloning of T cells. Long-term lines of mouse cytolytic T cells were developed in the following year (Gillis and Smith, 1977), and clones of T cells were described within a few more months (Nabholz *et al.*, 1978). Functional T cell hybrids were produced as an alternative approach for the clonal analysis of T cell function (Kontiainen *et al.*, 1978). As will be discussed in subsequent chapters, functional clones of each major mouse T lymphocyte subset have been developed. Although perhaps more difficult to obtain, human T cell clones also have been derived.

Experiments utilizing T lymphocyte clones have provided conclusive answers to several important immunological questions. For example, although it could be inferred using bulk cell populations that cytolytic and helper T lymphocytes could react with more than one antigen, this interpretation is clouded because of the presence of multiple cell types. Definitive proof for dual antigen reactivity requires analysis of responses of individual cells using a broad panel of antigens. Although methods are not available currently for studying the reactivity of single cells, analysis of the responses of clonal progeny of individual cells is a practical alternative approach. As will be discussed in Chapters 23 and 24, at least some cloned CTL which react with viral antigens in association with "self" histocompatibility antigens also can lyse target cells bearing other alloantigens. Other T cell clones which proliferate when stimulated by conventional antigens in the presence of cells expressing syngeneic I-A molecules also can be stimulated to divide by appropriate alloantigens (Chapter 31). The frequency of T cells having dual reactivity has not been determined, nor is it certain whether more than one receptor for antigen is involved in dual reactivity. However, answers to these questions will be possible using methods for clonal analysis of T cell function.

T cell clones also have been used to show that a large number of different antigenic determinants can be recognized by cytolytic T cells (Chapter 25), that some cytolytic T cells also can secrete biologically active materials usually produced by helper T cells (Chapter 28), and that helper T cells can secrete several different "factors" which modulate the function of other cells active in immune responses (Chapters 21 and 28). T cell clones confirmed definitively that there are unique antigenic determinants on cells from F_1 hybrid mice formed by the complementation of products from the two parental strains, and that these products are specified by genes in the *I* region (Chapter 26).

Other examples of the particular usefulness of T cell clones are reviewed elsewhere in this treatise which attempts to summarize current information concerning T lymphocyte clones. Part I includes chapters which deal with soluble factors, IL-1 (lymphocyte activating factor) and IL-2 (T cell growth factor), which influence the growth of cloned T cells. The use of T cell hybridomas for analysis of T cell functions is considered in Part II, with emphasis on the biochemical and functional properties of helper and suppressor factors. Analysis of T cell clones and T cell hybridomas using the techniques of somatic cell genetics is the topic of Part III. Clonal analysis by limiting dilution is reviewed in Part IV. The characteristics of murine T cell clones reactive with alloantigens and soluble antigens are discussed in Parts V and VI. Experience with human T cell clones is considered in Part VII. Part VIII deals with future perspectives and potential applications. Methods which the contributors have found useful in the isolation, characterization, and utilization of T lymphocyte clones are described in some detail in the Appendix.

T lymphocyte clones already have made considerable contributions to knowledge of the biology of immune responses, and it seems clear that they will make additional major contributions in the future.

REFERENCES

Archer, O. K., Pierce, J. C., Papermaster, B. W., and Good, R. A. (1962). Reduced antibody response in thymectomized rabbits. *Nature (London)* **195,** 191.

Bach, F., and Hirschhorn, K. (1964). Lymphocyte interaction; A potential histocompatibility test *in vitro*. *Science* **143,** 813.

Bain, B., Vas, M. R., and Lowenstein, L. (1964). The development of large immature mononuclear cells in mixed leukocyte cultures. *Blood* **23,** 108.

Bollman, J. C., Cain, J. C., and Grindlay, J. H. (1948). Techniques for the collection of lymph for the liver, small intestine, or thoracic duct of the rat. *J. Lab. Clin. Med.* **33,** 1349.

Boyse, E. A., Miyazawa, M., Aoki, T., and Old, L. J. (1968). Ly-A and Ly-B: Two systems of lymphocyte isoantigens in the mouse. *Proc. R. Soc. London, Ser. B* **170,** 175.

Cantor, H., and Boyse, E. A. (1975b). Functional subclasses of T lymphocytes bearing different Ly antigens. I. The generation of functionally distinct T-cell subclasses is a differentiative process independent of antigen. *J. Exp. Med.* **141,** 1376.

Cantor, H., and Boyse, E. A. (1975b). Functional subclasses of T lymphocytes bearing different Ly antigens. II. Cooperation between subclasses of Ly^+ cells in the generation of killer activity. *J. Exp. Med.* **141,** 1390.

Coons, A. H. (1961). The beginnings of immunofluorescence. *J. Immunol.* **87,** 499.

Coons, A. H., Leduc, E. H., and Connolly, J. M. (1955). Studies on antibody production. I. A method for the histochemical demonstration of specific antibody and its application to a study of the hyperimmune rabbit. *J. Exp. Med.* **102,** 49.

Gillis, S., and Smith, K. A. (1977). Long term culture of tumour-specific cytotoxic T cells. *Nature (London)* **268,** 154.

Glick, B., Chang, T. S., and Jaap, R. G. (1956). The bursa of Fabricus and antibody production. *Poult. Sci.* **35,** 224.

Gordon, J., and MacLean, L. D. (1965). A lymphocyte-stimulating factor produced *in vitro*. *Nature (London)* **208,** 795.

Gowans, J. L. (1957). The effect of continuous re-infusion of lymph and lymphocytes on the output of lymphocytes from the thoracic duct of unanesthetized rats. *Br. J. Exp. Pathol.* **38,** 67.

Gowans, J. L. (1959). The recirculation of lymphocytes from blood to lymph in the rat. *J. Physiol. (London)* **146,** 54.

Gowans, J. L., and Uhr, J. W. (1966). The carriage of immunological memory by small lymphocytes in the rat. *J. Exp. Med.* **124,** 1017.

Gowans, J. L., McGregor, D. D., Cowen, D. M., and Ford, C. E. (1962). Initiation of immune responses by small lymphocytes. *Nature (London)* **196,** 651.

Häyry, P., and Defendi, V. (1970). Mixed lymphocyte cultures produce effector cells: Model *in vitro* for allograft rejection. *Science* **168,** 133.

Hodes, R. J., and Svedmyr, E. A. J. (1970). Specific cytotoxicity of H-2 incompatible mouse lymphocytes following mixed culture *in vitro*. *Transplantation* **9,** 470.

Jankovic, B. D., Waksman, B. H., and Arnason, B. G. (1962). Role of the thymus in immune reactions in rats. I. The immunologic response to bovine serum albumin (antibody formation, Arthus reactivity, and delayed hypersensitivity) in rats thymectomized or splenectomized at various times after birth. *J. Exp. Med.* **116,** 159.

Kasakura, S., and Lowenstein, L. (1965). A factor stimulating DNA synthesis derived from the medium of leucocyte cultures. *Nature (London)* **208,** 794.

Kontiainen, S., Simpson, E., Bohrer, E., Beverley, P. C. L., Herzenberg, L. A., Fitzpatrick, W. C., Vogt, P., Torano, A., McKenzie, I. F. C., and Feldmann, M. (1978). T-cell lines producing antigen-specific suppressor factor. *Nature (London)* **274,** 477.

Kuhn, T. S. (1970). "The Structure of Scientific Revolutions." Univ. of Chicago Press, Chicago, Illinois.

McEndy, D. P., Boon, M. C., and Furth, J. (1944). On the role of thymus, spleen, and gonads in the development of leukemia in a high-leukemia stock of mice. *Cancer Res.* **4,** 337.

Miller, J. F. A. P. (1961a). Analysis of the thymus influence on leukemogenesis. *Nature (London)* **191,** 248.

Miller, J. F. A. P. (1961b). Immunological function of the thymus. *Lancet* **2,** 748.

Miller, J. F. A. P., and Osoba, D. (1967). Current concepts of the immunological function of the thymus. *Physiol. Rev.* **47,** 437.

Mitchell, G. F., and Miller, J. F. A. P. (1968). Cell to cell interaction in the immune response. II. The source of hemolysin-forming cells in irradiated mice given bone marrow and thymus or thoracic duct lymphocytes. *J. Exp. Med.* **128,** 821.

Morgan, D. A., Ruscetti, F. W., and Gallo, R. (1976). Selective *in vitro* growth of T lymphocytes from normal human bone marrows. *Science* **193,** 1007.

Nabholz, M., Engers, H. D., Collavo, D., and North, M. (1978). Cloned T-cell lines with specific cytolytic activity. *Curr. Top Microbiol. Immunol.* **81,** 176.

Nowell, P. C. (1960). Phytohemagglutinin: An initiator of mitosis in cultures of normal human leukocytes. *Cancer Res.* **20,** 462.

Nowell, P. C. (1977). Phytohemagglutinin: An initiator of mitosis in cultures of normal human leukocytes. *Curr. Contents* No. 42, p. 13.

Osgood, E. E., and Krippaehne, M. L. (1955). The gradient tissue culture method. *Exp. Cell Res.* **9,** 116.

Reif, A. E., and Allen, J. M. V. (1963). Specificity of isoantisera against leukemic and thymic lymphocytes. *Nature (London)* **200,** 1332.

Reif, A. E., and Allen, J. M. V. (1965). The AKR thymic antigen and its distribution in leukemias and nervous tissues. *J. Exp. Med.* **120,** 413.

Rich, A. R. (1936). Inflammation in resistance to infection. *AMA Arch. Pathol.* **22,** 228.

Ruscetti, F. W., and Gallo, R. C. (1981). Human T-lymphocyte growth factor: Regulation of growth and function of T lymphocytes. *Blood* **57,** 379.

Sanders, A. G., Florey, H. W., and Barnes, J. M. (1940). The output of lymphocytes from the thoracic duct in cats and rabbits. *Br. J. Exp. Pathol.* **21,** 254.

Schrek, R., and Donnelly, W. J. (1961). Differences between lymphocytes of leukemic and non-leukemic patients with respect to morphologic features, mobility and sensitivity to guinea pig serum. *Blood* **18,** 561.

Shiku, H., Kisielow, P., Bean, M. A., Takahashi, T., Boyse, E. A., Oettgen, H. F., and Old, L. J. (1975). Expression of T-cell differentiation antigens on effector cells in cell-mediated cytotoxicity *in vitro*. Evidence for functional heterogeneity related to the surface phenotype of T cells. *J. Exp. Med.* **141,** 227.

Stück, B., Boyse, E. A., Old, C. J., and Carswell, E. A. (1964). ML: A new antigen found in leukemias and mammary tumors of the mouse. *Nature (London)* **203,** 1033.

Trowell, O. A. (1958). The lymphocyte. *Int. Rev. Cytol.* **7,** 235.

2

Differentiation within the Immune System: The Importance of Cloning

N. A. Mitchison

I. Comparison with the Nervous System 11
II. Cloning Methods 13
III. Questions of the Day 14
References 16

I. COMPARISON WITH THE NERVOUS SYSTEM

Cloning is of the utmost importance in understanding the immune system for one very simple and very general reason: lymphocytes, the principal cells of the immune system, are organized as sets of clones. These sets are designated Bμ, Bγ, Bα, . . ., Th, Tc, Ts, . . ., a nomenclature which reflects in part their different patterns of development and in part their different functions. The number of these sets is probably near 20, and almost certainly in the range 10^2–10^3. Each set is made up of a very large number of clones ($> 10^6$) which are distinct from one another in the variable part of the structure of their receptors. These unique structures confer on each clone a unique ability to react with a particular range of antigens. The range of such structures is termed the receptor "repertoire." The repertoire is repeated, essentially in its entirety, in each set of lymphocytes; the sets exist, therefore, in parallel with one another (Mitchison, 1980). An arrangement of this sort poses many questions: how and when do the parallel sets differentiate from one another, just how many sets are there, to what extent do their repertoires overlap, what can we learn about the individual receptors of an isolated clone, what causes one set rather than another to engage in an immune response, how do the sets interact, and so on. It is the task of cloning to answer these questions.

There is a contrast here with the nervous system. These two systems, immune and nervous, have attained roughly comparable levels of complexity. Both show advanced integrative functions, such as memory and recognition-of-self, and

ISBN 0-12-249920-4

both show a flexibility and precision of response which far exceeds that of other body systems. In attaining these levels, both systems have had to generate enormous numbers of cells which are clearly different from one another. In man, the 10^{12} lymphocytes of the immune system actually exceed the number of neurons in the nervous system by a factor of 10–100. The contrast lies in the way that this differentiation has occurred. In the nervous system the differentiation is anatomical rather than molecular. That is to say, individual neurons are unique in the contact which they establish with one another: probably no single neuron exactly repeats the pattern of contacts established by another. Their molecular architecture, on the other hand, is remarkably repetitive; a generation of scientific work which has tried to place Sperry's chemoaffinity theory of retinotectal connections on a molecular basis has largely failed (Gaze and Straznicky, 1980).

In the immune system the balance of differentiation is reversed. Cell contacts are ephemeral, and lymphocytes to an extent behave like atoms in a perfect gas. The crucial differentiation is in molecular architecture, in antigen receptors, and in the other less well understood receptors which enable a lymphocyte to find its way to the right place at the right time in the immune response. The effect of this difference is to make cloning a matter of much less urgency in the nervous system. It is of course true that cell lines, clones, and somatic genetics are finding a place for themselves in neurobiology. However, it is debatable how much they have to offer in preference, say, to freshly isolated cells, and it is certain that for the foreseeable future the integrative functions of the nervous system will have to be studied *in situ*. This is not true of immunobiology.

At this point one ought to enter a qualification. Lymphocytes do not behave exactly like atoms in a gas. They traffic in a well-defined way, under constraints imposed by their own propensities coupled with the relatively fixed anatomical distribution of the other cells with which they interact, which are principally high epithelial cells, macrophages, and dendritic cells. The effect of these constraints is to divide the immune system into compartments, and this is a consideration which needs to be borne in mind when interpreting the outcome of *in vitro* experiments on clones.

Before leaving the comparison with the nervous system, there is one point which deserves further emphasis. This is the extent to which lymphocytes, like neurons, predominantly interact with one another rather than directly with the outside world. In immunobiology, this is a relatively recent discovery and where it has been one, arguably the most important theme of the T and B cell revolution in ideas. The discovery that most lymphocytes are engaged in regulatory activity is a great step forward. It has changed our thinking not only about how the immune system works but also about the nature of immunological diseases. Broadly, its effect has been to focus thinking about these diseases away from abnormalities in antigens or antibodies, and toward abnormalities in populations of regulatory lymphocytes (Reinherz *et al.*, 1979). Estimates of the fraction of regulatory lymphocytes vary; I calculate that some 70% of the total population are engaged in regulatory activity (Czitrom *et al.*, 1982).

Because the regulatory lymphocytes have as their primary target other lymphocytes, cloning has for them a special importance. We can hope to analyze their activity by isolating sets of clones, and recombining them *in vitro*. A system has already been described in which one clone of T lymphocytes suppresses the activity of another clone (Fresno *et al.*, 1981). This points the way to studies of an indefinite degree of elaboration, in which successive clones regulate one another.

We are in an era when new parallel sets of regulatory lymphocytes are being postulated one after another. Since these usually require special culture systems and serological reagents for their detection, they are greeted with some skepticism. Under these circumstances it is important to decide criteria of acceptibility in advance. One might well take a stringent position and decide that no hypothetical set of lymphocytes will be accepted until its existence has been demonstrated in a cloned population. This may be too inflexible a position because it does not take account of fluctuations in activity during the lifetime of a clone; for example, some activities may be characteristic only of cells which have undergone particular forms of activation. Even so one might reasonably ask that clones display these activities *in vitro,* with a switch from one activity to another after appropriate stimulation.

II. CLONING METHODS

Why is there so much excitement about cloning at the present time? This reflects not only the urgent need for testing ideas as outlined above, but also the possibilities opened up by technical advances. The situation at present is that remarkable advances have been made in somatic and molecular genetics which are in general terms bound to have an impact on cellular immunology. In the neighboring subject of B cell cloning, astonishing progress is being made which has already transformed entire areas of applied immunology, such as viral immunology and clinical radioimmunoassay. Within the field of T cell cloning an armamentarium of methods is accumulating and has already been applied on a fairly extensive scale. However, these methods are still under intensive development, and there is as yet little agreement on the methods which are appropriate for particular problems.

The possible approaches to cloning are dictated by the epigenetics of T cells. These cells, like other lymphocytes, live a life in which periods of division and differentiation alternate with periods of rest (if ceaseless recirculation can be so described). The periods of division and differentiation are brought about by antigen acting synergistically with still only partially understood antigen-nonspecific growth factors. One set of options therefore involves continuous or semicontinuous exposure of T cells to these natural stimuli. An alternative set circumvents these natural stimuli and instead involves altering the epigenetic state so that the cells proliferate independently. One option in this alternative set is simply to screen for suitable naturally occurring leukemias and lymphomas (Greaves, 1975). Another is to infect with a virus which derepresses growth and cell division (Finn *et al.*, 1979). A third is to fuse the desired T cell with a partner which has undergone malignant transformation and then permit selective segregation and loss of genetic material to take place so that the specific activity of the desired T cell remains behind in combination with the immortality of the transformed partner (Kontiainen *et al.*, 1978; Nabholz *et al.*, 1980a). There are many related options, few of which have yet been tested. Thus rather than infect with intact virus, it may be better to infect with defective virus, a genetically manipulated section of viral genome, or a synthetic viral-type strong promoter. All the options involving malignant transformation suffer from the drawback that normal T cell properties are lost to an unknown extent.

Historically, the first long-term cultures dependent on natural stimuli were simply mixed lymphocyte reactions in which fresh stimulator cells were added after an interval (MacDonald *et al.*, 1974). This established the principle, which was subsequently extended to long-term cell lines, that functionally active cytotoxic T cells could survive and proliferate provided that they received antigenic stimulation at intervals (Dennert and De Rose, 1976). Since then cloning of T cells has proceeded in two directions: the use of short-term clones to measure the frequency of various T cell sets by limiting dilution analysis, and the use of long-term clones to characterize individual properties more fully. Polyclonal mitogens, particularly concanavalin A (Eichmann *et al.*, 1980) and interleukin-2 (T cell growth factor) (Gillis and Smith, 1977) have proved useful in initiating and maintaining cultures. The subject has recently been comprehensively reviewed (MacDonald *et al.*, 1980; Nabholz *et al.*, 1980b; Wagner *et al.*, 1980; Schreier *et al.*, 1980).

III. QUESTIONS OF THE DAY

The uses of cloning is the subject of this entire treatise, which aims to present a representative selection of viewpoints on the subject. At this point, it is appropriate briefly to outline the kinds of purposes to which cloning has been put. These can be summarized under four headings.

First, cloning is being applied to the T cell receptor problem. In part, this is a matter of sorting out the fine specificities displayed by clones in relation to the major histocompatibility complex (von Boehmer *et al.*, 1979; Nabholz *et al.*, 1980a; Glasebrook and Fitch, 1980; Fathman and Hengartner, 1979). On the whole, there has been excellent agreement between specificities as defined by serology and those defined by T cell clones. Clones have been used to identify MHC determinants both as alloantigens and also as restriction elements. The agreement runs right down to the hybrid molecules formed by independent assortment of the α and β chains of the *A* and *E* loci. This agreement greatly strengthens the thesis of the unification of the MHC, that all the functions of each subregion of the complex are performed by the same molecule (Klein *et al.*, 1981). Only a few unexplained problems remain, for instance, the ability of hybrid T cell clones to recognize parental strain determinants (Nabholz *et al.*, 1980b).

Cloning permits study of the effect of background genes on MHC allospecificity, a matter of some theoretical interest. It has been proposed that allospecific T cells recognize not simply MHC antigens, but rather minor or background antigens which are restricted by the MHC (Matzinger and Bevan, 1977). Accordingly, one would expect to find on occasion clones that react with background antigens which are themselves polymorphic; such clones should react more strongly with an MHC molecule presented on the genetic background originally used to select the clone than with the same molecules when presented on another background. In a recent small survey, 60% of T helper cell clones behaved in this way (Yeh Ming *et al.*, 1982), although in another study $< 1\%$ of T cytotoxic cell clones did so (Langhorne and Fischer-Lindahl, 1982, but see also discussion in Mitchison, 1982).

Another area where clones can provide valuable information about the nature of the T cell receptor is in the study of idiotypes. Thus far antisera to T cell idiotypes have been raised using T cell populations selected by stimulation *in vitro,* using a variety of antigens Krammer *et al.*, 1980; Kees, 1981). To date the most recent findings have been interpreted as favoring a one-receptor rather than a two-receptor model, but it is agreed that at the present stage interpretation is uncertain.

Second, progress is being made with the effector functions of T cells by cloning. Thus far this has been mainly a matter of lining up functions and phenotypes defined by studies *in vitro* with functions *in vivo*. On the whole this has gone as expected. Thus, for example, all clones tested which display helper activity *in vitro* display the same activity *in vivo* (Tees and Schreier, 1980); all allo-H-2A-specific clones which proliferate *in vitro* display helper activity *in vivo* (Yeh Ming *et al.*, 1982; and helper clones mediate delayed-type hypersensitivity *in vivo* (Bianchi *et al.*, 1981). There have also been a few surprises, and no doubt there are more to come. One cytotoxic clone is claimed to mediate delayed-type hypersensitivity *in vivo* (Lin and Askonas, 1981). And among the first HLA-D-specific clones examined, the majority paradoxically displayed cytotoxic reactivity (Kornbluth and Dupont, 1980; for further discussion of this anomaly, see Mitchison, 1981). It has been suggested that the choice between helper and cytotoxic activity may be determined by the time at which the initial mixed lymphocyte reaction is subcultured: early subculture favors cytotoxic clones, while late subculture favours more proliferative cells and therefore helper clones (C. Mawas, personal communication).

Closely tied to effector function is the related area of regulatory functions. An important question here is the clonal basis of lymphokine production: do all clones produce all lymphokines, or is there some specialization of function? The answer is not yet known, but clonal methods capable of yielding an answer have been developed, and there is already evidence suggestive of heterogeneity (Krammer, 1981).

Another long-standing problem in regulatory functions which is yielding to clonal analysis is the relationship in *I* region restriction between T helper cell, macrophage, and B cell. It is becoming increasingly clear that restriction applies in the recognition of antigen by T cell clones on both macrophages and dendritic cells and also on small, unactivated B cells (Schreier *et al.*, 1980).

Undoubtedly the deepest problem in this area is to delineate populations of helper and suppressor cells and evaluate their importance in immunoregulation. One interesting approach is to examine, by limiting dilution analysis, just how many distinct populations of helpers and suppressors can be distinguished by their frequencies (Eichmann *et al.*, 1980; Simon *et al.*, 1981). Another, which has hardly begun but which is sorely needed, is to evaluate clones which would sample the various regulatory populations postulated to take part in regulatory circuits (Cantor and Gershon, 1979; Tada *et al.*, 1979a).

We come lastly to the uses of T cell clones and their products. In the immediate future clones are likely to provide aids to serology: the use of clones in the serological analysis of the family of *I-J* products is a good example (Tada *et al.*, 1979b). They provide also a convenient and reproducible source of lymphokines, at present particularly of interleukin-2 (Gillis and Watson, 1980) with γ-interferon as another lymphokine which is high on the agenda (Marcucci *et al.*, 1981). In the rather longer run, T cell clones are likely to find a use in the design and testing of vaccines. Finally, dare one speculate about the possible use of clones for intervention in clinical therapy? Much of the effort in bone marrow transplantation, for example, has been directed at eliminating T cells in order to avoid graft-versus-host disease. Should we not now be thinking in terms of isolating cytomegalovirus-reactive clones *in vitro,* in order to reconstitute the response in patients suffering from viral infection?

REFERENCES

Bianchi, A. T. J., Hoojikaas, H., Benner, R., Tees, R., Nordin, A. A., and Schreier, M. H. (1981). Clones of helper T cells mediate antigen-specific H-2-restricted, delayed-type hypersensitivity. *Nature (London)* **290,** 62.

Cantor, H., and Gershon, R. (1979). Immunological circuits: Cellular composition. *Fed. Proc., Fed. Am. Soc. Exp. Biol.* **38,** 2058.

Czitrom, A. A., Mitchison, N. A., and Yeh Ming (1982). Differentiation within the immune system: The importance of cloning. *In* "Differentiation in vitro" (M. M. Yeoman and D. E. S. Truman, eds.), pp. 253–265. Cambridge Univ. Press, London and New York.

Dennert, G., and De Rose, M. (1976). Continuously proliferating T killer cells specific for H-2^b targets: Selection and characterization. *J. Immunol.* **116,** 1601.

Eichmann, K., Falk, I., Melchers, I., and Simon, M. M. (1980). Quantitative studies on T cell diversity. I. Determination of the precursor frequencies for two types of streptococcus A-specific helper cells in non-immune, polyclonally activated spleen cells. *J. Exp. Med.* **152,** 477.

Fathman, C. G., and Hengartner, H. (1979). Cross-rective mixed lymphocyte reaction determinants, recognized by cloned allo-reactive T cells. *Proc. Natl. Acad. Sci. U.S.A.* **76,** 5863.

Finn, O. J., Boniver, J., and Kaplan, H. S. (1979). Induction, establishment *in vitro* and characterization of functional antigen-specific, carrier-primed murine T-cell lymphomas. *Proc. Natl. Acad. Sci. U.S.A.* **76,** 4033.

Fresno, M., Nabel, G., and Cantor, H. (1981). T-cell clones: Generation and analysis of antigen-specific molecules. *In* "Immunoglobulin Idiotypes" (C. Janeway, E. E. Sercarz, and H. Wigzell, eds.), pp. 373–386. Academic Press, New York.

Gaze, R. M., and Straznicky, C. (1980). Regeneration of optic nerve fibres from a compound eye to both ecta in *Xenopus:* Endemic relating to the state of specification of the eye and the tectum. *J. Embryol. Exp. Morphol.* **60,** 125.

Gillis, S., and Smith, K. A. (1977). Long term culture of tumour specific cytotoxic T cells. *Nature (London).* **268,** 154.

Gillis, S., and Watson, J. (1980). Biochemical and biological characterization of lymphocyte regulatory molecules. V. Identification on an interleukin-2-producing human leukaemia T cell line. *J. Exp. Med.* **152,** 1709.

Glasebrook, A. L., and Fitch, F. W. (1980). Alloreactive cloned T cell lines. I. Interactions between cloned amplifier and cytolytic T cell lines. *J. Exp. Med.* **151,** 876.

Greaves, M. F. (1975). "Cellular Recognition," Outline Series in Biology. Chapman & Hall, London.

Kees, U. (1981). Idiotypes on major histocompatibility complex-restricted virus-immune cytotoxic T lymphocytes. *J. Exp. Med.* **153,** 1562.

Klein, J., Juretic, A., Baxevanis, C. N., and Nagy, Z. A. (1981). The traditional and a new version of the mouse *H-2* complex. *Nature (London)* **291,** 455.

Kontiainen, S., Simpson, E., Bohrer, E., Beverley, P. C. L., Herzenberg, L. A., Fitzpatrick, W. C., Vogt, P., Torano, A., McKenzie, I. F. C., and Feldmann, M. (1978). T cell lines producing antigen-specific factor. *Nature (London)* **274,** 477.

Kornbluth, J., and Dupont, B. (1980). Cloning and functional characterization of primary alloreactive human T lymphocytes. *J. Exp. Med.* **152,** 164.

Krammer, P. H. (1981). Frequency of T cell growth factor producing cells in concanavalin A activated C57 BL/6 splenic T cells. *Immunobiology* **159,** 77.

Krammer, P. H., Rehberger, R., and Eichmann, K. (1980). Antigen receptors on major histocompatibility complex-restricted T lymphocytes. I. Preparation and characterization of syngeneic antisera against trinitrophenyl-activated T cell blasts and demonstration of their specificity for idiotypes on cytotoxic T lymphocytes. *J. Exp. Med.* **151,** 1166.

Langhorne, J., and Fischer-Lindahl, K. (1982). Role of non-H-2 antigens in the cytotoxic T cell response to allogeneic H-2. *Eur. J. Immunol.* (in press).

Lin, Y. L., and Askonas, B. A. (1981). Biological properties of an influenza A virus-specific killer T cell clone. Inhibition of virus replication *in vivo* are induction of delayed-type hypersensitivity reactions. *J. Exp. Med.* **154,** 225.

MacDonald, H. R., Cerottini, J.-C., Ryser, J.-E., Maryanski, J. L., Taswell, C., Widmer, M. B., and Brunner, K. T. (1980). Quantitation and cloning of cytolytic T lymphocytes and their precursors. *Immunol. Rev.* **51,** 93.

MacDonald, H. R. H., Engers, H. D., Cerottini, J.-C., and Brunner, K. (1974). Generation of cytotoxic T lymphocytes. II. Effect of repeated exposure to alloantigens on the cytotoxic activity of long-term mixed lymphocyte cultures. *J. Exp. Med.* **140,** 718.

Marcucci, F., Kirchner, H., and Krammer, P. H. (1981). Production of interferon-γ (IFN-γ) by a murine T cell clone from long term cultures. *Immunobiology* **159,** 89.

Matzinger, P., and Bevan, M. J. (1977). Why do so many lymphocytes respond to major histocompatibility antigens? *Cell. Immunol.* **29,** 1.

Mitchison, N. A. (1980). MHC molecules as guides for T lymphocyte parallel sets. In "Strategies of Immune Regulation" (E. E. Sercarz and A. J. Cunningham, eds.), pp. 121–133. Academic Press, New York.

Mitchison, N. A. (1981). Allospecific T cells. *Cell Immunol.* **62,** 258.

Mitchison, N. A. (1982). Information transfer between the minor antigen and T cell receptor repertoires. *Scand. J. Immunol.* **114,** 631.

Nabholz, M., Cianfriglia, M., Acuto, O., Conzelmann, A., Haas, W., von Boehmer, H., MacDonald, H. R., Pohlit, H., and Johnson, J. P. (1980a). Cytolytically active murine T-cell hybrids. *Nature (London)* **287,** 437.

Nabholz, M., Conzelmann, A., Acuto, O., North, M., Haas, W., Prohlit, H., von Boehmer, H., Hengartner, H., Mach, J.-P., Engers, H., and Johnson, J. P. (1980b). Established murine cytolytic T-cell lines as tools for a somatic genetic analysis of T-cell functions. *Immunol. Rev.* **51,** 125.

Reinherz, E. L., Rubinstein, A., Geha, R. S., Strelkauskas, A. J., Rosen, F. S., and Schlossman, S. F. (1979) Abnormalities of immunoregulatory T-cells in disorders of immune function. *N. Engl. J. Med.* **301,** 1018.

Schreier, M. H., Iscove, N. N., Tees, R., Aarden, L., and von Boehmer, H. (1980). Clones of killer and helper T cells: Growth requirements, specificity and retention of function in long-term culture. *Immunol. Rev.* **51,** 315.

Simon, M. M., Goronzy, J., and Eichmann, K. (1981). Comparison of the frequency of alloantigen specific T helper cell precursors in unselected and in selected T cell subpopulations after specific activation. *Immunobiology* **159,** 19.

Tada, T., Nonaka, M., and Okumura, K. (1979a). Ia antigens on suppressor, amplifier and helper T cells. *In* "Cell Biology and Immunology of Leukocyte Function" (M. R. Quastel, ed.), pp. 385–395. Academic Press, New York.

Tada, T., Taniguchi, M., Saito, T., and Matsuzawa, T. (1979b). Regulation of the antibody response by T-cell derived factors, their heterogeneity and genetics. *Monogr. Allergy* **14,** 45.

Tees, R., and Schreier, M. H. (1980). Selective reconstitution of nude mice with long-term cultured and cloned specific helper T cells. *Nature (London)* **283,** 780.

von Boehmer, H., Hengartner, H., Nabholz, W., Lenhardt, W., Schreier, M. H., and Haas, W. (1979). Fine specificity of a continuous growing killer cell clone specific for H-Y antigen. *Eur. J. Immunol.* **9,** 592.

Wagner, H., Hardt, C., Heeg, K., Pfizenmaier, K., Solbach, W., Bartlett, R., Stockinger, H., and Röllinghoff, M. (1980). T-T cell interactions during cytotoxic T lymphocyte (CTL) responses: T cell derived helper factor (interleukin 2) as a probe to analyse CTL responsiveness and thymic maturation of CTL progenitors. *Immunol. Rev.* **51,** 215.

Yeh Ming, Czitrom, A. A., and Mitchison, N. A. (1982). Allospecific T cell lines with functional activities. *Immunology* (in press).

I

IL-1 (Lymphocyte Activating Factor) and IL-2 (T Cell Growth Factor)

3

Biochemical Characterization of Interleukin-2 (T Cell Growth Factor)

Steven Gillis/James Watson/Diane Mochizuki

I.	IL-2 Microassay	24
II.	Purification of Human and Murine IL-2	24
III.	Temperature, Chemical, and Enzymatic Treatments of IL-2	26
IV.	Improved Cellular Sources for IL-2 Production and Characterization	26
V.	Polyacrylamide Gel Electrophoresis of IL-2	30
	A. Murine IL-2	30
	B. Human IL-2	33
VI.	Molecular Prospects for the Future	36
VII.	Conclusions	38
	References	38

The inability of cellular immunologists to obtain homogenous populations of effector T cells has hampered to a great extent rapid analysis of T cell function at the clonal level. Although several culture protocols, including repetitive antigen sensitization, mutagenesis, and even somatic cell hybridization, have been tested, clonable normal T lymphocytes could not be grown in exponential proliferative culture *in vitro*. An initial step toward this goal was taken approximately 5 years ago when workers in the laboratories of Robert Gallo at the National Cancer Institute noted, while attempting to culture acute myelogenous leukemia cells, that addition of conditioned medium harvested from cultures of T cell mitogen-stimulated human mononuclear leukocytes to normal and/or leukemic blood and bone marrow led to the exponential growth of a homogeneous population of cells. Although clearly not leukemic in nature, the proliferating cells were subsequently found to be E rosette positive and surface immunoglobulin and cytoplasm esterase negative (Morgan *et al.*, 1976). The cell population which proliferated also responded in mixed lymphocyte cultures but could not stimulate identical reactions; the cells also gave low but detectable proliferative responses to T cell mitogen activation (Ruscetti *et al.*, 1972). In short, these studies revealed the first successful method for the prolonged propagation of

ISBN 0-12-249920-4

normal functional T lymphocytes *in vitro*. However, the cells which proliferated in culture were acutely dependent on mitogen conditioned medium (CM) for their continuous replication.

Based on these studies, we adapted the use of CM to the mouse model system, and by using a tumor antigen stimulus (in contrast to lectin) for cultured cell activation developed the first continuous cultures of antigen specific effector cytolytic T cells (Gillis and Smith, 1977). Since this time, we (Baker *et al.*, 1979; Rosenberg *et al.*, 1978) and other investigators (whose reports are included in this treatise) have extended this culture technique to provide reproducible methods for the clonal isolation and maintenance of antigen-specific murine helper (Watson, 1979; Schreier and Tees, 1980) and cytolytic T cells (Nabholz *et al.*, 1978; von Boehmer *et al.*, 1979) as well as cloned antigen-specific human cytolytic T cells (Gillis *et al.*, 1978a; Strausser and Rosenberg, 1978). Critical for the various initiation and maintenance procedures recently standardized for the growth of human and murine T cell lines is the absolute and acute dependence of such cell lines on the continual presence of mitogen-stimulated mononuclear leukocytes.

Early investigation confirmed that the proliferation inducing agent present in CM was not the mitogen itself, in that exponential proliferation of either human peripheral blood leukocytes or murine spleen cells *in vitro* was not possible following repetitive phytohemagglutinin (PHA) or Concanavalin A (Con-A) stimulation (Gillis *et al.*, 1978b). Soon after (i) noting the acute dependence of proliferating effector T cells on CM and (ii) developing CM dependent methods for establishment of effector T cell lines, we became far more interested in determining the precise factor that was present in CM which could maintain indefinite T cell proliferation.

This curiosity has to a great extent shaped our research program over the past 4 years. Initially detailed as T cell growth factor (TCGF) (Gillis *et al.*, 1978b), we and other investigators have helped to identify a soluble protein factor which fuels T cell proliferation (Watson *et al.*, 1979; Farrar *et al.*, 1978). TCGF (now termed interleukin-2 or IL-2) is in fact a proliferation inducing lymphokine which controls T cell mitogenesis, antigen-induced proliferation witnessed in mixed lymphocyte cultures, and memory effector cell replication (Watson *et al.*, 1979; Aarden, 1979).

Basic studies *in vitro* quickly established the central role that IL-2 played in T cell proliferation. These experiments confirmed that the primary activation signal to a T cell population is delivered as a result of binding of antigen or mitogen to the cell membrane. It would seem then that a subset of activated mature T cells (Lyt-1^+ in the mouse and Okt-4^+ in the human model system) cooperates with macrophages to initiate IL-2 production. It has been confirmed recently in a number of laboratories that macrophages mediate their essential effect on IL-2 producer T cells via production and action of the monokine interleukin-1 (IL-1), formerly referred to as lymphocyte activating factor (Larsson *et al.*, 1980; Smith *et al.*, 1980). In fact, it would appear that IL-1 activity aids in the differentiation of antigen reactive IL-2 producer T cells (Gillis and Mizel, 1981). A separate set of activated T cells (IL-2 responders) simultaneously develops the capacity to react to IL-2 as a result of mitogen/antigen binding. This response capacity is presumably mediated by the acquisition of cell surface IL-2 receptors (Smith *et al.*, 1979). The signal inducing replication, originally thought to be mitogen or antigen, is actually mediated solely by IL-2. Once the primary activation is received, the responding cell population and presumably all subsequent daughter cells, given the ability of IL-2 to maintain indefinite effector T cell line replication, retain responsiveness to the proliferative stimulus provided by IL-2. The specificity of the response is mediated solely by the antigen-mitogen in that only those cells which have bound the ligand become responsive to IL-2. Obviously the proliferative signal (IL-2) itself is totally nonspecific and will promote the replicative expansion of any activated T cell clone. This fundamental biological principle, namely, that IL-2 drives the proliferation of ligand-activated lymphokine-responsive T cells, remains as the single mechanistic principle which explains the ability of IL-2 to promote positive responses in an overwhelming variety of immune response assays *in vitro* (Watson *et al.*, 1979; Farrar *et al.*, 1978; Gillis *et al.*, 1980a).

It is fairly straightforward to acknowledge that IL-2 functions as a proliferation-inducing agent to enhance thymocyte mitogenesis and the *in vitro* generation of cytolytic T cells (Watson *et al.*, 1979; Farrar *et al.*, 1978; Gillis *et al.*, 1980a). In fact, it is the relative paucity of IL-2-producing cells in nude mouse splenocyte or normal thymus cell preparations (IL-2-producing cells are present only in the peanut agglutinin negative, cortisone resistant, mature thymocyte subpopulation) which dictates the meager mitogen and CTL differentiation responses mediated by these cells *in vitro,* unless exogenous IL-2 is present (Watson *et al.*, 1979; Gillis *et al.*, 1979, 1980a; Wagner *et al.*, 1980). Similarly, it is the IL-2-dependent proliferation of pre/helper T cells present in nude spleen cell preparations (presumably replicating to the point where they in turn provide a helper effect to antigen triggered B-cells, perhaps mediated by a true T cell replacing factor) which results in the ability of IL-2 to augment plaque forming cell responses *in vitro* by nude mouse splenocytes in response to heterologous erythrocyte antigen stimulation (Watson *et al.*, 1979; Gillis *et al.*, 1980a). In fact based on the increased ability of poly(I:C)-stimulated normal and nude spleen cells to absorb IL-2, it would appear that IL-2 lymphokine–receptor interaction and subsequent proliferation may even be the mechanism behind the ability of IL-2 to augment natural killer cell (NK) functions (Henney *et al.*, 1981; Kuribayashi *et al.*, 1981).

The establishment of basic biological principles behind IL-2-mediated T cell proliferation, as well as experimentation detailing the ability of IL-2 to augment cell-mediated immune reactivity *in vitro*, has been dependent on the availability of biochemically characterized IL-2. In essence, no other single line of investigation, except for the development of multiple-cloned T cell lines of single antigen specificity, has done more to promote the understanding of lymphokine-mediated immune responses than the development of preparative purification schemes for the isolation and characterization of IL-2. In the following pages we have traced our research developments detailing the purification of IL-2 and have included a description of novel cellular reagents without which purification of IL-2 to possible homogeneity would not have been possible.

I. IL-2 MICROASSAY

Early in our attempts to approach the biochemical characterization of the factor present in CM which triggered T cell proliferation, we realized that our chances of success would be greatly enhanced if we could develop a rapid, quantitative assay for CM-induced T cell proliferation. The utility of such an assay, particularly from a biochemical standpoint, would be further enhanced if completion of the test required use of only a small amount of biochemically manipulated material. Essentially, the IL-2 microassay meets all of these requirements (Gillis *et al.*, 1978b). In addition to being instrumental for assessment of IL-2 activity following various biochemical separations and modifications, the IL-2 microassay remains as the only unequivocal assay for the presence of IL-2 activity.

The IL-2 assay is based solely on the factor requirement of cultured T cell lines. T cells harvested from IL-2-dependent culture, washed and placed back in culture in the absence of IL-2, invariably die within 24 hr. By using tritiated thymidine (^{3}H-TdR) incorporation as an index on cultured T cell replication, the IL-2 microassay provides a highly reproducible and quantitative indication of the amount of IL-2 activity present in a given sample of crude or biochemically manipulated CM.

II. PURIFICATION OF HUMAN AND MURINE IL-2

We used standard preparative purification techniques to begin initial biochemical characterization of human and murine T cell derived IL-2. A summary of the results from these studies is given in Table I. Twenty-four-hour serum-free supernates harvested from cultures of either 1% PHA-stimulated human peripheral blood lymphocytes (10^7 cells/ml) or Con-A-stimulated (2.5 μg/ml) murine spleen cells (5×10^6 cells/ml) were concentrated by ammonium sulfate precipitation at 80% saturation. Precipitated material was fractionated by AcA 54 gel filtration chromatography. A reproducible difference in size was found be-

TABLE I

Biochemical Characteristics of Murine and Human IL-2 Purified from Conventional Conditioned Medium Sources[a]

Property	Murine IL-2	Human IL-2
Size according to gel filtration chromatography	30,000 MW	15,000 MW
Salt concentration at elution point from DEAE-cellulose	185 m*M*	45 m*M*
Salt concentration at elution point from carboxymethyl-Sepharose	50 m*M*	225 m*M*
Isoelectric point	pH 4.3, 4.9	pH 6.5

[a] Murine: concanavalin A-stimulated spleen cell supernates. Human: phytohemagglutin-stimulated peripheral blood leukocyte supernates.

tween human and murine IL-2. Interleukin-2 activity fractionated from murine splenocyte CM chromatographed over a wide range of fractions and had a mean molecular weight of approximately 30,000 (Watson *et al.*, 1979), whcreas human IL-2 was detected in fractions which corresponded to mobility of molecules with a mean size range of 15,000 MW (Table I). Fractions with appreciable IL-2 titer were subjected to further separation using an ion exchange resin. However, pretreatment of DEAE-Sephacel was carried out to prevent nonspecific sticking of IL-2 to the resin. The matrix was incubated with 0.9% NaCl-HEPES containing 2% FCS and then washed with 0.1% Triton-X 100 to prevent hydrophobic interaction, and with 0.2 *M* sodium citrate to remove heavy metals. A fundamental difference was observed in charge characteristics of human and murine IL-2 activity. Although human IL-2 activity did not bind to DEAE-Sephacel (Gillis *et al.*, 1980b), murine IL-2 activity bound to the ion exchange resin and could be eluted with 185 m*M* salt (Table I). Even though human IL-2 activity did not bind DEAE, the use of this ion exchange step in the purification scheme was of some value in that the activity could be separated from negatively charged contaminant proteins which bound to the ion exchange resin in the equilibration buffer.

The inability of DEAE to act as an ion exchange affinity reagent for human IL-2 led us to examine the use of a negatively charged resin [carboxymethyl (CM)-Sepharose] as a second step ion-exchange procedure. After passage over DEAE-Sephacel, human IL-2 adhered to negatively charged carboxymethyl-Sepharose resin. Human IL-2 activity could be eluted from the negatively charged carboxymethyl-Sephadrose resin with 225 m*M* NaCl-HEPES. Following either one step (DEAE; murine) or two phase (DEAE-CM-Sepharose, human) ion exchange chromatography, active IL-2 fractions were subjected to preparative isoelectric focusing (IEF). Differences in basic physical characteristics between human and murine IL-2 continued to become apparent upon analysis of IEF data. Human IL-2 migrated upon isoelectric focusing with a predominant p*I* value of pH 6.8 and with a minor peak of activity at pH 7.1 (Gillis *et al.*, 1980a). Murine

IL-2, however, appeared to be more acidic in nature and migrated as two distinct peaks of activity at pH 4.3–4.5 and pH 4.9–5.1.

In summary, murine IL-2, as reflected by lower p*I* values and adherence to a positively charged ion exchange column, was more acidic in nature than human IL-2, although both sources of factor were capable of triggering murine T cell line proliferation to the same extent. One might speculate therefore that the domain of the molecule which gives murine IL-2 its more acidic character more than likely is not responsible for its biological activity.

III. TEMPERATURE, CHEMICAL, AND ENZYMATIC TREATMENTS OF IL-2

The yield of IL-2 activity following gel filtration, one or two cycle ion exchange chromatography and preparative flat-bed IEF was consistently less than 15%. Furthermore, only submicrogram quantities of material were available following the final IEF stage. Although such a low yield precluded further attempts at biochemical separation, the amount of material generated by the above separation scheme did provide sufficient murine and human IL-2 to allow testing of its sensitivity to various temperature and enzymatic treatments (Mochizuki *et al.*, 1980b). The suspected protein nature of IL-2 was confirmed by results of experiments summarized in Table II. IL-2 activity was destroyed by 24-hr 37°C incubation with 100 μg/ml trypsin or chymotrypsin or 200 μg/ml subtilisin. Exposure of IL-2 to leucine aminopeptidase (an enzyme which hydrolyzes N-terminal amino acids with free amino groups) resulted in approximately a 40% loss of biological activity. As expected, nucleic acid denaturing enzymes had no effect on IL-2 activity. Human and murine IL-2 activities were both stable after incubation at 37°C for 12 hr and at 56°C for a 1-hr period. Incubation at 70°C for 10 min also had little effect on IL-2 biological activity. However, 70°C incubation for 30 min or longer led to a significant loss of activity. The effects of SDS on biological activity were variable and determined by the conditions of the treatment. However, human and murine IL-2 activity were stable to treatment with 0.1% SDS at 70°C for 10 min. Increased incubation time led to a substantial loss of activity. IL-2 activity was remarkably stable after 4 hr exposure to either high or low pH solutions, urea, 2-mercaptoethanol (2Me), and dithiothreitol (DTT).

IV. IMPROVED CELLULAR SOURCES FOR IL-2 PRODUCTION AND CHARACTERIZATION

Using conventional sources of CM as starting material for biochemical characterization, literally hundreds of liters of CM would be required for isolation of

TABLE II

Susceptibility of IL-2 to Enzymatic/Physical Degradation

Treatment	% Control IL-2 activity remaining after treatment[a]	
	Murine IL-2	Human IL-2
Enzyme		
Control (salt solution dialysis, 37°C 12 hr)	100 (45 units)	100 (100 units)
Trypsin (37°C 12 hr)	0	0
Chymotrypsin (37°C 12 hr)	0	0
Subtilisin (37°C 12 hr)	0	0
Leucine aminopeptidase (40°C 12 hr)	38	22
DNase 1 (48°C 8 hr)	95	90
RNase A (48°C 8 hr)	86	98
Physical		
Control (pH 7.2 4.5 hr)	100	100
pH 7.2 (4°C 4.5 hr)	103	92
pH 10.5 (4°C 4.5 hr)	92	101
2 *M* urea (22°C 4.5 hr)	93	75
8 *M* urea (22°C 4.5 hr)	10	2
0.01% 2Me (pH 8 4.5 hr)	75	106
0.25 *M* 2Me (pH 8 4.5 hr)	94	102
0.05 *M* DTT (pH 8 4.5 hr)	90	85
37°C 12 hr	104	94
70°C 15 min	102	96
70°C 1 hr	0	0
0.1% SDS 70°C 10 min	87	97
0.1% SDS 70°C 15 min	82	62
0.1% SDS 70°C 30 min	54	32
0.1% SDS 70°C 45 min	0	0

[a] IL-2 as titer determined by standard microassay both before and after perturbant treatment.

pure IL-2 (see below). Because of the limitation that poor yields of IL-2 placed on further research, it became clear that more efficient means of factor production and recovery had to be developed.

Forty murine and human T cell leukemia and lymphoma cell lines were screened for both constitutive and mitogen-induced IL-2 production. Of the cell lines tested, only two (one each in both human and mouse systems) were found to produce high titer IL-2 upon mitogen stimulation. As shown in Table III, phytohemagglutinin (PHA) stimulation of cloned mouse LBRM-33 cells resulted in culture supernates which contained between 1000 and 5000 times the amount of biologically active IL-2 which was routinely generated by identical numbers (10^6 cells/ml) of optimally stimulated rat or mouse splenocytes (Gillis *et al.*, 1980b). Similarly, PHA and phorbol ester stimulation of the human leukemia T cell line Jurkat-FHCRC produced between 100 and 300 times the amount of

TABLE III

Screening of Leukemia and Lymphoma Cells for IL-2 Production

	IL-2 Activity (units/ml) present in 48-hr supernate following activation with		
Cell line	Medium[a]	Con-A (10 μg/ml)	PHA [1%(v/v)]
Murine T cell tumors			
RBL-5	0.0	0.0	0.0
EL-4	0.0	0.0	0.0
L51784	0.0	0.0	0.0
S49	0.0	0.0	NT[b]
BW5147	0.0	0.0	NT
RDM 4	0.0	0.0	0.0
ASL-1	0.0	0.0	0.0
RLo-1	0.0	0.0	0.0
HRST 34	0.0	0.0	0.0
LBRM-33	0.0	29.0	675.0
LBRM-33 1A5	0.0	0.0	0.0
LBRM-33 4C1	0.0	0.1	14.3
LBRM-33 5A4	0.0	45.0	1356.0
LBRM-33 4A2	0.0	62.0	929.0
LBRM-33 6B1	0.0	132.0	1266.0
Human T cell leukemias			
CEM-SK1	0.0	0.0	0.0
CEM-FHCRC	0.0	0.0	0.0
8402-FHCRC	0.0	0.0	0.0
HSB2-SK1	0.0	0.0	0.0
HSB2-FHCRC	0.0	0.0	0.0
MOLT-4-SK1	0.0	0.0	0.0
MOLT-4-FHCRC	0.0	0.0	0.0
Ke37-FHCRC	0.0	0.0	0.0
T-45-SK1	0.0	0.0	0.0
R-2-SK1	0.0	0.0	0.0
PEER-SK1	0.0	0.0	0.0
HPB-ALL-SK1	0.0	0.0	0.0
JURKAT-FHCRC	0.0	55.0	266.0

[a] RMP1 1640, 10% FCS.
[b] NT, not tested.

human IL-2 per milliliter normally generated by lectin-stimulated human PBL or spleen cells (Gillis and Watson, 1980). IL-2 activity derived from Jurkat-FHCRC was capable of sustaining the proliferation of both murine and human T cells *in vitro,* whereas CM generated from LBRM-33 cells proved effective only when tested on murine IL-2-dependent T cells. These results were consistent with our previous studies detailing the species specificity of IL-2 (Gillis *et al.*, 1978b) and confirmed that Jurkat-FHCRC CM was an excellent source of human IL-2 activity.

With both cell lines, peak levels of IL-2 were found in supernatants harvested from 24-hr cultures stimulated with either 1% PHA or 20 μg/ml Con-A. LBRM-33 cells stimulated in such a manner routinely generated conditioned medium containing greater than 1000 U/ml IL-2 activity, and Jurkat-FHCRC supernatants contained greater than 200 U/ml IL-2. It should be stressed that identical high titer IL-2 containing supernates could be produced by both Jurkat-FHCRC and LBRM-33 cells in the absence of serum.

Although the tumor cells produced CM containing high titers of IL-2, the mitogen required for induction of factor secretion was invariably accompanied by cell death. To avoid this problem, we attempted to generate constitutive IL-2-producing hybrid cell lines by fusing the IL-2-producing tumor cells with drug marked, mruine or human T cell lymphoma lines. Although attempts in the human system were not successful, fusion of cloned LBRM-33 cells with the BW5147 cell line, led to the establishment of a constitutive IL-2-producing mouse hybridoma. Although the IL-2 produced by the hybrid line appeared biochemically indistinguishable from that derived from LBRM-33 or murine spleen cells, the titer of the hybrid cell supernatant, even under optimal conditions, never approached that produced by parent IL-2 producer cells after mitogen stimulation (Stull and Gillis, 1981).

IL-2 derived from both human and murine tumor cell lines migrated somewhat differently in isoelectric focusing as compared to IL-2 from conventional

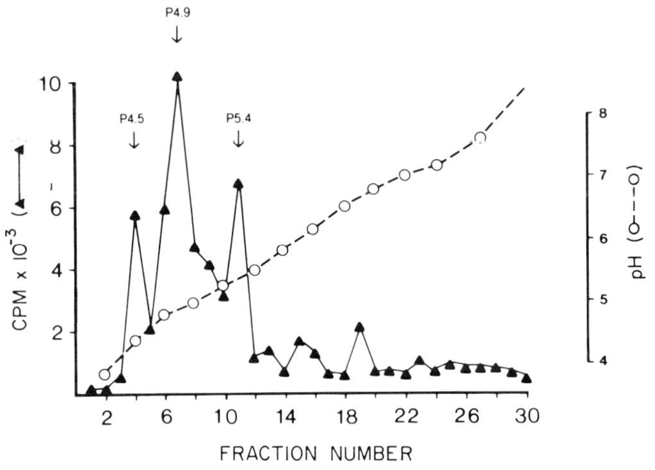

Fig. 1. IL-2 activity of fractions isolated by preparative IEF. Murine tumor cell line derived IL-2 was purified through DEAE-Sephacel and AcA54 gel filtration chromatography prior to isoelectric focusing. Five microliters of each fraction was assayed in a standard 200 μl IL-2 titration.

sources. For example, IL-2 from human PBL had a broad region of isoelectric points between pH 6 and 6.5. Isoelectric focusing of Jurkat-derived factor revealed a sharp peak of activity with a p*I* of 7.75 and a minor peak with a slightly more acidic p*I* (Frank *et al.*, 1981). Similarly, as shown in Fig. 1, in addition to the peaks (p*I* 4.5 and 5.4) observed with IL-2 from mouse spleen cells stimulated by mitogen, LBRM-derived IL-2 also contained an additional significant peak of activity which consistently migrated with a p*I* of 3.9–4.2 (Mochizuki *et al.*, 1980a). Nonetheless, the amount of activity and protein present in each peak separated by IEF was sufficient to warrant application of further separation techniques.

V. POLYACRYLAMIDE GEL ELECTROPHORESIS OF IL-2

A. Murine IL-2

Preparative polyacrylamide gel electrophoresis (PAGE) systems were developed for further separation of IL-2 obtained after IEF. The procedure was based in part on the application of a discontinuous, mono-Tris-bicene buffer system developed by Wiley and Wallace (Watson *et al.*, 1979), and is described in detail in the Appendix. Figure 2 shows the Coomassie blue staining pattern of LBRM-335A4-derived IL-2 subjected to preparative slab gel PAGE. This IL-2 preparation had been exposed to sequential gel filtration and ion exchange chromatography and preparative flatbed IEF, and the p*I* 4.9 peak was subjected to PAGE analysis. To our suprise, 7–9 protein bands were visible between the markers of soybean trypsin inhibitor (20,500 daltons) and carbonic anhydrase (30,000 daltons). Following electrophoretic elution, each band (2–6) was assayed for IL-2 activity, and the two bands corresponding to proteins of 25,000 daltons and 21,500 daltons contained large amounts of IL-2 activity. The recovery of biological activity was approximately 20% of the total number of IL-2 units applied to the slab gel. To reaffirm molecular homogeneity, these two bands were subjected to a second round of SDS-PAGE. The Commassie blue staining pattern of second cycle gels confirmed that each protein migrated as a well resolved band (Fig. 3). Each major IL-2 protein band had been separated successfully from minor contaminants which had migrated slightly ahead or behind the major activity peaks. Subsequent electroelution of the second set of gels confirmed that both proteins possessed significant IL-2 activity. It should be stressed that the starting material for the SDS-PAGE analysis was material obtained from IEF having a characteristic p*I* of 4.9.

SDS-PAGE separation of IEF peaks of murine IL-2 having p*I* of 4.5 and 5.4 (see Fig. 1) are depicted in Fig. 4. Although discrete stainable protein species having MW of 30–15,000 are visible in photographs of gels prepared with the

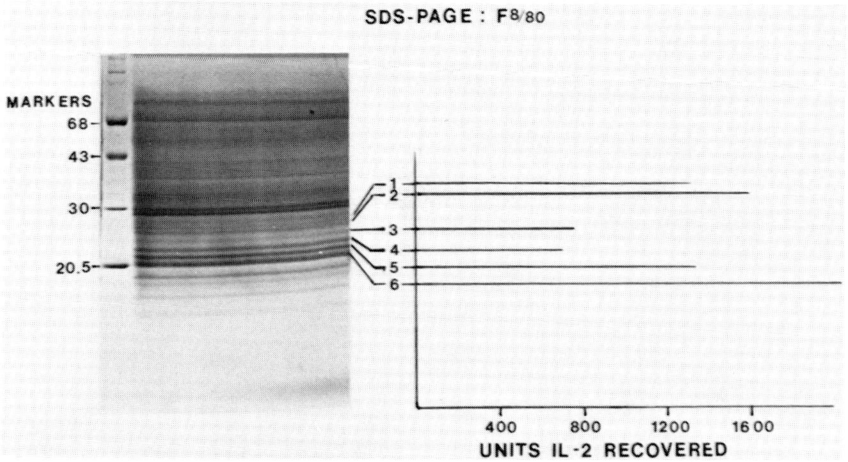

Fig. 2. The Coomassie blue protein staining pattern of LBRM IL-2 preparation F8/80 following 13% SDS-PAGE on 2-mm thick gels. The gel was loaded with 2×10^5 units of IL-2 which had been sequentially purified by AcA54 gel filtration, DEAE-Sephacel, and preparative IEF. The protein bands which migrated between the carbonic anhydrase (30,000 daltons) and SBT1 (21,500 daltons) markers were cut out, and the protein in a portion of the gel was eluted and titrated in an IL-2 microassay. The recovery of IL-2 activity from each band is also shown on the right. Recovery of biological activity after electrophoresis, staining/destaining of the slab gel, and subsequent elution was 21%. The apparent molecular weights of bands 2 and 6 were determined to be 25,000 and 21,000, respectively.

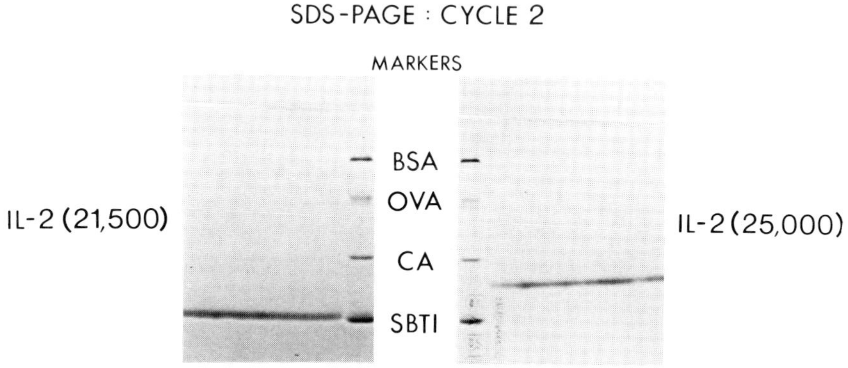

Fig. 3. The Coomassie blue protein staining pattern of LBRM IL-2 preparation F8/80 following a second cycle of SDS-PAGE on 11.6% acrylamide, 2-mm thick slab gels. The 25,000 and 21,000 MW species recovered from 2-mm thick slab gels (Fig. 2) were separately pooled and reelectrophoresed. The major 21,000 and 25,000 MW protein bands were cut out and the protein in a portion (8%) of the band was eluted and titrated in a TCGF microassay. Each apparently homogeneous protein band was found to contain IL-2 TCGF activity.

IEF peak having a p*I* of 4.5, these probably represent contaminant proteins since the majority of biological activity was associated with lightly stained bands having MW of 28,000 and 27,000, respectively. Similarily, although a major contaminant with a MW of 29,000 was seen in gels prepared with the p*I* 5.4 peak, the predominant protein which retained biological activity on subsequent electroelution had a MW of approximately 15,500. Such a relatively basic, low molecular weight, murine IL-2 may in fact be similar to the species with a MW of 15,000 suggested by the SDS-gel filtration chromatography data recently reported by Caplan *et al.* (1981).

The data presented in Figs. 2–4 suggests that there may exist for murine IL-2 some type of charge–size relationship in which more basic IL-2 species have a progressively lower molecular weight. Increase in the p*I* of the molecule may be accompanied by incremental increase in molecular weight which would be con-

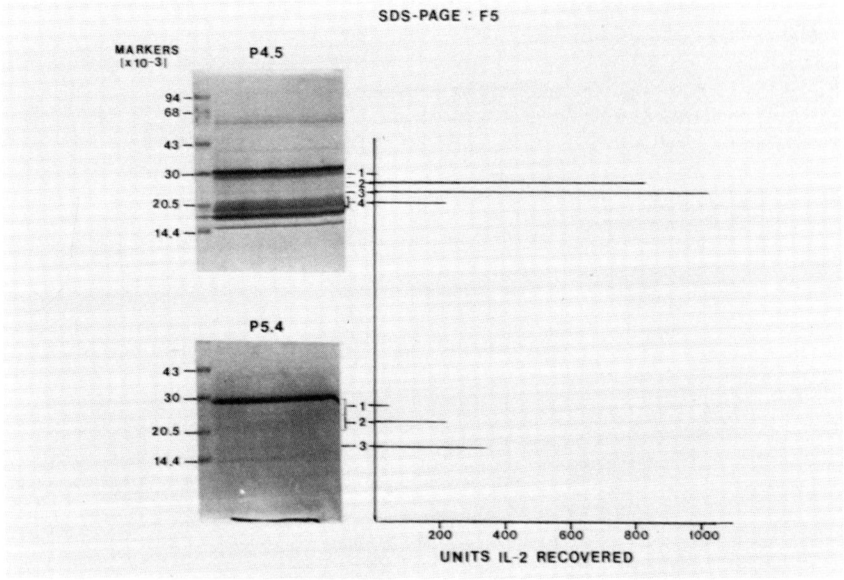

Fig. 4. The Coomassie blue protein staining pattern of IL-2 p*I* 4.5 species (upper panel) and p*I* 5.4 species (lower panel) following 13% SDS-PAGE on 2-mm thick gels. The gel in the upper panel was loaded with 3.9×10^4 units and the gel in the lower panel was loaded with 1.9×10^4 units of IL-2 which had been sequentially purified by gel filtration, DEAE-Sephacel, and preparative IEF (pH 2.5–6). The proteins which migrated between the carbonic anhydrase (30,000 daltons) and lactalbumin (14,000 daltons) markers were cut out, electrophoretically eluted, and titrated in an IL-2 assay. The apparent molecular weights of p*I* 4.5 (upper panel) bands 2, 3, 4 are 26,000, 24,000, and 21,000, respectively. The apparent molecular weights of the p*I* 5.4 (lower panel), bands 1, 2, 3 are 30,000, 21,500–25,500, and 16,500, respectively. The recovery of IL-2 activity was 6% for the p*I* 4.5 material and 3.5% for the p*I* 5.4 material.

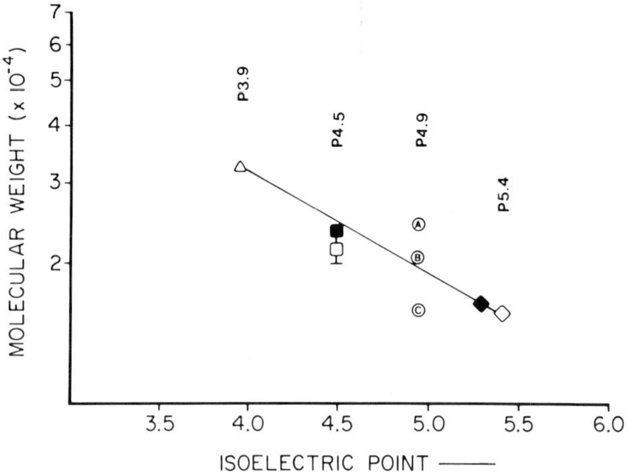

Fig. 5. Inverse relationship of size to charge of the different molecular forms of IL-2. The isoelectric point of the IL-2 species is plotted against the apparent molecular weight of the IL-2 species as determined by SDS-PAGE analysis. The open symbols represent IL-2 preparation F8 activity pools, p*I* 3.9 (△), p*I* 4.5 (□), p*I* 4.9 (Ⓐ, Ⓑ, Ⓒ), and p*I* 5.4 (◇). The closed symbols represent a separate preparation activity pools, p*I* 4.5 (■) and p*I* 5.4 (◆).

sistent with heightened posttranslational glycosylation. The relationship between molecular charge and size relationship is shown in Fig. 5. A species of murine IL-2 species having even lower p*I* (3.9) is often observed following processing of large volumes of CM from the IL-2 producing LBRM tumor cell line. On SDS-PAGE fractionation, this acidic IL-2 species has an apparent MW of 33,000, and therefore the highest molecular weight and lowest p*I* of any IL-2 species currently identified. In all cases, it seems plausible that SDS-PAGE fractionation followed by electrophoretic elution is successful in isolation of truly homogeneous IL-2. Preliminary amino acid sequence information obtained from identical, stained protein bands suggests the existence of only single N-terminal amino acids in each of the polypeptides detailed above.

B. Human IL-2

SDS-PAGE analysis of Jurkat-FHCRC-derived IL-2 activity, previously fractionated by sequential gel filtration, two-phase ion exchange chromatography, and preparative IEF, shows a simpler pattern of proteins associated with IL-2 biological activity (Fig. 6). Electrophoresis of human IL-2 with a p*I* of 7.75 led to visualization of some seven protein bands which migrated in the region between 10,000 and 20,000 daltons. Electroelution of each stainable band followed by microassay of eluted proteins clearly revealed that a single protein band

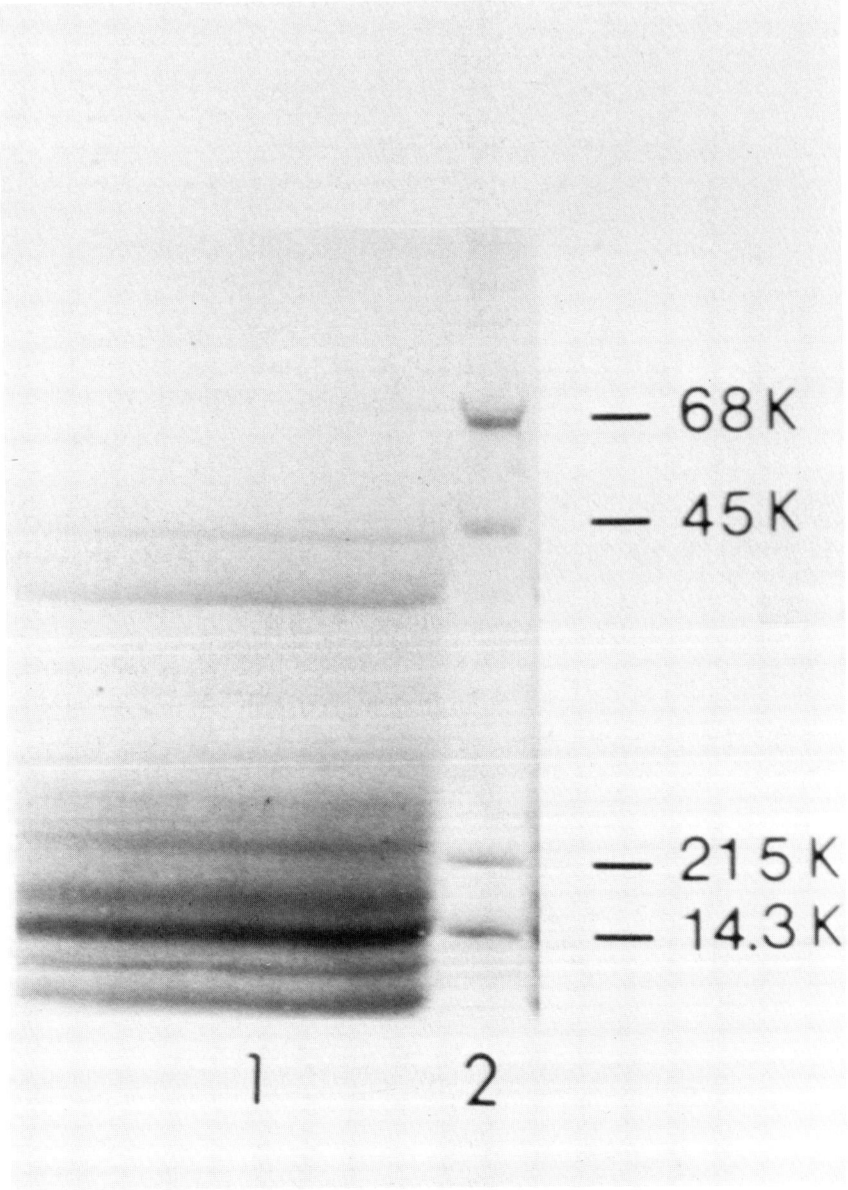

Fig. 6. A Coomassie blue stained polyacrylamide gel of protein present in Jurkat-FHCRC-derived IL-2. Prior to SDS-PAGE analysis, Jurkat-IL-2 had been subjected to sequential gel filtration, ion-exchange chromatography, and preparative IEF.

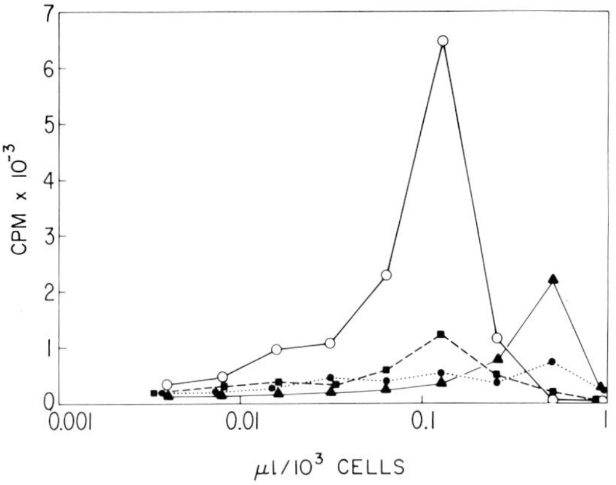

Fig. 7. Protein bands migrating within the region of 10,000–20,000 MW as detailed in Fig. 6 were cut from the gel and electroeluted. Reconstituted, eluted protein was then tested for IL-2 activity in a standard assay. The molecular weight of each respective band is 15,800 (▲), 14,800 (○), 13,500 (■), and 12,000 (●). ^{3}H-TdR incorporation in the absence of IL-2 was 500 cpm; maximum Il-2 induced thymidine incorporation in a 1 U/ml control sample was 7500 cpm. Based on these studies the concentration of IL-2 present in the 14,800 MW sample is in excess of 12,000 U/ml.

migrating between lysozyme and cytochrome *c*, with an apparent MW of 14,500, contained a majority of biological activity (Fig. 7). Some residual activity was detected in the two stained bands directly above that species. It is yet to be determined whether this pattern is due to separate molecular weight entities or whether elutable bands with lesser degrees of activity represent an artifactual trailing of smaller molecular weight proteins.

Several points are worth reiteration. Despite a five-step preparative purification scheme which includes isoelectric focusing, IL-2 preparations obtained using this procedure represent a heterogeneous group of proteins, of which only a minor portion consists of biologically active IL-2. Nevertheless using SDS-PAGE techniques, it is possible to isolate potentially homogeneous IL-2 in microgram quantities, corresponding to biological activities in excess of 10,000 units. Such calculations are suggestive that the molecule must function biologically in picomolar concentrations. It is rather remarkable that successive electrophoresis, staining, and destaining of slab gels allows for recovery of biologically active IL-2. Although the yield from this separation step is extremely poor (< 20%), the distinctive ability of the molecule to retain activity after such a harsh series of treatments, suggests that it may be exceptionally insusceptible to microenvironmental perturbation *in vivo,* a useful property if indeed IL-2 fuels the proliferation of activated T cells *in vivo* in areas of inflammation and immunological assault.

VI. MOLECULAR PROSPECTS FOR THE FUTURE

With the advent of recombinant DNA technology and its success in the cloning and bulk fermentation of other agents capable of modulating immune responses, most notably interferon, application of current molecular biology techniques to IL-2 may allow for more efficient production and more precise molecular characterization of this regulatory molecule.

We have begun experiments aimed at the isolation of messenger RNA coding for IL-2 and the development of detection systems that would be essential for cloning at the *Il-2* gene. In initial studies, total cellular RNA was extracted (using conventional phenol–chloroform extraction procedures) from mitogen-induced IL-2-producing Jurkat-FHCRC tumor cells. Translation of 5 μg of Jurkat poly(A^+) mRNA in a rabbit reticulocyte system *in vitro* yielded a biologically active product. Figure 8 depicts the results of IL-2 assays with this translation product. Less than 0.1 μl of translation product stimulated in excess of 4000 cpm of murine T cell line ^{3}H-TdR incorporation in a standard 24-hr IL-2 assay. These results, in addition to documenting successful isolation and translation of producer cell, human IL-2 message, also lend evidence that posttranslational processing may not be necessary for synthesis of biologically active IL-2, since glycosylation is not possible in reticulocyte systems. Despite the success of these studies, it is evident from the data displayed that the reticulocyte lysate probably contains several nonspecific inhibitors of IL-2 function, since concentrations of lysate greater than 1.25 μl (1.5% by volume) did not stimulate CTLL cell replication, whereas lesser concentrations did. The approach of using biological

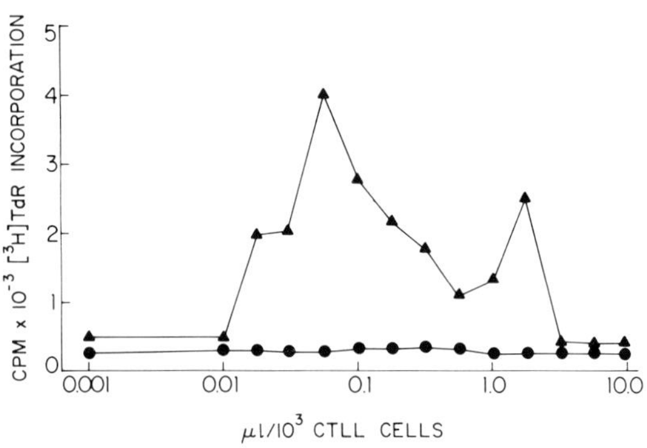

Fig. 8. IL-2 microassay data gathered from titration of rabbit reticulosate translation product (▲). Translation product was prepared from mitogen-induced Jurkat-FHCRC cell line poly(A^+) RNA. Maximum IL-2 induced thymidine incorporation by a 20 U/ml control sample was 19,000 cpm. Background ^{3}H-TdR incorporation in the absence of IL-2 was 500 cpm. Titration results were also depicted for microassay of a mock translation conducted with globin mRNA (●).

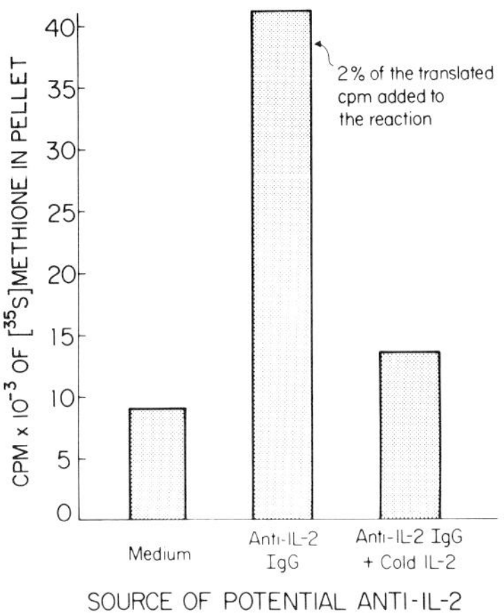

Fig. 9. Immune precipitation of [^{35}S]methionine-labeled Jurkat poly(A^+) mRNA translation product. Either 20 μl of tissue culture medium or 20 μl of monoclonal anti-IL-2 IgG (250 μg/ml) were mixed with 20 μl of radiolabeled translation product. After a 30-min incubation at 4°C, 200 μl of Igsorb (lyophilized *Staphylococcus aureus*) was added to the reaction mixture. Following an additional 90-min incubation at 4°C, Igsorb pellets were washed four times with 0.9% NaCl, resuspended in 3.5 ml of Biofluor liquid scintillation cocktail, and precipitated counts per minute counted by liquid scintillation. An additional reaction experiment contained 20 μl of 5 U/ml human IL-2 (cold IL-2) in addition to anti-IL-2 IgG and [^{35}S]methionine-labeled translation product.

activity as a screen for insertion of the *IL-2* gene in an appropriate vector and host may not always reveal an active product.

Therefore, we have sought alternative methods of detecting *IL-2* gene expression. We have attempted to use immune precipitation by monoclonal antibody against IL-2 (Gillis and Henney, 1981; Gillis *et al.,* 1981) to detect *IL-2* gene expression. As shown in Fig. 9, the reticulocyte lysate translation product of Jurkat poly(A^+) mRNA prepared in the presence of [^{35}S]methionine yielded a radioactive product. Incubation of this product with anti-IL-2 IgG and lyophilized *Staphyloccocus aureus* (Igsorb) resulted in precipitation of some 40,000 cpm of [^{35}S]methionine-labeled protein. When tissue culture medium was sustituted for anti-IL-2 IgG in a precipitation reaction, only 8000 cpm of radioactivity was associated with Igsorb precipitation pellet. The difference in radioactivity precipitated between these two reactions (approximately 35,000 cpm) represented approximately 2% of the total cpm added to the reaction mixture. Furthermore immune precipitation of [^{35}S]methionine-labeled translation product was totally abrogated by inclusion of a tenfold excess of biologically active human IL-2 in the reaction mixture. In addition to supplying preliminary evidence that IL-2 messenger RNA may represent 2% of the total Jurkat-poly(A^+) RNA pool, data presented in Fig. 9, suggest that radioimmune precipitation, either directly (using ^{35}S-labeled translation product) or in a competitive fashion, will be possible as an appropriate screening tool for monitoring antigenic IL-2 gene inclusion and expression in appropriate transfection vectors and bacterial or eukaryotic hosts.

VII. CONCLUSIONS

The results presented in the preceding pages have traced our involvement and experience in the area of biochemical and molecular characterization of IL-2. Obtaining potentially homogeneous purified material has been facilitated greatly by the identification of both murine and human tumor cells capable of producing high levels of IL-2. In addition, adaptation of SDS-gel electrophoresis techniques allows electroelution of single polypeptides with retention of biological activity. This approach has enabled production of what appears to be homogeneous IL-2 consisting of a single type of molecule. Large-scale SDS-PAGE processing of tumor cell line produced IL-2 has made it possible to begin to test the ability of the lymphokine to affect immune reactivity *in vivo*. Administration of biochemically characterized IL-2 *in vivo* has confirmed the ability of the factor to boost alloimmunity and natural killer cell responses (Conlon *et al.*, 1981). We hope that by continuing our studies in both biological and molecular arenas we will be able to provide significant data regarding the immunotherapeutic effect of IL-2 and perhaps, via application of recombinant DNA technology, unlock what may be a multi-gene family coding for soluble proteins which modify immune responses.

REFERENCES

Aarden, L. A. (1979). Revised nomenclature for antigen-nonspecific T cell proliferation and helper factors. *J. Immunol.* **123,** 2928.

Baker, P. E., Gillis, S., and Smith, K. A. (1979). Monoclonal cytotoxic T cell lines. *J. Exp. Med.* **149,** 273.

Caplan, B., Gibbs, C., and Paetkau, V. (1981). Properties of sodium dodecyl sulfate-denatured interleukin 2. *J. Immunol.* **126,** 1351.

Conlon, P. J., Hefeneider, S. H., Henney, C. S., and Gillis, S. (1981). The effects of interleukin 2 on primary *in vivo* immune responses. *In* "Immunotherapy of T Cell Lines" (E. A. Fefer, ed.). Raven, New York (in press).

Farrar, J. J., Simon, P. L., Koopman, W. J., and Fuller-Bonar, J. (1978). Biochemical relationship of thymocyte mitogenic factor and factors enhancing humoral and cell-mediated immune responses. *J. Immunol.* **121,** 1353.

Frank, M. B., Watson, J., and Gillis, S. (1981). Biochemical and biological characterization of lymphocyte regulatory molecules. VIII. Purification of interleukin 2 from a human T cell leukemia. *J. Immunol.* (in press).

Gillis, S., and Henney, C. S. (1981). The biochemical and biological characterization of lymphocyte regulatory molecules. VI. Generation of a B cell hybridoma whose antibody product inhibits interleukin 2 activity. *J. Immunol.* **126,** 1978.

Gillis, S., and Mizel, S. (1981). T cell lymphoma model for the analysis of interleukin-1 mediated T cell activation. *Proc. Natl. Acad. Sci. U.S.A.* **78,** 1133.

Gillis, S., and Smith, K. S. (1977). Long-term culture of tumor-specific cytocytic T cells. *Nature (London)* **268,** 154.

Gillis, S., and Watson, J. (1980). Biochemical and biological characterization of lymphocyte regulatory molecules. V. Identification of an interleukin 2 producer human leukemia T cell line. *J. Exp. Med.* **152,** 1709.

Gillis, S., Baker, P. E., Ruscetti, F. W., and Smith, K. A. (1978a). Long-term culture of human antigen-specific cytotoxic T cell lines. *J. Exp. Med.* **148,** 1093.

Gillis, S., Ferm, M. M., Ou, W., and Smith, K. A. (1978b). T cell growth factor: Parameters of production and a quantitative microassay for activity. *J. Immunol.* **120,** 2027.

Gillis, S., Union, N. A., Baker, P. E., and Smith, K. A. (1979). The *in vitro* generation and sustained culture of nude mouse cytolytic T-lymphocytes. *J. Exp. Med.* **149,** 1460.

Gillis, S., Smith, K. A., and Watson, J. D. (1980a). Biochemical and biological characterization of lymphocyte regulatory molecules. II. Purification of a class of rat and human lymphokines. *J. Immunol.* **124,** 1954.

Gillis, S., Scheid, M., and Watson, J. (1980b). The biochemical and biological characterization of lymphocyte regulatory molecules. III. The isolation and phenotypic characterization of interleukin 2 producing T cell lymphomas. *J. Immunol.* **125,** 2570.

Gillis, S., Gillis, A. E., and Henney, C. S. (1981). Monoclonal antibody directed against interleukin-2. I. Inhibition of T-lymphocyte mitogenesis, and the *in vitro* differentiation of alloreactive cytolytic T-cells. *J. Exp. Med.* (in press).

Henney, C. S., Kuribayashi, K., Kern, D. E., and Gillis, S. (1981). Interleukin-2 augments natural killer cell activity. *Nature (London)* **291,** 335.

Kuribayashi, K., Gillis, S., Kern, D. E., and Henney, C. S. (1981). Murine NK cell cultures: Effects of interleukin 2 and interferon on cell growth and cytotoxic reactivity. *J. Immunol.* **126,** 2321.

Larsson, E. L., Iscove, N. N., and Coutinho, A. (1980). Two distinct factors are required for induction of T cell growth. *Nature (London)* **283,** 664.

Mochizuki, D. Y., Watson, J., and Gillis, S. (1980a). The biochemical and biological characterization of lymphocyte regulatory molecules. IV. Purification of interleukin 2 from a murine T cell lymphoma. *J. Immunol.* **125,** 2579.

Mochizuki, D. Y., Watson, J., and Gillis, S. (1980b). Biochemical separation of interleukin 2. *J. Immunol. Methods* **39,** 185.

Morgan, D. A., Ruscetti, F. W., and Gallo, R. C. (1976). Selective *in vitro* growth of T lymphocytes from normal human bone marrows. *Science* **193,** 1007.

Nabholz, M., Enger, H. D., Collavo, D., and North, M. (1978). Cloned T cell lines with specific cytolytic activity. *Curr. Top. Microbiol. Immunol.* **81,** 176.

Rosenberg, S. A., Schwarz, S., and Spiess, P. J. (1978). *In vitro* growth of murine T cells. II. Growth of *in vitro* sensitized cells cytotoxic for alloantigens. *J. Immunol.* **121,** 1951.

Ruscetti, F. W., Morgan, D. A., and Gallo, R. C. (1977). Functional and morphological characterization of human T cells continuously grown *in vitro*. *J. Immunol.* **119,** 131.

Schreir, M. H., and Tees, R. (1980). Clonal induction of helper T cells: Conversion of specific into non-specific signals. *Int. Arch. Allergy Appl. Immunol.* **61,** 227.

Smith, K. A., Gillis, S., Baker, P. E., McKenzie, D., and Ruscetti, F. W. (1979). T cell growth factor-mediated T cell proliferation. *Ann. N.Y. Acad. Sci.* **332,** 423.

Smith, K. A., Lachman, L. B., Oppenheim, J. J., and Favata, M. F. (1980). The functional relationship of the interleukins. *J. Exp. Med.* **151,** 1551.

Strausser, J. L., and Rosenberg, S. A. (1978). *In vitro* growth of cytotoxic human lymphocytes. I. Growth of cells sensitized *in vitro* to alloantigens. *J. Immunol.* **121,** 1491.

Stull, D., and Gillis, S. (1981). Constitutive production of interleukin 2 activity by a T cell hybridoma. *J. Immunol.* **126,** 1680.

von Boehmer, H., Hengartner, H., Nabholz, M., Lernhardt, W., Schreier, M. H., and Haas, W. (1979). Fine specificity of a continuously growing killer cell clone specific for H-Y antigen. *Eur. J. Immunol.* **9,** 592.

Wagner, H., Hardt, C., Heeg, K., Rollinghoff, M., and Pfizenmaier, K. (1980). T cell derived helper factor (interleukin 2) allows *in vivo* induction of cytotoxic T cells in thymus deficient nu/nu mice. *Nature (London)* **284,** 278.

Watson, J. (1979). Continuous proliferation of murine antigen-specific helper T cells in culture. *J. Exp. Med.* **150,** 1510.

Watson, J., Gillis, S., Marbrook, J., Mochizuki, D., and Smith, L. (1979). Biochemical and biological characterization of lymphocyte regulatory molecules. I. Purification of a class of murine lymphokines. *J. Exp. Med.* **150,** 849.

4

Production and Assay of Interleukin-1 (IL-1)

Igal Gery

I. Production of IL-1 42
A. The Producing Cell 42
B. Stimulants of IL-1 43
C. The Relationship between Production and Release of IL-1 . . 43
D. Effects of Combined Agents on IL-1 Production and Release . 44
E. Role of Mϕ Damage in IL-1 Production 46
F. Production and Release of IL-1 by Activated Mϕ 47
G. Production and Release of IL-1 by Human Monocytes 48
II. IL-1 Assay 49
A. The Responding Cell 49
B. Mode of Action of IL-1 51
III. Conclusions 52
References 53

The essential role of macrophages (Mϕ) in supporting lymphocyte responses in culture was demonstrated by Mosier (1967) and Oppenheim *et al.* (1968) and has been well established since by numerous other studies (see Moller, 1978). The contribution of mediators produced by Mϕ was indicated subsequently by studies of Bach *et al.* (1970) and Dutton *et al.* (1970; Hoffman and Dutton, 1971), showing that Mϕ can apparently be substituted in certain *in vitro* systems by supernatants of their cultures. The discovery of lymphocyte activating factor (LAF), which was later designated interleukin 1 (IL 1) (see Aarden *et al.*, 1979), has further confirmed the role of Mϕ-derived mediators in the response of lymphocytes in culture. The detection of IL-1 activity was based on the unique responsiveness of murine thymocytes in culture: these cells react poorly to phytohemagglutinin (PHA), but this response is potentiated by very small numbers of monocytes or Mϕ or minute amounts of their product, IL-1 (Gery *et al.*, 1971, 1972). Larger amounts of IL-1 may also stimulate direct mitotic activity of the murine thymocytes (Gery *et al.*, 1972). These *in vitro* responses have thus provided a simple and sensitive assay for this Mϕ-derived mediator and have facilitated its characterization and, subsequently, its purification. The

ISOLATION, CHARACTERIZATION, AND
UTILIZATION OF T LYMPHOCYTE CLONES

ISBN 0-12-249920-4

physicochemical properties and multiple biological activities of IL-1 have been thoroughly reviewed by Rosenstreich and Mizel (1978), Unanue (1978), Oppenheim *et al.* (1979, 1982), and Farrar and Koopman (1979). The present chapter deals selectively with the production and assay of IL-1.

I. PRODUCTION OF IL-1

A. The Producing Cell

Interleukin-1 is produced by Mϕ of different tissues from a variety of animal species (Blyden and Handschumacher, 1977; Oppenheim *et al.*, 1979). In early studies, the cultures used for IL-1 production consisted of mixtures of Mϕ and other lymphoid cells, e.g., unfractionated white blood cells or whole spleen cell cultures (Gery *et al.*, 1971; Gery and Waksman, 1972). It may be assumed, therefore, that interleukin-2 [IL-2 or T cell growth factor (see Aarden *et al.*, 1979)] was also produced by these cultures and contributed to the "LAF activity" of their supernatants (Oppenheim *et al.*, 1979, 1982; Togawa *et al.*, 1979). The contamination of IL-1 preparations with IL-2 was minimized in later studies by the use of Mϕ monolayers for production of the mediator (Gery and Wiener, 1975; Calderon *et al.*, 1975) and was elminated in studies in which Mϕ cell lines were employed. The use of Mϕ cell lines was introduced by Lachman *et al.* (1977),and their usefulness has been well established by the elaborate studies of Mizel and co-workers (e.g., Mizel and Rosenstreich, 1979; Mizel and Mizel, 1981). It is noteworthy, however, that great variations were noted among the different murine Mϕ lines in their capacity to produce and release IL-1 (Lachman *et al.*, 1977; I. Gery, unpublished observations) and all human Mϕ lines examined so far have been found to produce only little or no activity (J. J. Oppenheim, personal communication).

Little is known about the production and release of IL-1 by Mϕ at various phases of maturation. Unfractionated bone marrow cells were found to produce high levels of "LAF activity" (Gery and Waksman, 1972), and more studies of these cells may prove to be productive. Changes in IL-1 production and release which follow Mϕ "activation" *in vivo,* or monocyte differentiation *in vitro,* are detailed below.

Most cells other than Mϕ do not produce or release IL-1 (Blyden and Handschumacher, 1977, and unpublished data). However, recent studies have shown that cultures of murine epidermal cells (Sauder *et al.*, 1981) and even keratinocyte cell lines (Luger *et al.*, 1981) may produce and release a molecule which carries identical properties to those of IL-1.

B. Stimulants of IL-1

The discovery of IL-1 activity has provided support for the hypothesis of Allison and Davies (1971), that adjuvants affect the immune system by stimulating Mϕ to produce and release T lymphocyte activating mediators; indeed, many of the agents which increase IL-1 production are well known adjuvants, such as lipopolysaccharide (LPS) (Gery and Waksman, 1972), or components of Mycobacteria [e.g., PPD (Mokyr and Mitchell, 1975), or muramyl dipeptide (Oppenheim *et al.*, 1980b)]. In addition to adjuvants, IL-1 release may be increased by a variety of other agents which were classified by Oppenheim *et al.* (1979) into the following classes: T cells and T cell mitogens; B cell mitogens, inducers of phagocytosis, inducers of cyclic GMP, and miscellaneous agents such as dimethyl sulfoxide (DMSO) or colchicine. The activities of these various agents are thoroughly reviewed by Oppenheim *et al.* (1979); the present chapter deals in detail only with the agents which were useful for further analysis of the production and release of IL-1.

C. The Relationship between Production and Release of IL-1

In most of the published studies on IL-1 activity, only the release of the mediator was measured, and no clear distinction was made between the production and release of IL-1. Recent studies have indicated, however, that the extracellular IL-1 activity and the total IL-1 production (extra- and intracellular) are not necessarily directly related. The first demonstration of a dissociation between the production and release of IL-1 was reported by Unanue and Kiely (1977) in unstimulated cultures of murine Mϕ. They observed a sharp increase in intracellular IL-1 activity within 1–2 hr of incubation, which peaked after about 4 hr in culture and declined rapidly to marginal levels 20 hr later. In contrast to these marked fluctuations in intracellular IL-1 levels, no significant changes were detected in the low level of extracellular activity. These findings of Unanue and Kiely were fully confirmed in a recent study in this laboratory (Gery *et al.*, 1981a). The stimulus for the increase in formation of intracellular IL-1 activity is not understood, but was attributed to the Mϕ attachment process (Unanue and Kiely, 1977).

Unanue and Kiely (1977) also tested the effects of latex beads on IL-1 levels, but found just minimal effects in this study. However, both intracellular and extracellular IL-1 levels were markedly increased in cultures of P388D1 cells when incubated with phorbol myristate acetate (PMA) (Mizel and Rosenstreich, 1979). The effects of various agents on intra- and extracellular IL-1 levels in monolayers of murine Mϕ were further studied in this laboratory (Gery *et al.*, 1981a). Clear differences were found between the effects of the tested agents,

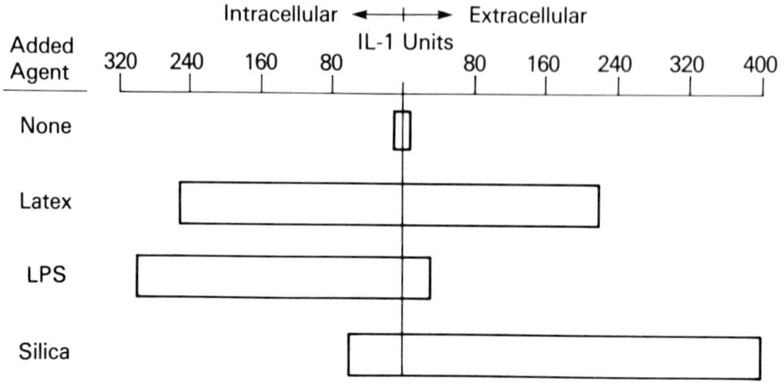

Fig. 1. Patterns of IL-1 production and release by murine Mϕ monolayers cultured with various agents. Resident peritoneal Mϕ were incubated with medium (none), latex (10^8 beads/ml), LPS (20 μg/ml) or silica particles (60 μg/ml) for 20 hr. Supernatants were collected and the monolayers were washed, frozen with fresh medium, thawed, scraped, and sonicated. The levels of IL-1 activities in the lysates (intracellular) and supernatants (extracellular) were determined by their capacity to potentiate the response of murine thymocytes (CBA/N) to PHA (see Appendix). The IL-1 unit values were assessed as described in Table I.

with three patterns being observed (Fig. 1): (a) both intracellular and extracellular activities were increased in response to high concentrations of latex beads; (b) a marked increase of intracellular IL-1, with just a minimal elevation of the extracellular activity, was stimulated by LPS; (c) a striking increase in IL-1 release, with a much smaller increment of the intracellular activity, was induced by silica particles. The effects of the added agents became clear as early as 4 hr after their addition, but reached maximal degrees after 20 hr of incubation. These data thus indicate that determination of both intracellular and extracellular IL-1 levels is essential to properly evaluate the effects of agents on the production of this mediator.

D. Effects of Combined Agents on IL-1 Production and Release

The difference in effect of LPS and silica on intracellular and extracellular IL-1 levels suggested that these agents differ in their mode of action on Mϕ. This notion was supported by the finding that silica and LPS synergize when added in combination to yield very high levels of IL-1, which exceed the activities produced and released by the individual agents (Table I). It is also of note that supernatants from Mϕ cultured with the combination of LPS and silica also exhibited high levels of direct mitogenic activity for murine thymocytes and had the capacity to potentiate antibody production by spleen cultures from nude mice; both reactions depend on high levels of IL-1 activity (Gery *et al.*, 1972; Wood, 1979). (The latter assay was kindly carried out by D. D. Wood, Merck Institute for Therapeutic Research.)

TABLE I

Synergy between LPS and Silica in Increasing IL-1 Production and Release by Murine Macrophages

Agent added to Mϕ cultures (μg/ml)	IL-1 in lysates (intracellular activity)			IL-1 in supernatants (extracellular activity)		
	[^{3}H]Thymidine uptake in samples diluted			[^{3}H]Thymidine uptake in samples diluted		
	1:40	1:640	IL-1 Units	1:40	1:640	IL-1 Units
None	710 ± 99[a]	339 ± 14	3[b]	2128 ± 448	353 ± 23	10
LPS (20)	58,305 ± 5389	7855 ± 495	500	10,651 ± 1134	1756 ± 230	50
Silica (60)	5963 ± 627	601 ± 101	30	37,038 ± 1342	5405 ± 71	300
LPS + Silica	61,206 ± 1281	12,528 ± 591	600	42,484 ± 2933	48,582 ± 5293	2000

[a] Mean counts per minute ± SEM of CBA/N thymocyte cultures incubated with the tested sample and PHA (0.05%) for 3 days and pulsed during the last 6 hr (0.5 μCi/well). Control thymocytes, cultured with medium and PHA, incorporated 294 ± 50 cpm.

[b] IL-1 units were evaluated by dilution analysis of the tested preparations and a standard sample containing 80 units/ml, as described by Mizel and Mizel (1981).

Using combinations of different stimulatory agents provides, therefore, a practical approach to obtain exceedingly high levels of IL-1. This approach was recently used by Mizel and Mizel (1981), who obtained large quantities of IL-1 from P388D1 cells by combining PMA, cycloheximide, actinomycin D, and sodium butyrate. These authors attributed the high yield of IL-1 to the "superinduction" phenomenon, in which the production of a cell product is increased as a result of inhibition of RNA or protein synthesis (see Unanue and Kiely, 1977). However, our results cannot be explained in this manner because none of the agents used in our study has known inhibitory effects on protein or RNA synthesis. We have suggested, therefore, an alternative explanation for the synergy between certain combined agents by relating the augmented IL-1 production to the injurious effect of at least one of the agents (Gery *et al.,* 1981a). This notion is further discussed below.

E. Role of Mϕ Damage in IL-1 Production

The effect of silica particles on IL-1 production deserves further analysis. These particles are cytotoxic to Mϕ (Allison *et al.,* 1966), and in our study (Gery *et al.,* 1981a), injury to Mϕ was noted in cultures incubated with silica at ≥ 25 μg/ml (by both microscopic observation and increased release of lactate dehydrogenase). In spite of the damage, our results showed that the elevated release of IL-1 by silica cannot be attributed merely to increased leakage of preformed IL-1, since both intra- and extracellular levels were increased in these cultures (see Fig. 1 and Table I). It is also noteworthy that silica particles increased both intra- and extracellular levels of IL-1 after 4 hr of incubation, when intracellular IL-1 activity reaches its peak. Furthermore, results similar to those with silica were obtained with another damaging agent, glucocerebroside (GL_1, the storage material of Gaucher's disease); cytotoxic doses of GL_1 increased both intracellular and extracellular IL-1 levels of Mϕ cultures (Gery *et al.,* 1981c). These data thus suggest that certain types of damage to Mϕ can increase the production of IL-1. This notion is in accord with reports showing that IL-1 release is increased by various other agents with damaging potential, such as DMSO (Blyden and Handschumacher, 1977), colchicine (Oppenheim *et al.,* 1979), or carrageenan (Stamenkovic *et al.,* 1979). Furthermore, it is possible that damage to Mϕ could play a role in the reported increase of both intra- and extracellular IL-1 levels of Mϕ cultured with cycloheximide (Unanue and Kiely, 1977). The effect of cycloheximide has been attributed to the "superinduction" phenomenon (Unanue and Kiely, 1977; Mizel and Mizel, 1981), but increased death rate was observed in Mϕ after 12 hr or more of incubation with this drug (Unanue and Kiely, 1977). Using the hypothetical framework of Unanue and Kiely (1977), one can propose, therefore, that Mϕ damage by any of the different agents may either enhance the process of conversion of the inactive precursor to active IL-1 or reduce the rate of degradation of the active molecule.

The injurious agents, silica or GL_1 particles, also caused a substantial increase in release of lysosomal enzymes (such as β-*N*-acetylglucosaminidase). However, unlike the increase in both intra- and extracellular levels of IL-1, the increase in enzyme release was accompanied by a matched decrease in levels of intracellular enzymatic activity, leaving the total activity unchanged (Gery *et al.*, 1981a). Thus, the mechanisms involved in IL-1 production seem to be fundamentally different from those which produce the lysosomal enzymes.

F. Production and Release of IL-1 by Activated Mϕ

Early studies had indicated that Mϕ activated *in vivo* by mycobacteria (Mitchell *et al.*, 1973; Meltzer and Oppenheim, 1977) or their components (Gery *et al.*, 1974) may release more IL-1 than nonactivated ("resident") Mϕ. In a more recent study (Barranger and Gery, 1981), we have found, however, that activated Mϕ actually produced less total IL-1 than did the control resident Mϕ. Thus, as shown in Fig. 2, monolayers of BCG-activated Mϕ released more IL-1 and a much larger proportion of their total IL-1 than the resident Mϕ when stimulated with LPS. However, the intracellular and total IL-1 activities were higher in the cultures of resident Mϕ. Activated Mϕ were also inferior to resident Mϕ in their IL-1 production and release when incubated with silica and were practically unaffected by GL_1. The increased release of IL-1 by activated Mϕ upon stimulation with LPS may be due to the high susceptibility of these cells to damage by

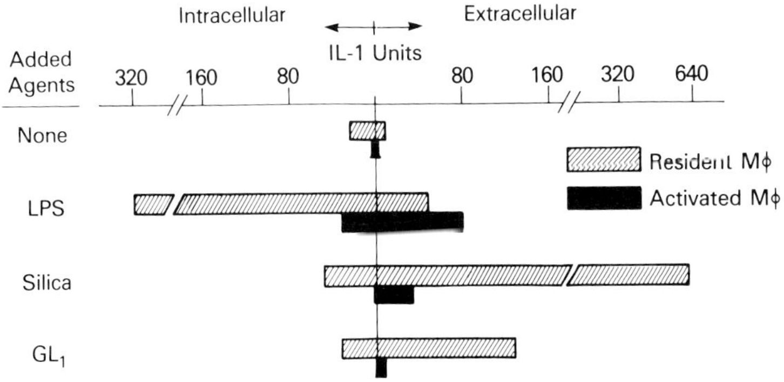

Fig. 2. IL-1 levels in lysates (intraceullular) and supernatants (extracellular) of resident or BCG-activated murine Mϕ. Activated Mϕ were collected 14 days after ip injection of 5×10^7 BCG living bacilli. Mϕ monolayers were cultured with medium (none), LPS (20 μg/ml), silica (50 μg/ml), or glucocerebroside (GL_1, 80 μg/ml) for 20 hr, and their lysates and supernatants were assayed for IL-1 levels as described in Fig. 1.

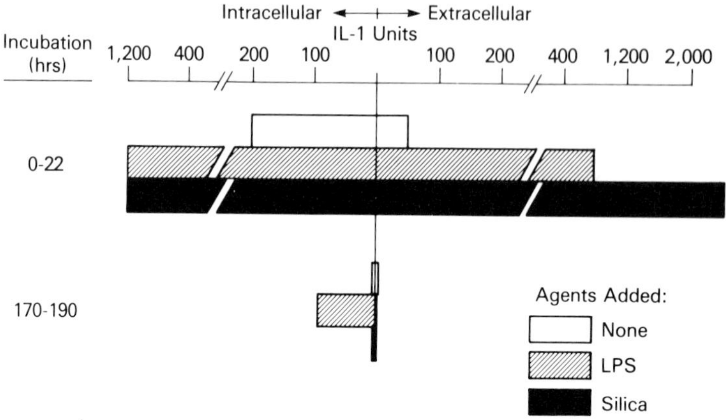

Fig. 3. Levels of IL-1 in lysates (intracellular) and supernatants (extracellular) of human blood monocyte monolayers stimulated at the time of culturing (0–22 hr), or after 7 days of preincubation (170–190 hr). The latter cells were transformed to "mature Mϕ" by the time the stimuli were added. LPS was added to 20 μg/ml and silica to 50 μg/ml. Supernatants and lysates were collected and their levels of IL-1 were determined as described in Fig. 1.

LPS (Peavy *et al.*, 1979; Vogel *et al.*, 1980). The decrease in total IL-1 production by activated Mϕ could be related to other metabolic changes that accompany the activation process, such as the decrease in secretion of prostaglandins or lysomsomal acid hydrolases (Humes *et al.*, 1980) or the reduced expression of certain surface structures (Ezekowitz *et al.*, 1981).

G. Production and Release of IL-1 by Human Monocytes

Human blood monocytes were found in numerous studies to be an excellent source of IL-1 (Gery *et al.*, 1971; Gery and Waksman, 1972; Blyden and Handschumacher, 1977; Togawa *et al.*, 1979). Recently, we have studied the intracellular and extracellular levels of IL-1 in human monocyte monolayers (Gery *et al.*, 1981b). Freshly cultured human monocytes are usually superior to murine peritoneal Mϕ in their production of IL-1 and were found to differ from these cells by two features (Figs. 1 and 3): (a) intracellular IL-1 levels in human monocytes increased relatively more slowly, and maximal levels were found in these cultures as late as after 20 hr of incubation; (b) LPS increased extracellular IL-1 in human cultures to levels similar to those of intracellular activity. Human monocytes transform in culture to "mature Mϕ" (Newman *et al.*, 1980). The transformed Mϕ differed from the freshly cultured monocytes by their lack of responsiveness to silica or GL_1 particles and by their only moderate levels of intracellular IL-1 and lack of extracellular activity when stimulated with LPS (Fig. 3). More studies are under way with human tissue Mϕ, in order to examine the role of differentiation per se in changing the pattern of IL-1 production and release by these cells.

II. IL-1 ASSAY

As mentioned above, the murine thymocyte culture provides a highly sensitive bioassay for IL-1 activity; it has been estimated that this assay may detect IL-1 at concentrations below 10^{-10} M (Mizel and Mizel, 1981). The highest sensitivity for IL-1 detection is achieved in the potentiation test, i.e., when IL-1 augments the mitotic response to PHA or suboptimal concentrations of concanavalin A (Con-A); higher levels of IL-1 are required for the direct mitogenic effect (Gery *et al.*, 1972; Oppenheim *et al.*, 1982).

A. The Responding Cell

The population of thymic lymphocytes is not homogeneous, and subsets of these cells were found to differ in their responsiveness to IL-1. The two major subsets of thymocytes, the medullary and cortical cells, may be readily separated according to their buoyant density or on the basis of the presence of receptors for peanut agglutinin (PNA) (Table II). Cortical thymocytes are more compact than the medullary cells, and the two subsets separate well on albumin gradients (Colley *et al.*, 1970). Using this method of separation, we showed (Gery *et al.*, 1972) that the fraction containing the more compact thymocytes did not respond to PHA and reacted just moderately to Con-A and to supernatants containing IL-1. The other cell fraction, consisting of the low density cells (i.e., enriched for medullary thymocytes), resembled peripheral T lymphocytes in its vigorous

TABLE II

Properties of Subsets of Thymocytes and Their Responses to IL-1 and Lectins

Properties	Cortical Cells	Medullary Cells
Proportion in thymus	80–90%	5–15%
Buoyant density	High	Low
PNA receptor	+	−
Ly 2	High	Low
Mitotic responsiveness		
Con-A	+	++++
PHA	0	++
IL-1	±	+++
IL-1 + PHA	+	++++

responses to both PHA and Con-A, but, unlike the peripheral lymphocytes, these thymocytes reacted strongly to the IL-1 stimulus.

The difference in PNA agglutinability of the subsets of thymocytes was demonstrated by Sharon's group (Reisner *et al.*, 1976) and was employed by Oppenheim *et al.* (1982) for further analysis of the mitotic responses of the different thymocyte subpopulations. The data obtained by this method of separation correlate well with those obtained by the albumin gradient fractionation, namely, PNA^+ thymocytes resemble the thymocytes of the high density fraction in their low mitotic responses, while PNA^- thymocytes react well to IL-1 and lectins, similarly to the fraction of low density.

Although the thymocytes which react well with either IL-1 or Con-A cannot be differentiated by their physical properties or surface markers (Table II), the possibility that different subpopulations are affected by these two stimuli should not be ruled out. As shown below, the responses to Con-A and IL-1 differ substantially in their susceptibility to the inhibitory effect of cyclosporin A, and this could be hypothetically attributed to the involvement of two subpopulations of thymocytes in the response to the two stimuli.

Thymocytes from all tested mouse strains were found to react to IL-1, but with a remarkable variability in their level of reactivity (Gery *et al.*, 1972). An inbred strain which has served in many studies as a source for thymocytes is the C_3H/HeJ. Lymphoid cells from this mouse do not react to LPS (see Vogel *et al.*, 1980), and, therefore, the presence of LPS in preparations tested for IL-1 does not affect the assay. [LPS may synergize with PHA to stimulate mitotic responses in murine thymocyte cultures (Gery and Waksman, 1972).] However, C_3H/HeJ thymocytes were found inferior to thymocytes from CBA mice (in particular CBA/N) in their sensitivity to IL-1 (I. Gery, unpublished data).

Thymocytes from species other than the mouse also react to IL-1, but with relatively lower levels of responsiveness; usually, only the potentiating IL-1 effect may be detected (Maizel *et al.*, 1981; I. Gery, unpublished data). IL-1 may also potentiate the mitotic responses of peripheral T lymphocytes to lectins or antigens (Gery *et al.*, 1972; Hoessli *et al.*, 1977; Mizel and Ben-Zvi, 1980). In addition, IL-1 can facilitate or augment the antibody production by B lymphocytes in culture, probably indirectly via its effect on T or pre-T helper lymphocytes (see reviews by Farrar and Koopman, 1979; Wood, 1982).

Recently, Gillis and Mizel (1981) have shown that IL-1 is also effective on lymphocyte cell lines. IL-1 was found to stimulate lymphocyte line LBRM-33 1A5 to release large amounts of IL-2 which can be assayed, in turn, on an IL-2-dependent cell line. This bicellular system provides, therefore, an assay for determining IL-1 activity and was reported to be about tenfold more sensitive than the conventional thymocyte assay (Gillis and Mizel, 1981).

In addition to its effect on lymphoid cells, IL-1 was found recently to stimulate a variety of other cells, including fibroblasts (Schmidt *et al.*, 1981), cells of the hypothalamus involved in fever induction (Rosenwasser *et al.*, 1979), liver cells which produce serum amyloid A (Sipe *et al.*, 1979), or rheumatoid synovial cells (Mizel *et al.*, 1981). This topic is thoroughly reviewed by Oppenheim *et al.* (1982).

B. Mode of Action of IL-1

Little is known about the biochemical processes induced by IL-1 in the target cells. An elevation in cyclic GMP was found by Katz *et al.* (1978) in rat lymphocytes incubated with rat IL-1 and PHA. In another study, IL-1 effect was reported to resemble closely that of enzymes such as carboxypeptidase or serine proteases (Katz *et al.*, 1980). The latter activity could be related, perhaps, to recent findings, that IL-1 may (a) increase the number of antigen binding sites and change membrane fluidity on murine lymphocytes (Lonai and Steinman, 1977), (b) change expression of Lyt markers on murine thymocytes (Oppenheim *et al.*, 1980a), or (c) increase the proportion of "stable" E-rosette forming cells among human blood lymphocytes (Ben-Zvi *et al.*, 1981).

The major pathway by which IL-1 may serve as a mediator of the immune response seems to be related to its capacity to stimulate the production of IL-2 by T lymphocytes. This function of IL-1 was suggested by Farrar and his collaborators (see Farrar and Koopman, 1979) and was recently established by the elegant studies of Smith *et al.* (1980a,b) Larsson *et al.* (1980), and Gillis and Mizel (1981). In fact, studies of Smith, *et al.* (1980b) and Oppenheim *et al.* (1982) have indicated that the expression of IL-1 effect on lymphocytes depends essentially on its capacity to induce IL-2 production. IL-2 is assumed to mediate the expansion of lymphocyte clones following antigenic stimulation (see Chapter 3 by Gillis *et al.*, and Chapter 6 by Chiller *et al.* in this treatise) and it is assumed, therefore, that IL-1 provides an essential signal in this amplification process.

An issue which has remained unresolved concerns the relationship between the direct mitogenic effect of IL-1 and its potentiating of mitotic responses to other stimuli (e.g., lectins). Data collected recently in this laboratory (I. Gery, unpublished observations) support the notion that the two effects may be basically different. These data were collected in experiments dealing with the effects of cyclosporin A (CSA) on responses of thymocytes to different stimuli. As shown in Table III, CSA at 0.2–1 μg/ml almost completely inhibited the thymocyte response to Con-A and abolished the synergistic activity of IL-1 and the lectins. On the other hand, CSA at these doses had practically no effect on the direct mitogenic activity of IL-1. These results may be interpreted in two ways: (a) that the biochemical processes in the two mitotic responses are not the same and are differently affected by CSA or (b) that two different subpopulations of thymocytes are stimulated by the mitogenic and potentiating activities of IL-1 and that

TABLE III

Cyclosporin A Dissociates between the Mitogenic and Potentiating Activities of IL-1

		Mitotic Response in Presence of	
Expt. No.	Stimulus Added	Medium	Cyclosporin A[a]
I	None	161 ± 7[b]	122 ± 34
	Con-A (3 μg/ml)	204,619 ± 14,080	1,495 ± 186
	IL-1 (5%)[c]	29,295 ± 1,058	23,998 ± 330
	Con-A + IL-1	185,505 ± 10,490	21,455 ± 894
II	None	214 ± 25	225 ± 43
	PHA (0.1%)	384 ± 46	298 ± 79
	IL-1 (5%)	26,090 ± 728	25.261 ± 590
	PHA + IL-1 (5%)	37,731 ± 108	16,080 ± 535
	IL-1 (0.5%)	8,104 ± 451	7,224 ± 362
	PHA + IL-1 (0.5%)	27,348 ± 1,099	3,037 ± 476

[a] Cyclosporin A was added to a final concentration of 1 μg/ml in Experiment I and 0.2 μg/ml in Experiment II.

[b] Mean cpm values ± SEM of triplicate cultures of murine thymocytes (CBA/N), harvested after 48 hr of incubation and pulsed with [^{3}H]thymidine (0.5 μCi/well) during the last 6 hr.

[c] A supernatant of human monocyte culture, stimulated with LPS.

CSA affects one subpopulation more than the other. Cyclosporin A is believed to inhibit the mitotic responses of T lymphocytes by blocking the expression of receptors of IL-2 (Larsson, 1980; Palacios, 1981), and it may be hypothesized that the thymocytes reacting to IL-1 alone carry these receptors at the time of culturing, while those reacting to IL-1 and PHA (or to Con-A) are "resting" cells, which do not express these receptors. The different hypotheses are currently being tested.

III. CONCLUSIONS

The accumulating data indicate that IL-1 may be considered a hormonelike molecule which is produced mainly by Mϕ and affects in minuscule amounts the metabolism of lymphocytes and other cells. As an immune mediator, IL-1 seems to play an important role in the amplification phase of the immune response by facilitating the production of another mediator, IL-2; this latter mediator is considered essential for the expansion of stimulated lymphocyte clones with defined specificities. The biologic role of the mitogenic activity of IL-1 on thymocytes is not clear and awaits further investigation. More studies are also needed to further analyze the *in vivo* activities of IL-1 and its mode of action on lymphocytes and other cells, such as fibroblasts, liver, or certain brain cells. All these cells may be involved in the inflammatory reaction, and a relationship between their response to IL-1 and biologic functions is an intriguing possibility. Recent studies by deWeck, Stadler, Oppenheim, and their colleagues (see Oppenheim *et al.*, 1982) have shown that monoclonal antibodies may be produced against IL-1. It may be assumed, therefore, that this powerful tool will prove useful in further investigating the various biological activities of IL-1.

ACKNOWLEDGMENTS

I am grateful to Dr. Joost J. Oppenheim for his constructive comments and to Mrs. Noreen Beavers for her invaluable secretarial assistance.

REFERENCES

Aarden, L. A. *et al.* (1979). Revised nomenclature for antigen-nonspecific T cell proliferation and helper factors. *J. Immunol.* **123,** 2928.

Allison, A. C., and Davies, A. J. S. (1971). Requirements of thymus-dependent lymphocytes for potentiation by adjuvants of antibody formation. *Nature (London)* **233,** 330.

Allison, A. C., Harington, J. S., and Birbeck, M. (1966). An examination of the cytotoxic effects of silica on macrophages. *J. Exp. Med.* **124,** 141.

Bach, F. H., Alter, B. J., Solliday, S., Zoschke, D. C., and Janis, M. (1970). Lymphocyte reactivity *in vitro*. II. Soluble reconstituting factor permitting response of purified lymphocytes. *Cell. Immunol.* **1,** 219.

Barranger, J. A., and Gery, I. (1981). Differences between resident and activated macrophages (Mϕ) in production of lymphocyte activating factor (LAF, or interleukin 1). *Fed. Proc., Fed. Am. Soc. Exp. Biol.* **40,** 1057.

Ben-Zvi, A., Mizel, S. B., and Oppenheim, J. J. (1981). Generation of human peripheral blood stable E-rosette-forming T cells by interleukin 1. *Clin. Immunol. Immunopathol.* **19,** 330.

Blyden, G., and Handschumacher, R. E. (1977). Purification and properties of human lymphocyte activating factor (LAF). *J. Immunol.* **118,** 1631.

Calderon, J., Kiely, J.-M., Lefko, J. L., and Unanue, E. R. (1975). The modulation of lymphocyte functions by molecules secreted by macrophages. I. Description and partial biochemical analysis. *J. Exp. Med.* **142,** 151.

Colley, D. G., Shih Wu, A. Y., and Waksman, B. H. (1970). Cellular differentiation in the thymus. III. Surface properties of rat thymus and lymph node cells separated on density gradients. *J. Exp. Med.* **132,** 1107.

Dutton, R. W., McCarthy, M. M., Mishell, R. I., and Raidt, D. J. (1970). Cell components in the immune response. IV. Relationships and possible interactions. *Cell. Immunol.* **1,** 196.

Ezekowitz, R. A. B., Austyn, J., Stahl, P. D., and Gordon, S. (1981). Surface properties of Bacillus Calmette-Guerin-activated mouse macrophages. Reduced expression of mannose-specific endocytosis, Fc receptors, and antigen F4/80 accompanies induction of Ia. *J. Exp. Med.* **154,** 60.

Farrar, J. J., and Koopman, W. J. (1979). Characterization of mitogenic factors and their effect on the antibody response *in vitro*. *In* "Biology of the Lymphokines" (S. Cohen, E. Pick, and J. J. Oppenheim, eds.), pp. 325-346. Academic Press, New York.

Gery, I., and Waksman, B. H. (1972). Potentiation of the T-lymphocyte response to mitogens. II. The cellular source of potentiating mediator(s). *J. Exp. Med.* **136,** 143.

Gery, I., and Wiener, E. (1975). Potentiation of the T-lymphocyte response to mitogens: Relationship between LAF production and "activation" of macrophages. *J. Reticuloendothel. Soc.* **18,** 252.

Gery, I., Gershon, R. K., and Waksman, B. H. (1971). Potentiation of cultured mouse thymocyte responses by factors released by peripheral leucocytes. *J. Immunol.* **107,** 1778.

Gery, I., Gerhson, R. K., and Waksman, B. H. (1972). Potentiation of the T-lymphocyte response to mitogens. I. The responding cell. *J. Exp. Med.* **136,** 128.

Gery, I., Baer, A., Stupp, Y., and Weiss, D. W. (1974). Further studies on the effects of the methanol extraction residue fraction of tubercle bacilli on lymphoid cells and macrophages. *Isr. J. Med. Sci.* **10,** 984.

Gery, I., Davies, P., Derr, J., Krett, N., and Barranger, J. A. (1981a). Relationship between production and release of lymphocyte activating factor (interleukin 1) by murine macrophages. I. Effects of various agents. *Cell. Immunol.* **64,** 293.

Gery, I., Seminara, D., Derr, J., and Barranger, J. A. (1981b). Production and release of lymphocyte activating factor (interleukin 1) by human monocytes and their derived macrophages. *In* "Mechanisms of Lymphocyte Activation" (K. Resch and H. Kirchner, eds.), pp. 541–543. Elsevier/North-Holland, Amsterdam.

Gery, I., Zigler, J. S., Jr., Brady, R. O., and Barranger, J. A. (1981c). Selective effects of glucocerebroside (Gaucher's storage material) on macrophage cultures. *J. Clin. Invest.* **68,** 1182.

Gillis, S., and Mizel, S. B. (1981). T-cell lymphoma model for the analysis of interleukin 1-mediated T-cell activation. *Proc. Natl. Acad. Sci. U.S.A.* **78,** 1133.

Hoessli, D. C., Jones, A. P., and Waksman, B. H. (1977). Potentiation of the T lymphocyte response to mitogens. IV. Serum-free production and testing of macrophage soluble products. *Cell. Immunol.* **30,** 310.

Hoffmann, M., and Dutton, R. W. (1971). Immune response restoration with macrophage culture supernatants. *Science* **172,** 1047.

Humes, J. L., Burger, S., Galavage, M., Kuehl, F. A., Jr., Wightman, P. D., Dahlgren, M. E., Davies, P., and Bonney, R. J. (1980). The diminished production of arachidonic acid oxygenation products by elicited mouse peritoneal macrophages: Possible mechanisms. *J. Immunol.* **124,** 2110.

Katz, S. P., Kierszenbaum, F., and Waksman, B. H. (1978). Mechanisms of action of "lymphocyte activating factor" (LAF). III. Evidence that LAF acts on stimulated lymphocytes by raising cyclic GMP in G_1. *J. Immunol.* **121,** 2386.

Katz, S. P., Shimamura, T., Dessaint, J.-P., Braverman, D., and Waksman, B. H. (1980). Mechanisms of action of "lymphocyte activating factor" (LAF). IV. Differential stimulation of T lymphocytes by induced macrophage enzymes (catheptic carboxypeptidase B and serine proteases). *Cell. Immunol.* **56,** 68.

Lachman, L. B., Hacker, M. P., Blyden, G., and Handschumacher, R. E. (1977). Preparation of lymphocyte activating factor from continuous murine macrophage cell lines. *Cell. Immunol.* **34,** 416.

Larsson, E.-L. (1980). Cyclosporin A and dexamethasone suppress T cell responses by selectively acting at distinct sites of the triggering process. *J. Immunol.* **124,** 2828.

Larsson, E.-L., Iscove, N. N., and Coutinho, A. (1980). Two distinct factors are required for induction of T-cell growth. *Nature (London)* **283,** 664.

Lonai, P., and Steinman, L. (1977). Physiological regulation of antigen binding to T cells: Role of a soluble macrophage factor and of interferon. *Proc. Natl. Acad. Sci. U.S.A.* **74,** 5662.

Luger, T. A., Stadler, B. M., Katz, S. I., and Oppenheim, J. J. (1981). Epidermal cell (keratinocyte)-derived thymocyte activating factor (ETAF). *J. Immunol.* **127,** 1493.

Maizel, A. L., Mehta, S. R., Ford, R. J., and Lachman, L. B. (1981). Effect of interleukin 1 on human thymocytes and purified human T cells. *J. Exp. Med.* **153,** 470.

Meltzer, M. S., and Oppenheim, J. J. (1977). Bidirectional amplification of macrophage-lymphocyte interactions: Enhanced lymphocyte activation factor production by activated adherent mouse peritoneal cells. *J. Immunol.* **118,** 77.

Mitchell, M. S., Kirkpatrick, D., Birnbaum-Mokyr, M., and Gery, I. (1973). On the mode of action of BCG. *Nature (London), New Biol.* **243,** 216.

Mizel, S. B., and Ben-Zvi, A. (1980). Studies on the role of lymphocyte activating factor (interleukin 1) in antigen-induced lymph node lymphocyte proliferation. *Cell. Immunol.* **54,** 382.

Mizel, S. B., and Mizel, D. (1981). Purification to apparent homogeneity of murine interleukin 1. *J. Immunol.* **126,** 834.

Mizel, S. B., and Rosenstreich, D. L. (1979). Regulation of lymphocyte-activating factor (LAF) production and secretion in $P388D_1$ cells: Identification of high molecular weight precursors of LAF. *J. Immunol.* **122,** 2173.

Mizel, S. B., Dayer, J.-M., Krane, S. M., and Mergenhagen, S. E. (1981). Stimulation of rheumatoid synovial cell collagenase and prostaglandin production by partially purified lymphocyte-activating factor (interleukin 1). *Proc. Natl. Acad. Sci. U.S.A.* **78,** 2474.

Mokyr, M. B., and Mitchell, M. S. (1975). Activation of lymphoid cells by BCG *in vitro*. *Cell. Immunol.* **15,** 264.

Moller, G., ed. (1978). Role of macrophages in the immune response. *Immunol. Rev.* **40.**

Mosier, D. E. (1967). A requirement for two cell types for antibody formation in vitro. *Science* **158,** 1573.

Newman, S. L., Musson, R. A., and Henson, P. M. (1980). Development of functional complement receptors during in vitro maturation of human monocytes into macrophages. *J. Immunol.* **125,** 2236.

Oppenheim, J. J., Leventhal, B. G., and Hersh, E. M. (1968). The transformation of column-purified lymphocytes with nonspecific and specific antigenic stimuli. *J. Immunol.* **101,** 262.

Oppenheim, J. J., Mizel, S. B., and Meltzer, M. S. (1979). Biological effects of lymphocyte and macrophage-derived mitogenic "amplification" factors. *In* "Biology of the Lymphokines" (S. Cohen, E. Pick, and J. J. Oppenheim, eds.), pp. 291–323. Academic Press, New York.

Oppenheim, J. J., Moore, R., Gmelig-Meyling, F., Togawa, A., Wahl, S., Mathieson, B. J., Dougherty, S., and Carter, C. (1980a). Role of cytokine and endotoxin induced monokines in lymphocyte proliferation, differentiation and immunoglobulin production. *In* "Macrophage Regulation of Immunity" (E. R. Unanue and A. S. Rosenthal, eds.), pp. 379–398. Academic Press, New York.

Oppenheim, J. J., Togawa, A., Chédid, L., and Mizel, S. B. (1980b). Components of Mycobacteria and muramyl dipeptide with adjuvant activity induce lymphocyte activating factor. *Cell. Immunol.* **50,** 71.

Oppenheim, J. J., Stadler, B. M., Siraganian, R. P., Mage, M., and Mathieson, B. (1982). Properties of interleukin 1 (IL-1). *Fed. Proc., Fed. Am. Soc. Exp. Biol.* **41,** 257.

Palacios, R. (1981). Cyclosporin A inhibits the proliferative response and the generation of helper, suppressor and cytotoxic T-cell functions in the autologous mixed lymphocyte reaction. *Cell. Immunol.* **61,** 453.

Peavy, D. L., Baughn, R. E., and Musher, D. M. (1979). Effects of BCG infection on the susceptibility of mouse macrophages to endotoxin. *Infect. Immun.* **24,** 59.

Reisner, Y., Linker-Israeli, M., and Sharon, N. (1976). Separation of mouse thymocytes into two subpopulations by the use of peanut agglutinin. *Cell Immunol.* **25,** 129.

Rosenstreich, D. L., and Mizel, S. B. (1978). The participation of macrophages and macrophage cell lines in the activation of T lymphocytes of mitogens. *Immunol. Rev.* **40,** 102.

Rosenwasser, L. J., Dinarello, C. A., and Rosenthal, A. S. (1979). Adherent cell function in murine

T-lymphocyte antigen recognition. IV. Enhancement of murine T-cell antigen recognition by human leukocytic pyrogen. *J. Exp. Med.* **150,** 709.

Sauder, D. M., Carter, C., Katz, S. I., and Oppenheim, J. J. (1981). Epidermal cell production of thymocyte activating factor. *Clin. Res.* **29,** 285A.

Schmidt, J. A., Mizel, S. B., and Green, I. (1981). A fibroblast proliferation factor isolated from human MLR supernatants has physical and functional properties similar to human interleukin 1 (IL-1). *Fed. Proc., Fed. Am. Soc. Exp. Biol.* **40,** 1084.

Sipe, J. D., Vogel, S. N., Ryan, L., McAdam, K. P. W. J., and Rosenstreich, D. L. (1979). Detection of a mediator derived from endotoxin-stimulated macrophages that induces the acute phase serum amyloid A response in mice. *J. Exp. Med.* **150,** 597.

Smith, K. A., Gilbride, K. J., and Favata, M. F. (1980a). Lymphocyte activating factor promotes T-cell growth factor production by cloned murine lymphoma cells. *Nature (London)* **287,** 853.

Smith, K. A., Lachman, L. B., Oppenheim, J. J., and Favata, M. F. (1980b). The functional relationship of the interleukins. *J. Exp. Med.* **151,** 1551.

Stamenkovic, M., Stosic-Grujicic, S., and Simic, M. M. (1979). Carrageenan-induced macrophage soluble factors with co-stimulatory effects in the proliferative response of T lymphocytes to mitogens. *Period. Biol.* **81,** 171.

Togawa, A., Oppenheim, J. J., and Mizel, S. B. (1979). Characterization of lymphocyte activating factor (LAF) produced by human mononuclear cells: Biochemical relationship of high and low molecular weight forms of LAF. *J. Immunol.* **122,** 2112.

Unanue, E. R. (1978). The regulation of lymphocyte functions by the macrophage. *Immunol. Rev.* **40,** 227.

Unanue, E. R., and Kiely, J.-M. (1977). Synthesis and secretion of a mitogenic protein by macrophages: Description of a superinduction phenomenon. *J. Immunol.* **119,** 925.

Vogel, S. N., Moore, R. N., Sipe, J. D., and Rosenstreich, D. L. (1980). BCG-induced enhancement of endotoxin sensitivity in C_3H/HeJ mice. I. *In vivo* studies, *J. Immunol.* **124,** 2004.

Wood, D. D. (1979). Mechanism of action of human B cell-activating factor. I. Comparison of the plaque-stimulating activity with thymocyte-stimulating activity. *J. Immunol.* **123,** 2400.

Wood, D. D. (1982). Antigen nonspecific factors elaborated by macrophages which stimulate lymphocytes; interleukin 1. *In* "The Reticuloendothelial System" (J. A. Bellanti and H. B. Herscowitz, eds.), Vol. 6. Plenum, New York (in press).

5

Production and Properties of Human IL-2

Elizabeth A. Grimm/Steven A. Rosenberg

I. Introduction 57
II. Culture Conditions for Generation of Human IL-2 58
A. Introduction 58
B. Tissues Used for IL-2 Production 58
C. Mitogens Effective in IL-2 Production 60
D. Mononuclear Cell Preparation and Culture Conditions 61
III. Testing of Culture Supernatant for IL-2 Content 63
A. Types of Assays Employed 63
B. Production of IL-2-Dependent Cells 64
C. Screening for IL-2 Activity by the Short-Term ^{3}H-TdR Uptake Assay 64
D. Determination of IL-2 Titer by the Long-Term Growth Test . . 65
IV. Removal of PHA from IL-2-Containing Culture Supernatants . . . 66
A. Introduction 66
B. Amnonium Sulfate Precipitation of Human IL-2 67
C. Removal of Residual PHA from SAS Preparations of IL-2 . . 67
V. Long-Term Growth of Cytotoxic T Lymphocytes in IL-2 69
A. Human T Lymphocytes Stop Growth after Two to Three Months in TCGF: The "Crisis" Problem 69
B. Selection of CTL by Expansion of *in Vitro* Sensitization Cultures (IVS) in Lectin-Free IL-2 70
C. Growth of Cytotoxic Cell Lines 72
D. Cloning of CTL in IL-2 74
VI. Use of IL-2-Containing Preparations for Activation of Cytolytic Lymphocytes: IL-2 Providing the Proliferative Stimulus Necessary for Allogeneic IVS 77
VII. Conclusions 79
References 79

I. INTRODUCTION

Since the discovery of human T cell growth factor (TCGF) by Morgan *et al.* in 1976, research on TCGF production and utilization has had important impact on immunologic studies in human and murine systems. In 1977, Ruscetti *et al.*

ISOLATION, CHARACTERIZATION, AND UTILIZATION OF T LYMPHOCYTE CLONES

ISBN 0-12-249920-4

reported long-term growth of human PBL in TCGF, and in 1978 our laboratory (Strausser and Rosenberg, 1978) reported long-term growth of human cytotoxic T lymphocytes (CTL) with maintenance of lytic function and specificity.

T cell growth factor is also referred to as interleukin-2 (IL-2), a name given to a variety of functionally defined factors thought to be represented by the same molecular entity (Aarden 1979). While the terms TCGF and IL-2 are currently used interchangeably, crude TCGF refers to a soluble lymphokine defined by its ability to support the long-term growth of activated lymphocytes.

Our continuing interest in the use of TCGF or IL-2 is in both the activation and long-term growth of target specific cytotoxic lymphocytes, and is aimed at achieving large numbers of antitumor-specific CTL for use in adoptive immunotherapy. We have investigated a variety of aspects concerned with IL-2 production, partial purification, and the use of TCGF in the activation of cytotoxic lymphocytes. This chapter presents our data concerning these aspects in human systems, along with a review of the relevant literature.

II. CULTURE CONDITIONS FOR GENERATION OF HUMAN IL-2

A. Introduction

To produce human IL-2, a variety of human lymphoid cell populations can be cultured with PHA for 1–3 days, and the supernatant collected and used as a crude preparation of human IL-2. Many investigators have reported variations of this basic protocol in order to optimize IL-2 production. Most of these reports (Table I) have only provided information on enhanced ^{3}H-TdR uptake in the short-term IL-2 assay and have not provided information showing that long-term growth of human lymphocytes can be supported (see Section III). Therefore, we will present in detail our simplified procedure which consistently produces ample quantities of IL-2 functional in long-term growth of human lymphocytes (see Appendix for specific protocol). A variety of conditions reported to affect human IL-2 production are presented in Table I.

B. Tissues Used for IL-2 Production

Several types of human lymphoid tissues can be used for generation of IL-2. We have found that peripheral blood mononuclear leukocytes (PBL), spleen cells, and thoracic duct cells (TDL) are all capable of producing IL-2. While the majority of researchers and commercial sources prepare IL-2 from PBL, others have successfully used human spleen cells (Moretta *et al.*, 1981), human bone marrow and lymph node (Ruscetti and Gallo, 1980) tonsils (Kurnick *et al.*, 1979;

TABLE I

Conditions Affecting PHA-Stimulated Human IL-2 Production

Condition	Reference
1. Use of single versus pooled donor cells	Bonnard and Alvarez (1980)
	Ruscetti *et al.* (1980)
	Alvarez *et al.* (1981)
2. Lymphoid cell concentration	Alvarez *et al.* (1981)
3. Monocyte concentration	Alvarez *et al.* (1979)
	Inouye *et al.* (1979)
	Bach (1980)
	Bonnard *et al.* (1980)
4. Serum type and concentration	Alvarez *et al.* (1979)
	Bonnard *et al.* (1980)
	Fabricius *et al.* (1980)
	Mier and Gallo (1980)
	Ruscetti *et al.* (1981)
	Warren and Pembry (1981)
5. Time of incubation	Bonnard *et al.* (1980)
	Ruscetti *et al.* (1980, 1981)
	Moretta *et al.* (1981)
	Strausser and Rosenberg (1978)
6. Culture vessels	See this chapter
7. Addition of LBL- or HLA-D-positive cells	Inouye *et al.* (1979)
	Ruscetti *et al.* (1980)
	Bach (1980)
	Bonnard *et al.* (1980)
8. Irradiation of lymphoid cells	Bonnard *et al.* (1979)
	Inouye *et al.* (1979)
	Bach (1980)

Warren and Pembrey, 1981; Robb and Smith, 1981), and thoracic duct lymphocytes (E. A. Grimm, unpublished).

IL-2 production requires the presence of E-rosette-positive T cells (Bonnard and Alvarez, 1980; Ruscetti and Gallo, 1980), probably T helper cells. Malignant lymphoid cells from patients with Sezary syndrome, thought to be a malignancy of helper cells, have been reported to produce IL-2 (Solbach *et al.*, 1980). Monocytes are also necessary in the producer cell population and from 1 to 5% is considered optimal (Bonnard *et al.*, 1980; Fagnani and Bonnard, 1980; Ruscetti *et al.*, 1980). The addition of greater than 10% adherent cells was found to slightly suppress IL-2 production (Alvarez *et al.*, 1980; Bach, 1980), as measured in the short-term ^{3}H-TdR uptake assay. Initial procedures for human IL-2 production included passage of PBL over nylon wool columns to remove most of the monocytes and B cells (Strausser and Rosenberg, 1978; Ruscetti *et al.*, 1980; Bonnard *et al.*, 1980; Alvarez *et al.*, 1980); however, we believe that this step is unnecessary, since the percentage of monocytes in normal mononuclear cell populations is normally not much greater than 10%. Glucocorticosteroids have also been shown by Gillis *et al.* (1979) to suppress IL-2 production.

Fagnini and Bonnard (1980) have reported that human IL-2 can be produced by purified T cells, only if monocytes are added to the culture. T lymphocyte lines also will produce IL-2 if either adherent cells or the macrophage product, lymphocyte activating factor (LAF, also called interleukin-1) is added. Ruscetti *et al.* (1980) reported that addition of HLA-D-positive cells or their plasma membranes to nylon wool purified single donor T cells significantly enhances IL-2 production. The HLA-D-positive cell line, Daudi was found to support IL-2 production, while MOLT-4, an HLA-D-negative line, does not. Therefore, it appears that both IL-1 and HLA-D are involved in IL-2 production. Recently, a number of constitutive producers of human IL-2 have been found. A human leukemia line, Jurkat-FHCRC (Gillis *et al.*, 1980, 1981), cultured Sezary cells (Solbach *et al.*, 1980), and several human cutaneous T cell lymphoma-leukemias (Gootenberg *et al.*, 1981) have been reported to produce IL-2. As of yet these lines have not gained wide usage, nor has their IL-2 quantity been directly compared to that produced by whole lymphoid populations.

Therefore to produce IL-2, any whole lymphoid population that contains T cells and adherent cells should suffice. While the T cells are the IL-2 producers, the role(s) of the adherent cell is not known, and possibilities include HLA-D expression, mitogen processing, and LAF production. Human PBL, spleen, thoracic duct cells, and tonsils are all competent for IL-2 production.

C. Mitogens Effective in IL-2 Production

Phytohemagglutinin (PHA) is the preferred mitogen for stimulation of IL-2 production by human lymphoid cell cultures. PHA-M and PHA-P (Difco; Detroit, Michigan) have been used by us at 1.0 and 0.2%, respectively. PHA-P has also been used at 0.08% when cells were at the lower concentration of 1×10^6/ml (Strausser and Rosenberg, 1978). The more purified PHA from Wellcome (Burroughs-Wellcome Co., Research Triangle Park, North Carolina) has been used at 0.5 μg/ml (Bonnard *et al.*, 1980) or 1.0 μg/ml (Kurnick *et al.*, 1979), and leukoagglutinin (Pharmacia Chemicals, Uppsala, Sweden) at 1 μg/ml (Ruscetti *et al.*, 1980) has also been used. Concanavalin A (Con-A) has not been widely used because some investigators have found no IL-2 induced (Bonnard *et al.*, 1980; J. L. Strausser, unpublished) or low levels of IL-2 produced (Alvarez *et al.*, 1979; Warren and Pembry, 1981) in Con-A-stimulated cultures. One group of investigators has reported IL-2 production in response to Con-A (Northoff *et al.*, 1980) if phorbol myristic acetate (PMA) is added to the cultures (Stadler *et al.*, 1980); however, there was no comparison of the quantities induced by Con-A versus that obtained with PHA. The mitogenic stimulus provided by oxidizing cells with the enzymes neuraminidase and galactose oxidase (NaGO) has also been found to generate human IL-2 (Novogrodsky *et al.*, 1980). Stimulation by NaGO appears to be a reasonable alternative for IL-2 production when the presence of PHA is undesirable. Mixed leukocyte culture (MLC) (Alvarez *et al.*, 1980) and pokeweed mitogen (Ruscetti *et al.*, 1980) have been found to stimulate weak IL-2 activity, and may also prove useful if PHA is undesirable. Limited experiments by us have clearly shown PHA stimulation to yield higher levels of IL-2 activity than those induced by Con-A (J. L. Strausser, unpublished), MLC supernatants (Lotze and Rosenberg, 1981), or by the NaGO supernatants (E. A. Grimm, unpublished). Each of the four major types of PHA commercially available (PHA-M and PHA-P from Difco; purified PHA, Burroughs-Wellcome; leukoagglutinin, Pharmacia) is an excellent stimulus. The choice of which PHA to use rests more on cost and availability, since no direct comparison of the four has been reported. We currently favor the 0.2% PHA-P, since it is less expensive than the Wellcome PHA and is purer, with less agglutinating activity than the PHA-M.

D. Mononuclear Cell Preparation and Culture Conditions

Slight variations in the exact procedures used successfully by many investigators suggest that most of the cell preparation details are not critical. Studies performed to compare techniques and conditions have found that the original methods were unnecessarily complex (Bonnard *et al.*, 1980). We also have simplified our original procedure (Strausser and Rosenberg, 1978). Similar conditions are optimal for IL-2 production from PBL, human spleen, and human TDL. Mononuclear cells are obtained by LSM (Litton Bionetics, Kensington, Maryland) or Ficoll–Hypaque gradient centrifugation of heparinized whole blood, heparanized thoracic duct drainage, or single cell suspensions of spleen tissue prepared by mincing with scissors in a balanced salt solution (BSS). Residual red blood cell (RBC) contamination was found to have no effect on IL-2 production. Lymphoid cells are collected from the gradient interface, washed in BSS, and used at 5×10^6/ml PBL will produce IL-2 at 1×10^6/ml when the donor is a known "high producer" (Bonnard *et al.*, 1980); however, 5×10^6/ml is now favored, since this concentration appears to overcome individual donor variation (Alvarez *et al.*, 1981). Both spleen and TDL cells produce IL-2 optimally at 5×10^6/ml.

Pooling of cells from several donors is not required. Initially the concomitant MLC was believed to enhance IL-2 production, but recent studies using 5×10^6/ml have not found this to be true. Alvarez *et al.* (1981) using PBL and our own results using spleen cell mixtures have found no advantage of mixing two or more donors' cells. If the PHA stimulus is optimal, then all potential IL-2 producers should be activated; however, if the PHA cell concentration or monocyte presence is suboptimal, it is possible that an MLC could contribute to IL-2 production.

RPMI 1640 (Gibco, Grand Island, New York) medium is most widely used in IL-2 production. We routinely supplement the medium with fresh glutamine (2%), antibiotics (penicillin, 100 U/ml; streptomycin 100 μg/ml; NIH Media Unit) and 2% heat decomplemented human AB serum (KC Biologicals, Lenexa, Kansas). While many investigators employ fetal calf serum (FCS), it was found to be deleterious to IL-2 production (Bonnard *et al.*, 1980) and is not recommended.

Though Fabricius *et al.* (1980) have reported that specific serum proteins are needed for IL-2 production, it is not clear how much serum if any is absolutely required, since many investigators routinely generate IL-2 using serum-free conditions (Mier and Gallo, 1980; Warren and Pembry, 1981; Alvarez *et al.*, 1979; Novogrodsky *et al.*, 1980; Ruscetti and Gallo, 1981; Bonnard *et al.*, 1980).

Incubation of cultures for IL-2 production has been reported for 18 hr (Moretta *et al.*, 1981) to 72 hr (Strausser and Rosenberg, 1978; Ruscetti *et al.*, 1980). Incubation for as long as 72 hr is acceptable if serum is employed (J. L. Strausser, unpublished; Bonnard *et al.*, 1980), though 38–44 hr provides optimal levels of IL-2 and is convenient.

A variety of sizes and shapes of culture vessels have been used to culture cells during IL-2 production. As long as the cell concentration is 5×10^6/ml and PHA concentration is optimal, no differences have been noted; however, no study has yet reported a comparison of culture vessels. Standard incubation conditions of 5% CO_2, humidified atmosphere at 37°C is used.

Harvesting of crude IL-2-containing supernatants is best done by two sequential contrifugations. Initial centrifugation of the culture contents at 1500 rpm is performed to pellet the cells. The supernatant can then be ultracentrifuged to pellet subcellular debris or should be frozen immediately. [Cells from the IL-2 production culture can be saved and recultured for 12 more days for use as dependent cells (see Section III,B).]

Several modifications of the basic IL-2 production protocol have gained some popularity and deserve further mention. As discussed earlier in Section II,B, excess adherent cells have been reported to suppress IL-2 production. One mechanism of IL-2 suppression by adherent cells was reported by Inouye *et al.* (1979) and Bach (1980) to be due to prostaglandins produced by adherent cells, since the addition of the prostaglandin synthetase inhibitor, indomethacin, to IL-2 production cultures can cause augumented IL-2 production.

Several groups of investigators who remove adherent cells from the IL-2 production population find that addition of Epstein-Barr virus transformed lymphoblastoid cells (LBL) also increases IL-2 production up to threefold (Inouye *et al.*, 1979; Bach, 1980; Bonnard *et al.*, 1980; Ruscetti *et al.*, 1980), most likely attributable to the enhancing property of HLA-D expression (Ruscetti *et al.*, 1980). In these situations, the LBL may be providing the HLA-D stimulus normally supplied by the removed nylon adherent monocytes or B cells.

Interleukin-2 production was reported to be enhanced threefold if the PBL used for culture were initially irradiated (Bonnard *et al.*, 1979; Inouye *et al.*, 1979; Bach, 1980). Up to 3000 R has been found effective, with 1000 R considered optimal (Bach, 1980). Since IL-2 is produced during the G_1 phase of the cell cycle (Stadler *et al.*, 1980) and is absorbed by blast cells (Bonnard *et al.*, 1979), probably in the S phase, irradiation is hypothesized to permit a greater accumulation of IL-2 in the culture supernatant, but inhibiting lymphocyte entry into S phase. This hypothesis is supported by the data of Ruscetti *et al.* (1980) that DNA synthesis inhibitors colchicine or cystosine arabinoside had no effect on IL-2 release, while the protein synthesis inhibitors puromycin and cyclohexamide profoundly inhibited IL-2 production.

III. TESTING OF CULTURE SUPERNATANT FOR IL-2 CONTENT

A. Types of Assays Employed

Two types of tests are employed for measurement of IL-2 activity. One is the short-term stimulation of IL-2-dependent cells with dilutions of culture supernatants, quantified by an end pulse of ^{3}H-TdR (Gillis *et al.*, 1978; Ruscetti *et al.*, 1980). The second test is a longer-term growth assay in which dependent cells are cultured for 5–7 days (one passage) with varying growth factor dilutions. Cultures are then counted for cell number and viability, and the actual cell growth is determined.

Though the short-term ^{3}H-TdR assay is widely used, it may not always correlate with the ability to support prolonged cell growth. It, thus, is primarily useful for screening purposes and not for determining growth factor titers that are then to be used in long-term lymphocyte propagation. The only reliable means to determine IL-2 content is to determine directly the dilution of the putative IL-2-containing preparation that will best grow previously activated cells. In our experience, some growth factor preparations that appeared positive in the ^{3}H-TdR uptake test have been unable to support cell growth. The reverse situation has also been observed in which preparations appeared to contain an inhibitory activity at high concentrations so that poor ^{3}H-TdR uptake was observed, but such preparations were excellent for long-term growth of cells. It is likely that factors other than IL-2 stimulate ^{3}H-TdR uptake but are incapable of stimulating continuous growth. Therefore, we urge that continued growth of dependent cells, in addition to ^{3}H-TdR uptake be used to determine IL 2 content.

B. Production of IL-2-Dependent Cells

The IL-2-dependent cells used in these tests are critical. If the dependent cells contain any lymphocytes responsive to mitogens, then false positive results may be observed in mitogen-containing IL-2 preparations. We prepare IL-2-dependent cells by initially culturing 1×10^5/ml fresh PBL in crude growth factor preparations containing PHA. On day 4 or 5, the cells are counted, washed, and split back to 1×10^5/ml and recultured. This count, split, and feed procedure is then repeated on day 8 or 9. By day 14, all growing cells are unresponsive to PHA and therefore are dependent only on IL-2. Cells prepared in this manner are split and fed weekly, and can be maintained for at least 1 month, at which time new lines should be initiated. Dependent cells to be used in IL-2 assays should not be taken from the cultures immediately after a split and feed, but rather toward the end of the week's growth when they are not rapidly proliferating in response to the IL-2 used for feeding.

In either the ^{3}H-TdR uptake, or the long-term growth assay, it is important to test whether the "dependent cells" are truly dependent, by including serial dilutions of a PHA solution as a control. This is especially important for these investigators attempting to use 5 to 7 day PHA blasts as dependent cells.

Human IL-2 is known to stimulate mouse lymphocytes (Gillis *et al.*, 1978a), and many investigators use mouse-dependent cells to test for human IL-2 activity. It is not known, however, whether mouse and human cells require similar concentrations of IL-2 or other factors present in the supernatant for long-term growth.

C. Screening for IL-2 Activity by the Short-Term ^{3}H-TdR Uptake Assay

Serial twofold 100-μl dilutions of the culture supernatant or PHA are prepared in 96-well microtiter plate wells (Costar, Cambridge, MA) in RPMI 1640 medium containing 10% human AB serum, called complete medium (CM). Dilutions are usually performed horizontally across the microplate to the tenth row, and the eleventh and twelfth rows are then filled with CM and used for controls of dependent cells plus CM in row 11, and CM only in row 12. Dependent cells are then added to the wells in 100-μl volumes at 1×10^4 cells/well. The plates are incubated for 30–34 hr, at which time each well is pulsed with 1 μCi ^{3}H-TdR (New England Nuclear, Boston, Massachusetts), in 10 μl. After 6 more hours of incubation, the well contents are harvested using an automated sample harvester onto filter papers and counted (Fig. 1). A titer can be defined as the reciprocal of the dilution causing one-half maximum [^{3}H]thymidine incorporation. It has not yet become widely popular to convert the ^{3}H-TdR uptake data into units (Ruscetti *et al.*, 1980) as is now commonly done with murine IL-2.

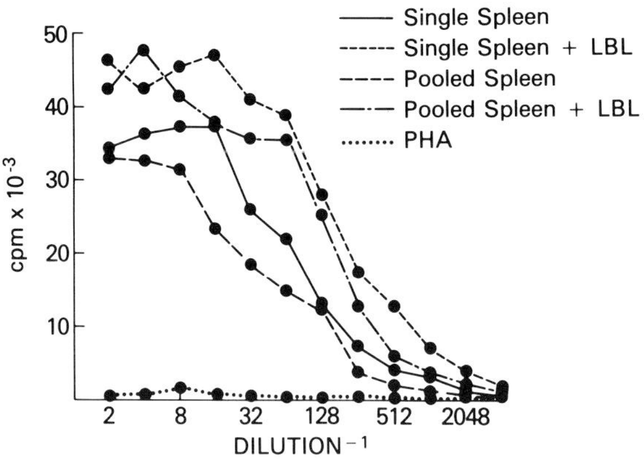

Fig. 1. Short-term ^{3}H-TdR assay results of IL-2 activity from PHA-stimulated spleen cell cultures, from single and pooled donors, and in the absence and presence of an irradiated B cell lymphoblastoid line 8866 (Rogentine and Gerber, 1969). Culture supernatants were harvested and used directly in both the short-term and long-term (Fig. 2) growth assay. Factor from the pooled spleen appears to be no better than the single spleen; however the factors produced by addition to the B cell line appears to contain two- to fourfold more activity, though this was not found to be true in the long-term assay.

D. Determination of IL-2 Titer by the Long-Term Growth Test

Dilutions of culture supernatants are prepared in 1-ml volumes in 24-well Costar plates, to which 1 ml containing 10^5 dependent cells in CM is added. Controls are dependent cells with media only, and when available a positive control of a known IL-2-containing preparation is used. Plates are incubated for 7 days, and then the well contents are suspended and counted in trypan blue to determine the dilution supporting optimal expansion of the dependent cells. Figure 2 shows the expansion and growth kinetics of PBL in the same unpurified IL-2-containing supernatants used in the short-term ^{3}H-TdR assay reported in Fig. 1.

The data in Figs. 1 and 2 illustrate the lack of correlation between the short-term and long-term IL-2 assays. In the short-term assay, Fig. 2, all four IL-2 preparations appeared positive, with those prepared in the presence of a B cell line having a two- to fourfold higher titer. The dependent cells did not respond to PHA, so they are assumed to be dependent on IL-2. The growth assay in Fig. 2 illustrates several points. All preparations were able initially to stimulate fresh PBL to proliferate. By week 1, the PHA could no longer support growth, and presumably IL-2 stimulated all further growth of activated cells. For weeks 2 and 3, growth was essentially equivalent by all factors, but on week 4, the factors produced by the LBL supplemented culture no longer supported growth. The factors produced in the absence of LBL which by the short-term assay would be assumed to contain fewer units and less IL-2, was functional in continuing

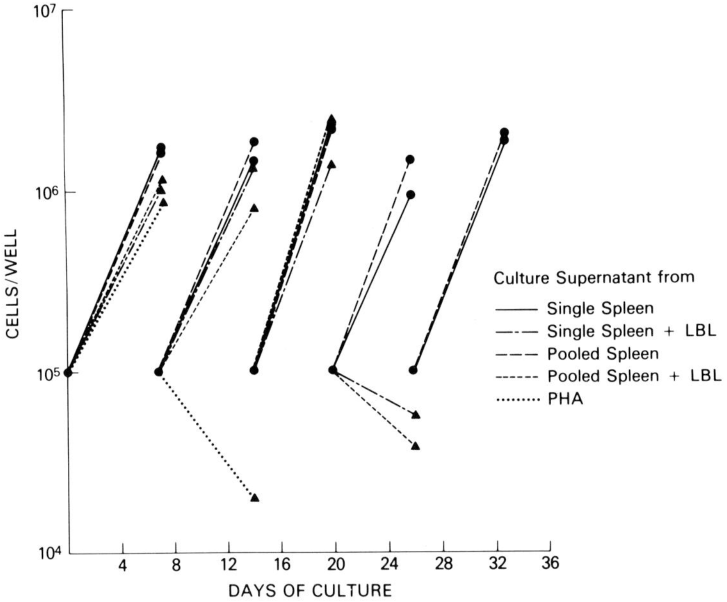

Fig. 2. Long-term growth assay of PHA-stimulated spleen cell IL-2 from single and pooled donors in the absence and in the presence of an irradiated B cell line 8866 (Rogentine and Gerber, 1969). Culture supernatants were harvested and used directly to initiate and support long-term dependent cell growth. Fresh lymphocytes use cultured at 1×10^5 per well, and split back to 1×10^5 as shown. The supernatant from LBL supplemented cultures did not support growth beyond the third week; however, supernatants from both the single and pooled spleen preparations were equivalent in supporting long-term growth.

growth, and was, therefore, superior. This finding of enhanced ^{3}H-TdR uptake, but deficient growth supporting activity from LBL supplemented cultures has been consistently observed by us in three experiments. These data also show that pooling of spleen cells does augment IL-2 production; pooling of PBL (Alvarez *et al.*, 1981) was also found not to increase IL-2 production.

IV. REMOVAL OF PHA FROM IL-2-CONTAINING CULTURE SUPERNATANTS

A. Introduction

Since both polyclonal activation and nonspecific lytic interactions can be caused by lymphocyte interaction with the lectin PHA, it is often desirable to remove PHA from the culture supernatants containing IL-2. Our preferred method is that developed by Lotze and Rosenberg (1981) using saturated ammonium sulfate precipitation (SAS) followed by passage over an anti-PHA affinity column. The use of anti-PHA columns was introduced by Kurnick *et al.* (1979). We have also found that absorption of the SAS preparation with chicken red blood cells (CRBC) originally described by Alvarez *et al.* (1981) is effective for removal of PHA-P and PHA-M. Affinity chromatography on porcine thyroglobulin has been reported by Fagnani and Braatz (1980) to remove PHA, and a preculture "pulse" and wash of PHA from tonsil cells has been reported by Warren and Pembrey (1981) to result in production of PHA-free culture supernatants.

B. Ammonium Sulfate Precipitation of Human IL-2

Ammonium sulfate precipitation of human IL-2 occurs at 75% SAS, while PHA and a number of other proteins precipitate at 50% SAS and lower. To remove PHA, an IL-2-containing supernatant is brought to 50% as saturation by slowly adding 312 g of crystalline ammonium sulfate per liter of culture supernatant. The resultant slurry is slowly stirred for 2 hr at room temperature, then centrifuged at 9000 rpm for 20 min. The supernatant is collected (pellet discarded), and this 50% SAS supernatant is then brought to 75% SAS by slow addition of 172 g of ammonium sulfate per liter. After a final 2 hr of mixing at room temperature, the slurry is centrifuged again at 9000 rpm for 20 min. This time the supernatant is discarded and the pellet resuspended with deionized water at one-tenth the volume of the starting supernatant. This SAS preparation is then dialyzed versus water with two changes, and then versus either phosphate-buffered saline or a BSS solution with two changes for a minimum 24 hr each at 4°C. Dialysis tubing should have a molecular weight cutoff no greater than 10,000. This SAS procedure eliminates 50–70% of the non-IL-2 protein, and removes 92% of the PHA with at least a 77% yield of IL-2.

C. Removal of Residual PHA from SAS Preparations of IL-2

In order to remove the small amount of PHA remaining in the SAS–IL-2 preparations, we used an anti-PHA immunoadsorbent column. The column is prepared by coupling the γ-globulin fraction of rabbit anti-PHA antisera with cyanogen bromide-activated Sepharose 4B (Pharmacia, Uppsala, Sweden). Lotze and Rosenberg (1981) coupled 10 mg of antibody to 5 ml of the gel, and then packed the coupled gel in a 14×0.9 cm column. Using an ^{125}I-labeled PHA tracer, this column was found to remove greater than 99.8% of the PHA from an initial 1500-ml IL-2 culture supernatant. After adsorption, no PHA was detectable in the functional assay. Therefore, as determined by both biochemical and functional tests, SAS precipitation followed by passage over an anti-PHA column removed greater than 99% of the PHA initially employed to stimulate IL-2 production. The column is then washed, and bound PHA is eluted by running a solution of 0.2 *M* glycine HC1, pH 3.0, containing 0.5 *M* NaCl through for several hours, and then regenerated by running PBS for at least another hour. Such a column can be kept and reused indefinitely when stored at room temperature in PBS containing 0.01 *M* sodium azide. We have maintained and used our current anti-PHA column for greater than 12 months with no noticeable loss of activity.

Since human IL-2 has been reported to have a molecular weight of 13,000–17,000 (Gillis *et al.*, 1980; Mier and Gallo, 1980) and PHA to be much higher at 150,000 (Leavitt *et al.*, 1977) it seemed logical to attempt a simple size separation of PHA and IL-2. Lotze and Rosenberg (1981), however, were unable to achieve sufficient PHA removal by either gel filtration on Sephadex G-100, or using ultrafiltration by Amicon membrane (Amicon Corporation, Lexington, Massachusetts) with 30,000 or 50,000 molecular weight cutoffs. Neither were we able to absorb the PHA with human red blood cells or sheep red blood cells. Recently we have tested the ability of chicken red blood cells (CRBC) to absorb PHA (Alvarez *et al.*, 1981) and have found the procedure to be as efficient as the anti-PHA column for PHA-P and PHA-M (Difco). However, this procedure does not work for the Burroughs-Wellcome PHA (E. A. Grimm, unpublished). The CRBC adsorption requires a large amount of fresh chicken blood and is more tedious than running the column. Chicken red blood cells also apparently do not bind purified PHA and absorb only the PHA-M or PHA-P which contain agglutinnating moitics.

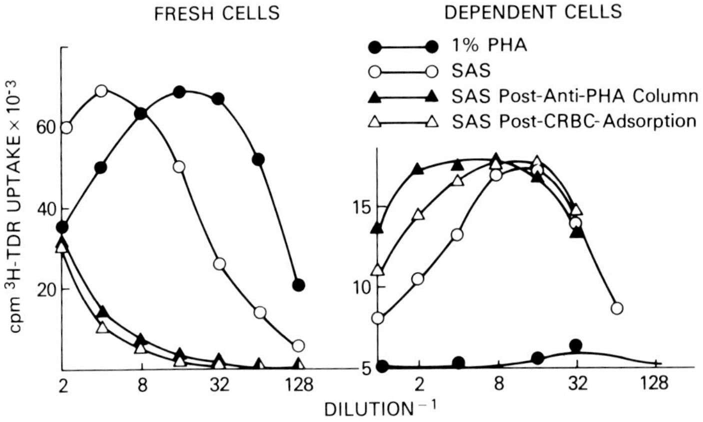

Fig. 3. Removal of mitogenic PHA from IL-2-containing culture supernatants. Crude culture supernatants prepared using 0.2% PHA-P were precipitated with SAS, and adjusted to one-tenth the original volume. A sample of the SAS–IL-2 was saved for testing, and the remainder either adsorbed to the anti-PHA column or to CRBC. All three IL-2 preparations were then tested for PHA content by stimulation of dependent cells in both the short-term ^{3}H-TdR uptake assay and the long-term growth assay. Both the anti-PHA column and CRBC absorption were found to remove PHA.

Figure 3 shows the testing for residual PHA and IL-2 by ^{3}H-TdR uptake assays. Phytohemagglutinnin is measured by an assay identical to the one described for IL-2 except that fresh PBL are used at 1×10^5 per well. The fresh PBL responds to the 1% PHA, and the IL-2-dependent cells do not. According to the ^{3}H-TdR counts in the fresh cells, the SAS preparation has about 10% of the functional PHA remaining, while the anti-PHA or CRBC-absorbed SAS preparation has less than 1%. The small amount of ^{3}H-TdR uptake by fresh cells to high concentrations of PHA-free preparations has been noted by many investigators and occurs even when an IL-2-containing MLC supernatant is tested (Lotze and Rosenberg, 1981). Presumably some fraction of fresh PBL are "activated" and can respond to IL-2, though the response is negligible when compared to that caused by PHA.

V. LONG-TERM GROWTH OF CYTOTOXIC T LYMPHOCYTES IN IL-2

A. Human T Lymphocytes Stop Growth after Two to Three Months in TCGF: The "Crisis" Problem

Optimal conditions for long-term growth of lymphocytes have not been established. Though some workers have grown cell lines and clones for periods up to 13 months (Ruscetti *et al.*, 1977), these reports are the exception rather than the rule. After approximately 30 to 60 days of growth in TCGF, cells cease to respond to IL-2. This has been referred to as the "crisis period." We have observed this phenomenon in cultures of both sensitized and unsensitized lymphocytes, both with and without filler cells. The reason for the "crisis" in growth is not known. Since IL-2 is reported to cause continuous proliferation of suppressor cells for MLC and mitogen stimulation (Maca *et al.*, 1979), it is possible that some cells grow in IL-2 with the property of limiting the growth of other lymphocytes. This might represent a homeostatic mechanism or an "immune surveillance" guarding against rapidly dividing lymphocytes. Such a mechanism should be overcome by cloning, but we have found that most human lymphoid clones also exhibit limited cell growth.

Another possible means to overcome the crisis period is suggested in the report by Boylston and Anderson (1980) who grew lymphocytes for 9 months utilizing a double chamber culture system. One chamber was used to produce continuously fresh IL-2 which was immediately available via a porous membrane to the lymphocyte line growing in the other chamber. The accompanying exchange of fresh media also helps dilute cell waste products and toxins and may foster better nutrition of the cells. The loss of growth potential during the crisis may reflect the finite life span of most nonmalignant cells, that would be limited at approximately the 15 generations that occurs during 30 days of growth in IL-2; however, this crisis period is not observed in cultures of murine lymphocytes (Rosenberg *et al.*, 1978). Such information argues against the human lymphocyte crisis period representing a common homeostatic or suppressor cell function and suggests it is due to inadequate IL-2 or other culture conditions. Such an explanation still does not account for the fact that occasionally a few of identically cultured lines survive the crisis. The mechanism(s) responsible for this crisis period is currently unknown, and discovery of reliable means to overcome the crisis would be a significant contribution to lymphocyte culture research.

B. Selection of CTL by Expansion of *in Vitro* Sensitization Cultures (IVS) in Lectin-Free IL-2

Figure 4 depicts our model based on much data from ourselves and others concerning the role of IL-2 in both activation and expansion of CTL. If PBL are activated by a specific alloantigen, IL-2 will cause further expansion of the cytolytic cells. Only previously activated lymphocytes can absorb IL-2 and grow in its presence (Bonnard *et al.*, 1979). The use of lectin-free IL-2 preparations to initiate long-term lines of CTL for IVS results in a selective advantage for growth of the CTL activated during the IVS (Lotze and Rosenberg, 1981). If IL-2-containing PHA is used resting lymphocytes responsive to PHA will also be activated to grow and will dilute the concentration of specifically activated CTL. Data presented by Lotze and Rosenberg (1981) shown in Table II illustrates this point. After either a primary or secondary IVS, the specific lytic units per 10^6 lymphocytes was usually much greater from cultures expanded in lectin-free IL-2 than that found in cultures expanded in crude IL-2.

While we and many others have been successful in initiating CTL lines in crude PHA and IL-2-containing culture supernatants, data such as ours in Table II, or

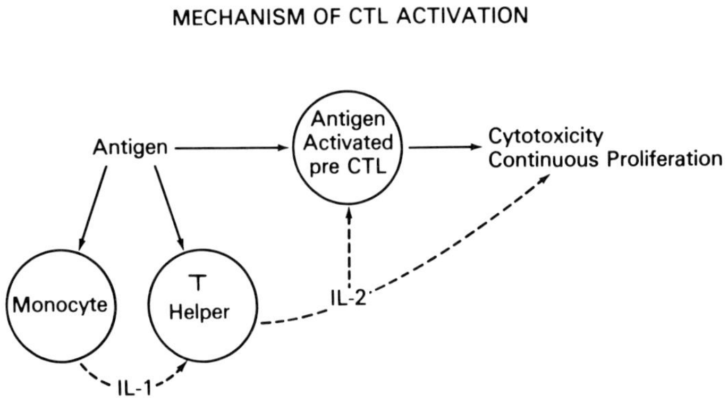

Fig. 4. Current model for the action of human IL-2 in selection of CTL for continuous growth, and to provide the proliferative stimulus functional in CTL generation *in vitro*.

TABLE II

Increased Lytic Specificity after Growth in Lectin-Free IL-2 Compared to Crude IL-2[a]

		Lectin-free IL-2			Crude IL-2[c]		
Allostimulation	Day	Specific L.U./10^6 cells[b]	Cells/well[c] $\times 10^5$	Specific L.U./culture	Specific L.U./10^6 cells	Cells/well $\times 10^5$	Specific L.U./culture
Y anti-Z	Primary MLC, day 4	263.0	1.3	34.2	12.5	20.0	25.0
	Primary MLC, day 6	250.0	2.2	55.0	10.0	1.8	1.8
	Primary MLC, day 10	667.0	8.0	533.6	10.0	2.0	2.0
A anti-Y	Primary MLC, day 4	220.0	6.3	126.0	3.1	5.3	1.6
	Primary MLC, day 6	22.7	14.3	32.5	17.9	1.5	2.7
	Secondary MCL, day 10 (2)	500.0	5.0	250.0	50.0	6.0	30.0

[a] From Lotze and Rosenberg (1981).

[b] Lytic units (L.U.) defined as the number of cells required to lyse 1×10^4 target cells at 20% specific lysis.

[c] All cultures were initiated at 1×10^5 cells/well in PP-TCGF or crude TCGF and grown for 8 days (day 4), 6 days (day 6), or 5 days [day 10(2)] before harvest and assay.

similar findings by Moretta *et al.* (1981) using IL-2 from spleen cells indicates that selection of CTL from IVS cultures using lectin-free IL-2 presents a very efficient first step for initiating long-term CTL lines or clones.

C. Growth of Cytotoxic Cell Lines

The first report of IL-2-dependent long-term human CTL lines was by Strausser and Rosenberg (1978). While Ruscetti *et al.* (1977) had previously grown nonsensitized lymphocytes for greater than 13 months, the cells were not reported to exhibit any cytolytic effector functions. Strausser and Rosenberg reported that both allogeneic target cell specificity and growth was maintained for up to 92 days (Table III), and that nonsensitized cells grown in the same crude IL-2 preparation did not develop cytotoxic activity. The allosensitized cells increased 10^{10}-fold their original number. While Gillis *et al.* (1978b) also reported growth and maintenance of human CTL in crude IL-2 preparations for 3 months, the inability to grow cells for prolonged periods and the expression of nonspecific lytic activities (Schendel *et al.*, 1980a) have plagued many other attempts.

It has been reported that non-CTL cytolytic effector cells, such as natural killer ADCC effectors (K cells), grow well in IL-2 (Alvarez *et al.*, 1978; Timonen *et al.*, 1981; Ortaldo *et al.*, 1980) and that these cells may obscure target specific cytolytic activities. Lotze *et al.* (1981) reported that PBL from tumor bearing individuals, when cultured in IL-2, became lytic for fresh autologous human

TABLE III

Lysis in ^{51}Cr Assay ± S.D.[a,b]

Effectors	Days Grown on HCM	X^2	Y	Z
X (Nonsensitized)	0	−1.5 ± 0.8	0.9 ± 0.1	2.7 ± 1.0
	30	0.5 ± 0.5	3.6 ± 0.7	4.4 ± 2.0
	44	1.5 ± 1.1	3.4 ± 1.1	4.6 ± 0.1
	57	4.6 ± 1.2	7.4 ± 0.9	6.2 ± 0.5
	92	0.7 ± 1.0	7.2 ± 2.3	—
X (Sensitized to Y)	0	−0.1 ± 0.8	39.3 ± 3.3	22.4 ± 3.3
	30	0.4 ± 1.3	19.3 ± 1.4	13.7 ± 0.7
	44	0.7 ± 0.9	15.3 ± 0.7	6.4 ± 2.5
	57	1.0 ± 0.5	36.5 ± 1.5	16.5 ± 2.4
	92	5.4 ± 1.0	26.3 ± 2.2	—

[a] From Strausser and Rosenberg (1978).

[b] Percent lysis ± S.D. determined. Freshly thawed effector lymphocytes were added to ^{51}Cr-labeled target lymphocytes in Linbro round bottom microtiter plates and incubated for 4 hr at 37°C and 5% CO_2 at 10:1 effector to target ratios. Supernatants from these cultures were harvested with the Skatron-Titertek system and counted for γ particle emission.

TABLE IV

Specificity of IL-2-Induced Antitumor Lysis[a]

Target cells	Effector cells[b]		
	PBL cultured 5 days in IL-2	PBL cultured 5 days in CM	Fresh PBL
Autologous fresh leiomyosarcoma	35.0 ± 1.8[c]	4.1 ± 2.1	−0.8 ± 1.2
	22.3 ± 1.4	−3.5 ± 2.1	NT[d]
	12.6 ± 0.6	8.2 ± 10.8	NT
Autologous fresh PBL	1.6 ± 1.1	4.2 ± 2.2	−3.0 ± 1.7
	0.7 ± 1.4	1.7 ± 0.2	NT
	1.5 ± 3.3	1.1 ± 1.5	NT
Con-A lymphoblasts	8.0 ± 1.0	2.8 ± 1.0	−0.8 ± 0.4
	6.1 ± 0.4	2.0 ± 0.7	NT
	6.1 ± 0.5	1.7 ± 0.5	NT
K562	84.4 ± 1.2	14.8 ± 0.3	26.4 ± 1.3
	71.1 ± 1.4	9.3 ± 0.9	NT
	49.6 ± 0.9	4.9 ± 0.1	NT
Daudi	75.5 ± 0.4	6.1 ± 0.2	3.9 ± 0.5
	50.0 ± 0.6	3.9 ± 0.4	NT
	34.0 ± 0.2	2.4 ± 0.5	NT

[a] Percent specific lysis ± SEM.

[b] Melanoma patients PBL were obtained by leukophoresis and cryopreserved. Some PBL were then thawed and cultured for 5 days in lectin-free IL-2 or used uncultured as fresh PBL.

[c] Effector–target ratios = 50.1, 25.1, 12.5.

[d] NT, not tested.

tumor cells, as measured in a 4-hr chromium-51 release assay. These experiments have revealed that cells cultured in IL-2 expressed a broad range of lytic activities. The susceptible target cells included all tissue cultured cells, and occasionally fresh PBL. Table IV gives an example of the IL-2-stimulated antitumor and nonspecific lysis patterns.

Culture of PBL in either crude or lectin-free IL-2 preparations resulted in the generation of this broad range of activities. In a report by Spits *et al.* (1981) and in preliminary cloning experiments by us, not all cells grown in Il-2 expressed or maintained expression of this broad range of lytic activities. However, expression of nonspecific lytic activities is a consistent phenomenon in all early cultures of cell lines and must be considered when specific lysis patterns are desired. Ortaldo *et al.* (1980) have reported that nonspecific lytic functions are lost when cells growing in IL-2 are incubated in IL-2-free medium for 24 hr prior to testing. Since autologous anti-solid tumor human cytotoxicity is evident in IL-2 cultured cell lines, we are continuing to study the possible biologic relevance of this phenomenon.

Growth of allosensitized target-specific CTL has been reported by a number of investigators. Kurnick *et al.* (1979) cultured target-specific CTL for 30 days by first selecting the lymphoblasts from the IVS culture using a Percoll gradient, and then culturing in the presence of irradiated syngeneic filler cells. These cultures were fed every 3 days with fresh IL-2-containing medium, Kurnick *et al.* (1979) also suggested that lectin-free IL-2 preparations were preferable for maintaining specific CTL function. Use of lectin-free IL-2 eliminates the lectin-dependent cellular cytotoxicity (LDCC) reported to be expressed by cells grown in PHA-containing IL-2 preparations (Alvarez *et al.,* 1978). Addition of irradiated ''feeder'' or ''filler'' cells appears to be important for maintenance of specificity of cell lines as well as clones. Reiss *et al.* (1980) cultured allospecific long-term cytotoxic lines for 6–8 months in IL-2 and showed that weekly addition of irradiated, stimulator allogeneic lymphocytes were required to maintain cytolytic activity. Cultures fed only with IL-2 and no feeder cells for 16 days lost lytic activity but continued growth. The importance of the type of feeder cell was not explored. Spits *et al.* (1981) grew target-specific CTL for longer than 1 year, also by including irradiated stimulator cells with IL-2 in the culture, and also showed that nonspecific lytic activities to either Daudi or K562 cells remained low. Spits performed multiple antigen stimulation for 20 months prior to initiating growth in IL-2.

Therefore, long-term growth of CTL with maintenance of specificity may be favored by preselection of blasts (Kurnick *et al.,* 1979) or use of post-tertiary stimulated cultures (Spits *et al.,* 1981), addition of either syngeneic or allogeneic filler cells (Kurnick *et al.,* 1979; Lotze and Rosenberg, 1981).

D. Cloning of CTL in IL-2

Cloning of human target specific CTL was reported by Lotze *et al.* (1980) using soft agar as well as limiting dilution techniques. While Lotze identified significant polymorphism in the lytic activity of the clones grown in lectin-containing IL-2 preparations, clones from a secondary MLC in which irradiated stimulator cells (JC) were included during each feeding with IL-2 resulted in a stable target-specific cytotoxic clone (Fig. 5). Lytic activity of the 5A2 + JC clone from an ET anti-JC IVS was tested for lytic activity in parallel to the parent cell line 10(2) and a nonlytic control clone, 5A5. The parent line lost lytic activity by day 45, while the 5A2 + JC clone maintained lytic activity and specificity for JC target cells up to 63 days. Figure 6 shows the growth of the parent line and the two clones, and all grew well, though the lytic 5A2 + JC clone grew somewhat slower.

In recent experiments, we have also determined that the partially purified and lectin-free IL-2 preparations were excellent in initiating and supporting growth of CTL clones (E. A. Grimm, unpublished data). Cells from a secondary allogenic

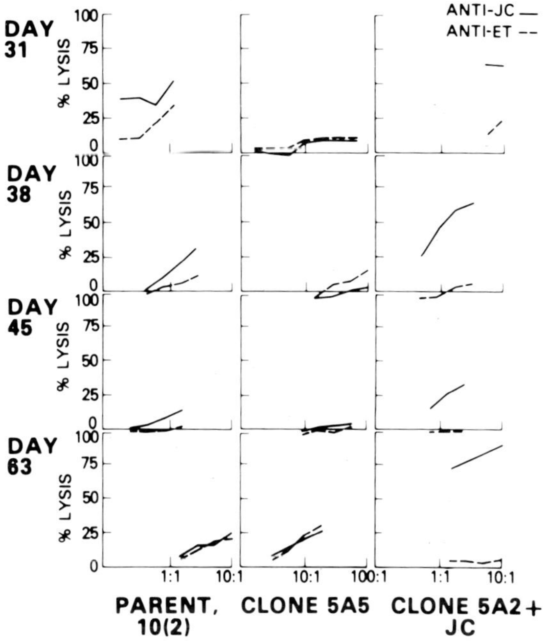

Fig. 5. Sequential cytotoxicity data of parent culture and two clones from ET anti-JC IVS. The parent culture and two clones were grown continuously in IL-2. On the days indicated, aliquots of the cells were collected and cryopreserved. The cells were then thawed simultaneously and tested for lysis to JC, the specific target, and to ET, and autologous target. The parent line maintained cytotoxic activity past day 38, but this activity was later lost. Clone 5A5 was never cytotoxic and did not gain this activity during culture. Clone 5A2 + JC continuously maintained very high cytotoxic activity for the duration of the culture (Lotze *et al.*, 1980).

IVS were cloned by limiting dilution in the presence of irradiated stimulator filler cells in both crude and lectin-free IL-2 preparations. By day 14, 27% (52/192 wells) of the cultures plated at 1 cell/well in crude IL-2 were growing, and only 6% (11/192) of the cultures of 100 cells/well in the lectin-free IL-2 preparation contained growing cells. Therefore, approximately 450 times more clones grew in the lectin-containing IL-2 than in the lectin-free IL-2. However, tests for cytotoxic function in these clones revealed that about half of the clones from lectin-free cultures were cytotoxic, whereas less than 10% of the clones from the crude IL-2 preparation expressed cytolytic activity to the specific allogeneic targets. Several "clones" from each set were selected to grow continuously, with weekly feeding and addition of irradiated stimulator lymphocytes. While about half of the cultures ceased to grow between days 25 and 36, several stable clones grew with a doubling time of 1.5 days until day 74 at which time they were cryopreserved. Repeated tests for cytotoxic activity revealed two of the

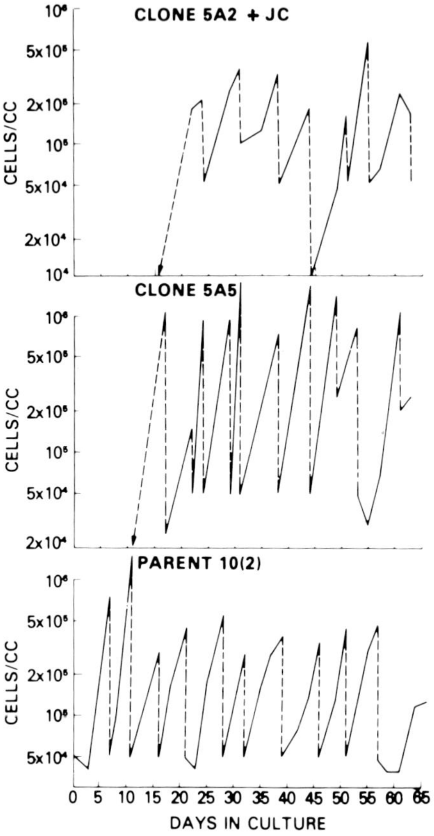

Fig. 6. Growth of parent culture and clones for which cytotoxicity data are shown in Fig. 4. The parent culture and the noncytolytic clone 5A5, and cytolytic clone 5A2 + JC were maintained in continuous culture, reaching densities up to 1×10^6/ml. Cells were counted and split to 5×10^4/ml every 5 to 7 days in fresh medium containing IL-2 (Lotze *et al.*, 1980).

clones from the lectin-free cultures were highly cytotoxic, with $49.2 \pm 8.2\%$ specific lysis at an effector to target ratio of 0.5 : 1. When these cytolytic clones, P1 and P6, were analyzed in parallel with several of the noncytolytic clones for surface phenotype, using the fluorescence activated cell sorter, only the cytolytic clones were found to express extremely high levels of Leu 2a, and were negative for Leu 3a (E. A. Grimm, A. Frankel, J. Ledbetter, and S. A. Rosenberg, unpublished). All clones expressed Leu 1, 4, 5, 6 and human Ia, and were therefore T cells. It is hoped that selection against Leu 3 and for Leu 2a, and growth in lectin-free preparations of IL-2 will significantly enhance our ability to acquire stable, long-lived target specific cytolytic T cell clones.

VI. USE OF IL-2-CONTAINING PREPARATIONS FOR ACTIVATION OF CYTOLYTIC LYMPHOCYTES: IL-2 PROVIDING THE PROLIFERATIVE STIMULUS NECESSARY FOR ALLOGENEIC IVS

In addition to the previously recognized function of supporting continuous culture of activated lymphocytes, we recently reported that lectin-free IL-2 preparations both augmented the production of human allospecific CTL during IVS and provided a proliferative signal which restored the development of CTL to nonimmunogenic alloantigen (Grimm and Mazumder, 1980; Grimm *et al.*, 1981). We have developed three model systems employing weakly immunogenic or nonimmunogenic allogeneic stimulator cells, and in each system addition of lectin-free preparations of IL-2 (also called PP-TCGF, for partially purified T cell growth factor) restores the production of CTL. The most thoroughly studied system is that employing suboptimal and weakly stimulatory numbers of stimulator cells in IVS cultures. If the stimulator cell number is reduced to 1/10 to 1/120 of the optimal, very little CTL activity develops under standard culture conditions. As shown in Fig. 7, if

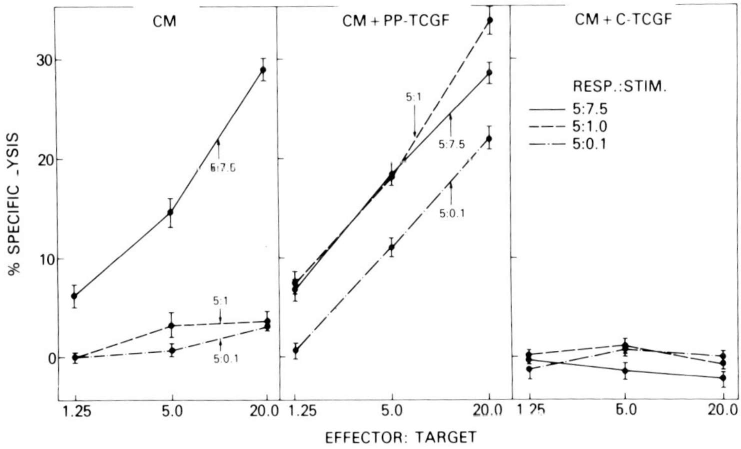

Fig. 7. IL-2 augments of IVS cultures employing minimal stimulator cell numbers. Allogeneic IVS cultures were initiated on day 0 at three responder to stimulator (R : S) ratios: 5 : 7.5, 5 : 1, and 5 : 0.1, in triplicate. One set was incubated in standard culture medium (CM), the second set in CM supplemented with PP-TCGF, and the third set supplemented with C-TCGF. On day 7 all cultures were harvested and cytotoxicity tested to the stimulating cell as shown above, and to control targets (data not shown)., in a 4-hr ^{51}Cr release assay. Cultures in CM developed CTL only when the 5 : 7.5 R : S ratio was used. If the cultures were supplemented with PP-TCGF, CTL developed at all R : S. Crude TCGF was not functional in IVS augmentation. Therefore PP-TCGF contains an activity which augments CTL development in IVS cultures employing suboptimal numbers of stimulator cells.

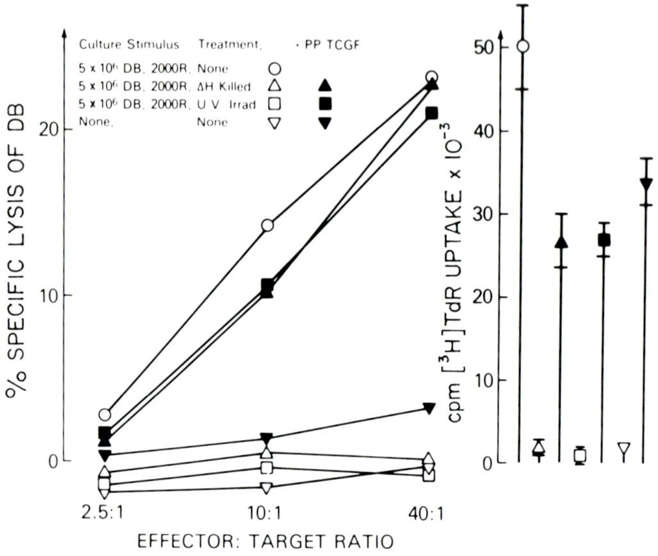

Fig. 8. To determine whether PP-TCGF augments IVS by providing the required proliferative stimulus (second signal?) we treated allogeneic D. B. stimulator PBL by means known to eliminate their function (heat killing at 56°C for 10 min, and uv irradiation at 20 cm for 4 min). Allogeneic MR anti-DB IVS and ^{3}H-TdR tests were incubated, and on day 5 the ^{3}H-TdR cultures were pulsed and harvested, and on day 7 the IVS cultures harvested and tested for lysis of fresh D. B. lymphocytes. Both the uv irradiated and the heat killing of stimulator cells eliminated their proliferative and IVS stimulatory activity. Addition of PP-TCGF to the ^{3}H-TdR cultures was found to stimulate proliferation. Addition of PP-TCGF to the IVS cultures was able to cause generation of CTL, thereby substituting for the proliferative stimulus normally supplied by a competent stimulator cell.

such cultures are supplemented with PP-TCGF, then lytic activity is generated. Lectin-containing IL-2 preparations (called C-TCGF) suppressed the development of CTL, indicating that PHA was not responsible for this augmentation of CTL development. In other experiments, we have shown that CTL derived from IL-2 augmented cultures employing nonimmunogeneic numbers of stimulator cells are target specific; IL-2 can be added up to day 4 of the 7-day IVS, and the amount of IL-2 added regulates the amount of cytolytic activity generated. To test whether augmentation in IVS was due to a proliferative stimulus contributed by IL-2, we adapted two murine systems in which allogeneic stimulator cells had been made nonimmunogenic by either uv irradiation or heat killing at 56°C. Both treatments also abolished the ability of the cells to stimulate allogeneic responder cells to proliferate. Figure 8 shows IVS of human PBL employing uv- or heat-killed stimulator cells in the absence or presence of lectin-free IL-2 (PP-TCGF). The control ^{3}H-TdR uptake data shows that the treated cells did not stimulate proliferation. Also, IVS cultures of the treated cells with responders in regular medium showed no development of lytic activity. However, addition of PP-TCGF to the cultures did cause the responder cells to proliferate and did restore the generation of CTL. Therefore, nonimmunogenic alloantigen activates lymphocytes to the IL-2 responsive state, and as depicted in Fig. 3, IL-2 is then required for final differentiation into CTL. In summary, lectin-free IL-2 preparations do contain a factor(s) functional as the proliferative stimulus in allogeneic IVS.

VII. CONCLUSIONS

Human IL-2 can be prepared using simple procedures employing a variety of human lymphoid tissues. Phytohemagglutinin is the preferred mitogen, and incubation is performed for approximately 40 hr. Proper testing of putative IL-2-containing culture supernatants is critical for identifying the preparations which will support long-term growth of human lymphocytes. While the short-term ^{3}H-TdR uptake assay seems most popular, direct determination of the IL-2 dilution supporting long-term growth of dependent cells is the only reliable assay for testing the ability of preparations to support cell growth.

Removal of PHA from crude IL-2-containing culture supernatants can be achieved by a variety of means including ammonium sulfate precipitation, followed by immunoadsorption by an anti-PHA column. Use of lectin-free IL-2-containing preparations is shown to have many advantages over the crude supernatants including: (1) selection and expansion of CTL from IVS cultures for long-term growth, (2) more selective cloning of CTL from IVS cultures, and (3) activation of CTL during IVS employing subimmunogenic or nonimmunogenic stimuli. Growth of human PBL leads to the generation of a variety of cytolytic functions including the ability to lyse fresh autologous tumor cells.

REFERENCES

Aarden, L. A. *et al.* (1979). Letter to the Editor. Revised nomenclature for antigen-nonspecific T cell proliferation and helper factors. *J. Immunol.* **123,** 2928.

Alvarez, J. M., deLandazuri, M. O., Bonnard, G. D., and Herberman, R. B. (1978). Cytotoxic activities of normal cultured human T cells. *J. Immunol.* **121,** 1270.

Alvarez, J. M., Silva, A., and deLandazuri, M. O. (1979). Human T cell growth factor. I. Optimal conditions for its production. *J. Immunol.* **123,** 977.

Alvarez, J. M., Rodriguez, J., Lopez-Botet, M., Silva, A., and deLandazuri, M. O. (1981). Removal of PHA from supernatants containing T cell growth factor. *J. Immunol. Methods* **40,** 289.

Bach, F. H. (1980). T cell growth factor—Production and use with bulk or cloned cell populations. *Behring Inst. Mitt.* **67,** 235.

Bach, F. H., Inouye, H., Hank, J. A., and Alter, B. J. (1979). Human T lymphocyte clones reactive in primed lymphocyte typing and cytotoxicity. *Nature (London)* **281,** 307.

Bonnard, G. D., and Alvarez, J. M. (1980). Conditions and cellular requirements for the production of human interleukin 2. A review. *Behring Inst. Mitt.* **67,** 230.

Bonnard, G. D., Yasaka, K., and Jacobson, D. (1979). Ligand-activated T cell growth factor—induced proliferation: Absorption of T cell growth factor by activated T cells. *J. Immunol.* **123,** 2704.

Bonnard, G. D., Yasaka, K., and Maca, R. D. (1980). Continued growth of functional human T lymphocytes: Production of human T cell growth factor. *Cell. Immunol.* **51,** 390.

Boylston, H. W., and Anderson, R. L. (1980). Continuous culture of human lymphocytes. *J. Immunol. Methods* **39,** 39.

Fabricius, H. A., Kottgen, E., Stahn, R., Macke, S., and Osswald, B. (1980). The role of serum proteins in PHA-induced production of interleukin 2 by human peripheral blood lymphocytes. *Behring Inst. Mitt.* **67,** 249.

Fagnani, R., and Bonnard, G. D. (1980). Accessory cells reconstitute human cultured T cells response to PHA. *Clin. Res.* **28,** 345A.

Fagnani, R., and Braatz, J. A. (1980). Removal of phytohemagglutinin from conditioned medium by affinity chromatography. *J. Immunol. Methods* **33,** 313.

Gillis, S., and Watson, J. (1981). Biochemical and biological characterization of lymphocyte regulatory molecules. V. Identification of an interleukin 2 producing human leukemia T cell line. *J. Exp. Med.* **152,** 1709.

Gillis, S., Ferm, M. M., Ou, W., and Smith, K. A. (1978a). T-cell growth factor: Parameters of production and a quantitative microassay for activity. *J. Immunol.* **120,** 2027.

Gillis, S., Baker, P. E., Ruscetti, F. W., and Smith, K. A. (1978b). Long-term culture of human antigen-specific cytotoxic T cell lines. *J. Exp. Med.* **148,** 1093.

Gillis, S., Crabtree, G. R., and Smith, K. A. (1979). Glucocorticoid-induced inhibition of T cell growth factor production. I. The effect on mitogen-induced lymphocyte proliferation. *J. Immunol.* **123,** 1624.

Gillis, S., Smith, K. A., and Watson, J. (1980). Biochemical characterization of lymphocyte regulatory molecules. II. Purification of a class of rat and human lymphokines. *J. Immunol.* **124,** 1954.

Gootenberg, J. E., Ruscetti, F. W., Mier, J. W., Gazdar, A., and Gallo, R. C. (1981). Human cutaneous T cell lymphoma and leukemia cell lines produce and respond to T cell growth factor. (Submitted for publication.)

Grimm, E. A., and Mazumder, A. (1981). Augmentation of human *in vitro* sensitization (IVS) by the addition of lectin free T cell growth factor: Applications to allogeneic and autologous antitumor systems. *Proc. Am. Assoc. Cancer Res.* **22,** 314.

Grimm, E. A., Mazumder, A., and Rosenberg, S. A. (1981). *In vitro* growth of cytotoxic human lymphocytes. V. Generation of allospecific cytotoxic lymphocytes to nonimmunogenic antigen by supplementation of *in vitro* sensitization with partially purified T cell growth factor (PP-TCGF). (Submitted for publication.)

Inouye, H., Hank, J. A., Alter, B. J., and Bach, F. H. (1979). TCGF production for cloning and growth of functional human T lymphocytes. *Scand. J. Immunol.* **12,** 149.

Kurnick, J. T., Gronuik, K. O., Kimura, A. K., Lindblom, J. B., Skoog, V. T., Sjobug, O., and Wigzell, H. (1979). Long term growth *in vitro* of human T cell blasts with maintenance of specificity and function. *J. Immunol.* **122,** 1255.

Leavitt, R. D., Felsted, R. L., and Bachur, N. R. (1977). Biological and biochemical properties of *Phaseolus vulgaris* isolectins. *J. Biol. Chem.* **252,** 2961.

Lotze, M. T., and Rosenberg, S. A. (1981). *In vitro* growth of cytotoxic human lymphocytes. III. The preparation of lectin-free T cell growth factor (TCGF) and an analysis of its activity. *J. Immunol.* **126,** 2215.

Lotze, M. T., Strausser, J. L., and Rosenberg, S. A. (1980). *In vitro* growth of cytotoxic human lymphocytes. II. Use of T cell growth factor (TCGF) to clone human T cells. *J. Immunol.* **124,** 2972.

Lotze, M. T., Grimm, E. A., Mazumder, A., Strausser, J. L., and Rosenberg, S. A. (1981). *In vitro* growth of cytotoxic human lymphocytes. IV. Lysis of fresh and cultured antologous tumor by lymphocytes cultured in T cell growth factor (TCGF). *Cancer Res.* **41,** 4425.

Maca, R. D., Bonnard, G. D., and Herberman, R. (1979). The suppression of mitogen and alloantigen-stimulated peripheral blood lymphocyte by cultured human T lymphocytes. *J. Immunol.* **125,** 246.

Mier, J. W., and Gallo, R. C. (1980). Purification and some characteristics of human T cell growth factor from phytohemagglutinin-stimulated lymphocyte conditioned media. *Proc. Natl. Acad. Sci. U.S.A.* **77,** 6134.

Moretta, A., Colombatti, M., and Chapius, B. (1981). Human spleen as a source of T cell growth factor. *Clin. Exp. Immunol.* **44,** 262.

Morgan, D. A., Ruscetti, F. W., and Gallo, R. C. (1976). Selective *in vitro* growth of T lymphocytes from normal human bone marrows. *Science* **193,** 1007.

Northoff, H., and Oppenheim, J. J. (1979). The molecular basis of immune cell function. *In* (J. G. Kaplan, ed.), pp. 700–703. Elsevier/North Holland, New York.

Northoff, H., Hooks, J. J., Jordan, G., and Oppenheir, J. J. (1980). Direct correlation between the production of interleukin 2 (IL-2) and immune interferon (IF) by human mononuclear cells (MNL). *Behring Inst. Mitt.* **67,** 90.

Novogrodsky, A., Suthanthiran, M., Saltz, B., Newman, D., Rubin, A. L., and Stengel, K. H. (1980). Generation of a lymphocyte growth factor by treatment of human cells with neuraminidase and galactose oxidase. *J. Exp. Med.* **151,** 755.

Ortaldo, J. R., Timonen, T. T., Vose, B. M., and Alvarez, J. A. (1980). Human natural killer cells as well as T cells maintained in continuous culture with IL-2. *Behring Inst. Mitt.* **67,** 258.

Ortaldo, J. R., Timonen, T. T., Vose, B. M., and Alvarez, J. M. (1981). Human natural killer as well as T cells maintained in continuous culture with IL-2. *In* "The Potential Role of T Cell Subpopulations in Cancer Therapy" (A. Fefer, ed.). Raven, New York (in press).

Reiss, C. S., Hemler, M. F., Englehard, U. H., Mier, J. W., Strominger, J. L., and Burakoff, S. J. (1980). Development and characterization of allospecific long-term human cytolytic T cell lines. *Proc. Natl. Acad. Sci. U.S.A.* **77,** 5432.

Robb, R. J., and Smith, K. A. (1981). Heterogeneity of human T cell growth factor(s) due to variable glycosylation. *Mol. Immunol.* (in press).

Rogentine, G. N., Jr., and Gerber, P. (1969). HLA antigens of human lymphoid cells in long term tissue culture. *Transplantation* **8,** 28.

Rosenberg, S. A., Schwartz, S., and Spiess, P. J. (1978). *In vitro* growth of murine T cells. II. Growth of *in vitro* sensitized cells cytotoxic for alloantigens. *J. Immunol.* **121,** 1951.

Ruscetti, F. W., and Gallo, R. C. (1980). Production of T cell growth factor by cultured human T lymphocytes. *Behring Inst. Mitt.* **67,** 240.

Ruscetti, F. W., and Gallo, R. C. (1981). Human T lymphocyte growth factor: Regulation of growth and function of T lymphocytes. *Blood* **57,** 379.

Ruscetti, F. W., Morgan, D. A., and Gallo, R. C. (1977). Functional and morphologic characterization of human T cells continuously grown *in vitro*. *J. Immunol.* **119,** 131.

Ruscetti, F. W., Mier, J. W., and Gallo, R. C. (1980). Human T cell growth factor: Parameters for production. *J. Supramol. Struct.* **13,** 547.

Schendel, D. J., Wank, R., and Bonnard, G. D. (1980a). Genetic specificities of primary and secondary proliferative and cytotoxic responses of human lymphocytes grown in continued culture. *Scand. J. Immunol.* **11,** 99.

Schendel, D. J., Wank, R., and Bonnard, G. D. (1980b). Proliferative and cytotoxic human cultured

T cell lines specific for major histocompatibility complex (HLA) antigens. *Behring Inst. Mitt.* **67,** 252.

Solbach, W., Barth, S., Graubner, M., Rollinghoff, M., and Wagner, H. (1980). Sezary Syndrome: Evidence for malignant proliferation of T cells producing interleukin 2. *Behring Inst. Mitt.* **67,** 265.

Spits, H., deVries, J. E., and Terhorst, C. (1981). A permanent human cytotoxic T cell line with high killing capacity against a lymphoblastoid B-cell line shows preference for HLA A, B target antigens and lacks spontaneous cytotoxic activity. *Cell. Immunol.* **59,** 435.

Stadler, B. M., Farrar, J. J., and Oppenheim, J. J. (1980). Cell cycle dependent production of human interleukin 2. *Behring Inst. Mitt.* **67,** 245.

Strausser, J. L., and Rosenberg, S. A. (1978). *In vitro* growth of cytotoxic human lymphocytes. I. Growth of cells sensitized *in vitro* to alloantigens. *J. Immunol.* **121,** 1491.

Timonen, T. T., Ortaldo, J. R., Stadler, B. M., Bonnard, G. D., and Herberman, R. B. (1981). Cultures of purified human natural killer cells: Growth in the presence of interleukin 2. (Submitted for publication.)

Warren, H. S., and Pembrey, R. G. (1981). A method for the production and quantitative assay of human lymphokine preparations. *J. Immunol. Methods* **41,** 9.

Zarling, J. M., and Bach, F. H. (1979). Continuous culture of T cells cytotoxic for autologous human leukemia cells. *Nature (London)* **280,** 685.

6

Signal Requirement For T Lymphocyte Activation

Jacques M. Chiller/Elaine C. DeFreitas/
Robert W. Chesnut/Howard M. Grey/Barry J. Skidmore

I. T Lymphocyte Propagation 83
II. T Lymphocyte Activation 86
References 89

Immune function is mediated by a web of interacting cells and molecules responding, on one hand, to external stimuli and regulated, on the other hand, by internal signals and pathways. This chapter will analyze one of these processes, namely, antigen-induced, accessory cell-dependent T cell activation.

I. T LYMPHOCYTE PROPAGATION

Antigen- or mitogen-induced T cell proliferation has provided our best experimental systems by which to study accessory cell–lymphocyte interaction. A set of general conclusions emanating from a large number of studies of antigen-induced T cell proliferation can be summarized as follows: Antigen-dependent T cell activation requires accessory cells (Ia^+ macrophages) whose function is essential as antigen-presenting cells (Seeger and Oppenheim, 1970; Rosenthal and Shevach, 1973; Thomas and Shevach, 1977; Yano *et al.,* 1978; Schwartz and Paul, 1976; Cowings *et al.,* 1978; Farr *et al.,* 1979; Kammer and Unanue, 1980). Furthermore, there is a requirement for compatibility at the *I* region of the MHC between the interacting sets of cells, a conclusion which is also applicable to other interactions involving lymphocytes, for example, T-B collaboration (Kindred and Schreffler, 1972; Katz *et al.,* 1973), cytotoxic T cell–target interactions (Zinkernagel and Doherty, 1974), and T cell activity leading to delayed-type hypersensitivity (DTH) (Vadas *et al.,* 1977). In essence, it appears that most T lymphocytes must recognize specific antigen in the context of self

ISBN 0-12-249920-4

molecules coded by regions of the MHC, either I in the case of T cell proliferation, T-B collaboration and DTH, or K or D in the case of cytotoxic T cells. Suppressor cells may be an example of one T cell subpopulation that may be an exception to this rule (Ishizaka and Adachi, 1976; Feldmann and Kontiainen, 1976; Pierres and Germain, 1978), although it is still not well established whether it is the activation of these cells or their mode of action which reflects lack of restriction.

Recent experiments have provided further understanding of the mechanisms by which accessory cell-dependent T cell activation occurs. Although the process of T cell proliferation per se requires a cell growth factor, recently termed interleukin-2 (IL-2) (Morgan *et al.*, 1976; Gillis and Smith, 1977), such factors do not induce growth in resting T cells (Coutinho *et al.*, 1979). However, the latter can be rendered sensitive to IL-2 by a short pulse of specific ligands in the form of either mitogens (Larsson and Coutinho, 1979) or antigen (Schrier *et al.*, 1979), a process which apparently leads to T cell activation and the expression of putative receptors for IL-2 (Larsson *et al.*, 1980). Our own efforts have focused on defining those elements which are necessary to render T cells sensitive to IL-2 (DeFreitas *et al.*, 1981). The conclusions from studies to be detailed in this chapter are that the process requires macrophage–T cell *H-2* restricted cooperation which can be divided into two signals, namely, the recognition by T cells of antigen/Ia presented by accessory cells (signal 1) and the action on T cells of a macrophage product in the form of lymphocyte-activating factor (signal 2), more recently termed interleukin-1 (IL-1). IL-1 was described some years ago as a monokine which augments proliferative response to lectins (Gery *et al.*, 1972; Lachmann *et al.*, 1977), promotes T cell-dependent *in vitro* antibody responses (Koopman *et al.*, 1977), and enhances the development of cytotoxic T cells (Farrar *et al.*, 1980).

A major factor which has hampered the progress and interpretation of studies relating to lymphocyte activation and regulation has been the fact that the cellular components of the immune system are extremely heterogeneous, not only from the standpoint of distinct populations of functional cells but also from the perspective of the clonal spectrum within each subpopulation. Recent developments in a number of laboratories have provided the potential means by which to overcome this problem in the capacity to obtain lines of enriched or clonally derived specific T cells (Nabholz *et al.*, 1978; Fathman and Hengartner, 1978; Baker *et al.*, 1979; Bach *et al.*, 1979; von Boehmer *et al.*, 1979; Schreier and Tees, 1980; Hengartner and Fathman, 1980; Lotze *et al.*, 1980; Sredni *et al.*, 1981; Chiller *et al.*, 1981). Derivation of T cell hybridoma lines whose induction is antigen-specific and MHC-restricted (Kappler *et al.*, 1981) provides an additional experimental tour de force in that specific activation can be quickly and readily monitored. Coupled to the availability of lines of cells which produce quantities of cytokines, such as IL-1 (Mizel *et al.*, 1978) or IL-2 (Harwell *et al.*,

1980), conditions now exist which permit a more precise analysis of specific T lymphocyte activation/recognition.

We have previously described methodologies by which to enrich and propagate antigen-specific murine T lymphocytes which possess specific function. A brief description of such procedures is as follows: Mice are primed subcutaneously at the base of the tail with 50 to 100 μg of antigen emulsified in complete Freund's adjuvant (CFA), and 7 days later the paraaortic and inguinal lymph nodes are harvested (Corradin *et al.*, 1977). These lymph node cells are cultured at 4×10^6/ml in Click's medium containing 0.5% to 1.0% fresh syngeneic normal mouse serum and 10 to 100μg/ml of antigen (Schrier *et al.*, 1979). After 4 days of culture, the live cells are recovered on Ficoll–Hypaque gradients and cultured for an additional 3–4 days in RPMI medium supplemented with 5% fetal calf serum (FCS) and IL-2 obtained either from a concanavalin A (Con-A)-induced T cell hybridoma (Harwell *et al.*, 1980) or as the supernatant fluid (SUP) from normal mouse spleen cells incubated with a mitogenic concentration of Con-A for 24 hr, then supplemented with α-methyl mannoside to neutralize residual Con-A. This procedure yields a population of cells with the following physical and functional characteristics.

1. The cells are > 99% *Thy-1*$^+$, *Lyt-1*$^+$, *Lyt-2,3*$^-$.
2. They proliferate *in vitro* in response to challenge with specific antigen in the presence of *I* region-compatible macrophages.
3. They function as specific helper cells for hapten-primed histocompatible B cells in a modified *in vitro* Mishell-Dutton system.
4. Such proliferative and helper activities are profoundly (> 100-fold) enriched as a consequence of *in vitro* propagation when compared to cells tested directly from primed animals.

Using this methodology, cells specific for the following antigens have been cultured: OVA, HGG, KLH, beef apocytochrome *c*, (T,G)-A--L, and Sendai virus. The methods can be applied to obtain not only short-term propagated T lymphocytes, but, in addition, T cells which can be maintained for prolonged periods (up to 12 months). Further, the technology can be extended to obtain clonally derived lines of antigen-specific, functional T cells in the following fashion. Propagated lines, which after 5–8 weeks in culture show proper specificity and restriction, are utilized for cloning by seeding into wells of microtiter plates 100 μl of a suspension containing 5×10^5 accessory cells and an appropriate concentration of IL-2. Each well is then supplemented with 100 μl of a suspension containing IL-2 and propagated T cells (averaging less than 1 cell/well). Plates are incubated for 1 week at 37°C, 2% CO_2, after which time 100 μl of the supernatant fluid is removed and replaced with 100 μl of fresh medium–IL-2 solution. Positive growth usually becomes evident by 10 to 14 days. Next 100 to 150 μl of the content of the positive wells are tranferred to larger vessels

(Costar plates) with a 1-ml suspension containing fresh IL-2, antigen, and accessory cells (5×10^6). Growth is then followed and cultures are further expanded to flasks under the same conditions.

II. T LYMPHOCYTE ACTIVATION

Thus T cells from lymph nodes of immunized animals, after activation *in vitro* with antigen, can be propagated in the following conditions: (1) with specific antigen and a source of irradiated syngeneic accessory cells, (2) in the absence of antigen and accessory cells but in the presence of a source of IL-2, or (3) using the combination of both approaches. Such cells can be maintained in culture for prolonged periods of time and show enriched function, defined either by the capacity to proliferate specifically to antigen in the context of *H-2* (Ia)-restricted accessory cells or by the ability to provide carrier-specific T help in the response of hapten-primed B cells of haptenated carrier proteins. Those T lymphocytes propagated in a source of IL-2 without either antigen or accessory cells provide an exquisite means by which to study accessory cell-dependent antigen stimulation since, when such cells are removed from the IL-2 source, they will continue to proliferate only when supplemented with specific antigen and syngeneic spleen or LN accessory cells which can be defined as plastic-adherent, Ig^-, $Thy\ 1^-$, esterase-staining, and 50% to 60% Ia^+. Thus, the technique of *in vitro* enrichment and propagation of such T lymphocytes provides not only a source of cells whose activation obeys requirements similar to those previously described by others using cells from immune tissues, but, in addition, populations which can be markedly enriched for specific activity, even cloned so as to permit analysis of the activation of small numbers of cells.

In experiments aimed at delineating the requirement for the specific activation of propagated T lymphocytes, it was observed that whereas antigen and either nontreated or γ-irradiated accessory cells supported T cell proliferation, antigen and uv-irradiated cells did not. These data are compatible with previous observations by others that uv is capable of incapacitating antigen presenting function (Lafferty and Woolnough, 1977; Letvin *et al.*, 1980). Further, the same relationship held when accessory cells were pulsed with antigen prior to treatment with either γ or uv irradiation. However, antigen-pulsed, uv-irradiated accessory cells were capable of stimulating T cells when supplemented with a source of IL-1, usually obtained as the supernatant fluid from a murine macrophage line, $p388D_1$ (Table I). It should be stressed that the T cells used in these experiments were those which were propagated in IL-2 to a point when further growth on IL-2 alone did not occur. Such cells could only be restimulated with antigen-pulsed accessory cells. Additional relevant observations in this system were that (1) IL-1 alone failed to stimulate, (2) stimulation was dependent on specific antigen, and

TABLE I

Activation of Propagated T Cells[a]

Accessory Cell Treatment	Response (cpm ± SEM × 10^{-3})
None	0.2 (0.1)
OVA	37.6 (6.8)
OVA-pulsed, γ-irradiated (4000 rads)	24.7 (3.8)
OVA-pulsed, uv-irradiated	0.7 (0.3)
OVA-pulsed, uv-irradiated + Con-A SUP	17.6 (1.9)
Con-A SUP alone	2.6 (1.1)
OVA-pulsed, uv-irradiated + IL-1	11.3 (1.9)
HGG-pulsed, uv-irradiated + IL-1	0.7 (0.4)
IL-1 alone	0.4 (0.1)

[a] Lymph node cells obtained from BDF_1 mice, primed at the base of tail 7 days previously with OVA in CFA, were cultured with OVA for 4 days. Following Ficoll separation, viable cells were re-seeded with antigen and syngeneic irradiated (4000 rads) cells for another 4 days, at which time Ficoll separated cells were cultured in the *absence* of antigen and accessory cells, but in the presence of a source of IL-2 (designated as Con-A SUP and representing supernatant fluids obtained following a 24-hr incubation of BDE, spleen cells, and Con-A, then supplemented with α-methyl mannoside). Such cells were propagated for 7–11 days to a stage where they no longer grew in IL-2 alone. Then 10^4 cells were seeded in microtiter wells with accessory cells (splenic adherent cells) and treated in the conditions described in the table. The source of IL-1 was treated supernatant fluid from the murine macrophage line $p388D_1$, utilized at a final concentration of 20%. Irradiation consisted of exposure to 4000 rads (γ) or 5 min, 20 cm from a 30 W germicidal lamp (uv). Cells were incubated for 3 days, pulsed 24 hr with ^{3}H-TdR, harvested, and uptake of label quantified by scintillation counting.

(3) the source of antigen-pulsed uv accessory cells needed to be homologous with the T lymphocytes, restriction mapping to the *Ia* region of the MHC (Table II). Further, fractionation of the IL-1 source revealed that the activity resided primarily within a peak having a molecular weight of 14,000–16,000, a size compatible with that previously described for murine IL-1. Finally, it should be stressed that uv irradiation does not have a direct effect on the activity of preformed IL-1. This is supported by the fact that (a) the induction of IL-1 by LPS in peritoneal cells is markedly reduced when the cells are treated with uv prior to, but not after, mitogen, (b) uv treatment of the macrophage line $p388D_1$, a constitutive producer of IL-1, actually increases the amount of activity recoverable from supernatant fluids, and (c) uv treatment of fluids containing IL-1 has no effect on IL-1 activity.

In order to place the observations dealing with the requirements for T cell activation in some coordinated perspective, the following hypothetical scheme is offered as a basis underlying the process of antigen-triggered T cell activation. T lymphocytes, more specifically T cells functionally tested for help or for proliferation, require two obligatory signals for activation: the recognition on mac-

TABLE II

Restriction of Stimulation of Propagated T Cells Using OVA-Pulsed, uv-Treated Filler Cells and IL-1[a]

uv-Treated accessory cells	Response (cmp ± SE × 10^{-3})	
	−IL-1	+IL-1
B10.A	1.2 (0.6)	12.3 (0.1)
B10	0.5 (0.1)	0.2 (0.1)
B10.A (4R)	1.8 (1.0)	21.6 (2.3)
B10.A (5R)	1.0 (0.3)	5.4 (0.7)
B10.TL	2.6 (1.0)	24.9 (3.4)
B10.S (7R)	0.1 (0.1)	0.3 (0.1)
None	0.1 (0.1)	0.2 (0.1)

[a] The methods are similar to those described in Table I, with the exception that T cells specific to OVA were obtained from B10.A-primed mice. The data shown represent those derived when 10^4 propagated B10.A T cells were incubated with IL-1 (p388D_1-derived; 25% final concentration) and accessory cells (normal spleen cells) from the sources listed. Such cells were pulsed with OVA (1 mg/ml) for 3 hr, then washed and irradiated with uv light.

rophages of antigen presented in the context of self Ia (signal 1) and the binding of IL-1 (signal 2), itself produced by macrophages as a consequence of back stimulation by T cells. Signal 1 also leads to the expression of IL-1 acceptor sites on T cells. Unless signal 2 (IL-1) is available to signal 1-induced T cells (expressing IL-1 acceptor sites), such cells will not become activated but may become specifically anergic. The sum total of signal 1–signal 2 results in T cell activation, i.e., differentiation to a stage where IL-2 acceptor sites are expressed. In the presence of IL-2, T cell proliferation and amplification proceed. In the absence of IL-2, activated cells revert to a "resting" stage, and subsequent triggering once again requires the same sequence of signals. Thus three stages can be envisioned in the process of T cell proliferation, namely, induction, requiring the interaction with antigen-self and leading, on one hand, to the expression of IL-1 acceptor sites on T cells and, on the other hand, to back stimulation of the interacting macrophages; activation, requiring the interaction with IL-1 and leading to the expression of IL-2 acceptor sites; and proliferation, requiring the interaction with IL-2 and leading to cell replication. Of significant interest is the question of whether signal 1 in the absence of signal 2 may, as implied here and originally predicted by Bretcher and Cohn (1970), lead to tolerance. Although formal proof for this possibility is not yet available, preliminary data demonstrating that exposure of T cells to antigen Ia in the absence of IL-1 can lead to specific anergy (Skidmore *et al.*, 1981) are certainly compatible with that notion.

ACKNOWLEDGMENTS

This is publication No. 2583 from the Department of Immunopathology, Scripps Clinic and Research Foundation, LaJolla, California. This research was supported by USPHS Grants AI-13131 and CA-21825. Barry J. Skidmore is supported by NIH Young Investigator Award AI-16573.

REFERENCES

Bach, F. H., Inouye, H., Hank, J. A., and Alter, B. J. (1979). Human T lymphocyte clones reactive in primed lymphocyte typing and cytotoxicity. *Nature (London)* **281,** 307.

Baker, P. E., Gillis, S., and Smith, K. (1979). Monoclonal cytolytic T-cell lines. *J. Exp. Med.* **149,** 273.

Bretcher, P. A., and Cohn, M. (1970). A theory of self-nonself discrimination. *Science* **169,** 1042.

Chiller, J. M., Julius, M. H., and Sidman, C. L. (1981). MHC-restricted cellular interaction determining B cell activation. (In preparation.)

Corradin, G., Etlinger, H. M., and Chiller, J. M. (1977). Lymphocyte specificity to protein antigens. I. Characterization of the antigen-induced *in vitro* T cell-dependent proliferative response with lymph node cells from primed mice. *J. Immunol.* **119,** 1048.

Coutinho, A., Larsson, E. L., Gronvik, K. O., and Andersson, J. (1979). Studies on T lymphocyte activation. II. The target cells for concanavalin A-induced growth factors. *Eur. J. Immunol.* **9,** 587.

Cowings, C., Pincus, S. H., Sachs, D., II., and Dickler, H. B. (1978). A subpopulation of adherent accessory cells bearing both I-A and I-E or C sub-region antigens is required for antigen-specific murine T lymphocyte proliferation. *J. Immunol.* **121,** 1680.

DeFreitas, E. C., Chesnut, R. W., Grey, H. M., and Chiller, J. M. (1981). Macrophage activation of antigen specific T cells: separation into two phases. (Submitted for publication.)

Farr, A. G., Kiely, J. M.,and Unanue, E. R. (1979). Induction of cytocidal macrophages after *in vitro* interactions between *Listeria*-immune T cells and macrophages. *J. Immunol.* **122,** 2405.

Farrar, W. L., Mizel, S. B., and Farrar, J. J. (1980). Participation of lymphocyte activating factor (interleukin 1) in the induction of cytotoxic T cell responses. *J. Immunol.* **124,** 1371.

Fathman, C. G., and Hengartner, H. (1978). Clones of alloreactive T cells. *Nature (London)* **272,** 617.

Feldmann, M., and Kontiainen, S. (1976). Suppressor cell induction *in vitro*. *Eur. J. Immunol.* **6,** 302.

Gery, I., Gershon, R. K., and Waksman, B. H. (1972). Potentiation of the T-lymphocyte response to mitogens. I. The responding cell. *J. Exp. Med.* **136,** 128.

Gillis, S., and Smith, D. A. (1977). Long term culture of tumor-specific cytotoxic T cells. *Nature (London)* **268,** 154.

Harwell, L., Skidmore, B., Marrack, P., and Kappler, J. (1980). Concanavalin A-inducible, interleukin-2-producing T cell hybridoma. *J. Exp. Med.* **152,** 893.

Hengartner, H., and Fathman, C. G. (1980). Clones of alloreactive T cells. I. A unique homozygous MLR-stimulating determinant present on B6 stimulators. *Immunogenetics* **10,** 175.

Ishizaka, K., and Adachi, T. (1976). Generation of specific helper cells and suppressor cells *in vitro* for the Ig E and Ig G antibody responses. *J. Immunol.* **117,** 40.

Kammer, G. M., and Unanue, E. R. (1980). Accessory cell requirement in the proliferative response of T lymphocytes to hemocyanin. *Clin. Immunol. Immunopathol.* **15,** 434.

Kappler, J. W., Skidmore, B. J., White, J., and Marrack, P. (1981). Antigen-inducible, H-2-restricted, interleukin-2-producing T cell hybridomas. *J. Exp. Med.* **153,** 1198.

Katz, D. H., Hamaoka, T., and Benacerraf, B. (1973). Cell interactions between histoincompatible T and B lymphocytes. II. Failure of physiologic cooperative interactions between T and B lymphocytes from allogeneic donor strains in humoral response to hapten-protein conjugates. *J. Exp. Med.* **137,** 1405.

Kindred, B., and Shreffler, D. C. (1972). H-2 dependence of cooperation between T and B cells *in vivo*. *J. Immunol.* **109,** 940.

Koopman, W. J., Farrar, J. J., Oppenheim, J. J., Fuller-Bonar, J., and Dougherty, S. (1977). Association of a low molecular weight helper factor(s) with thymocyte proliferative activity. *J. Immunol.* **119,** 55.

Lachmann, L. B., Hacker, M. P., and Handschumaker, R. E. (1977). Partial purification of human lymphocyte-activating factor (LAF) by ultrafiltration and electrophoretic techniques. *J. Immunol.* **119,** 2019.

Lafferty, K. J., and Woolnough, J. A. (1977). The origin and mechanism of the allograft reaction. *Immunol. Rev.* **35,** 231.

Larsson, E. L., and Coutinho, A. (1979). The role of mitogenic lections in T-cell triggering. *Nature (London)* **280,** 239.

Larsson, E. L., Iscove, N. N., and Coutinho, A. (1980). A suggested mechanism for T lymphocyte activation: Implications of the acquisition of functional reactivities. *Immunol. Rev.* **51,** 61.

Letvin, N. L., Greene, M. I., Benacerraf, B., and Germain, R. N. (1980). Immunologic effects of whole-body ultraviolet irradiation: Selective defect in splenic adherent cell function *in vitro*. *Proc. Natl. Acad. Sci. U.S.A.* **77,** 2881.

Lotze, M. T., Strausser, J. L., and Rosenberg, S. A. (1980). *In vitro* growth of cytotoxic human lymphocytes. II. Use of T cell growth factor (TCGF) to clone human T cells. *J. Immunol.* **124,** 2972.

Mizel, S. B., Oppenheim, J. J., and Rosenstreich, D. L. (1978). Characterization of lymphocyte-activating factor (LAF) produced by the macrophage cell line, P388D. I. Enhancement of LAF production by activated T lymphocytes. *J. Immunol.* **120,** 1497.

Morgan, D. A., Ruscetti, F. W., and Gallo, G. (1976). Selective *in vitro* growth of T lymphocytes from normal human bone marrows. *Science* **193,** 1007.

Nabholz, M., Engers, H. D., Collaro, D., and North, M. (1978). Cloned T-cell lines with specific cytolytic activity. *Curr. Top. Microbiol. Immunol.* **81,** 176.

Pierres, M., and Germain, R. N. (1978). Antigen-specific T cell-mediated suppression. IV. Role of macrophages in generation of L-glutamic acid-L-alanine-L-tyrosine (GAT)-specific suppressor T cells in responder mouse strains. *J. Immunol.* **121,** 1306.

Rosenthal, A., and Shevach, E. (1973). Function of macrophages in antigen recognition by guinea pig T lymphocytes. *J. Exp. Med.* **138,** 1194.

Schreier, M. H., and Tees, R. (1980). Clonal induction of helper T cells: Conversion of specific signals into nonspecific signals. *Int. Arch. Allergy Appl. Immunol.* **61,** 227.

Schrier, R. A., Skidmore, B. J., Kurnick, J. T., Goldstine, S. N., and Chiller, J. M. (1979). Propagation of antigen-specific T cell helper function *in vitro*. *J. Immunol.* **123,** 2525.

Schwartz, R. H., and Paul, W. E. (1976). T-lymphocyte enriched murine peritoneal exudate cells. II. Genetic control of antigen-induced T-lymphocyte proliferation. *J. Exp. Med.* **143,** 529.

Seeger, R. C., and Oppenheim, J. J. (1970). Synergistic interaction of macrophages and lymphocytes in antigen-induced transformation of lymphocytes. *J. Exp. Med.* **132,** 44.

Skidmore, B. J., White, J., DeFreitas, E. C., Kappler, J., Marrack, P., and Chiller, J. M. (1981). Exposing T cells *in vitro* to antigen-pulsed ultraviolet light treated macrophages induced specific unresponsiveness. *Fed. Proc. Fed. Am. Soc. Exp. Biol.* **40,** 1060.

Sredni, B., Tse, H. Y., Chen, C., and Schwartz, R. H. (1981). Antigen-specific clones of proliferating T lymphocytes. I. Methodology, specificity, and MHC restriction. *J. Immunol.* **126,** 341.

Thomas, D. W., and Shevach, E. M. (1977). Nature of the antigenic complex recognized by T lymphocytes: Specific sensitization by antigens associated with allogeneic macrophages. *Proc. Natl. Acad. Sci. U.S.A.* **74,** 2104.

Vadas, M. A., Miller, J. F. A. P., Whitelaw, A., and Gamble, J. (1977). Regulation by the *H-2* gene complex of delayed type hypersensitivity. *Immunogenetics* **4,** 137.

von Boehmer, H., Hengartner, H., Nabholz, M., Lenhardt, W., Schreier, M. H., and Haas, W. (1979). Fine specificity of a continuously growing killer cell clone for H-Y antigen. *Eur. J. Immunol.* **9,** 592.

Yano, A., Schwartz, R. H., and Paul, W. E. (1978). Antigen presentation in the murine T lymphocyte proliferative response. II. Ir-GAT-controlled T lymphocyte responses require antigen presenting cells from a high responder donor. *Eur. J. Immunol.* **8,** 344.

Zinkernagel, R. M., and Doherty, P. C. (1974). Immunological surveillance against altered self components by sensitized T lymphocytes in lymphocytic choriomeningitis. *Nature (London)* **251,** 547.

II

T Cell Hybridomas and Their Products

7

An Overview

Tomio Tada/Makoto Nonaka

I.	A Catalog	97
II.	Problems	99
III.	Lessons	101
	A. What Did We Learn About the Antigen-Binding Structure of T Cells?	102
	B. Are There New *I* Region Loci Expressed Exclusively on T Cells?	103
IV.	Conclusions	105
	References	105

The success of making hybridomas secreting monoclonal antibodies by somatic hybridization between normal B cells and nonsecreter myeloma cell lines (Köhler and Milstein, 1975) resulted in an unprecedented fruitful age of immunology. Dr. Yoshio Okada, who first described the cell fusion phenomenon with Sendai virus (Okada *et al.*, 1957), mentioned to us that this phenomenon has been most wisely applied in immunology to achieve an unpredicted success. The method is now being widely used to produce extremely specific reagents which have unlimited potentials in immunological research.

The same principle has been applied to make T cell hybrids with specific functions that are borne by parental T cells. One of the most important applications in this regard is the analysis of antigen recognition units of T cells (i.e., the T cell receptor). This has been pursued by two different approaches using normal T cells, i.e., the analysis of isolated antigen-binding molecules (reviewed by Rajewsky and Eichmann, 1977; Binz and Wigzell, 1977) and the characterization of antigen-specific T cell factors (reviewed by Tada and Okumura, 1979). Biochemical studies suggesting the presence of membrane-bound Ig-like molecules on T cells also have been reported (Marchalonis and Warr, 1979). Unfortunately, the definitive answer to the T cell receptor question has not been provided up to the present time. This is due in large part to the difficulty in obtaining antigen-specific materials from heterogenous populations of T cells in an amount sufficient for biochemical analyses. Thus, the technique of cell fusion

ISBN 0-12-249920-4

was quickly introduced to the study of T cell antigen receptors with the expectation of obtaining T cell hybrids that secrete homogeneous materials with antigen-binding abilities. Since there exist reagents capable of detecting the expression of immunoglobulin variable region idiotypes, it should be possible to analyze the receptor sites on T cell hybrids with much greater accuracy and resolution than on mixtures of conventional T cells. Furthermore, analysis of the constant structure of the T cell receptor molecule(s) may be greatly facilitated by the use of T cell hybrids.

Another meaningful application of hybridization of T cells is the analysis of the origin of the genetic restrictions in cell interactions. It has been well established that T cells recognize antigen in "association" with self cell surface components (e.g., H-2 and Ia antigens). Some of the T cell factors also show MHC or Ig allotype restricted effects in the regulation of immune responses. It is predictable that hybrid T cells exhibiting antigen restricted recognition should allow us to analyze this problem with much greater accuracy than using heterogeneous T cells.

The third important use of T cell hybrids is the study of T lymphocyte physiology. Many of the hybrids secrete biologically active substances such as IL-2 (and other T cell factors) without external stimulus, while in other cases, such activities are inducible by stimulation. Receptors and transmembrane signals can be studied with such inducible hybrids to define the mechanisms and genetic requirements for a particular T cell activation.

One further problem, which we will discuss later, is the nature of *I* region determinants expressed on T cells. Although some reports indicate that T cells, especially blastoid T cells, express Ia antigens indistinguishable from those of B cells, the existence of unique *I* region-encoded determinants on functional subsets of T cells has also been reported (Murphy *et al.*, 1976; Okumura *et al.*, 1976; Tada *et al.*, 1976; Hayes and Bach, 1978, 1979; Tokuhisa *et al.*, 1978; Rich *et al.*, 1979). The nature of such determinants, associated with certain functions of T cells, is still unknown. It has been suggested that these T cell-specific *I* region determinants are probably distinct from class II antigens composed of α and β chains. T cell hybrids with suppressor or helper functions associated with *I* region expression provide a unique opportunity to examine the genetics and biochemical structure of such unknown *I* region products.

For these reasons, the T cell fusion technique has been introduced to make functional T cell hybrids. Although the results are not yet as fruitful as the results have been in B cell fusions, important information has been obtained during the past few years. Since many of the achievements are described by individual authors in this volume, in this chapter we shall discuss some of the problems in studying T cell hybrids, with emphasis on examining the antigen-binding structure and *I* region determinants on antigen-specific T cell hybrids.

I. A CATALOG

Early reports on T cell hybrids made by fusion between unselected T cells and an enzyme-deficient mutant cell line of a thymoma (BW5147) of AKR origin established that the same cell hybridization method used in B cell fusion was applicable to T cells. Despite the fact that these cell lines were made with T cells from allotype-suppressed or antigen-primed mice, their stability and functional characteristics were not fully described (Goldsby *et al.*, 1977; Hämmerling, 1977). Taniguchi and Miller (1978) reported the first successful fusion between selected functional T cells and a mutant EL-4 of C57BL/6 origin. They used two advantageous procedures: (1) selection of antigen-binding T cells from spleen cells of CBA mice tolerized to human γ-globulin (HGG) by adsorption to and elution from HGG-coated plastic dishes, and (2) sorting of functional hybrids by fluorescence-activated cell sorting (FACS) after staining with antibodies against products of the *I-J* subregion of the murine major histocompatibility complex (MHC). The principle of these procedures has been adopted by others in later fusion experiments.

Although they were successful in producing several clones with expression of products encoded within the *I-J* subregion, associated with antigen-specific and nonspecific suppressor functions, many of the clones quickly lost such properties probably due to chromosomal loss. Such instability of T cell hybrids has been repeatedly experienced by others and has forced investigators to reclone laboriously the cells in order to maintain activities. This is a limitation of T cell hybrids and constitutes a major obstacle in the biochemical analysis of T cell receptor molecules from such hybrids.

Kontiainen *et al.* (1978) and Taniguchi *et al.* (1979) were successful in making more stable suppressor hybridomas by fusion between keyhole limpet hemocyanin (KLH)-specific suppressor T cells and Bw5147. Of special interest is that such hybridomas secrete a molecule with antigen-specific suppressor function (TsF) carrying an apparent antigen-binding site and determinants controlled by genes in *I-J* subregion. The products of hybrids made by Taniguchi *et al.* (1979) show a rigid genetic restriction in which TsF can suppress the responses only of syngeneic and semisyngeneic animals. It is probable that TsF from these hybridomas activates comparable cellular consequences to those induced by normal suppressor T cells, by selecting the specific T cells as their targets (Taniguchi and Tokuhisa, 1980). These findings are of interest in the context of the structure of antigen-specific T cell factors as will be discussed below.

Similar types of antigen-specific suppressor hybridomas have been reported by several other investigators (Ruddle *et al.*, 1980; Kapp *et al.*, 1980; Okuda *et al.*, 1981), some of which will be reviewed in this treatise. A somewhat different

TABLE I

A Catalog of Some Selected T Cell Hybrids[a]

Hybrid Cell Line	Parental T Cell	Comments	Reference
Allotype-specific Ts?	Allotype suppressed	No further characterization	Goldsby *et al*. (1977)
Functions unknown	NP-CGG-primed	No further characterization	Hämmerling (1977)
Antigen-specific Ts	KLH-primed	Ia^+, suppresses primary IgM antibody response	Kontiainen *et al*. (1978)
Antigen-specific Ts	HGG tolerant	$I\text{-}J^+$, unstable, suppresses IgG antibody response	Taniguchi and Miller (1978)
Antigen-specific Ts	SRBC-primed	Ia^+ (not I-J or I-A), directly suppresses B cells	Taussig and Holliman (1979)
Antigen-nonspecific Ts	DNP-Tbc-primed	Suppresses IgE antibody response	Watanabe *et al*. (1978)
Delayed type Ts	SRBC-primed	Ia^+, suppresses footpad reaction	Hewitt and Liew (1979)
Antigen-specific Ts	KLH-primed	$I\text{-}J^+$, VH^+, suppresses IgG response antibody	Taniguchi *et al*. (1979)
Antigen-nonspecific Ts	KLH-primed	$I\text{-}J^+$, nonspecifically suppresses antibody response	Taniguchi *et al*. (1979)
Antigen-specific Th	(T,G)-A--L-primed	$I\text{-}A^+$, VH^+, helps B cell response	Eshhar *et al*. (1980)
Antigen-specific Ts	GAT or GT-primed nonresponder	$I\text{-}J^+$, id^+, suppresses antibody and proliferative responses	Kapp *et al*. (1980)
Alloreactive T cell	Allostimulated	Produces AEF	Katz *et al*. (1980)
Antigen-specific Ts	ABA-primed	Suppresses antibody response	Ruddle *et al*. (1980)
Antigen-specific Ta	KLH-primed (A/J)	$I\text{-}A^+$, VH^+, augments helper T cell	Hiramatsu *et al*. (1981)
Antigen and H-2 reactive T cell	TNP-HGG-primed	Produces IL-2 by antigen plus *H-2*	Kappler *et al*. (1981)
Antigen-specific Ts	Pc-Tbc-primed	Ia^+, id^+, suppresses IgE antibody response	Kishimoto *et al*. (1981)
Antigen-specific Ts	NP-primed	$I\text{-}J^+$, id^+, suppresses antibody response	Kontiainen *et al*. (1981)
Antigen-specific Th	NP-CGG-primed	$I\text{-}A^+$, VH^+, *H-2* restricted, helps B cell response	Lonai *et al*. (1981)
Antigen-specific Ts	NP-primed	$I\text{-}J^+$, id^+, induces Ts_2 to suppress antibody response	Okuda *et al*. (1981)
Idiotype-specific Ts	NP-primed	$I\text{-}J^+$, anti-idiotypic	Minami *et al*. (1981)
Antigen-specific Ts	NP-primed	$I\text{-}J^+$, id^+, VH^+, produces heteroclitic suppressor factor	Suzuki (unpublished) cited in Tada *et al*. (1981)

[a] Abbreviations: Ts, suppressor T cell; NP, 4-hydroxy-3-nitrophenyl acetyl; CGG, chicken γ-globulin; KLH, keyhole limpet hemocyanin; HCG, human γ-globulin; SRBC, sheep red blood cells; DNP, 2,4-dinitrophenyl; Tbc, killed-tubercule bacillus; Th, helper T cell; (T,G)-A--L, poly(L-tyrosine, L-glutamic acid)-poly(DL-alanine)--poly(L-lysine) GAT, L-glutamic acid-L-alanine-L-tyrosine; id, idiotype; AEF, allogeneic effect factor; Ta, augmenting T cell; TNP, 2,4,6-trinitrophenyl; IL-2, interleukin-2; Pc, phosphorylcholine.

suppressor hybridoma was reported by Taussig and Holliman (1979). Their hybridoma A1 was made by fusion between sheep red blood cell (SRBC)-primed splenic T cells and BW5147. The culture supernatant contained a factor specifically suppressing the SRBC antibody response without *H-2* restriction. The factor also contained determinants controlled by the *H-2* complex, but the subregion controlling this determinant was not *I-J*. The molecular weight of the factor was much larger than those of others, and the direct target was determined to be B cells, unlike other suppressor factors which had been characterized previously. Hewitt and Liew (1979) also obtained clones which produce a suppressor factor for delayed type hypersensitivity. Some comparison can be made in Table I.

There are reports of the establishment of helper T cell hybrids (Eshhar *et al.*, 1980; Lonai *et al.*, 1981). These hybrids produce antigen-specific factors which can replace helper T cells (ThF). One interesting observation made by Lonai *et al.* (1981) is that the hybridoma cell can bind antigen only in the presence of macrophage-derived Ia molecules (reviewed in Chapter 8 by Lonal *et al.* this treatise). This suggests that their helper factor has a structure which recognizes self Ia antigen.

Another type of antigen-specific T cell hybrid is one which produces an augmenting T cell factor (TaF). Hiramatsu *et al.* (1981) recently obtained hybrid clones by hybridization of KLH-binding T cells of A/J mice with BW5147. A/J is known to be a nonproducer of KLH-specific TsF, and accordingly KLH-binding T cells obtained from A/J spleen cells were augmenting T cells. The materials extracted from these hybrids had KLH-specific augmenting activity, which was associated with *I* region determinants encoded in the *I-A* subregion, whereas this molecule was entirely different from conventional B cell Ia antigens (see below). TaF was not helper T cell-replacing, but augmented the antibody response only in the presence of KLH-specific helper T cells.

There are several other important fields in which T cell hybridomas serve as important tools to analyze antigen-nonspecific mediators and receptors. These include class-specific regulators (Kishimoto *et al.*, 1981; Watanabe *et al.*, 1978), antigen-nonspecific suppressor factor with or without Fc receptors, and interleukin-2, some of which have been extensively reviewed (in Lymphokine Report V, 1981).

II. PROBLEMS

The efficiency of cell fusion techniques between T cells and thymoma cells is probably comparable to that in making B cell hybridomas. BW5147 is a stable cell line, and we have had no problems with any of the HAT-sensitive sublines obtained from different sources. Many of the hybrids with BW5147 divide rapidly, and, therefore, one must be aware of the potential overgrowth of the cells.

One notorious problem with T cell hybrids is the instability of their chromosomes during long-term maintenance of cell lines. We have encountered a case in which the karyotype of a clone was heptaploid at first yet became nearly diploid within a week of cultivation (see Chapter 15 by Johnson *et al.*). Thus, we sometimes have to reclone the cells repeatedly within short intervals. At this time, it seems that it is only a matter of luck to obtain a very stable cell line. In addition, many of the procedures to select functional T cell clones are extremely tedious, since karyotype, function, and phenotypic expression have to be examined.

The only way to avoid this problem is to select a cell line which initially has stable function. Otherwise, one should keep aliquots of cells frozen at a time when they are fully functional and express cell surface products of interest. It is then easy to revive the frozen clone whenever the cultured cells lose any of the properties of interest. As an example, a freshly thawed clone from our stock of idiotype-bearing T cell hybrids usually expresses idiotype on about 70% of cells. By the seventh to eighth generation in semisynchronized culture, only 20% of the cells are idiotype positive. This creates a serious problem when we perform biochemical and functional studies, since a large number of homogeneous cells are required.

The expression of a certain phenotype appears to be dependent on the stage of cell cycle. The idiotype expression in our cell lines is maximal in M phase rather than G phase (G. Suzuki, unpublished). Ia expression is somewhat more stable, but increases also in M phase (M. Taniguchi, unpublished). As an extreme case, the expression of an idiotype was almost negligible 8 hr after its maximal expression in culture. It is thus suggested that one should harvest the cells at the appropriate time in cell cycle for biochemical and biological analyses. Although some cell lines are reported to be stable over a long period of time (Kapp *et al.*, 1980), this is not true for all T cell hybrids.

The third problem we have observed is the presence of a large amount of viral products both on hybrids and in culture supernates. BW5147 produces gp-70, p-30, and other virus-associated antigens. Since many of the alloantibodies contain appreciable anti-viral antibodies, it is difficult to define the surface phenotype of such hybrids. It is our own experience that after absorption with other virus-producing lymphomas, e.g., E♂G2, AKSL-2, and EL-4, some of the alloantisera often lose their reactivity to T cell hybrids. On the other hand, this type of absorption frequently diminishes the specific reactivity of alloantisera with low cytotoxic titers. This may be the major reason why none of us have been able to characterize unequivocally the biochemistry of antigen-specific T cell factors from hybridomas. Even after repeated purification over antigen and antibody columns, the purity of such material is not guaranteed.

We can expect several other unforeseen problems after hybridization. For example, Thy-1 antigens are often lost after long-term cultivation, which obscures the origin of parental partner cells. Several clones that we maintain in our laboratory have no Thy-1.2 antigen from parental normal T cells. Nevertheless, the clones preserve the original parental T cell functions. Another typical case is the loss of Lyt antigens. A number of hybrids do not have any Lyt antigens regardless of the functions known to be associated with Lyt phenotypes. Many of our suppressor hybrids have no Lyt-2 antigens, which argues that the Lyt-2 antigen itself is not directly involved in the antigen receptor of these T cells.

Kanno *et al.* (1981) have shown that neuraminidase treatment of T cell hybrids increases their sensitivity to the cytotoxic effects of alloantibodies and complement. This may be due to the fact that glycolipid is more abundant on tumor cell lines than normal counterparts.

Some peculiar gene activations have been reported after cell hybridization of T cells. Kontiainen *et al.* (1978) showed that one of their hybrids made by fusion between BW5147 and a CBA T cell expressed Lyt-1.2 antigen of AKR origin, which was not expressed in BW5147 before hybridization. They suggested that a gene from the CBA T cell activated the silent *Lyt-1.2* gene of BW5147 after cell fusion. Similarly, Kontiainen *et al.* (1981) reported that a product controlled by the $I\text{-}J^k$ allele was expressed on hybrids made by fusion between B10 ($H\text{-}2^b$) suppressor T cells and BW5147 ($H\text{-}2^k$), in which the silent $I\text{-}J^k$ allele seemed to be activated by an I-J^b positive partner cell after hybridization, even though such cells did not express the parental I-J^b product. These hybrids were 4-hydroxy-3-nitrophenyl acetyl (NP)-specific suppressor cell lines with idiotype expression linked to $Igh\text{-}1^b$. Since the allotype-linked idiotypic properties were unaltered, these investigators suggested that antigen-binding site and *I* region expression are separately controlled. If such epigenetic alterations are prevalent among T cell hybrids, we must be alert for many unexpected events.

On the contrary, the studies of Kappler and co-workers (see Chapter 9 by Marrack *et al.* in this treatise) demonstrated the solid association of antigen and restriction specificities after hybridization between two T cells having different antigen and Ia specificities. This latter example serves as an important clue for studying the antigen recognition unit of T cells with H-2 restriction. The problem, however, remains unsolved until biochemical probes become available.

III. LESSONS

Although we have heretofore discussed problems rather than advantages of T cell hybridomas in studying T cell receptors and regulatory molecules, we have gained some important knowledge from these hybrids during the past few years.

We shall discuss here some of the issues which have been extensively studied with T cell hybridomas in various laboratories.

A. What Did We Learn about the Antigen-Binding Structure of T Cells?

Antigen-binding molecules from T cell hybridomas have been studied with various reagents. It has been established that these molecules have identical antigen-binding properties to those obtained from normal antigen-specific T cells. With semipurified materials from T cell hybridomas, several investigators have demonstrated that antigen-binding structures react with antibodies directed at the framework structure of immunoglobulin heavy chain V region (anti-V_H) but not to those reactive with the light chain V region (anti-V_L) (Eshhar *et al.*, 1980; Tada *et al.*, 1980; Lonai *et al.*, 1981). We have tested two batches of anti-V_H independently prepared from M315 myeloma by Drs. D. Givol and H. Eisen, and both of these were equally effective in killing and staining two different T cell hybrids, a NP-specific, I-J^+ suppressor hybridoma, and a KLH-specific I-J^-, I-A^+ (see below) augmenting hybridoma. Thus, even though participation of V_L is not formally excluded, the antigen-binding structure on T cells has determinants in common with V_H framework determinants. Information obtained with regard to V_H-J gene rearrangement is reported by Hood and his collaborators in Chapter 39 by Krenenberg *et al.* in this treatise).

Several attempts have also been made to detect idiotypic determinants and their factors on T cell hybridomas. These include idiotypes associated with antibodies to the synthetic copolymer, glutaminic acid-alanine-tyrosine (GAT) by Kapp (see Chapter 11 by Kapp and Araneo in this treatise), phosphorylcholine (PC) by Kishimoto *et al.* (1981), and NP by Tada *et al.* (1981), Okuda *et al.* (1981), and Kontiainen *et al.* (1981). Since most of these idiotypes are heavy chain allotype-linked, it has been presumed that antigen receptors on T cell hybridomas are determined in part by V_H genes.

Noteworthy, is the NP^b idiotype on T cell hybrids. Our laboratory examined one interesting hybridoma with NP^b idiotype (7C3), and determined the following properties: (1) Binding of anti-idiotype of 7C3 was inhibited by 10-7 *M* 4-hydroxy-3-iodo-5-nitrophenyl acetyl (NIP), while 10-5 *M* NP was required for partial inhibition (heteroclicity). (2) The receptor material was photoaffinity labeled by [^{125}I]NIP-arylazide. (3) The suppressor factor derived from 7C3 could suppress the response by spleen cells of Igh^b compatible but *H-2* incompatible strains. The last observation indicates that the molecule might be involved in network type regulation. In addition, Dr. M. Cramer of the University of Cologne was able to isolate a receptor material with extremely high haptenated phage-neutralizing ability from 7C3 hybridoma by their hapten-coupled nylon mesh method. The material, with a molecular weight of 80,000, showed a definite heteroclicity in that two log scale higher molar concentrations of NP than NIP were required for 50% inhibition of haptenated phage inhibition (unpublished). Although biochemical studies are still in progress, these results compel us to conclude that T cells possess antigen-binding sites with essentially identical idiotypic properties to those of antibody molecules. More recently, Minami *et al.* (1981) reported the successful derivation of anti-idiotypic hybrid T cells that recognize NP^b idiotype.

Since all these T cell hybrids expressed idiotype, we were encouraged to attempt to separate and characterize the antigen-binding receptors of T cells (despite disimilar molecular size and antigenic determinants). Representative molecular weights of the antigen-binding polypeptides are 80,000 (Taussig *et al.*, 1979), 60,000 to 70,000 (Lonai *et al.*, Chapter 8 in this treatise), 24,000 (Kapp *et al.*, 1980), and 54,000 (Kishimoto *et al.*, 1981). Our own results indicated a MW of 27,000 for the hapten-binding moiety of an NP-specific suppressor hybridoma as determined by photoaffinity labeling (Y. Kumagai, unpublished) and 34,000 for KLH-specific augmenting T cell factor by external labeling (S. Miyatani, unpublished). Some investigators claim that these antigen-binding sites are associated with *I* region-encoded determinants together with idiotype on a single polypeptide chain, while others show an additional chain of MW 24,000–34,000 that is separately controlled by *I* region genes. Although we can expect some heterogeneity among antigen-binding molecules of T cells having different functions, the substantial differences listed above in molecular weight of such products do not allow us to deduce any meaningful prototypic structure of antigen-binding molecule of T cells. We have to await further biochemical analysis having better accuracy and resolution.

B. Are There New *I* Region Loci Expressed Exclusively on T Cells?

Many of the T cell hybrids express Ia antigen detected by conventional anti-Ia antisera. As the T cell factors produced from them also carry *I* region determinants, the question was raised as to whether the Ia antigens associated with T cell factors are the same as or different from known B cell Ia antigens.

The subregions which control Ia antigens on hybrids have certain characteristics depending on functions. Many of the suppressor hybridomas carry *I-J* subregion gene products, while the one reported by Taussig *et al.* (1979) has a product of a gene mapped to the right of *I-J*. The helper hybridoma reported by Lonai *et al.* (1981) express Ia determinants controlled by *I-A* and *I-E* subregions. We also reported a hybridoma augmenting the antibody response, which carried determinants coded for by an *I-A* subregion gene (Hiramatsu *et al.*, 1981).

Since *I-J* subregion genes are not expressed on B cells, it is presumed that Ia antigens on suppressor hybridomas are different from known B cell Ia antigens.

I. Takei (unpublished) made a survey on the heterogeneity of *I-J* subregion gene products on functionally different hybridomas. They have identified three distinct types of I-J$^+$ hybrids: KLH-specific suppressor hybridomas, antigen-nonspecific hybridomas, and nonfunctional ones (reviewed by Tada *et al.*, 1979). By adsorption of a conventional anti-I-J^b antiserum with antigen-specific or nonspecific hybrids and testing the residual cytotoxic activity against the other, they were able to show that at least two different molecules were expressed on these functionally different hybridomas. Neither of them were detectable on B cells. In addition, Taniguchi *et al.* (1981) showed that the *I-J* subregion gene product is covalently bound to the antigen-binding structure by a disulfide bond, a fact which is contradictory to the prototype of the conventional B cell Ia antigen.

Our laboratory has been concerned with the nature of Ia determinants on the augmenting T cell factor (TaF) from a hybrid with I-A^k expression (FL10) (Hiramatsu *et al.*, 1981). This factor differs from the helper factor, since TaF cannot replace helper T cell function but augments the antibody response only in the presence of helper T cells with the same carrier specificity to TaF. Hiramatsu *et al.* (1981) extensively absorbed the conventional anti-Ia (A.TH anti-A.TL) and anti-I-A^k [(B10.S(9R) × ATFR 5)F_1 anti-A.TL] antisera with B cells until no cytotoxic activity against *H-2^k* B cells were detected. The resultant antiserum was still capable of killing the TaF-producing hybridoma. Furthermore, two well-defined monoclonal anti-Ia antibodies directed against private (Ia.2) and public (Ia.17) specificities of the B cell Ia molecule did not react with the hybridoma. These results indicate that Ia antigens on T cell hybridomas are entirely different molecules from known class II MHC antigens.

Hiramatsu *et al.* (1982) further made monoclonal antibodies reactive with FL10 but not with B cells of *H-2^k* mice by hybridization between A.TH spleen cells from mice immunized with A.TL spleen and myeloma cells. *I-A* subregion specificities were confirmed by absorption studies using H-2 recombinant spleen cells. Regardless of their inability to kill *H-2^k* B cells including nu/nu spleen cells, these monoclonals were capable of killing FL10. In addition, many of these monoclonals were able to kill normal augmenting T cells and to absorb TaF produced by *H-2^k* mice. Some others showed a striking reactivity to normal helper T cells. Both B cells and macrophages were unable to absorb the antibody activity.

These results compel us to conclude that Ia antigens on functional T cell hybrids are distinct from known B cell Ia antigens (class II), regardless of subregion assignments, and that there are probably multiple loci within the *I* region that encode for a family of molecules on functionally different T cell subsets. Since the boundaries of *I-A, I-J,* and *I-E/C* subregions have been only arbitrarily assigned by the occurrence of recominant events which separate *Ia-1, Ia-4,* and *Ia-5* loci, the potential presence of multiple *I* region determinants exclusively expressed on T cells urges us to reconsider the organization and function of *I* region genes.

These results are reminiscent of the findings that certain T cell subsets and their factors have Ia antigens which differ from B cell Ia antigens (Hayes and Bach, 1978, 1979; Okumura *et al.*, 1976; Tokuhisa *et al.*, 1978). Since several monoclonal anti-I-J and anti-I-A antibodies are now available, some of the controversies on Ia antigenic structures associated with T cell factors will be resolved by these reagents.

IV. CONCLUSIONS

There is no doubt that T cell hybridomas still have great potential for understanding several outstanding issues in current immunology. On reflection, however, most of the findings are reminiscent of the results obtained with normal functional T cells. For instance, we thought that the problem of the T cell antigen receptor would be quickly solved when antigen-specific T cell hybridomas were produced. This is clearly not true. Although some important materials and clues have been provided, the application of T cell hybridomas is still only a starting point. There now exist the problems of the biochemistry and molecular genetics of T cell components, which may only be answered with well-defined T cell hybridomas. Studies on the regulation of cell interactions with T cell hybrids also may have great significance. We anticipate a fruitful age when artificial cells solve the enigma of natural cells.

ACKNOWLEDGMENTS

The authors wish to thank Drs. K. Hiramatsu, S. Miyatani, Y. Kumagai, and G. Suzuki for their dedicated work which is cited herein. They are also grateful to Ms. Yoko Yamaguchi for her expert secretarial assistance. These studies were supported by grants from the Ministry of Education, Science, and Culture, Japan.

REFERENCES

Binz, H., and Wigzell, H. (1977). Antigen-binding, idiotypic T-lymphocyte receptors. *Contemp. Top. Immunobiol.* **7,** 113.

Eshhar, Z., Apte, R. N., Lowy, I., Ben-Neriah, Y., Givol, D., and Mozes, E. (1980). T-cell hybridoma bearing heavy chain variable region determinants producing (T,G)-A—L-specific helper factor. *Nature (London)* **286,** 270.

Godsby, R. A., Osborne, B. A., Simpson, E., and Herzenberg, L. A. (1977). Hybrid cell lines with T-cell characteristics. *Nature (London)* **267,** 707.

Hämmerling, G. J. (1977). T lymphocyte tissue culture lines produced by cell hybridization. *Eur. J. Immunol.* **7,** 743.

Hayes, C. E., and Bach, F. H. (1978). T-cell-specific murine Ia antigens: Serology of *I-J* and *I-E* subregion specificities. *J. Exp. Med.* **148,** 692.

Hayes, C. E., and Bach, F. H. (1979). Murine T cell Ia antigens. II. Further studies on an *I-J* subregion specificity. *J. Immunol.* **123,** 1678.

Hewitt, J., and Liew, F. Y. (1979). Antigen-specific suppressor factors produced by T cell hybridomas for delayed-type hypersensitivity. *Eur. J. Immunol.* **5,** 572.

Hiramatsu, K., Miyatani, S., Kim, M., Yamada, S., Okumura, K., and Tada, T. (1981). Unique T cell Ia antigen expressed on a hybrid cell line producing antigen-specific augmenting T cell factor. *J. Immunol.* **127,** 1118.

Hiramatsu, K., Ochi, A., Miyatani, S., Segawa, A., and Tada, T. (1982). Monoclonal antibodies specific for *I* region determinants uniquely expressed on T cells with helper and augmenting functions. *Nature* (*London*) (in press).

Kanno, M., Kobayashi, S., Tokuhisa, T., Takei, I., Shinohara, N., and Taniguchi, M. (1981). Mopnoclonal antibodies that recognize the product controlled by a gene in the *I-J* subregion of the mouse *H-2* complex. *J. Exp. Med.* **154,** 1290.

Kapp, J. A., Aranes, B. A., and Clevinger, B. L. (1980). Suppression of antibody and T cell proliferative responses to L-glutamic acid $_{60}$-L-alinine $_{30}$-L-tyrosine $_{10}$ (GAT) by a specific monoclonal T cell factor. *J. Exp. Med.* **152,** 235.

Kappler, J. W., Skidmore, B., White, J., and Marrack, P. (1981). Antigen-inducible, *H-2*-restricted interleukin-2-producing T cell hybridomas. Lack of independent antigen and *H-2* recognition. *J. Exp. Med.* **153,** 1198.

Katz, D. H., Bechtold, T. E., and Altman, A. (1980). Construction of T cell hybridomas secreting allogeneic effect factor. *J. Exp. Med.* **152,** 956.

Kishimoto, T., Suemura, M., Sugimura, K., Okada, M., Nakanishi, K., and Yamamura, Y. (1981). Characterizations of T cell-derived immunoregulatory molecules from murinc or human T hybridomas. *Lymphokine Rep.* **5** (in press).

Köhler, G., and Milstein, C. (1975). Continuous cultures of fused cells secreting antibody of predefined specificity. *Nature (London)* **256,** 495.

Kontiainen, S., Simpson, E., Bohrer, E., Beverley, P. C. L., Herzenberg, L. A., Fitzpatrick, W. C., Vogt, P., Torano, A., McKenzie, I. F. C., and Feldmann, M. (1978). T-cell lines producing antigen-specific suppressor factor. *Nature (London)* **274,** 477.

Kontiainen, S., Culbert, E. J., Cecka, M., Simpson, E., McKenzie, I. F. C., and Feldmann, M. (1981). T cell hybridomas producing hapten specific suppressor factors. *Immunology* **43,** 747.

Lonai, P., Puri, J. and Hammerling, G. J. (1981). *H-2* restricted antigen binding by a hybridoma clone that produces antigen-specific helper factor. *Proc. Natl. Acad. Sci. U.S.A.* **78,** 549.

Marchalonis, J. J., and Warr, G. W. (1979). Antigen receptors on thymus-derived lymphocytes: *In* "Cancer Biology Reviews" (J. J. Merchalonis, M. G. Hanna, Jr., and I. J. Fidler, eds.), p. 1. Dekker, New York.

Minami, M., Okuda, K., Furusawa, S., Benacerraf, B., and Dorf, M. E. (1981). Analysis of T cell hybridomas. I. Characterization of *H-2* and *Igh* restricted monoclonal suppressor factors. *J. Exp. Med.* **154,** 1390.

Murphy, D. B., Herzenberg, L. A., Okumura, K., Herzenberg, L. A., and McDevitt, H. O. (1976). A new *I* subregion (*I-J*) marked by a locus (*Ia-4*) controlling surface determinants on suppressor T lymphocytes. *J. Exp. Med.* **144,** 699.

Okada, Y., Suzuki, T., and Hosaka, Y. (1957). Interaction between influenza virus and Ehrlich's tumor cells. III. Fusion phenomenon of Ehrlich's tumor cells by the action of HVJ Z strain. *Med. J. Osaka Univ.* **7,** 709.

Okuda, K., Minami, M., Ju, S.-T., and Dorf, M. E. (1981). Functional association of idiotypic and *I-J* determinants on the antigen receptor of suppressor T cells. *Proc. Natl. Acad. Sci. U.S.A.* (in press).

Okumura, K., Herzenberg, L. A., Murphy, D. B., McDevitt, H. O., and Herzenberg, L. A. (1976). Selective expression of *H-2* (*I*-region) loci controlling determinants on helper and suppressor T lymphocytes. *J. Exp. Med.* **144,** 685.

Rajewsky, K., and Eichmann, K. (1977). Antigen receptors of T helper cells. *Contemp. Top. Immunobiol.* **7,** 69.

Rich, S., David, C. S., and Rich, R. (1979). Regulatory mechanisms in cell mediated immune responses. VII. Presence of *I-C* subregion determinants on mixed leukocyte reaction suppressor factor. *J. Exp. Med.* **149,** 114.

Ruddle, N. H., Beezley, B., Lewis, G. K., and Goodman, J. W. (1980). Antigen-specific T cell hybrids. III. T cell hybrids which bind asobenzen arsonate. *Mol. Immunol.* **17,** 925.

Tada, T., and Okumura, K. (1979). The role of antigen-specific T cell factors in the immune response. *Adv. Immunol.* **28,** 1.

Tada, T., Taniguchi, M., and David, C. S. (1976). Properties of the antigen-specific suppressive T cell factor in the regulation of antibody response in the mouse. IV. Special subregion assignment of the gene(s) which codes for the suppressive T cell factor in the *H-2* histocompatibility complex. *J. Exp. Med.* **144,** 713.

Tada, T., Taniguchi, M., Saito, T., and Matsuzawa, T. (1979). Regulation of the antibody response by T cell-derived factors: Their heterogeneity and genetics. *Monogr. Allergy* **14,** 45.

Tada, T., Hayakawa, K., Okumura, K., and Taniguchi, M. (1980). Coexistence of variable region of immunoglobulin heavy chain and I region gene products on antigen-specific suppressor T cells and suppressor T cell factor: A minimal model of functional antigen receptor of T cells. *Mol. Immunol.* **17,** 867.

Tada, T., Okumura, K., Hayakawa, K., Suzuki, G., Abe, R., and Kumagai, Y. (1981). Immunological circuitry governed by MHC and V_H gene products. *In* Immunoglobulin Idiotypes" (C. Janeway, E. E. Sercarz, and H. Wigzell, eds.), p. 563. Academic Press, New York.

Taniguchi, M., and Miller, J. F. A. P. (1978). Specific suppressive factors produced by hybridomas derived from the fusion of enriched suppressor T cells and a T lymphoma cell line. *J. Exp. Med.* **148,** 373.

Taniguchi, M., and Tokuhisa, T. (1980). Cellular consequences in the suppression of antibody response by the antigen-specific T-cell factor. *J. Exp. Med.* **151,** 517.

Taniguchi, M., Saito, T., and Tada, T. (1979). Antigen-specific suppressive factor produced by a transplantable *I-J* bearing T-cell hybridoma. *Nature (London)* **278,** 555.

Taniguchi, M., Saito, T., Takei, T., and Tokuhisa, T. (1981). Presence of interchain disulfide bonds between two gene products that compose the secreted form of an antigen-specific suppressor factor. *J. Exp. Med.* **153,** 1672.

Taussig, M. J., and Holliman, A. (1979). Structure of an antigen-specific suppressor factor produced by a hybrid T-cell line. *Nature (London)* **277,** 308.

Taussig, M. J., Corvalan, J. R. F., and Holliman, A. (1979). Characterization of an antigen-specific factor from a hybrid T-cell line. *Ann. N.Y. Acad. Sci.* **332,** 316.

Tokuhisa, T., Taniguchi, M., Okumura, K., and Tada, T. (1978). An antigen-specific I region gene product which augments the antibody response. *J. Immunol.* **120,** 414.

Watanabe, T., Kimoto, M., Maruyama, S., Kishimoto, T., and Yamamura, Y. (1978). Regulation of antibody response in different immunoglobulin classes. V. Establishment of T-hybrid cell line secreting IgE class-specific suppressor factor. *J. Immunol.* **121,** 2113.

8

Factors, Receptors, and Their Ligands: Studies with *H-2* Restricted Helper Hybridoma Clones

Peter Lonai/Esther Arman/Huub F. C. Savelkoul/
Varda Friedman/Joseph Puri/Günter Hämmerling

I.	Ia-Associated Antigen Complex	109
II.	Isolation of T Hybridomas	111
III.	Characterization of the Hybridoma Clones	111
IV.	Analysis of the Altered Self–Dual Recognition Problem	112
V.	Isolation of Helper Factors	116
	References	116

The mechanism of *H-2* restriction is one of the central problems of immunology today. The structure and function of both the T cell receptor and the ligand recognized by T cells will have to be analyzed to understand this mechanism. Our laboratory has studied this question using a previous finding which suggests that macrophages release a part of the antigen which they have taken up as a genetically restricted Ia-associated antigen complex (IAC), which is bound by T cells and is immunogenic (Puri and Lonai, 1980). Thus, in our model, we study IAC as the ligand of T cells. As a source of receptors and antigen-specific factors, we use T hybridoma clones which were selected according to their IAC binding property (Lonai *et al.*, 1981a). In this chapter, we will discuss some of our recent reports and will describe preliminary results to illustrate our approach to the problem.

I. IA-ASSOCIATED ANTIGEN COMPLEX

Some years ago Erb and Feldmann (1975) reported that there is no need for direct contact between T cells and macrophages for the *in vitro* generation of

ISOLATION, CHARACTERIZATION, AND
UTILIZATION OF T LYMPHOCYTE CLONES

ISBN 0-12-249920-4

helper cells. A soluble, genetically restricted, Ia-containing factor (GRF) can replace adherent cells. We have "rediscovered" this factor while studying the binding of protein antigens to T cells by microscopic autoradiography.

According to our studies, two operationally separated phases can be distinguished in antigen binding by *Lyt-1⁺,2,3⁻* (T cells (T-ABC). First, as a preparatory step, they need a genetically nonrestricted monokine which is present in peritoneal macrophage cultures (Lonai and Steinman, 1977), or in cultures of lipopolysaccharide (LPS)-treated P388D1 macrophage-like tumor cells (Puri *et al.,* 1980). This monokine is most likely identical with Interleukin-1 (IL-1) (Mizel, 1980), and its effect on T-ABC, a 3- to 10-fold increase in the number of ABC, appears to be connected to an induced increase of plasma membrane viscosity (Puri *et al.,* 1980). IL-1 is necessary for antigen binding both in normal helper cells (*Lyt-1⁺,2,3⁻*) (Puri and Lonai, 1980), and in helper hybridoma cells (Lonai *et al.,* 1981a). Its effect, however, could not be observed with *Lyt-1⁻,2,3⁺* normal T-ABC and with a suppressor hybridoma clone (a gift of Drs. Taniguchi and Tada).

The second step in antigen binding involves the production of IAC and its binding by IL-1-treated T cells. We incubate different protein antigens, in the presence of IL-1, with splenic or bone marrow-derived macrophages (grown with lung colony stimulating factor) at 37°C for 1 hr. These contain *Ia⁺* macrophages. $p388D_1$, other *Ia⁻* macrophage tumor lines, and peritoneal exudate cells did not produce IAC. In our hands, peritoneal exudates contain 5–10% *Ia⁺* cells, whereas bone marrow-derived macrophages contained 20–30% *Ia⁺* cells. The supernatant of such cultures contains IAC, in a concentration not higher than around 1% of the original antigen concentration (10–20 μg/ml). IAC binds to T-ABC or T hybridoma cells in an *H-2* restricted manner (Puri and Lonai, 1980; Lonai *et al.,* 1981a). It is immunogenic in limiting amounts *in vivo,* radioactive IAC "suicides" helper cells *in vitro;* and it induces antigen-dependent prolifera-

TABLE I

***H-2*-Restricted Stimulation Induced by IAC-Ovalbumin *in Vitro*[a]**

Addition	Stimulation (cpm)
No addition	194 ± 64
100 g ovalbumin	5005 ± 331
1 g ovalbumin	300 ± 19
1 g C57BL/10-IAC-ovalbumin	1280 ± 207
1 g B10.BR-IAC-ovalbumin	291 ± 46

[a] C57BL/10 mice were immunized by 100 μg/ovalbumin in complete Freund's adjurant into the tail base. Proliferation assay performed according to Corradin *et al.* (1977). Maximal stimulation with soluble ovalbumin was obtained at a concentration of 100 μg/ml.

tion of T cells *in vitro* (Table I). All these functional parameters are *H-2* restricted, and the restriction maps to the *I-A* subregion of *H-2* (Puri and Lonai, 1980). Recent experiments have demonstrated that IAC can be produced by bone marrow-derived macrophages which contain over 95% phagocytic esterase-positive cells, and that the presence of IL-1 also is necessary for this function (Friedman and Lonai, 1982).

II. ISOLATION OF T HYBRIDOMAS

Splenic T cells of C57BL/6 ($H\text{-}2^b$) or B10.BR ($H\text{-}2^k$) mice immunized with NP-chicken globulin (NP-CGG) were fused with the AKR ($H\text{-}2^k$) lymphoma BW-5147. Fusion lines were screened for activity by an IAC-CGG binding assay (Lonai *et al.*, 1981a). From 530 lines 11 were found to be positive. Six of six antigen-binding positive lines now available secrete helper factors specific to CGG as carrier. These lines were cloned by limiting dilution cloning. Most of the clones produce *H-2* restricted helper factors and bind IAC-CGG in an *H-2* restricted manner. The extent to which our methods are responsible for obtaining such functionally homogeneous lines is not clear. Different long-term lines and hybridoma clones, also described in this volume, have quite different functional properties. Besides representing the major functional classes, some produce factors, some do not; some factors are *H-2* restricted, but others not. While this could represent the natural heterogeneity of T lymphocytes, the solution of this problem must await further information.

III. CHARACTERIZATION OF THE HYBRIDOMA CLONES

The helper factors of our clones are carrier (CGG) specific and can be purified on CGG-Sepharose affinity columns. They also contain Ia determinants controlled by the *A* and probably also by the *E* subregion of *H-2* (Lonai *et al.*, 1981a,b). The most interesting functional characteristic of these factors is their genetic restriction. They provide help only to those B cell sources (spleen cells from animals immunized with 4-hydroxy-5-iodo-3-nitrophenyl)acetyl(NIP)-ovalbumin which share the *H-2K-I-A* interval with the hybridoma cells. In addition, the factors can be absorbed on normal spleen cells syngeneic at *I-A*. This suggests that the factors, similarly to *H-2* restricted T cells, may have anti-self H-2 recognition units (Lonai *et al.*, 1981b).

The antigen-binding characteristics of the hybridoma clones are similar to those of normal T cells (Lonai *et al.*, 1981a, and Table III). They require pretreatment with IL-1, and they bind CGG processed by macrophages which are syngeneic in *H-2* with the hybridoma cells. Approximately 20–40% of the cells bind antigen. *H-2* allogeneic IAC, or irrelevant antigens, like HGG or

(T,G)-A--L, are bound by 0.1–5% of the cells. It is possible that we detect binding only by a portion of the cells in these cloned populations because antigen binding may depend on cell cycle, or that the low concentration of IAC in our crude preparation (0.1–0.2 μg/ml) allows binding only by a minority of the available receptors.

IV. ANALYSIS OF THE ALTERED SELF–DUAL RECOGNITION PROBLEM

One of the simplest questions which can be analyzed by these hybrid cells is whether one or more loci are responsible for antigen recognition. This is in connection with the central question of the dual recognition–altered self controversy (for review, see Zinkernagel and Doherty, 1979). In simplified terms, dual recognition suggests that the specificity of *H-2* restricted T cells is controlled by two loci, whereas altered self requires one locus. It is important to distinguish this problem from the genetic regulation of the antibody molecule, where specificity is defined by two loci, but the V_H and V_L products form a combining site specific for one ligand, whereas the dual recognition hypothesis predicts recognition of two different determinants.

As an initial step toward a somatic genetic analysis, we studied *H-2* restricted T cell factors secreted by *H-2* heterologous hybridoma cells. We assumed that a helper hybridoma constructed from a CGG-specific C57BL/6 ($H\text{-}2^b$) T cell and the BW-5147 ($H\text{-}2^k$) lymphoma contains only one carrier-specific locus, that of the normal partner cell, but may contain two self Ia-specific loci. Our reasoning was that BW-5147 has no known antigen specificity, and does not produce CGG-specific helper factors or bind CGG (Lonai *et al.*, 1981a). If such a clone secretes two CGG-specific helper factors, one restricted to $H\text{-}2^b$, the other to $H\text{-}2^k$, this would indicate that the anti-carrier and the anti-self loci are independent. Such independence suggests that the specific site of *H-2* restricted helper factors is controlled by two independent loci, and supports the validity of dual recognition concepts.

Our results with a number of CGG-specific *H-2* heterologous hybridoma clones suggested that these cells produce two helper factors. They could be separated either by absorption on normal $H\text{-}2^b$ or $H\text{-}2^k$ spleen cells or on monoclonal anti-Ia affinity columns, into a factor specific for CGG + H-2^b and a factor specific for CGG + H-2^k (Lonai *et al.*, 1981c, and Table II). Hence, these results suggested that in the factors restricted to $H\text{-}2^k$, a CGG-specific unit deriving from the BW-5147 parental cell, cooperate in defining dual specificity. It follows that the specificity of these factors is controlled by two separate loci, which is in support of the dual recognition hypothesis for *H-2* restricted helper factors.

TABLE II

Separation of Two Helpers Factors from the Culture Supernatant of an *H-2*^{b} + *H-2*^{k} Hybridoma Clone on Monoclonal I-A^k- and I-A^b-Specific Affinity Columns

		PFC/10^6 B cell sources	
Factor		(C3H × BALB/c)F_1	(B6 × BALB/c)F_1
B cell control		130 ± 30	150 ± 25
T cell help		469 ± 15	612 ± 55
Helper factor		746 ± 18	728 ± 86
Helper factor	Anti-I-A^k-Sepharose effluent	173 ± 46	677 ± 9
Helper factor	Anti-I-A^k-Sepharose eluate	661 ± 30	136 ± 11
Helper factor	Anti-I-A^b-Sepharose effluent	885 ± 66	143 ± 24
Helper factor	Anti-I-A^b-Sepharose eluate	115 ± 53	648 ± 88

Six such double producer clones were detected from ten. Three of the ten clones were chosen from a large number of clones for "double binding" by our autoradiographic antigen binding assay. Six of the ten were subclones of a clone which was detected by chance as being double producer. Hence, the sampling was not random, and the frequency of this phenomenon is not yet known. Contrasting reports were published by Kappler *et al.* (1981). They have used a system of antigen-inducible IL-2 production by T hybridoma cells. Fusion of hybridomas which had different antigen plus self specificities did not result in clones of "mixed" stimulator specificity (Kappler *et al.*, 1981), neither could they detect double sensitive cultures among eleven *H-2* heterologous IL-2-producing hybridoma clones and uncloned F_1 plus BW5147 lines. Additional studies in both systems will be necessary to resolve the problem. Because the actual frequency of double helper factor producers in our sample is not yet known, at present it is not clear whether the two sets of data are indeed at variance.

The relationship of antigen-specific T cell factors and T cell receptors is not unequivocal (Tada and Okumura, 1979; Lonai *et al.*, 1982). Recent preliminary antigen-binding experiments have shown that *H-2* heterologous (*H-2*^{b} + *H-2*^{k}) hybridoma cells bind the carrier in the form of IAC processed by macrophages of either parental *H-2* haplotype, but not when it was processed by macrophages of a foreign *H-2* haplotype (Table III). This suggests that the hybridoma clones express both parental anti-self specificities not only in the helper factors but also in their cellular antigen-binding receptors. Hence, our working hypothesis for future experiments is that the membrane-bound receptor and the antigen-specific factor of these hybridomas may be quite similar, and the dual specificity of both may be controlled by two genes.

TABLE III

Cells of an *H-2* Heterologous Helper Hybridoma Clone (T77-146-C3) Bind Carrier Material Processed by Macrophages of Either Parental *H-2* Type

IL-1	Antigen[a]	Antigen-Binding Cells (%)
−	Soluble CGG	5
−	H-2^b-IAC CGG	3
−	Soluble NIP-OVA	5
−	H-2^b-IAC NIP-OVA	6
+	Soluble-CGG	1
+	H-2^b-IAC-CGG	25
+	H-2^k-IAC-CGG	42
+	H-2^f-IAC-CGG	1
+	Soluble NIP-OVA	6
+	H-2^b-IAC-NIP-OVA	4

[a] Antigens: CGG, chicken gamma globulin; NIP-OVA, (4-hydroxy-3-nitrophenyl)acetyl-ovalbumin; IAC, Ia-associated antigen couples. The *H-2* types indicate the haplotype of the macrophages used for production of IAC.

The identity of the self Ia and CGG specific loci in our hybridoma cells is not clear. It is possible that both are V_H products. In this case the Ia antigens of the factor may be functionally irrelevant, and their presence in the helper factor may be explained by being bound by the anti-self site. Alternatively self recognition may be mediated by the Ia antigens in the factor. This is consistent with the anti-Ia column separation experiment, which suggests that anti-self specificity is associated with Ia alloantigens of the helper factor (Table III). In this case, either the Ia moiety of the factor recognizes determinants on the B cells or macrophages or they themselves are recognized by determinants on these cells. Finally it has to be taken into consideration that antigen-specific T cell factors and T cell receptors may be different. This conclusion is supported by studies which did not find Ia antigens associated with antigen receptors isolated from T cells (Binz *et al.*, 1979; Cramer *et al.*, 1978). Therefore, it is possible that the T cell receptor could contain only two V_H-like products (Janeway *et al.*, 1976), whereas the factor includes a carrier-specific V_H moiety coupled with Ia (Droege, 1981).

Taken together, our results suggest that the specificity of *H-2* restricted helper factors, and possibly also of cellular receptors of the hybridoma cells, is controlled by independent loci. The identity of these loci is not clear, but could be clarified by defining whether such hybridoma cells contain both parental *H-2* and *Igh* chromosomes.

Our experiments with helper factors support the dual recognition hypothesis.

Dual recognition concepts are consistent either with two independent receptors which recognize two separate ligands or with two closely associated receptors which recognize a complex. If the first alternative is valid, then an *H-2* restricted T cell would bind soluble antigen in the absence of MHC products. Our results do not support this alternative. We have shown for normal T-ABC (Lonai *et al.*, 1981d), and also for the hybridoma clones (Lonai *et al.*, 1981a), that cold

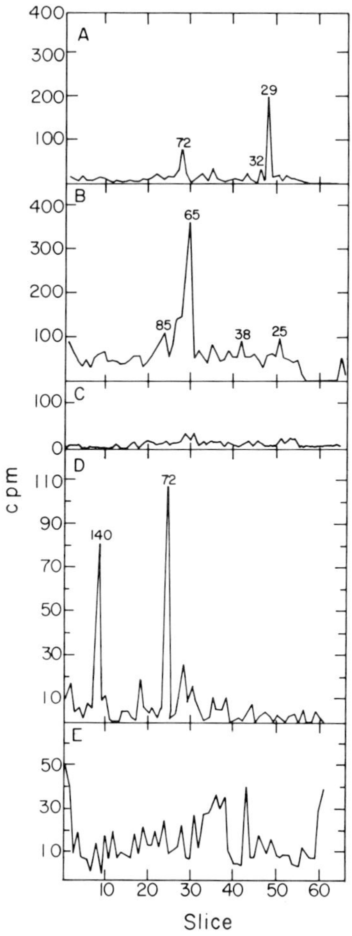

Fig. 1. Isolation of helper factor from the culture fluid of an *H-2* homologous hybridoma clone. SDS-PAGE 7–15%, reduction with 2-mercaptoethanol. Labeling 250 μCi/ml [^{35}S]methionine overnight. (A) CGG-Sepharose eluate. (B) Anti-V$_H$-Sepharose eluate. (C) HGG-Sepharose eluate. (D) HGG-Sepharose effluent anti-I-A^k (monoclonal) precipitate. (E) Anti-V$_H$ effluent anti-I-A^k (monoclonal) precipitate. (A)–(C) and (D)–(E) were separate experiments.

soluble antigen does not inhibit the binding of homologous ^{125}I-labeled IAC even at a 10^3-fold excess. It follows that both the self Ia and the nominal antigen specific sites of the receptor, as well as the antigen and Ia portions of the ligand, may be closely associated.

V. ISOLATION OF HELPER FACTORS

Three serological parameters, defined by functional studies, were used to isolate biosynthetically labeled ([^{35}S]methionine) materials from the culture fluid of the helper hybridoma clones described above. They were isolated either by affinity separation on CGG-Sepharose, by immunoprecipitation with rabbit anti-$V_{H\text{-}315}$ antibodies (Ben-Neriah *et al.*, 1978), or with monoclonal anti-Ia antibodies (Fig. 1). Analysis was performed by SDS polyacrylamide gel electrophoresis in reducing conditions. The major component of these factors is a polypeptide of 60,000–70,000 MW. In most experiments two additional peaks of approximately 35,000 and 30,000 MW can be also detected. In cultures of high cell density, quite frequently the major specific product, or part of it, appears at higher molecular weights (140,000 or 300,000 apparent molecular weight), which may be aggregates (Fig. 1D). The specificity of these peaks is supported by the fact that the same pattern is obtained by antigen affinity separation and by anti-V_H or anti-Ia precipitation or affinity separation experiments. Additional studies are necessary to define whether the V_H, and Ia markers of the factor are situated on the same or on separate molecules. The major component of the *H-2* restricted helper factors is similar in apparent molecular weight to that described for a suppressor factor derived from a long-term T cell clone (Fresno *et al.*, 1981) described recently. It is possible that this material of approximately 60,000 daltons represents the immunoglobulin gene product of T cell factors.

We think that the most important aspect of these very recent results with T hybridoma clones is the ease by which one can construct experiments for the study of questions which were indeed difficult to approach with classic cellular immunological techniques. It appears to us that the various T cell cloning methods coupled with somatic genetic and biochemical techniques will help to solve many of the controversial problems in basic immunology.

REFERENCES

Ben-Neriah, Y., Wuilmart, C., Lonai, P., and Givol, D. (1978). Preparation and characterization of anti-framework antibodies to the heavy chain variable region (V_H) of mouse immunoglobulins. *Eur. J. Immunol.* **8,** 797.

Binz, H., Frischknecht, H., Mercolli, C., Dunst, S., and Wigzell, H. (1979). Binding of purified soluble major histocompatibility complex polypeptide chains onto isolated T cell receptors. I. Reactivity against cells- and self-determinants. *J. Exp. Med.* **150,** 1084.

Corradin, G., Ettinger, H. M., and Chiller, J. M. (1977). Lymphocyte specificity to protein antigens. *J. Immunol.* **119,** 1048.

Cramer, M., Krawinkel, K., Hämmerling, G., Black, S. J., Berek, C., Eichmann, K., and Rajewsky, K. (1978). Antigen receptors on T lymphocytes. *In* "Ir Genes and Ia Antingens" (H. O. McDevitt, ed.), pp. 583–595. Academic Press, New York.

Droege, W. (1981). Theoretical considerations and probability models for the somatic development of the T cell repertoire. *Cell. Immunol.* **57,** 251.

Erb, P., and Feldmann, M. (1975). The role of macrophages in the generation of T helper cells. III. Influence of macrophage derived factors in helper cell induction. *Eur. J. Immunol.* **5,** 759.

Fresno, M., McVay-Boudreau, L., Nabel, G., and Cantor, H. (1981). Antigen specific T lymphocyte clones. II. Purification and biological characterization of an antigen specific suppressive protein synthetized by cloned T cells. *J. Exp. Med.* **153,** 1260.

Friedman, V., and Lonai, P. (1982). In preparation.

Janeway, C. A., Jr., Wigzell, H., and Binz, H. (1976). Two different V_H gene products make up the T cell receptor. *Scand. J. Immunol.* **5,** 993.

Kappler, J. W., Skidmore, B., White, J., and Marrack, P. (1981). Antigen inducible, *H-2* restricted interleukin-2-producing T cell hybridomas. Lack of independent antigen and *H-2* recognition. *J. Exp. Med.* **153,** 1198.

Lonai, P., and Steinman, L. (1977). Physiological regulation of antigen binding to T cells, role of a soluble macrophage factor and of interferon. *Proc. Natl. Acad. Sci. U.S.A.* **74,** 5662.

Lonai, P., Puri, J., and Hämmerling, G. J. (1981a). *H-2* restricted antigen binding by a hybridoma clone which produces specific helper factor. *Proc. Natl. Acad. Sci. U.S.A.* **78,** 549.

Lonai, P., Puri, J., Bitton, S., Ben-Neriah, Y., Givol, D., and Hämmerling, G. J. (1981b). *H-2*-restricted helper factor secreted by cloned hybridoma cells. *J. Exp. Med.* **154,** 942.

Lonai, P., Bitton, S., Savelkoul, H. F. J., Puri, J., and Hämmerling, G. J. (1981c). Two separate genes regulate self-Ia and carrier recognition in *H-2*-restricted helper factors secreted by hybridoma cells. *J. Exp. Med.* **154,** 1910.

Lonai, P., Steinman, L., Friedman, V., Drizlikh, G., and Puri, J. (1981d). Specificity of antigen binding by T cells; competition between soluble and Ia associated antigen. *Eur. J. Immunol.* **11,** 382.

Lonai, P., Puri, J., and Hämmerling, G. J. (1982). T hybridoma cells which produce genetically restricted helper factors and bind the carrier in association with Ia. *Lymphokine Rep.* **5,** (in press).

Mizel, S. B. V. (1980). Studies on the purification and structure-function relationship of murine lymphocyte activating factor (Il-1). *Mol. Immunol.* **17,** 571.

Puri, J., and Lonai, P. (1980). Mechanism of antigen binding by T cells. *H-2* (*I-A*) restricted binding of antigen plus Ia by helper cells. *Eur. J. Immunol.* **10,** 273.

Puri, J., Shinitzky, M., and Lonai, P. (1980). Concomitant increase in antigen binding and in T cell membrane lipid viscosity by the lymphocyte activating factor, LAF. *J. Immunol.* **124,** 1937.

Tada, T., and Okumura, K. (1979). The role of antigen-specific T cell factors in the immune response. *Adv. Immunol.* **28,** 1.

Zinkernagel, R. M., and Doherty, P. C. (1979). MHC-restricted cytotoxic T cells: Studies on the biological role of polymorphic major transplantation antigens determining T-cell restriction-specificity, function and responsiveness. *Adv. Immunol.* **27,** 51.

9

Properties of Antigen-Specific *H-2* Restricted T Cell Hybridomas

Philippa Marrack/Sam D. Graham, Jr., /H. James Leibson/ Neal Roehm/Dale Wegmann/John W. Kappler

I.	Factor Production by T Cell Hybridomas	120
II.	Use of T Cell Hybridomas to Examine Properties of the T Cell Receptor	122
III.	T Cell Hybridomas Do Not Express Unexpected H-2 Specificities .	123
IV.	Karyotypic Analysis of T Cell Hybridomas	124
	References	126

Cloned T cell lines with various activities and with the property of *H-2*-associated antigen (Ag/H-2) recognition have been available for some time. These have been extremely useful as manifested by many of the other papers in this treatise. However, they are not suitable for all purposes. For example, it is laborious to grow very large quantities of this type of cell for biochemical and immunochemical studies. Moreover, they are not amenable to certain kinds of manipulations, for example, those associated with somatic cell genetics.

Although techniques are available for making useful B cell and suppressor T cell hybridomas, it has not been so easy to make T cell hybridomas which have the property of simultaneous antigen and H-2 recognition. The primary reason for this, in retrospect, seems to have been lack of a suitable assay. T cell hybridomas of this type do not bind free antigen or H-2 products and therefore cannot be assayed by these criteria. Although they do bind to antigen pulsed presenting cells of the appropriate haplotype (see below), we have found this assay to be too laborious for routine use. In our experience these hybridomas are most easily studied by following their ability to secrete lymphokines in response to Ag/H-2 challenge. Although such hybridomas secrete many different lymphokines, interleukin-2 (IL-2) production has been used most often in our laboratory, since it is produced by the hybridomas within 24 hr after challenge, and has a rapid (24 hr) and reliable assay (Kappler *et al.*, 1981). In fact, however, the choice of lymphokine for assay may depend upon the convenience of the labora-

ISOLATION, CHARACTERIZATION, AND
UTILIZATION OF T LYMPHOCYTE CLONES

ISBN 0-12-249920-4

tory using it. Techniques for production of these hybridomas are described in the Appendix. In this chapter, we will describe some of their properties and briefly outline some of what we hope will be their future uses.

I. FACTOR PRODUCTION BY T CELL HYBRIDOMAS

When these experiments were begun, Ag/H-2-specific T cells were fused to a T cell hybridoma which already had the property of Concanavalin A (Con-A)-inducible IL-2 production (Kappler *et al.*, 1981). This was because we were concerned that Ag/H-2-specific, IL-2-secreting T cell blasts might be so rare that hybrids with these properties might not be detected after fusion of T cell blasts to apparently nonfunctional T cell tumors such as BW5147. Our results have shown, however, either that cells producing IL-2 are very frequent among normal T cells or T cell blasts, or that they fuse with BW5147 preferentially, since we have obtained a high percentage of inducible IL-2-secreting hybrids in fusions to this cell line. As shown in Table I, between 70 and 90% of hybrids from such a fusion responded to appropriate challenge by secreting IL-2. By comparison, in some fusions to FS6-14.13.AG2, which already bears the property of inducible IL-2 secretion, 100% of hybrids responded to appropriate Ag/H-2 challenge with IL-2 secretion.

We were encouraged by these results to screen hybridomas for production of other factors, including interferon, macrophage Ia recruiting factor (MIRF), macrophage activating factors, and lymphokines with stimulatory activity in B cell antibody responses. Hybridomas were challenged with Con-A for these experiments to avoid complications due to production of factor by "filler" cells in antigen presenting cultures. So far we have little or no evidence for constitu-

TABLE I

Production of Inducible, Interleukin-2 Secreting Hybridomas by Fusion to BW5147

Fusion Name	Specificity of T Cell Parent	Number of Hybrids Tested	Stimulus	Percent Responding by IL-2 Production
FS-7	Normal spleen and lymph node T cells	90	Con-A	73
FS-8	Normal spleen and lymph node T cells	18	Con-A	39
2Rb	$H\text{-}2^b$ + KLH[a]	17	$H\text{-}2^b$ + KLH	70
AS4	$H\text{-}2^a$ + Sendai	98	$H\text{-}2^a$ + Sendai	78
BDK	$H\text{-}2^{b \times d}$ + KLH	57	$H\text{-}2^{b \times d}$ + KLH	82

[a] KLH, keyhole limpet hemocyanin.

tive (i.e., noninduced) production of any factors by long-term, stabilized T cell hybridomas. Active supernatants have only been found after Con-A (or Ag/H-2) induction. This result contrasts with some, but not all, other reports (Kontiainen *et al.*, 1978; Katz *et al.*, 1980; Harwell *et al.*, 1980; Schrader *et al.*, 1981).

Preliminary data are encouraging. For example, supernatants of certain stimulated hybridomas contain MIRF, others contain factors which stimulate tumoricidal activity of macrophages, and others have factors which are active in B cell responses. So far we have found no T cell hybrids which secrete interferon in response to Con-A. Many of the hybridomas secrete several factors. Whether this is because they contain portions of the genome from several different cells or whether this reflects the properties of the normal T cell parent remains to be seen, although data with cell clones would suggest the latter is a possible explanation (Nabel *et al.*, 1981).

The fact that these somatic cell hybrids are somewhat unstable can be used to advantage in selecting clones which secrete only desired factors. For example, we have been working with factors which contribute to B cell plaque forming cell (PFC) responses to sheep red blood cells (SRBC). One of these appears to be IL-2 (Harwell *et al.*, 1980). Another factor contributing to the response is distinct from IL-2 (Liebson *et al.*, 1981) but acts synergistically with this lymphokine. Past endeavors to distinguish these factors have depended on the removal of IL-2 from Con-A-induced supernatants by absorption with T cell blasts. This is laborious, expensive, and subject to artifacts, since T cells blasts may secrete additional factors into supernatants. To avoid this, we have used one hybridoma, FS7-20, which secreted IL-2 and the other, synergizing factor in response to Con-A. Clones of this hybrid were tested for IL-2 and synergizing factor production. Examples of the results are shown in Table II. The clones displayed all possible combinations of response. Some secreted large quantities

TABLE II

Segregation of IL-2 and Synergizing Factor Production in Response to Con-A by Cloned by Cell Lines

Cell line	Units IL-2 produced[a]	Synergizing factor production[b]
FS7—20.1	80	±
FS7—20.3	<10	−
FS7—20.9	<10	±
FS7—20.11	640	−
FS7—20.13	640	+
FS7—20.14	<10	+

[a] Assayed as in Kappler *et al.*, 1981. <10 units = no detectable IL-2.
[b] Assayed by synergy with IL-1 and IL-2 in anti-SRBC PFC response of purified B cells (Leibson *et al.*, 1981).

of both factors, some secreted IL-2 alone, while others secreted the synergizing factor without IL-2. Some made much smaller amounts of both lymphokines. FS7-20.14 was chosen for further production of the synergizing factor since it made large quantities of this factor without IL-2 production. Although we do not know why factor production segregates in the different clones, we presume it is due to chromosome loss. These hybrids contain many chromosomes, some of which are lost on subcloning (see below).

II. USE OF T CELL HYBRIDOMAS TO EXAMINE PROPERTIES OF THE T CELL RECEPTOR

We started to prepare Ag/H-2-specific hybridomas with the intention of deriving a cloned cell which simultaneously expressed specificities for two different antigens and two different *H-2* haplotypes. We assumed that such a cell would necessarily be the product of multiple fusions and, therefore, difficult to prepare and unstable. Nevertheless, we felt the effort worthwhile because success would allow us to distinguish among some of the main theories concerning how T cells recognize simultaneously Ag and H-2 products. For example, dual receptor theories which postulate independent receptors that independently recognize antigen and H-2 products on a cell surface would predict that a cell which inherited two different Ag/H-2 specificities from two different parents would also recognize the scrambled Ag/H-2 combinations, i.e., Ag from parent A plus *H-2* from parent B and vice versa. Single receptor theories, on the other hand, would predict that a hybrid with two Ag/H-2 specificities would not recognize the mixtures.

We have prepared such hybrids. Their properties have been described in some detail elsewhere (Kappler *et al.*, 1981) and will simply be reviewed here. From three different fusions, we were able to test the specificities of 27 uncloned hybridomas. Of these, four had lost the ability to recognize Ag/H-2 in any combination. Seven hybrids retained the Ag/H-2 specificity of one of the T cell parents but not the other. Sixteen hybrids inherited the Ag/H-2 specificites of both T cell parents. Interestingly, in no case was a hybrid observed which could recognize any mixture of parental antigen and H-2 specificities. From this result, we concluded that simple dual receptor theories which predicted that antigen and *H-2* would be recognized independently by their receptors could not be correct. In order to be sure of this conclusion, it was necessary to clone one of the hybridomas with two Ag/H-2 specificities. One hybridoma, AOFK-11.11.1, was cloned twice. This hybridoma recognized $I\text{-}A^k$ plus ovalbumin (OVA) and $I\text{-}A^f$ plus keyhole limpet hemocyanin (KLH), as did its parents, but did not recognize either mixed combination, i.e., $I\text{-}A^k$ plus KLH or $I\text{-}A^f$ plus OVA.

In our view such a result is compatible with any theory which predicts that

Ag/H-2 are recognized by a single receptor on the T cell surface. It is also compatible with certain dual receptor models, particularly those which predict that Ag and H-2 interact on the Ag-presenting cell surface, in such a manner that the *H-2* haplotype affects the Ag determinants presented or vice versa.

III. T CELL HYBRIDOMAS DO NOT EXPRESS UNEXPECTED H-2 SPECIFICITIES

We have examined Ag/H-2-specific T cell hybridomas for reactivity toward allogeneic H-2, and in some cases for unexpected Ag/H-2 reactivity. Of some 200 hybridomas obtained from fusions both to BW5147 and FS6-14.13.AG2.1 which have been examined, we have identified only six hybridomas with reactivity for allogeneic H-2. In every case, this was for $H\text{-}2^b$. The reasons for this preponderance of $H\text{-}2^b$-reactive hybridomas are not clear. It would be fair to point out, however, that we have only screened for reactivity on a panel of six independent *H-2* haplotypes (*b,d,f,k,g,s*), and that only about half the hybridomas have so far been screened on this full panel.

As far as unexpected Ag/H-2 specificities are concerned, again our screening techniques have not been overwhelmingly thorough. We were particularly interested, however, in the report by Lonai *et al.* (see Chapter 8, this treatise) that chicken γ-globulin (CGG)/$H\text{-}2^b$ T cell fusions to BW5147 yielded hybridomas which secreted factors which specifically stimulated both $H\text{-}2^b$ and $H\text{-}2^k$ cells to respond to CGG. Lonai *et al.* conclude that an $H\text{-}2^k$ specificity was inherited from BW5147 and that this could combine with a CGG specificity inherited from the normal T cell parent to yield an $H\text{-}2^k$ plus CGG stimulating factor. This result is at apparent odds with our own data, discussed above in Section II, which would suggest that such scrambling does not occur, at least in the 16 doubly specific hybrids we could test. As an additional check we have examined some of our hybrids produced by fusion of T cell blasts to BW5147 for unexpected reactivity with $H\text{-}2^k$ plus antigen. Our results are listed in Table III. Of three cloned lines with Ag/H-2 reactivity from the BDK fusion, none responded to $H\text{-}2^k$ plus KLH. Hybrids from the SKK fusion have not yet been cloned. Of the 24 Ag/H-2 reactive lines so far obtained, six responded to $H\text{-}2^s$ plus KLH and showed no signs of $H\text{-}2^k$ plus KLH reactivity. Sixteen responded to $H\text{-}2^k$ plus KLH alone and yielded no information for the present discussion, since this reactivity was probably inherited from the $H\text{-}2^{(s \times k)}$ normal T cell blast parent. One cell line responded to KLH presented by either $H\text{-}2^s$ or $H\text{-}2^k$ cells, a result in apparent agreement with that of Lonai *et al.* However, SKK was a particularly successful fusion. Hybrids grew in all 500 wells into which the cells were aliquoted immediately after fusion, and 60% of wells tested contained antigen-reactive hybridomas. Since not all the lines have yet been cloned, it is possible

TABLE III

Antigen Reactivities of Hybridomas Prepared by Fusion to BW5147

Fusion	Normal T cell parent/Ag	Number of hybrids	Hybrid reactivity		
			$H\text{-}2^b$ + KLH	$H\text{-}2^d$ + KLH	$H\text{-}2^k$ + KLH
BDK	BDF_1/KLH	2^a	+	−	−
	($H\text{-}2^{b \times d}$)/KLH	1^a	−	+	−
			$H\text{-}2^s$ + KLH	$H\text{-}2^k$ + KLH	
SKK	SJL × B10.BR/KLH	16^b	−	+	
	($H\text{-}2^{s \times k}$)/KLH	6^b	+	−	
		1^b	+	+	

[a] Cloned T cell hybridomas.

[b] Uncloned T cell hybridomas from a fusion in which all initially plated wells were positive for cell growth.

that the line reacting to $H\text{-}2^k$ or $H\text{-}2^s$ plus KLH is actually a mixture of two different hybridomas. We, therefore, doubt that in any of these cases $H\text{-}2^k$ reactivity has been inherited from the BW5147 parent.

In general, therefore, our results do not support the idea that T cells have independent receptors for Ag/H-2. Moreover we have not observed, at least as a common phenomenon, the result reported by Lonai *et al.* that $H\text{-}2^k$ specificity can be inherited from BW5147. Since our hybrids and those of Lonai *et al.* are assayed in different fashions, ours by response to Ag/H-2 and theirs by production of Ag/H-2-specific factors, it is possible that two completely different phenomena are being examined in the two series of experiments. For example, we have been unable to identify any antigen-specific helper material shed or secreted by our hybridomas. Moreover there is no indication that our hybridomas or their products bind free antigen, although they do bind to Ag-pulsed cells of the appropriate *H-2* haplotype. The properties of the receptors that we and Lonai *et al.* are examining thus seem to be completely different, and perhaps this accounts for the differences between our results.

IV. KARYOTYPIC ANALYSIS OF T CELL HYBRIDOMAS

Because hybridoma cells have more than a diploid number of chromosomes they offer a number of advantages. As described above, various properties can be segregated in subclones, presumably because of chromosome loss. These properties include not only production of various factors but also antigen recognition. Thus the instability of these lines has allowed us to produce negative subclones of various Ag/H-2 reactive clones which lack specific characteristics. These are useful in demonstrating that particular properties of the cells are related to a specific characteristic such as the presence or absence of an Ag/H-2 receptor. These variant clones should be useful in the future for biochemical and immunochemical studies on receptor material, and for karyotype analysis in mapping the gene(s) responsible for the T cell receptor for Ag/H-2.

Preliminary experiments with variants of the hybridoma clone AODH 7.1 are summarized in Table IV. The clone was passaged in tissue culture for 6–10 weeks before recloning. The subclones and their parent were tested in various assays, and the number of chromosomes in each cell line was determined. All of the cell lines shown here responded to Con-A by producing IL-2. Four of the subclones apparently expressed the HGG/H-2^d-specific receptor from their parent, since they responded to this combination by secreting IL-2, and they also bound to antigen-pulsed, spleen cell monolayers of this type. All four of these subclones also demonstrated antigen-specific, *H-2* restricted helper activity in B cell responses to TNP-HGG. In contrast four other subclones had lost all three antigen-specific, *H-2* restricted properties, but still retained the capacity for IL-2 production as manifested by their response to Con-A.

These results suggest that the presence of the same antigen receptor was

TABLE IV
Properties of AODH 7.1 and Its Subclones

Clone	Mean chromosome number (± S.E.M.)	Titer of IL-2 in response to[a]: H-2^d+HGG	Con-A	Specific binding to HGG/H-2^d cells[b]	HGG/H-2^d-specific helper activity[c] PFC/culture ± S.E.M.
AODH 7.1	74.6 ± 0.8	80	320	+	16,360 ± 340
Subclones					
7.1.3	75.9 ± 0.5	640	640	+	16,840 ± 320
7.1.5	72.8 ± 0.3	640	ND[d]	+	15,950 ± 260
7.1.6	75.0 ± 1.1	0	640	−	−440 ± 20
7.1.7	72.3 ± 0.7	0	640	−	−10 ± 60
7.1.8	73.7 ± 0.3	320	640	+	19,960 ± 590
7.1.9	ND	0	640	−	−110 ± 100
7.1.12	72.6 ± 0.4	0	640	−	110 ± 250
7.1.14	75.2 ± 0.9	320	640	+	27,960 ± 6240

[a] As described in Kappler *et al.*, 1981.
[b] Assayed by specific binding of ^{3}H-TdR labeled T cell hybridoma cells to antigen pulsed splenic adherent cells (Marrack *et al.*, 1982).
[c] Assayed by ability of hybridoma cells to cooperate specifically in anti-TNP-HGG responses of splenic B cells and macrophages of appropriate *H-2* haplotype (Roehm *et al.*, 1981). Results are expressed in terms of the number of anti-TNP PFC/10^6 hybridoma cells/culture.
[d] ND, not done.

necessary for all the three specific activities of these cells. We have not yet found subclones that have lost other cell functions required for production of these factors. For example, we have not been able to identify a subclone that can bind to antigen-pulsed presenting cells, but cannot secrete IL-2 in response to this stimulus.

From 30 to 67% of the subclones of AODH7.1 have lost the ability to recognize Ag/H-2. This high frequency suggested that these negative variants arose because of loss of the chromosome(s) which bear the genes coding for the HGG/H-2^d receptor(s). It is possible that detailed karyotypic analysis of the positive and negative subclones might reveal which chromosome(s) bear T cell receptor genes.

In summary, T cell hybridomas which recognize antigen in association with *H-2* products will facilitate the biochemical and immunochemical analysis of the receptor(s) for these materials and will also allow the use of somatic cell genetics to probe not only these receptor(s) but also other properties of T cells.

ACKNOWLEDGMENTS

The authors would like to thank Ella Kushnir for her excellent technical assistance in these experiments. This work was supported by ACS Grant IM-49, and USPHS Grant A1-17134. It was performed during the tenure of an established investigatorship by one of us (PM) from the America Heart Association with funds supplied in part by the Colorado Heart Association, and during the tenure of a Faculty Research Award from the American Cancer Society, Inc. by another of us (JWK).

REFERENCES

Harwell, L., Skidmore, B., Marrack, P., and Kappler, J. W. (1980). Concanavalin A-inducible interleukin-2-producing T cell hybridomas. *J. Exp. Med.* **152,** 893.

Kappler, J. W., Skidmore, B., White, J., and Marrack, P. (1981). Antigen-inducible, *H-2*-restricted interleukin-2-producing T cell hybridomas. Lack of independent antigen and H-2 recognition. *J. Exp. Med.* **153,** 1198.

Katz, D. H., Bechtold, T. E., and Altman, A. (1980). Construction of T cell hybridomas secreting allogeneic effect factor. *J. Exp. Med.* **152,** 956.

Kontianen, S., Simpson, E., Bohrer, E., Beverly, P. C. L., Herzenberg, L. A., Fitzpatrick, W. C., Vogt, P., Torano, A., McKenzie, I. F. C., and Feldman, M. (1978). T cell lines producing antigen-specific suppressor factor. *Nature (London)* **274,** 477.

Liebson, J., Marrack, P., and Kappler, J. W. (1981). B cell helper factors. I. Requirement for both interleukin-2 and another 40KD factor. *J. Exp. Med.* **154,** 1681.

Marrack, P., Skidmore, B., and Kappler, J. W. (1982). In preparation.

Nabel, G., Fresno, M., Chessman, A., and Cantor, H. (1981). Use of cloned populations of mouse lymphocytes to analyze cellular differentiation. *Cell* **23,** 19.

Roehm, N., Kappler, J., and Marrack, P. (1982). Use of T cell hybridomas in the analysis of helper T cell functions in B cell responses. *In* "Second International Symposium on the Immunobiology of Proteins and Peptides" (M. Z. Atassi, ed.). Plenum, New York (in press).

Schrader, J., Arnold, B., and Clark-Lewis, I. (1981). A Con A-stimulated T-cell hybridoma releases factors affecting colony-forming cells and B-cell antibody responses. *Nature (London)* **283,** 197.

10

Studies on an Antigen-Specific Suppressor Factor Produced by a T Hybrid Line

Michael J. Taussig

I.	Derivation and Specificity of the A1 Suppressor Line	128
II.	B Cells as the Targets for A1 Factor	129
III.	Genetic Control of Suppression	130
IV.	Interaction between Suppressor Factor and Monoclonal Antibodies in Regulation of the Immune Response	132
V.	Conclusion	134
	References	135

T cell hybrids are now a widely used source of antigen-binding T cell products, including antigen-specific helper and suppressor factors (Taussig, 1980; Eshhar *et al.*, 1980; Lonai *et al.*, 1981; Kapp *et al.*, 1980; Kontiainen *et al.*, 1978; Taniguchi *et al.*, 1979; Taussig *et al.*, 1979a,b,c; and contributions to this treatise). We have studied a suppressor factor with specificity for sheep red blood cells (SRBC) produced by a T hybrid line designated A1 and present in culture supernatants of the A1 cells. In general properties, it resembles the immunoregulatory molecules associated with suppressor T cells (Tada and Okumura, 1979) and other T cell hybrids. Namely, it shows antigen specificity in its action, binds to its specific antigen, is not classic immunoglobulin (Ig) in nature, and is partially coded by the major histocompatibility complex (MHC). On the other hand, the A1 suppressor factor shows several distinct features. For example, the *H-2* contribution seems to be from a gene mapping between *I-J* and *H-2D* rather than in *I-J* itself (Taussig *et al.*, 1979b); it does not show a strict self-H-2 restriction in its action, but does display an *H-2*-determined selectivity in its suppression of different mouse strains; the target of suppression appears to be a B cell; and its molecular weight of about 200,000 is higher than reported for most specific factors (Taussig and Holliman, 1979). Hence, there is some justifi-

ISOLATION, CHARACTERIZATION, AND
UTILIZATION OF T LYMPHOCYTE CLONES

ISBN 0-12-249920-4

cation for considering this molecule to be a member of a class of suppressor molecules which have not been recognized hitherto using more conventional material.

In this chapter, I will review some recent studies on the mechanism of suppression by the factor. The principal references to the published work on this line are Taussig *et al.* (1979a,b,c) and Taussig and Holliman (1979), and are more fully reviewed in Taussig (1982).

I. DERIVATION AND SPECIFICITY OF THE A1 SUPPRESSOR LINE

The line was a result of fusion between cells of the AKR thymoma BW 5147 and spleen cells of a C57BL/10ScSn mouse which had been injected with SRBC 5 days earlier (Taussig *et al.*, 1979c). The supernatants of T hybrid lines were screened by adding them to primary or secondary microcultures of spleen cells or TDL responding to SRBC. The supernatant of the A1 line was able to produce complete inhibition of both the primary (IgM) and secondary (IgM and IgG)

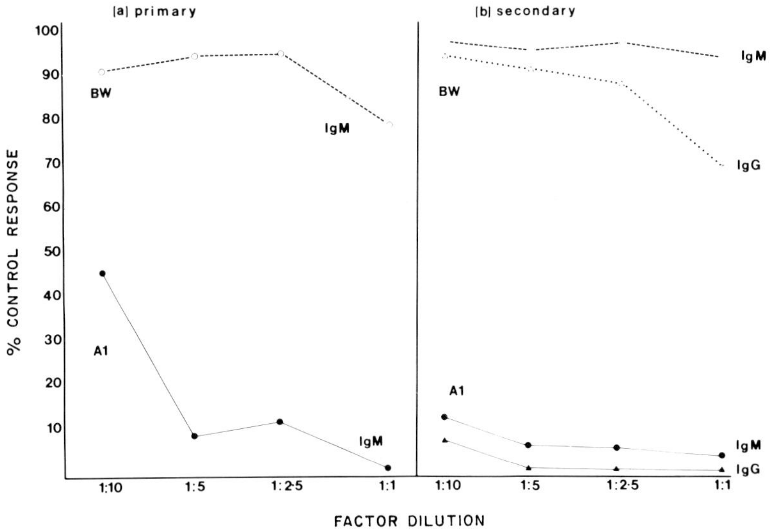

Fig. 1. Suppression of (a) primary IgM response of thoracic duct lymphocytes (TDL) and (b) secondary IgM and IgG responses of spleen cells (C57BL/10) to SRBC *in vitro* by Al supernatant (closed symbols) with BW5147 supernatant as control (open symbols). Factor dilutions shown are before addition to cultures; 1 : 1 indicates undiluted supernatant. Mean positive control responses were 212 PFC/culture for primary IgM, 970 PFC/culture for secondary IgM, and 760 PFC/culture for secondary IgG (5 × 10^5 cells/cultures, volume 225 μl).

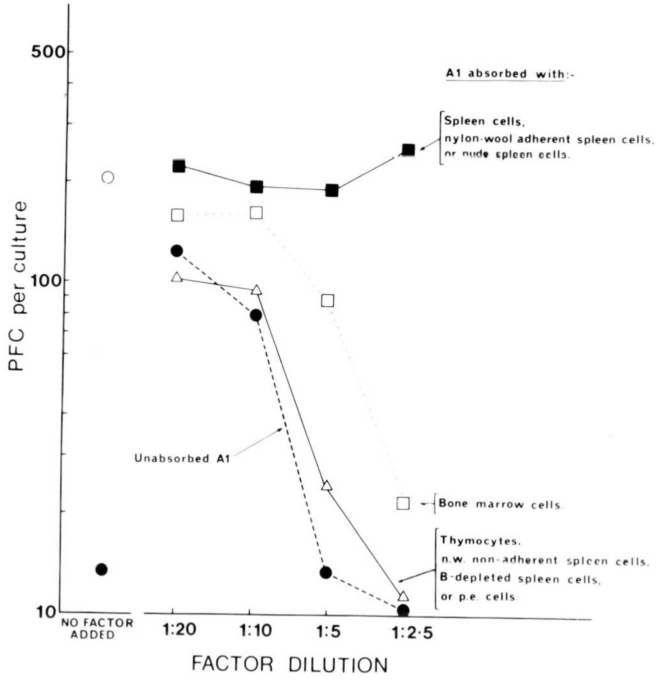

Fig. 2. Absorption of A1 factor by different cell populations. The figure shows the primary anti-SRBC response of CBA mouse TDL in the presence of unabsorbed A1 supernatants (●—●) or of A1 supernatant following its absorption by the cell populations indicated. n.w. nylon wool; p.e. peritoneal exudate. Positive control response (○) in the absence of A1 factor, and background (●) are shown. Data from Taussig *et al.* (1979b).

anti-SRBC responses *in vitro,* as shown in Fig. 1. The suppression only affected responses to SRBC and haptens, such as trinitrophenyl (TNP), coupled to SRBC; moreover, suppression was prevented by absorbing the A1 supernatant with SRBC. The completeness of suppression produced by this supposedly determinant specific material argues against antigen blocking as the mechanism, and the experiments described below support a cellular action of the factor, particularly on B cells.

II. B CELLS AS THE TARGETS FOR A1 FACTOR

A variety of possible mechanisms for the action of antigen-specific suppressor factors can be envisaged, and indeed several different mechanisms have been described. Apart from the blocking of antigen recognition by specific T or B cells, they include the direct action of the factor on a target T cell, B cell, or

TABLE I

Dual Genetic Control of Suppression: Mapping Genes for Absorption of A1 Factor and Suppression of Response[a]

		I									
Strain	K	A	B	J	E	C	S	G	D	Absorbs?	Suppressed?
B10.BR	k	k	k	k	k	k	k	k	k	+	+
B10.S	s	s	s	s	s	s	s	s	s	−	−
B10.S(7R), A.TH	s	s	s	s	s	s	s	s	d	−	−
B10.HTT	s	s	s	s	k	k	k	k	d	+	−
						1					
B10.S(9R)	s	s	—	k	k	d	d	d	d	+	−
A.TL	s	k	k	k	k	k	k	k	d	+	+
		2									

[a] Spleen cells of different strains of mice were tested for ability to absorb A1 factor and for suppressibility by A1 factor. The table shows the haplotypes of the strains used and summarizes the absorption or suppression characteristic of each. "*1*" indicates the location of a gene controlling the absorption trait (acceptor gene), while "2" is a gene controlling suppressibility by A1 (see also Fig. 3).

macrophage, with effects such as inhibition of helper cell action, induction of further suppressor T cells, or liberation of nonspecific mediators from specifically "armed" macrophages (see Taussig, 1980). It is envisaged that a target cell would carry surface "acceptor sites" through which the factor could be bound and that in the presence of antigen the factor would be focused onto the acceptors of antigen-specific cells (in the case of T or B cells). Since acceptor-bearing cells can often be detected by their ability to absorb out a factor in the absence of antigen, we attempted to define the cell types reacting with the A1 factor by absorbing A1 supernatants with different cell populations. Standard aliquots of A1 supernatant were absorbed with equal number of spleen cells (normal or nude); spleen cells depleted of B cells by a rosetting technique; thymocytes; nylon wool adherent or nonadherent spleen cells; peritoneal exudate cells; or bone marrow cells. As Fig. 2 shows, complete absorption was only obtained by populations containing B cells, namely, normal and nude spleen cells and nylon wool adherent spleen cells, while populations lacking B cells failed to absorb. These results suggested that the acceptor-bearing target for the A1 factor was neither a T cell nor a macrophage, but a B cell.

III. GENETIC CONTROL OF SUPPRESSION

When the ability of spleen cells of different mouse strains to absorb the A1 factor were compared, some interesting differences were observed, the cells of some strains being able to absorb much more efficiently than those of others. Moreover the absorption trait is determined by the *H-2* complex. For example, spleen cells of B10 (*H-2*^{b}) mice are 5–10 times more efficient at removing A1 factor than spleen cells of B10.S (*H-2*^{s}); since the strains are congenic, the gene(s) controlling this difference is in *H-2*. At least two other independent haplotypes are "high absorbers," similar to *H-2*^{b}, namely, *H-2*^{k} and *H-2*^{d}. By using recombinant congenic strains derived from the "low absorber" haplotype *H-2*^{s}, an absorption or acceptor gene has been mapped to the right-hand side of *H-2*, as shown in Table I; the acceptor locus, marked "*1*," lies between *I-J* and *H-2D*. This is a similar mapping to the factor itself (Taussig *et al.*, 1979b), a finding reminiscent of the close linkage of factor and acceptor genes for other specific helper and suppressor factors (Munro and Taussig, 1975; Taussig and Munro, 1976; Tada and Okumura, 1979; Tada *et al.*, 1979).

We then asked whether the spleen cells of strains which were relatively inefficient in absorbing the factor (low absorbers) could be suppressed by the factor *in vitro*, anticipating that if the acceptor sites were less able to interact with the

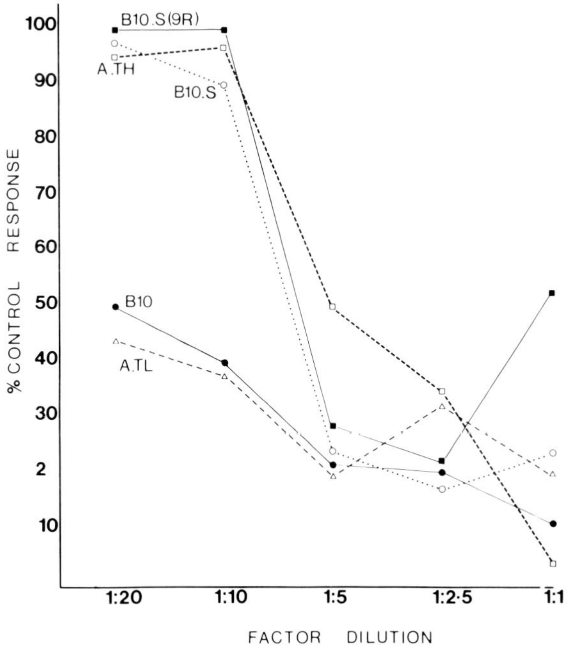

Fig. 3. Suppression of response of different strains by A1 factor. SRBC-primed spleen cells of the mouse strains shown were cultured *in vitro* with SRBC and A1 supernatant at different dilutions. Result as percent of response without A1 factor. (Result for B10.HTT not shown, but similar to B10.S).

factor, the target cells would be more difficult to suppress. A comparison of the action of A1 factor on spleen cells of high and low absorber strains is shown in Fig. 3. B10 and A.TL, high absorbers, were indeed more sensitive to suppression by A1 factor than the low absorbers B10.S and A.TH. Nevertheless, both the latter could be suppressed by high levels of A1 factor, though the 50% end point of activity of A1 was 4–5 times lower than against high absorber strains. However, this experiment also showed that some high absorber strains, notably B10.HTT and B10.S(9R) were as poorly suppressed as the low absorbers B10.S and A.TH (Fig. 3). Thus, the ability to absorb the suppressor factor does not guarantee suppression. When the suppression characteristics of these strains are compared with haplotype, as in Table I, it is apparent that a gene in the *I-A* or *I-B* subregion controls differences in suppressibility; this gene is marked "*2*" in Table I. In fact, these experiments did not answer the question of whether the absorption trait is related to functional suppression, though this could be solved with further recombinants, such as B10.S(8R), which should possess the suppression gene (*2*) while lacking the absorption gene (*1*). Our interim view is that suppression is probably controlled by two MHC genes: gene *1* controls absorption of the suppressor factor to B cells but does not ensure suppression, while gene *2* may control suppression by the factor and antigen bound at the B cell surface. However, although this is an attractive hypothesis, there is yet no evidence that gene *2* is also expressed in B cells, and the involvement of other cell types cannot be excluded.

IV. INTERACTION BETWEEN SUPPRESSOR FACTOR AND MONOCLONAL ANTIBODIES IN REGULATION OF THE IMMUNE RESPONSE

We have recently found that the action of the factor is modified by the presence of anti-SRBC antibodies. The latter were monoclonal products of hybridomas designated D3 (produced locally) and Spl (Köhler and Milstein, 1976), the D3 product being an IgG_2 and Sp1 an IgM antibody. Antibody was added together with A1 supernatant to cultures responding to SRBC. Figure 4 shows that in the presence of the D3 antibody the suppression produced by the factor was markedly enhanced; in the result shown, the concentration of D3 in the culture was well below the level at which it alone had any significant effect on the response. This synergistic effect was also found with higher concentrations of D3, which on their own are partially suppressive. Absorption of the D3 antibody with SRBC prevented the enhancement of suppressor activity. In contrast, the Spl antibody tended to abolish the suppressive activity of A1 factor. As Fig. 5 shows, the magnitude of the effect was dependent on the concentration of Spl antibody. Spl alone partially suppressed at a 1 : 1 initial concentration, but inhi-

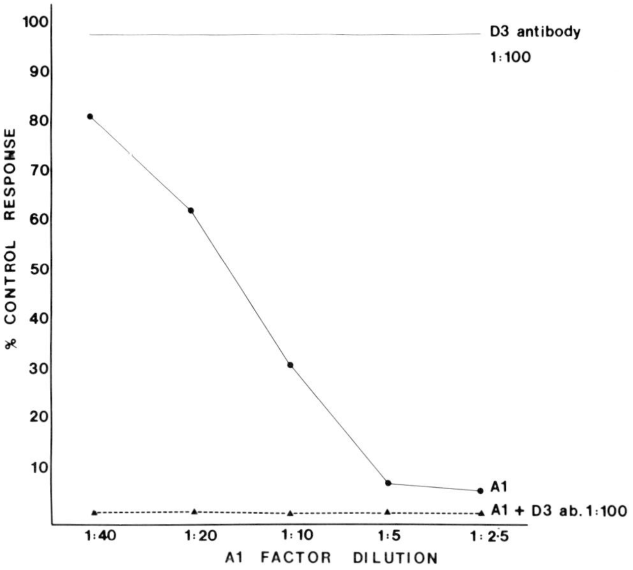

Fig. 4. An IgG monoclonal anti-SRBC antibody enhances suppression by A1 supernatant factor. A1 factor was titrated for suppressive activity in the presence or absence of the D3 IgG anti-SRBC monoclonal antibody (25 μl of a 1 : 100 dilution of D3 supernatant per 225 μl culture). The topmost line shows the effect of D3 alone. Mean positive control response (A1 and D3 omitted) was 342 PFC/culture (5×10^5 spleen cells).

bition was negligible at 1 : 10 and 1 : 100. Once again, the absorption of the monoclonal antibody by SRBC negated its effects. Interestingly, there seems to be mutual reversal of suppression here: at the 1 : 1 level of Sp1, its own partial suppressive effect was no longer operative in the presence of A1 factor.

The modulation of the activity of the A1 suppressor factor by antibody suggests this type of interaction may have physiological importance. Although the results suggest that antibody class may be important in the phenomenon, it must first be established that more trivial explanations do not apply, e.g., that the Sp1 antibody and A1 factor compete for a common site on the red cell. However, it would be logical and advantageous for the activity of T cell factors to be responsive to antibody levels and class. For example, early in a response it may be necessary to circumvent the action of suppressor T cells in order that the response be established; it seems appropriate, therefore, that the IgM anti-SRBC antibody (Sp1) did indeed abolish suppression by the factor. Conversely, later in the response IgG antibody may aid the termination of antibody production through cooperative interaction with suppressor factors as in Fig. 4. Indeed the dependence of antibody feedback on antibody class is recognized (e.g., Henry and Jerne, 1968; Möller, 1980).

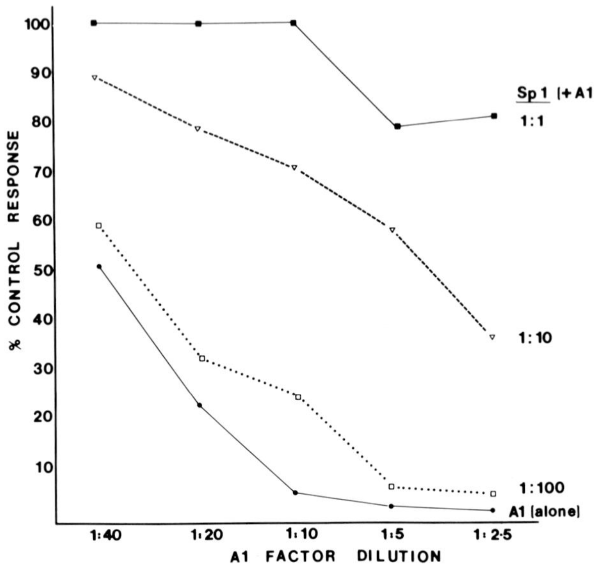

Fig. 5. An IgM monoclonal anti-SRBC antibody abolishes suppression by A1 supernatant factor. A1 suppressive activity was titrated in the presence of Sp1 IgM anti-SRBC antibody (25 μl of different dilutions, from 1 : 1 to 1 : 100, of Sp1 supernatant per 225 μl culture). Sp1 alone produced 65% inhibition at response of 1 : 1, but at 1 : 10 and 1 : 100 was without effect. Mean positive control response (without addition of A1 or Sp1) was 310 PFC/culture.

Our observation also suggests that assays for suppressor factors, as when screening supernatants of T hybrid lines, for instance, might with advantage be carried out in the presence of a small amount of added IgG antibody.

V. CONCLUSION

T cell hybrids clearly have important advantages in the study of antigen-specific T cell factors in terms of a stable supply of material and reproducibility of experimental results—qualities which have not always been prominent features of factors from more conventional sources. They should also help to sort out some of the contradictions which have appeared when factor molecules are studied in different systems if, as seems likely, these contradictions are the result of a fair degree of heterogeneity among factors and the cells producing them. On the other hand, it is only to be expected that the active products of the cloned T hybrid lines, while recognizably factor-like in their major properties, should display idiosyncrasies which may not have been noticed in the extracts or supernatants of antigen-primed T cells. This seems to be the case with the suppressor factor described here. The A1 product is marked out as a T cell factor by its combination of SRBC-specific activity and binding, its non-Ig nature, and its MHC derivation, properties which suggest that its parent cell was a suppressor T cell with specificity for SRBC. However, there are sufficient differences between this factor and others described from suppressor T cells or lines to suggest that it represents a "new" class of factor. A summary of the properties of this class would be as follows.

1. Antigen-specific in suppression and antigen-binding
2. Nonimmunoglobulin
3. High molecular weight
4. MHC component coded between *I-J* and *H-2D*
5. Capable of acting late in the immune response
6. Acts on B cells via an MHC-coded acceptor site

As the other contributions to this treatise illustrate, there are certainly other classes of suppressor factor; T cell hybrids are a means of defining the properties of each one and the functional and structural relationships of the classes to one another.

ACKNOWLEDGMENTS

Sp1 cells were a kind gift of Dr. C. Milstein. I thank Andrew Holliman for his assistance in these experiments and Joan Payne for typing the manuscript.

REFERENCES

Eshhar, Z., Apte, R. N., Löwy, I., Ben-Neriah, Y., Givol, D., and Mozes, E. (1980). T-cell hybridoma bearing heavy chain varible region determinants producing (T,G)-A—L-specific helper factor. *Nature (London)* **286,** 270.

Henry, C., and Jerne, N. K. (1968). Competition of 19 S and 7 S antigen receptors in the regulation of the primary immune response. *J. Exp. Med.* **128,** 133.

Kapp, J. A., Araneo, B. A., and Clevinger, B. L. (1980). Suppression of antibody and T cell proliferative responses to L-glutamic acid^{60}-L-alanine^{30}-L-tyrosine^{10} by a specific monoclonal T cell factor. *J. Exp. Med.* **152,** 235.

Köhler, G., and Milstein, C. (1976). Derivation of specific antibody-producing tissue culture and tumor lines by fusion. *Eur. J. Immunol.* **6,** 511.

Kontiainen, S., Simpson, E., Bohrer, E., Beverley, P. C. L., Herzenberg, L. A., Fitzpatrick, W. C., Vogt, P., Torano, A., McKenzie, I. F. C., and Feldmann, M. (1978). T-cell lines producing antigen-specific suppressor factor. *Nature (London)* **274,** 477.

Lonai, P., Puri, J., and Hammerling, G. J. (1981). H-2 restricted antigen binding by a hybridoma clone that produces antigen specific helper factor. *Proc. Natl. Acad. Sci. U.S.A.* **78,** 549.

Möller, G., ed. (1980) Regulation of the immune response by antibodies against the immunogen. *Immunol. Rev.* **49.**

Munro, A. J., and Taussig, M. J. (1975). Two genes in the major histocompatibility complex control immune response. *Nature (London)* **256,** 103.

Tada, T., and Okumura, K. (1979). The role of antigen-specific T cell factors in the immune response. *Adv. Immunol.* **28,** 1.

Tada, T., Nonaka, M., Okumura, K., Taniguchi, M., and Tokuhisa, T. (1979). Ia antigens on suppressor, amplifier and helper T cells. *In* "Cell Biology and Biochemistry of Leukocyte Function" (M. R. Quastel, ed.), p. 385. Academic Press, New York.

Taniguchi, M., Saito, T., and Tada, T. (1979). Antigen-specific suppressive factor produced by a transplantable I-J-bearing T cell hybridoma. *Nature (London)* **278,** 555.

Taussig, M. J. (1980). Antigen-specific T-cell factors. *Immunology* **41,** 759.

Taussig, M. J. (1982). Studies on an antigen-specific suppressor factor produced by a T-hybrid line. *Lymphokines* **5** (in press).

Taussig, M. J., and Holliman, A. (1979). Structure of an antigen-specific suppressor factor produced by a hybrid T-cell line. *Nature (London)* **277,** 308.

Taussig, M. J., and Munro, A. J. (1976). Cell co-operation mediated by products of genes in the major histocompatibility complex. *In* "Leukocyte Membrane Determinants Regulating Immune Reactivity" (V. P. Eijsvoogel, D. Roos, and W. P. Zeijlemaker, eds.), p. 255 Academic Press, New York.

Taussig, M. J., Corvalan, J. R. F., Binns, R. M., and Holliman, A. (1979a). Production of an H-2 related suppressor factor by a hybrid T-cell line. *Nature (London)* **277,** 305.

Taussig, M. J., Corvalan, J. R. F., and Holliman, A. (1979b). Characterization of an antigen-specific factor from a hybrid T-cell line. *Ann. N.Y. Acad. Sci.* **332,** 316.

Taussig, J. J., Corvalan, J. R. F., Binns, R. M., Roser, B., and Holliman, A. (1979c). Immunological activity of a T hybrid line. I. Production of an H-2 related suppressor factor with specificity for sheep red blood cells. *Eur. J. Immunol.* **9,** 768.

11

Characterization of Antigen-Specific Suppressor Factors from T Cell Hybridomas

Judith A. Kapp/Barbara A. Araneo

I.	Experimental Systems Used to Identify Suppressor T Cells and Their Products	138
	A. Nature of Immune Regulation in Nonresponder Mice	138
	B. Nature of Immune Regulation in Responder Mice	139
II.	Characterization of GAT- and GT-Specific TsF	140
	A. Development of a Panel of Suppressor T Cell Hybridomas	140
	B. Characterization of T Cell Hybridoma Products	140
	C. Expression of Cell Surface Antigens by T Cell Hybridomas	143
III.	Comparison of GAT-TsF and GT-TsF to Other Suppressor T Cell Factors	144
	References	145

One of the biggest problems in immunology today is the nature of the T cell receptor(s) for antigen. The extreme functional heterogeneity of T cell subsets and the number of different antigenic specificities that each T cell subset can recognize suggests that only a few copies of each T cell exist at any given time in normal lymphoid tissues. Perhaps then it is no wonder that T cell receptors have yet to be isolated and characterized. We anticipate that the hybridoma technology that was so successful in the study of B cells by Kohler and Milstein (1975) and now being applied to T cells is one method that will provide sufficient numbers of cells to resolve the T cell receptor problem in the near future. Techniques for maintenance of long-term cultures of normal T cells (MacDonald *et al.*, 1980; Kimoto and Fathman, 1980; Nabel *et al.*, 1981; Fresno *et al.*, 1981) represent an alternative approach, but an approach that we feel will be more useful for the study of physiological mechanisms of cell interactions.

The first of the T cell subsets to be hybridized reproducibly were suppressor T cells (Kontiainen *et al.*, 1978; Taniguchi and Miller, 1978; Kapp *et al.*, 1980).

ISOLATION, CHARACTERIZATION, AND
UTILIZATION OF T LYMPHOCYTE CLONES

ISBN 0-12-249920-4

Using this technology, we have begun characterization of suppressor T cell products specific for the synthetic polymers L-glutamic acid^{60}-L-alanine^{30}-L-tyrosine^{10} (GAT) and L-glutamic acid^{50}-L-tyrosine^{50} (GT).

I. EXPERIMENTAL SYSTEMS USED TO IDENTIFY SUPPRESSOR T CELLS AND THEIR PRODUCTS

For the past 10 years, our studies have focused on the mechanisms by which *Ir* genes control development of responses to GAT and GT. In mice, immune responses to GAT are controlled in an all or none fashion; GAT stimulates development of antibody responses and primes T cells for subsequent proliferative responses in mice bearing the $H\text{-}2^{a,b,d,k}$ haplotypes, but not in mice bearing the $H\text{-}2^{p,q,s}$ haplotypes (Kapp *et al.*, 1973a,b; Schwartz and Paul, 1976; Araneo and Kapp, 1980a). However, GAT complexed to methylated bovine serum albumin (GAT-MBSA) stimulates GAT-specific antibody responses and primes for GAT-specific T cell proliferative responses in both nonresponder and responder mice, suggesting that nonresponsiveness is not the result of a complete absence of GAT-specific T cells or B cells (Kapp *et al.*, 1973a,b; Araneo and Kapp, 1980a).

A. Nature of Immune Regulation in Nonresponder Mice

Although soluble GAT does not stimulate immunity in nonresponders, it does stimulate the development of GAT-specific suppressor T cells that inhibit the development of GAT-specific plaque forming cell (PFC) responses to GAT-MBSA in mice of all three nonresponder haplotypes (Kapp *et al.*, 1974). This observation led to detailed studies of the immunobiology of specific suppressor T cells which demonstrated that a GAT-specific T cell-derived factor (GAT-TsF) obtained from cell extracts mimics suppressor T cell activity *in vivo* and *in vitro* (Kapp *et al.*, 1976, 1977). The active mediator in these extracts is a protein that binds to insolubilized antigen and bears determinants encoded by the *I-J* subregion of the *H-2* gene complex, but does not bear detectable determinants encoded by *IgCH* genes (Thèze *et al.*, 1977a). Nevertheless, GAT-TsF bears idiotypic determinants that cross-react with certain murine GAT-specific antibodies (Germain *et al.*, 1979; Kapp *et al.*, 1981). Lymphoid cell extracts containing GAT-TsF inhibit PFC responses to GAT-MBSA and T cell proliferative responses to GAT, but not MBSA, by lymph node cells from GAT-MBSA primed nonresponder mice (Araneo and Kapp, 1980b). Inhibition of these responses by GAT-TsF does not require syngenicity at *H-2* between donor and acceptor mice (Kapp, 1978), and inhibition of PFC responses by GAT-TsF is mediated by the induction of a new class of suppressor T cells (Germain and Benacerraf, 1978).

All nonresponder mice bearing the $H\text{-}2^{p,q,s}$ haplotypes produce GAT-TsF, and all nonresponder strains are suppressed by GAT-TsF from all other nonresponder strains (Kapp, 1978). That is, there are no known strains that express a genetically controlled defect in the GAT-specific suppressor T cell pathway. Therefore, to further dissect the cellular interactions that occur in the suppressor T cell pathway, we have turned to the related polymer GT and investigated the genetics of suppression by GT-TsF. This system was chosen because antibody responses to GT-MBSA can be suppressed by GT in all strains tested except $H\text{-}2^a$ and $H\text{-}2^b$ mice (Debre *et al.*, 1975a,b). These haplotypes show different defects in the suppressor pathway, since GT induces production of GT-TsF by all strains tested except $H\text{-}2^a$, and all strains except $H\text{-}2^b$ can be suppressed by GT-TsF (Germain *et al.*, 1980). More importantly, the defects manifest in $H\text{-}2^a$ and $H\text{-}2^b$ mice are complementing defects as shown by the fact that GT suppresses the response to GT-MBSA in (B6 × A)F_1 mice (Debre *et al.*, 1975b); thus the F_1 hybrid of two nonsuppressor strains can produce GT-TsF and is sensitive to GT-TsF. GT-TsF, like GAT-TsF, is an antigen-specific, $I\text{-}J^+$ protein that inhibits GT-specific antibody and T cell proliferative responses (Theze *et al.*, 1977b; Araneo and Kapp, 1981). Recent data demonstrate that no allogeneic barrier to GT-TsF-mediated suppression exits but that two complementing genes encoded by the *H-2* gene complex are required for susceptibility to suppression by GT-TsF (Araneo and Kapp, 1981).

B. Nature of Immune Regulation in Responder Mice

In responder ($H\text{-}2^{a,b,d,k}$) mice GAT stimulates PFC responses and primes for radioresistant helper T cells and T cells that can undergo a proliferative response, but fails to stimulate detectable GAT-specific suppressor T cells under conditions where specific suppressor T cells are observed in nonresponder mice (Kapp *et al.*, 1974). Nevertheless, we have identified a GAT-specific suppressor T cell system in responder strain that develops after the peak, primary immune response to GAT. This suppressor T cell subset was identified in studies designed to investigate why virgin responder spleen cells develop antibody responses to GAT-pulsed syngeneic or allogeneic macrophages (Mϕ), whereas immune spleen cells respond preferentially to the GAT-Mϕ used for priming *in vivo* (Pierce *et al.*, 1976, 1977). When spleen cells from normal mice were cocultured with T cells from primed mice, antibody responses to GAT developed only in the presence of GAT-Mϕ syngeneic with the Mϕ used for priming. Moreover, the lack of responses in cultures stimulated with inappropriate GAT-Mϕ was due to the activity of GAT-specific suppressor T cells (Pierce and Kapp, 1978) or suppressor T cell promotor cells (Pierce *et al.*, 1982). Thus, the genetic restriction observed in responses of immune spleen cells is dominant and is associated with regulatory activity of GAT-specific T cells. Development of GAT-specific suppressor T cells appears to be a natural consequence of the immune response to

GAT in responder mice as well as nonresponder mice. The immunobiology of this T cell subset is currently under investigation.

II. CHARACTERIZATION OF GAT- AND GT-SPECIFIC TsF

A. Development of a Panel of Suppressor T Cell Hybridomas

Further analysis of the biochemistry, serology, and biology of specific suppressor T cell factors has been hampered by the small amount of material that can be extracted from or is secreted by primed lymphoid cells. Thus, 3 years ago we initiated experiments to produce stable T cell hybridomas that synthesize suppressor factors constitutively. Supernatants from such T cell hybridomas provide a rich source of suppressor factor compared with extracts of lymphoid cells as demonstrated by the fact that each milliliter of supernatant from 258C4-4, the prototype suppressor factor, contains 20 to 40 times the amount of suppressor material that can be obtained in an extract of the lymphoid cells in an entire mouse (Kapp *et al.*, 1980). To date we have produced T cell hybridomas by individually fusing the AKR thymoma BW5147 with suppressor T cells from GAT-primed nonresponders bearing the $H\text{-}2^{q}$ or $H\text{-}2^{s}$ haplotypes or GT-primed nonresponders bearing the $H\text{-}2^{b,d,k}$ or $H\text{-}2^{s}$ haplotypes. Several hybridomas have been cloned from each haplotype, including some that do not make TsF to be used as controls. The suppressor mediators produced by these T cell hybridomas are proteins that have antigen-binding activity, determinants encoded by the *I-J* subregion, and idiotypic determinants that cross-react with certain murine antibodies specific for GAT (Kapp *et al.*, 1981). In addition, two hybridomas have been derived from GAT-primed responder C57BL/10 T cells by fusion during the time in which suppressor T cells associated with genetic restriction were detectable.

Our strategy for the analysis of suppressor T cell products was to develop a panel of T cell hybridomas from different haplotypes expressing distinct fine antigenic specificities. A partial list of T cell hybridomas currently available is shown in Table I. In most fusions, more than one active hybridoma was obtained and saved, but as yet only one cloned hybridoma per fusion has been well characterized.

B. Characterization of T Cell Hybridoma Products

1. *Isolation and Purification of Monoclonal GAT-TsF*

In collaboration with Drs. David Webb and Stanley Stein at the Roche Institute of Molecular Biology we have purified GAT-TsF from hybridoma clone 258C4-4 ($H\text{-}2^{q}$). This has been accomplished by a sequence of affinity

TABLE I

Currently Available T Cell Hybridomas

				TsF Activity in Supernate			
Clone	Strain	*H-2*	Priming Antigen	S_{50} U/ml[a]	Ia	CGAT[b]	GA-1[c]
258C4-4	DBA/1	*q*	GAT	20,000	I^q	+	+
258C4-5	DBA/1	*q*	GAT	<1,000[d]	—	−	−
342B1-11	B10.S	*s*	GAT	35,000	$I\text{-}J^s$	+	−
365A1-1	B10.S	*s*	GAT	<1,000[d]	—	−	−
365A2-4	B10.S	*s*	GAT	8,400	$I\text{-}J^s$	NT[e]	NT
359C1-12	B10	*b*	GAT	10,000	NT	NT	NT
366D3-2	B10	*b*	GT	30,000	$I\text{-}J^b$	+	−
368B1-5	BALB/c	*d*	GT	27,000	NT	+	−
367A5-2	CBA	*k*	GT	17,000	$I\text{-}J^k$	NT	NT
395A4-4	B10.S	*s*	GT	36,000	$I\text{-}J^s$	±	−

[a] S_{50} U is the inverse dilution of supernate causing 50% suppression of specific PFC response.

[b] Common idiotypic determinant expressed by anti-GAT antibodies that bind GT as well as GAT.

[c] Common idiotypic determinant expressed by anti-GAT antibodies that bind GA as well as GAT.

[d] No detectable suppressive activity in clones which were isolated from the same fusion as 285C4-4 or 365A2-4, therefore these clones serve as negative controls in many experiments.

[e] NT, not tested.

chromatography, three cycles of reverse phase high performance liquid chromatography (HPLC), and ion exchange HPLC which resulted in a final purification factor of 5.2×10^7 as monitored by bioactivity. Based on the fact that we have isolated a protein that has antigen-specific suppressive activity and that the protein and biological activity copurify as a single moiety by both reverse phase and DEAE-HPLC, we conclude that GAT-TsF has been purified to homogeneity (Krupen *et al.*, 1982 in press). From 6000 ml of culture supernate, approximately 2 μg of purified protein was obtained. However, since only fractions containing the peak suppressive activity were selected at each step of the purification scheme, this recovery could be as low as 50% of the actual bioactive material. Therefore, the original supernatant fluids probably contain 0.5 to 1.0 ng GAT-TsF per ml. If the specific activity (7.8×10^4 S_{50}U/ng) of this hybridoma product is a close approximation of the specific activity of factors produced *in vivo,* then extracts of the lymphoid cells from GAT-primed mice would yield about 0.013 ng GAT-TsF per mouse. Clearly, only the application of hybridoma technology to the production of these T cell-derived mediators could have provided sufficient material for purification and subsequent biochemical and structural analysis.

The purified factor is composed of a single polypeptide chain that has a molecular weight of approximately 24,000 by SDS-PAGE under reducing or nonreducing conditions; it suppresses both antibody and T cell proliferative responses specifically (Krupen *et al.*, 1982; in press). This estimated size conflicts with the previous estimates of 50,000 MW obtained by Sephadex chromatography of GAT-TsF in extracts (Thèze *et al.*, 1977a) and in the crude supernatant from this clone 258C4-4 (Kapp *et al.*, 1980). The original estimates could have been erroneous if GAT-TsF is not a globular protein. Alternatively, under physiological conditions GAT-TsF may exist as a complex composed of two noncovalently linked 24,000 dalton subunits or even as a complex with other proteins that are not essential for biological activity. Experiments to resolve this discrepancy are in progress.

We are convinced that the procedures developed for purifying this TsF will be generally applicable to other TsF, since GAT-TsF produced by the T cell hybridoma, 342B1-11, has been purified using the same methods, and only minor variations in elution volumes were detected between the $H\text{-}2^q$ and $H\text{-}2^s$ TsF (Healy *et al.*, 1982). We anticipate that biochemical and structural comparison of several purified monoclonal TsF molecules will provide information concerning the degree of homology between members of a family of closely related T cell products from responder and nonresponder mice.

2. *Mechanism(s) of Action of TsF*

The demonstration that monoclonal GAT-TsF inhibits both PFC and proliferation responses suggests that a single mediator is capable of inhibiting two different GAT-specific responses. We consider the possibility that individual hybrids are producing two functionally distinct, GAT-specific factors unlikely because the factor which has been purified to apparent homogeneity is also capable of suppressing both antibody and proliferative responses.

Since it had been demonstrated earlier that GAT-TsF (Germain and Benacerraf, 1978) and GT-TsF (Waltenbaugh *et al.*, 1977) mediated suppression by activation of a new class of suppressor T cells, we examined the ability of monoclonal GT-TsF to induce suppressor T cells. Induction of suppressor T cells by TsF contained in extracts required a minute amount of antigen. Therefore, we injected 0.5 ml of supernate containing monoclonal GT-TsF from the BALB/c hybridoma 368B1-5 with or without 10 ng GT iv into DBA/2 recipients. Seven days after injection, spleen cells were cultured, and those mice receiving TsF plus 10 ng GT were unresponsive to GT-MBSA but capable of developing normal PFC responses to SRBC; recipients of TsF or GT alone responded normally to both GT-MBSA and SRBC (data not shown). More importantly, this specific unresponsiveness was associated with suppressor cells, as demonstrated by the ability of spleen cells from these treated mice to inhibit the response to GT-MBSA by spleen cells from normal, syngeneic mice (Table II). Suppression was abrogated by treating spleen cells with anti-Thy-1.2 and complement suggesting that TsF induced suppressor T (Ts2) cells. Experiments are currently underway to characterize the DBA/2 Ts2 cells by characterizing the T cell hybrids produced by fusing Ts2 to BW5147.

TABLE II

Induction of Suppressor Cells by Injection of Monoclonal GT-TsF + 10 ng GT

Normal DBA/2 spleen cells ($\times 10^6$)	2×10^6 DBA/2 spleen cells from mice injected with[a]	IgC PFC/culture[b]	
		GT-MBSA	SRBC
5	—	555	500
7	—	895	885
5	GT-TsF	505	1895
5	10 ng GT	420	820
5	GT-TsF + 10 ng GT	5	1970

[a] Mice injected iv with 0.5 ml culture supernate or 10 ng GT or both.

[b] Spleen cells were cultured for 5 days using modified Mishell-Dutton culture conditions and assayed for PFC responses using GAT-SRBC or SRBC as indicator cells.

Several Ts2 hybridomas that produce specific suppressive factors have been cloned and preliminary characterization of the soluble factor (GT-TsF2) indicates that it is antigen-specific in activity, has antigen-specific binding site(s), and is I-J^+ and MHC-restricted (Kapp and Araneo, 1982, submitted for publication). Thus, GT-TsF2 closely resembles the carrier-specific, I-J^+, genetically restricted suppressor factor described by Tada, *et al.* (1976). Since GT-TsF2 was induced by GT-TsF1, we suggest that cells producing GT-TsF1 are an early cell in the suppressor pathway and that this cell is required for the activation of antigen-specific, MHC-restricted TsF-producing cells. Hybridoma Ts2 cells should provide the opportunity to characterize TsF products and subsequently to determine if there are additional cells in the suppressor pathway as suggested by Germain and Benacerraf (1981). We believe that the use of monoclonal hybridoma products sequentially to activate additional cells in the suppressor T cell pathway may result in the identification of a complete set of cells essential to one pathway. Such studies will begin to address the issues of how complex are the pathways of suppression and what is the relationship among the T cells and/or T cell products of a given sequence.

C. Expression of Cell Surface Antigens by T Cell Hybridomas

In addition to providing a stable source of suppressor factor, these T cell hybridomas can be useful for detecting new cell surface alloantigens and mapping new *I* region encoded determinants such as *I-J*. In collaboration with Drs. Donald C. Shreffler, Vera Haupfeld, and JoAnn Trial, we have begun to characterize cell surface antigens expressed by these T cell hybridomas using cytotoxicity and immunofluorescence techniques. Alloantisera were first used to examine the expression of serologically detectable determinants controlled by genes within the *H-2* gene complex by the T cell hybridomas. It soon became clear that it would be very difficult to interpret any data obtained with alloantisera for three reasons: (1) the suppressor hybridomas, as well as the BW5147 thymoma, express the murine leukemia virus product, gp70 (Tung and Fleissner, 1980), and many alloantisera contain anti-gp70 activity (Nowinski and Kaehler, 1974); (2) there is an endless variety of recombinant forms of gp70 that potentially may be expressed by hybridomas (Elder *et al.*, 1977); and (3) the relative expression of gp70 and MHC gene products is not constant throughout the cell cycle (J. Trial, unpublished observations). Some alloantisera repeatedly exhibited the expected pattern of reactivities on a panel of hybridoma cells, but many antisera reacted more broadly than expected, and often inappropriately based on the known genetic constitution of the cells. Given such ambiguities, we do not believe it is valid to conclude that the expected reactivities are of relevance, whereas the unexpected are not. Although absorption with BW5147 removes most of the unexpected reactivities, one cannot reigorously conclude that residual positive reactions with the hybridomas are due to the expression of *H-2* gene products, rather than to the expression on the hybridomas of gp70 molecules that are *different* from those on BW5147.

A more clear-cut approach which avoids the problem of anti-gp70 activity has been the use of monoclonal antibodies derived from hybridoma supernatant fluids to characterize the surface phenotypes of suppressor T cell hybridomas. Our preliminary studies demonstrate that these hybridomas do bear the Lyt 1^+2^+ phenotype and I-J determinants using monoclonal anti-I-J antibodies prepared and donated by Dr. Carl Waltenbaugh, Northwestern University (Waltenbaugh, 1980). These T cell hybridomas are also being used as immunogens to produce alloantisera against new antigenic determinants and to screen B cell hybridoma products produced by fusion of B cells from mice immunized with cells disparate at the *I-J* subregion in order to determine whether the *I-J* subregion encodes multiple distinct proteins.

In collaboration with Dr. Susan E. Cullen, we are asking whether the suppressor factor found in the supernate is represented on the cell surface as suggested by the observation that the T cell hybridomas bear serologically detectable I-J determinants. If membrane-bound factor is demonstrated, then we will ask whether it represents an antigen-specific receptor (analogous to the relationship between membrane-bound and secreted IgM) or whether it represents soluble factor transiently associated with membrane enroute to secretion.

III. COMPARISON OF GAT-TsF AND GT-TsF TO OTHER SUPPRESSOR T CELL FACTORS

Comparison of antigen-specific suppressor factors from extracts, T cell hybridomas, and cloned T cell lines reveals a large number of shared characteristics as well as some disparities. All of these factors bind antigen specifically and most bear determinants encoded by the *I-J* subregion of the MHC. Nevertheless, there are substantial differences in the molecular weights of these factors ranging from 24,000 to 100,000 (Krupen *et al.*, 1982, in press; Thèze *et al.*, 1977a,b; Taniguchi *et al.*, 1981; Taussig and Holliman, 1979; Fresno *et al.*, 1981). More importantly, some of these factors appear to be single polypeptide chains (Krupen *et al.*, 1982; Fresno *et al.*, 1981), whereas others are composed of two different polypeptide chains (Taniguchi *et al.*, 1981). Some of these factors are genetically restricted and require that factor donors and recipients share MHC encoded genes, some of which have been mapped to the *I-J* subregion (Tada *et al.*, 1976; Deitz *et al.*, 1981); other factors bearing *I-J* encoded determinants have no genetic restrictions in activity (Kapp, 1978; Deitz *et al.*, 1981). Furthermore, some TsF even show restrictions that are allotype- and/or idiotype linked (Hirari and Nisonoff, 1980; Weinberger *et al.*, 1980). Although some of the apparent differences among these antigen-specific, T cell-derived suppressor factors may be trivial experimental variations, it seems clear that some differences are real. In our opinion, these differences most likely reflect differences in products produced by different T cell subsets. Whether these suppressor T cell subsets all can be organized into a "consensus" pathway as proposed by Germain and Benacerraf (1981) or whether different subsets interact in different pathways remains an issue to be resolved. Elucidation of the structure of these diverse TsF should provide insight into the relationship of the various suppressor T cell subsets.

ACKNOWLEDGMENTS

We thank Yvette Fulcher and John Hauenstein for technical assistance; Barbara Wollberg for secretarial assistance; and our colleagues for helpful criticism and encouragement. This investigation was supported by U.S. Public Health Service Grants AI-13987 and AI-15353 from the National Institute of Allergy and Infectious Diseases and Grant PCM 80-21809 from The National Science Foundation. Judith Kapp is the recipient of U.S. Public Health Service Research Career Development Award AI-00361 from the National Institute of Allergy and Infectious Diseases.

REFERENCES

Araneo, B. A., and Kapp, J. A. (1980a). *H-2*-linked *Ir* gene control of T cell proliferative responses to the synthetic terpolymer L-glutamic acid^{60}-L-alanine^{30}-L-tyrosine^{10} (GAT). I. Requirements for T cell activation in responder and nonresponder mice. *J. Immunol.* **124**, 1492–1497.

Araneo, B. A., and Kapp, J. A. (1980b). Immunosuppressive factor(s) from lymphoid cells of nonresponder mice primed with L-glutamic acid^{60}-L-alanine^{30}-L-tyrosine^{10} (GAT). V. Inhibition of T cell proliferative responses. *J. Immunol.* **125**, 118–123.

Araneo, B. A., and Kapp, J. A. (1981). Genetic analysis of immune suppression. I. Gene complementation is required for suppression of antigen-specific proliferative responses by T cell derived factors. *Immunogenetics* **14,** 221–230.

Debre, P., Kapp, J. A., and Benacerraf, B. (1975a). Genetic control of specific immune suppression. I. Experimental conditions for the stimulation of suppressor cells by the copolymer L-glutamic acid^{50}-L-tyrosine^{50} (GT) in BALB/c mice. *J. Exp. Med.* **142,** 1436.

Debre, P., Kapp, J. A., Dorf, M. E., and Benacerraf, B. (1975b). Genetic control of specific immune suppression. II. *H-2* linked dominant genetic control of immune suppression by the random copolymer L-glutamic acid^{50}-L-tyrosine^{50} (GT). *J. Exp. Med.* **142,** 1447.

Deitz, M. H., Sy, M.-S., Benacerraf, B., Nisonoff, A., Greene, M. I., and Germain, R. N. (1981). Antigen-and receptor-driven regulatory mechanisms. VII. *H-2* restricted anti-idiotypic suppressor factor from efferent suppressor T cells. *J. Exp. Med.* **153,** 450.

Elder, J. H., Jensen, F. C., Bryant, M. L., and Lerner, R. A. (1977). Polymorphism of the major envelope glycoprotein (gp 70) of murine C-type viruses: Virus-associated and differentiation antigens encoded by a multi-gene family. *Nature (London)* **267,** 23.

Fresno, M., McVay-Boudreau, L., Nable, G., and Cantor, H. (1981). Antigen-specific T lymphocyte clones. II. Purification and biological characterization of an antigen-specific suppressive protein synthesized by cloned T cells. *J. Exp. Med.* **153,** 1260.

Germain, R. N., and Benacerraf, B. (1978). Antigen-specific T cell-mediated suppression. III. Induction of antigen-specific suppressor T cells (Ts2) in L-glutamic acid^{60}-L-alanine^{30}-L-tyrosine^{10} (GAT-responder mice by nonresponder-derived GAT-suppressor factor (GAT-TsF). *J. Immunol.* **121,** 608.

Germain, R. N., and Benacerraf, B. (1981). A single major pathway of T-lymphocyte interactions in antigen-specific immune suppression. *Scand. J. Immunol.* **13,** 1–10.

Germain, R. N., Ju, S.-T., Kipps, T. J., Benacerraf, B., and Dorf, M. E. (1979). Shared idiotypic determinants on antibodies and T-cell-derived suppressor factor specific for the random terpolymer L-glutamic acid^{60}-L-alanine^{30}-L-tyrosine^{10}. *J. Exp. Med.* **149,** 613.

Germain, R. N., Waltenbaugh, C., and Benacerraf, B. (1980). Antigen-specific T cell mediated suppression. V. *H-2* linked genetic control of distinct antigen-specific defects in the production and activity of L-glutamic acid^{50}-L-tyrosine suppressor factor (GT-TsF). *J. Exp. Med.* **151,** 1245.

Healy, C., Araneo, B. A., Kapp, J. A., and Webb, D. R. (1981). In preparation.

Hirari, Y., and Nisonoff, A. (1980). Selective suppression of the major idiotypic component of an anti-hapten responses by soluble T cell-derived factors with idiotypic or anti-idiotypic receptors. *J. Exp. Med.* **151,** 1213.

Kapp, J. A. (1978). Immunosuppressive factor(s) from lymphoid cells of nonresponder mice primed with L-glutamic acid^{60}-L-alanine^{30}-L-tyrosine^{10} (GAT). IV. Lack of strain restrictions among allogeneic nonresponder donors and recipients. *J. Exp. Med.* **147,** 997.

Kapp, J. A., and Araneo, B. A. (1982). Antigen-specific suppressor T cell interactions, I. Induction of an MHC-restricted suppressor factor specific for L-glutamic acid^{50}-L-tyrosine^{50}. *J. Immunol.* (In press.)

Kapp, J. A., Pierce, C. W., and Benacerraf, B. (1973a). Genetic control of immune responses *in vitro*. I. Development of primary and secondary plaque-forming cell responses to the random terpolymer L-glutamic acid^{60}-L-alanine^{30}-L-tyrosine^{10} (GAT) my mouse spleen cells *in vitro*. *J. Exp. Med.* **138,** 1107.

Kapp, J. A., Pierce, C. W., and Benacerraf, B. (1973b). Genetic control of immune responses *in vitro*. II. Cellular requirements for the development of primary plaque-forming cell responses to the random terpolymer L-glutamic acid^{60}-L-alanine^{30}-L-tyrosine^{10} (GAT) by mouse spleen cells *in vitro*. *J. Exp. Med.* **138,** 1121.

Kapp, J. A., Pierce, C. W., Schlossman, S., and Benacerraf, B. (1974). Genetic control of immune responses *in vitro*. V. Stimulation of suppressor T cells in nonresponder mice by the terpolymer L-glutamic acid^{60}-L-alanine^{30}-L-tyrosine^{10} (GAT). *J. Exp. Med.* **140,** 648.

Kapp, J. A., Pierce, C. W., DaLaCroix, F., and Benacerraf, B. (1976). Immunosuppressive factor(s) extracted from lymphoid cells of nonresponder mice primed with L-glutamic acid^{60}-L-alanine^{30}-L-tyrosine^{10} (GAT). I. Activity and antigenic specificity. *J. Immunol.* **116,** 305.

Kapp, J. A., Pierce, C. W., and Benacerraf, B. (1977). Immunosuppressive factor(s) extracted from lymphoid cells of nonresponder mice primed with L-glutamic acid^{60}-L-alanine^{30}-L-tyrosine^{10} (GAT). II. Cellular source and effects on responder and nonresponder mice. *J. Exp. Med.* **145,** 828–838.

Kapp, J. A., Araneo, B. A., and Clevinger, B. L. (1980). Suppression of antibody and T cell proliferative responses to L-glutamic acid^{60}-L-alanine^{30}-L-tyrosine^{10} (GAT) by a specific monoclonal T cell factor. *J. Exp. Med.* **152,** 235.

Kapp, J. A., Araneo, B. A., Ju, S.-T., and Dorf, M. E. (1981). Immunogenetics of monoclonal suppressor T cell products. (In press.)

Kimoto, M., and Fathman, C. G. (1981). Antigen-reactive T cell clones. I. Transcomplementating hybrid *I-A*-region gene products function effectively in antigen-presentation. *J. Exp. Med.* **152,** 759.

Kohler, G., and Milstein, C. (1975). Continuous cultures of fused cells secreting antibody of predefined specificity. *Nature (London)* **256,** 495.

Kontiainen, S., Simpson, E., Bohrer, E., Beverley, P. E. L., Herzenberg, L. A. Fitzpatrick, W. C., Vogt, P., Torano, A., McKenzie, I. F. C., and Feldmann, M. (1978). T cell lines producing antigen-specific suppressor factor. *Nature (London)* **274,** 477.

Krupen, K., Araneo, B. A., Brink, L., Kapp, J. A., Stein, S., Wieder, K. J., and Webb, D. R. (1982). Purification of a monoclonal T cell suppressor factor specific for L-glutamic acid^{60}-L-alanine^{30}-L-tyrosine^{10} (GAT). *Proc. Natl. Acad. Sci.,* in press.

MacDonald, H. R., Cerottini, J. C., Ryser, J. E., Maryanski, T. L., Taswell, C., Widmer, M. B., and Brunner, K. Y. (1980). Qualtitation and cloning of cytolytic T lymphocytes and their precursors. *Immunol. Rev.* **51,** 93.

Nabel, G., Fresno, M., Chessman, A., and Cantor, H. (1981). Use of cloned populations of mouse lymphocytes to analyze cellular differentiation. *Cell* **23,** 19–28.

Nowinski, R. C., and Kaehler, S. L. (1974). Antibody to leukemia virus: Widespread occurrence in inbred mice. *Science* **185,** 869.

Pierce, C. W., and Kapp, J. A. (1978). Suppressor T-cell activity in responder × nonresponder (C57BL/10 × DBA/1)F_1 spleen cells responsive to L-glutamic acid^{60}-L-alanine^{30}-L-tyrosine^{10}. *J. Exp. Med.* **148,** 1282.

Pierce, C. W., Kapp, J. A., and Benacerraf, B. (1976). Regulation by the *H-2* gene complex of macrophage-lymphoid cell interactions in secondary antibody responses *in vitro*. *J. Exp. Med.* **144,** 371.

Pierce, C. W., Germain, R. N., Kapp, J. A., and Benacerraf, B. (1977). Secondary antibody responses *in vitro* to L-glutamic acid^{60}-L-alanine^{30}-L-tyrosine^{10} (GAT) by (responder × nonresponder)F_1 spleen cells stimulated by parental GAT-macrophages. *J. Exp. Med.* **146,** 1827.

Pierce, C. W. *et al.* (1982). In preparation.

Schwartz, R. H., and Paul, W. E. (1976). T-lymphocyte-enriched murine peritoneal exudate cells. II. Genetic control of antigen-induced T-lymphocyte proliferation. *J. Exp. Med.* **143,** 529.

Tada, T., Taniguchi, M., and David, C. S. (1976). Properties of the antigen-specific suppressive T cell factor in the regulation of antibody response in the mouse. IV. Special subregion assignment of the gene(s) which codes for the suppressive T cell factor in the *H-2* histocompatibility complex. *J. Exp. Med.* **144,** 713.

Taniguchi, M., and Miller, J. F. A. P. (1978). Specific suppressive factors produced by hybridomas derived from the fusion of enriched suppressor T cells and a T lymphoma cell line. *J. Exp. Med.* **148,** 373.

Taniguchi, M., Saito, T., Takei, I., and Takuhisa, T. (1981). Presence of interchain disulfide bonds between two gene products that compose the secreted form of an antigen-specific suppression factor. *J. Exp. Med.* **153,** 1672.

Taussig, M. J., and Holliman, A. (1979). Production of an *H-2*-related suppressor factor by a hybrid T cell line. *Nature (London)* **277,** 305.

Thèze, J., Kapp, J. A., and Benacerraf, B. (1977a). Immunosuppressive factor(s) extracted from lymphoid cells of nonresponder mice primed with L-glutamic acid^{60}-L-alanine^{30}-L-tyrosine^{10} (GAT). III. Immunochemical properties of the GAT-specific suppressive factor. *J. Exp. Med.* **145,** 839.

Thèze, J., Waltenbaugh, C., Germain, R. N., and Benacerraf, B. (1977b). Immunosuppressive factor(s) specific for L-glutamic acid^{50}-L-tyrosine^{50} (GT). IV. *In vitro* activity and immunochemical properties. *Eur. J. Immunol.* **7,** 705.

Tung, J. and Fleissner, E. (1980). Amplified *env* and *gag* products on AKR cells. origins from different murine leukemia virus genomes. *J. Exp. Med.* **151,** 975.

Waltenbaugh, C. (1981). Regulation of immune responses by I-J gene products. I. Production and characterization of anti-I-J monoclonal antibodies. *J. Exp. Med.* **154,** 1570.

Waltenbaugh, C., Thèze, J., Kapp, J. A., and Benacerraf, B. (1977). Immunosuppressive factor(s) specific for L-glutamic acid^{50}-L-tyrosine^{50} (GT). III. Generation of suppressor T cells by a suppressive extract derived from GT-primed lymphoid cells. *J. Exp. Med.* **146,** 970–985.

Weinberger, J. Z., Germain, R. N., Benacerraf, B., and Dorf, M. E. (1980). Hapten-specific T-cell responses to 4-hydroxy-3-nitrophenyl acetyl. V. Role of idiotypes in the suppressor pathway. *J. Exp. Med.* **152,** 161.

12

Suppression of Antibody Responses by a T Cell Hybridoma-Derived Haplotype-Specific Suppressor Factor

Craig M. Sorensen/Carl W. Pierce

I.	Properties of TsF-H	150
II.	Mechanism of Action of TsF-H	152
III.	Conclusions	153
	References	155

Injection of neonatal C57BL/10 (B10) mice with 2×10^7 semiallogeneic (B10 × B10.D2)F_1 spleen cells results in the generation of a population of haplotype-specific suppressor T cells which suppress primary, but not secondary, antibody responses and fail to suppress mixed lymphocyte and cytotoxic lymphocyte responses (Sorensen and Pierce, 1981a). Restimulation of these T cells with B10.D2 macrophages (Mϕ) results in the production of a soluble suppressor factor, TsF-H, which substitutes for the haplotype-specific suppressor T cell in causing abrogation of primary plaque-forming cell (PFC) responses by syngeneic spleen cells to a variety of T cell-dependent and -independent antigens. TsF-H fails to suppress secondary antibody responses and T cell responses to conventional antigens and alloantigens (Sorensen and Pierce, 1981b).

Detailed analysis of this suppressor T cell factor, as well as other suppressor factors, has been hampered by the inability to obtain sufficiently large quantities of material for study. Amounts of material secreted into culture supernatant fluids are often sufficient only for functional biological characterization and do not allow detailed biochemical or structural analysis. This problem has been overcome by the successful fusion of the TsF-H producing cell with the AKR thymoma, BW5147, to produce a hybridoma cell line which secretes TsF-H in a constitutive basis. In this chapter, we describe some of the properties of TsF-H and present some data on possible mechanism(s) of action.

ISOLATION, CHARACTERIZATION, AND
UTILIZATION OF T LYMPHOCYTE CLONES

ISBN 0-12-249920-4

I. PROPERTIES OF TsF-H

The fusion of activated B10 haplotype-specific suppressor cells with BW5147 resulted in 30 primary fusion wells showing growth (Sorensen and Pierce, 1981b,c). Cloning of cells from the seven wells that showed suppression of primary PFC responses by B10 spleen cells yielded two clones with significant suppressive activity in the culture supernatant fluids. One of these clones, 267.A4.A1, was chosen for further analysis and characterization; the negative clone from the same fusion 267.C4.C4 was the source of control factor. Similar to the findings made with conventional supernatant fluids from haplotype-specific Ts cells, supernatant fluid from 267.A4.A1 was capable of suppressing *in vitro* primary PFC responses in an antigen nonspecific manner. Significant suppression (> 50%) was demonstrated at final dilutions as great as 1/100,000 in culture; at no dilution was significant suppression (> 15%) seen by supernatant fluids from BW5147 or 267.C4.C4. Suppression was limited to primary PFC responses to a wide variety of antigens; no demonstrable effect on secondary PFC responses, cytotoxic T lymphocyte (CTL) responses, or mixed lymphocyte responses (MLR) was observed (Sorensen and Pierce, 1981b,c). More recent data suggest that both conventional and hybridoma-derived TsF-H are unable to suppress antigen-specific proliferation of T cells (C. M. Sorensen and C. W. Pierce,

TABLE I

Serological Characterization of 267.A4.A1

		% Control response GAT-specific PFC/culture[a]	
Immunoabsorbent	Specificity	Effluent[b]	Eluate[b]
None		16	
(B10.A × A)anti-B10.A(5R)	(KAB)^b	100	5
(B10.MBR × A/Sn)anti-B10.A(5R)	(A)^b	125	6
(B10.A × B10)anti-B10.D2	(KABJE)^d	12	88
B10.A(5R)anti-B10.A(3R)	(J)^b	6	94
(A.TL × B10.S(9R))anti-B10.HTT	(J)^s	7	93
RαMIg	"C_H"	10	89
BSA		8	96
PNA	D-GAL	107	7

[a] B10 spleen cells (5 × 10^6) were cultured with 2 μg GAT and TsF-H (1/1000 final dilution) under Mishell-Dutton conditions; IgG GAT-specific PFC/culture were determined on day 5. Data are presented as percent control responses; control response was 485 IgG GAT-specific PFC/culture.

[b] Effluents from immunoabsorbents were tested directly; eluates were obtained with 2.0 *M* KCl and dialyzed prior to assay.

TABLE II

Activity of Hybridoma-Derived TsF-H *in Vivo*

Treatment of animals[a]	Day 5 PFC/culture[a] GAT	SRBC
None	510	20,410
10 μg GAT	498	16,100
200 μl PBS	463	15,800
200 μl PBS + 10 μg GAT	513	17,510
200 μl 267.A4.A1	10	5,460
200 μl 267.A4.A1 + 10 μg GAT	10	2,500
200 μl 264.C4.C4	485	16,700
200 μl 264.C4.C4 + 10 μg GAT	440	17,750

[a] B10 mice were injected ip with phosphate buffer (PBS) or affinity purified (eluted from anti-A^b immunoabsorbent) 267.A4.A1 or 267.C4.C4 (control hybridoma) 24 hr prior to ip immunization with 10 μg GAT in Maalox-pertussis. Seven days later spleens were removed and were cultured at 5 × 10^6/culture with 2 μg GAT or with SRBC under Mishell-Dutton conditions; IgG GAT-specific PFC/culture or IgM PFC/culture versus SRBC were determined on day 5.

unpublished observations, 1981). Examination of the ability of the 267.A4.A1 supernatant fluids to suppress primary PFC responses by spleen cells from congenic strains of mice showed that suppression was restricted to those mice that were syngeneic at the *I-A* subregion of *H-2* with the normal fusion partner and source of the haplotype-specific Ts cell, B10 (Sorensen and Pierce, 1981b).

Serological analysis showed that hybridoma-derived TsF-H could be absorbed by and eluted from (B10.A × A) anti-B10.A(5R), anti-$(KAB)^b$, and (B10.MBR × A/Sn) anti-B10.A(5R), anti-(A^b), immunoabsorbents, but failed to be absorbed by (B10.A × B10) anti-B10.D2, anti-$(KABJE)^d$; B10.A(5R) anti-B10.A(3R), anti-(J^b); or (A.TL × B10.S(9R)) anti-B10.HTT, anti-J^S, immunoabsorbents (Table I). No binding by an anti-Ig or BSA immunabsorbent was detected. These data show that TsF-H (267.A4.A1) bears determinants encoded by the *I-A* subregion of the *H-2* complex, but fails to express classical immunoglobulin constant region or *I-J* subregion determinants. Data also presented in Table I show that hybridoma-derived TsF-H is absorbed by and can be eluted from a peanut agglutinin (PNA) immunoabsorbent.

The ability of hybridoma-derived TsF-H to mediate suppression *in vivo* was examined by administering 200 μl of affinity purified (eluted from anti-A^b immunoabsorbent) intraperitoneally in B10 mice 24 hr before challenge with GAT in Maalox-*pertussis*. Data in Table II show that administration of 267.A4.A1 TsF-H prior to challenge with antigen prevented priming for a secondary response to GAT *in vitro* and also prevented the stimulation of a primary response *in vitro* to an unrelated antigen, SRBC, by spleen cells from treated mice. Injection of control factor (267.C4.C4) failed to affect subsequent PFC responses *in vitro* following antigenic challenge. Similar results were seen with conventional TsF-H (data not shown).

II. MECHANISM OF ACTION OF TsF-H

The mechanism of action of TsF-H has been probed in preliminary experiments. B10 spleen cells were cultured with 267.A4.A1 TsF-H or control factor 267.C4.C4 for 24 hr. The cells were harvested, extensively washed to remove excess factor and added to fresh cultures of B10 spleen cells stimulated with GAT or SRBC to test their ability to suppress. The data in Table III show that spleen cells incubated with 267.A4.A1 TsF-H were able to suppress generation of primary PFC responses by naive spleen cells, while 267.C4.C4 control factor-treated cells mediated no significant suppression. Similar results were obtained when spleen cells from B10 mice injected 7 days earlier with 267.A4.A1 TsF-H were added to fresh spleen cell cultures (data not shown). Further characterization of these second-order suppressor cells is in progress.

TABLE III

Induction of Second Order of Suppressor Cells by 267.A4.A1

		Day 5 PFC/culture[b]	
Culture 1[a]	Number of culture 1 cells added	GAT	SRBC
None	None	403	1200
267.C4.C4	10×10^5	340	1100
267.C4.C4	5×10^5	375	1200
267.C4.C4	1×10^5	363	1300
267.A4.A1	10×10^5	70	105
267.A4.A1	5×10^5	180	260
267.A4.A1	1×10^5	333	800
None	267.A4.A1	8	425

[a] B10 spleen cells (5×10^6) were cultured for 24 hr with 267.C4.C4 control factor or 267.A4.A1 TsF-H (1/1000 final dilution). Cells were collected, washed and adjusted to the desired concentration of viable cells.

[b] B10 spleen cells (5×10^6) were cultured with 2 μg GAT or 10^7 SRBC and the indicated number of cells from culture 1 under Mishell-Dutton conditions; IgG GAT-specific PFC or IgM PFC versus SRBC were determined on day 5. Data are expressed as PFC/culture.

III. CONCLUSIONS

B10 mice neonatally injected with semiallogeneic (B10 × B10.D2)F_1 spleen cells as neonates contain a population of haplotype-specific suppressor T cells which after stimulation with the appropriate allogeneic (B10.D2) macrophages suppress primary PFC responses by syngeneic spleen cells through release of a soluble haplotype-specific suppressor factor, TsF-H (Sorensen and Pierce, 1981b,c). Functional and structural analysis of this factor has been facilitated by the generation of a T cell hybridoma which produces TsF-H on a constitutive basis (Sorensen and Pierce, 1981b,c). Comparison of hybridoma-derived and conventional TsF-H shows no detectable differences functionally or serologically. Suppression is limited to primary PFC responses to a variety of antigens by spleen cells syngeneic at *I-A* with the TsF-H producing T cell in the hybridoma and is mediated by a non-Ig-bearing protein with serologically detectable I-A determinants. TsF-H fails to suppress mixed lymphocyte or cytotoxic lymphocyte responses or secondary PFC responses.

An important and interesting feature of TsF-H is the lack of serologically detectable I-J determinants, and the presence instead of *I-A* subregion encoded determinants. Expression of I-A determinants has been demonstrated by antisera potentially directed against $(KAB)^b$ determinants, as well as with an $I\text{-}A^b$ specific reagent. Currently experiments are in progress using monoclonal anti-I-A reagents to specifically absorb factors and determine the identity of the I-A determinants on TsF-H more precisely. The lack of I-J determinants on TsF-H or lack of genetic restrictions governed by the *I-J* subregion at the TsF-H target cell interaction level is in contrast to previous reports with antigen-specific suppressor T cell factors (Kapp and Araneo, this volume, Chapter 11; Tada and Okumura, 1980). The lack of I-J determinants on a T cell suppressor factor has been demonstrated previously by Rich *et al.* (1979); *I-C* subregion determinants were detected on the MLR suppressor factor (MLR-TsF). A major difference between TsF-H and MLR-TsF and the antigen-specific suppressor T cell factors is the nature of the stimulating antigenic determinants; the former are stimulated by cell surface alloantigens, while the latter are stimulated by nonalloantigen particulate or protein antigens. A possible interpretation is that the *I* subregion responsible for genetic control of T cell-mediated regulation is determined at least in part by the nature of the stimulating antigen.

A further interesting feature of hybridoma-derived TsF-H is the ability to absorb activity using a peanut agglutinin (PNA) immunoabsorbent. PNA, a lectin with specificity for D-Gal-β(1 → 3)-GalNAc, has recently been reported to selectively agglutinate suppressor T cells (Nakano *et al.*, 1980). The ability to bind TsF-H would suggest a glycoprotein nature for this factor. Analysis of both hybridoma-derived and conventional TsF-H for carbohydrate and the nature of such carbohydrates is currently in progress.

Induction of a second population of suppressor T cells by a suppressor factor has been reported previously in several systems (Germain *et al.*, 1978; Germain and Benacerraf, 1981). The preliminary data from this system as well as from the other antigen-specific systems suggests that suppression is not a simple one-step process, but instead is the result of a series of specific interactions among multiple cell populations, many of which are restricted by *I* subregion products. This is not to say that T cell-mediated suppression proceeds by a single or common pathway, but more probably by a number of parallel and/or interacting pathways. An initial formulation of this concept has been presented already by Germain and Benacerraf (1981). If and how haplotype-specific Ts cells and TsF-H fit into this concept requires further study, as does the physiological relevance of these Ts cells and their factor in the regulation of antibody responses. The demonstration of activity *in vivo* suggests this not a tissue culture artifact.

A further point to be made concerns the role, if any, of I-J determinants in mediating suppression. As previously mentioned, both TsF-H and MLR-TsF do not bear serologically detectable I-J determinants. This is not to say that the suppressor T cells themselves do not bear suface I-J determinants. The presence of I-J determinants has, in fact, been demonstrated on the MLR suppressor T cell (Rich and David, 1979), and I-J determinants have been detected in preliminary experiments on the haplotype-specific suppressor T cell(s) (C. M. Sorensen and C. W. Pierce, unpublished observations, 1981). These data suggest that I-J serves as a membrane marker for functional subpopulations of T cells. The I-J determinants on suppressor factors and cell surface I-J determinants on T cells and non-T, non-B cells are not necessarily the product defined by the Ia.4 specificity (Murphy *et al.*, 1976), suggesting that the *I-J* subregion is a more complex locus which may encode several gene products that may be displayed on cells other than T cells (Murphy *et al.*, 1981).

Finally, it is important to note that the findings with hybridoma-derived TsF-H, previously reported from *in vitro* systems (Sorensen and Pierce, 1981b), occur *in vivo,* suggesting that the pathway of suppression involving TsF-H may represent a physiologically relevant immunological control mechanism in the intact animal. The availability of hybridomas producing TsF-H constitutively should enable us to characterize this molecule biochemically and structurally. Initial studies have indicated a molecular weight in the 50,000 range, like most other Ts cell factors. Moreover, activity is destroyed by low pH, high temperature, and proteolytic enzymes. The serological analysis and genetic restrictions on action of TsF-H have provided the novel aspects of this factor and its parent T cell. The tasks ahead are numerous and, in addition to characterization of this molecule, include determining the parameters of TsF-H action *in vivo,* the nature of the second-order suppressor cells generated and their mode of action, and the reasons for limited activity of TsF-H on primary antibody responses. It will be essential to determine if other lymphokine activities are produced by these hybridomas in addition to TsF-H. This suppressor T cell system is novel; its significance and biological relevance are not fully understood, and the path ahead is uncharted. The next series of experiments could be quite exciting.

ACKNOWLEDGMENTS

This investigation was supported by USPHS Research Grants AI-13915 and AI-15353. We thank Dr. D. Shreffler for providing special mice and antisera, Dr. C. David for antisera to I-A^b, and Mr. John Mulkie of the Hybridoma Facility for assistance in generating hybridomas used in these studies. We thank Paula Ryan for expert and patient secretarial assistance.

REFERENCES

Germain, R. N., and Benacerraf, B. (1981). A single major pathway of T-lymphocyte interactions in antigen-specific immune suppression. *Scand. J. Immunol.* **13,** 1–10.

Germain, R. N., Thèze, J., Waltenbaugh, C., Dorf, M., and Benacerraf, B. (1978). Antigen specific T cell mediated suppression. II. *In vitro* induction by *I-J* coded L-glutamic acid^{50}-L-tyrosine^{50}(GT)-specific T cell suppressor factor (GT-TsF) of suppressor T cells (Ts_2) bearing distinct *I-J* determinants. *J. Immunol.* **121,** 602–607.

Murphy, D., Herzenberg, L., Okumura, K., Herzenberg, L., and McDevitt, H. (1976). A new *I*-subregion (*I-J*) marked by a locus (*Ia4*) controlling surface determinants on suppressor T lymphocytes. *J. Exp. Med.* **144,** 699–712.

Murphy, D., Yamauchi, K., Habu, S., Eardley, D., and Gershon, R. (1981). T cells in a suppressor circuit and non-T non-B cells bear different I-J determinants. *Immunogenetics* **13,** 205–213.

Nakano, T., Imai, Y., Naiki, M., and Osawa, T. (1980). Characterization of mouse helper and suppressor T cell subsets separated by lectin. *J. Immunol.* **125,** 1928–1932.

Rich, S., and David, C. (1979). Regulatory mechanisms in cell mediated immune responses. VIII. Differential expression of *I*-region determinants by suppressor cells and their targets in suppression of mixed leukocyte reactions. *J. Exp. Med.* **150,** 1108–1121.

Rich, S., David, C., and Rich, R. (1979). Regulatory mechanisms in cell mediated immune responses. VII. Presence of *I-C* subregion determinants on mixedleukocyte reaction suppressor factor. *J. Exp. Med.* **149,** 114–126.

Sorensen, C. M., and Pierce, C. W. (1981a). Haplotype-specific suppression of antibody responses *in vitro*. I. Generation of genetically restricted suppressor T cells by neonatal treatment with semiallogeneic spleen cells. *J. Exp. Med.* **154,** 35–47.

Sorensen, C. M., and Pierce, C. W. (1981b). Haplotype-specific suppression of antibody responses *in vitro*. II. Suppressor factor produced by T cells and T cell hybridomas from mice treated as neonates with semiallogeneic spleen cells. *J. Exp. Med.* **154,** 48–59.

Sorensen, C. M., and Pierce, C. W. (1981c). Characterization of a monoclonal haplotype specific suppressor factor produced by a T cell hybridoma. *In* "Monoclonal Antibodies and T Cell Hybridomas" (G. J. Hammerling, U. Hammerling, and J. F. Kearney, eds.), pp. 497–502. Elsevier/North-Holland Biomedical Press, Amsterdam.

Tada, T., and Okumura, K. (1979). The role of antigen specific T cell factors in the immune response. *Adv. Immunol.* **28,** 1–88.

13

Soluble Immune Response Suppressor (SIRS) Derived from T Cell Hybridomas

Thomas M. Aune/Carl W. Pierce

I. Characteristics of SIRS 158
II. Speculations 161
References 161

Soluble mediators produced by lymphocytes (lymphokines) have been shown to play a significant role in regulating immune responses. Although the biology of many lymphokines is reasonably well understood, little is known about their chemical nature or about the precise mechanism by which they act. In the past, biochemical investigation of lymphokines has been hampered by the presence of multiple lymphokine activities in cuture supernatant fluids and by the relatively low concentrations of lymphokines present in biologically active fluids (Cohen *et al.*, 1979). The generation of hybrid T cell lines offers the potential to circumvent both of these problems. Although it is not certain whether a hybrid T cell line produces only one product, as appears to be the case with B cell hybrids producing monoclonal antibody, this technology will certainly make available to the investigator sufficient material to begin purification and characterization of the particular lymphokine of interest.

We have investigated the mechanism of action of concanavalin A (Con-A)-activated suppressor T cells (Pierce and Kapp, 1976; Rich and Pierce, 1973); their mediator, soluble immune response suppressor (SIRS) (Rich and Pierce, 1974; Pierce *et al.*, 1979; Tadakuma *et al.*, 1976); and the active factor produced by SIRS-treated macrophages [macrophage derived-suppressor factor (Mϕ-SF)] (Aune and Pierce, 1981a,b; Tadakuma and Pierce, 1978). This suppressor T cell pathway suppresses a variety of immune responses, including T cell and B cell proliferative responses to mitogens, primary and secondary antibody responses to T cell-dependent and -independent antigens, mixed lymphocyte responses, and generation of cytotoxic T lymphocytes (Aune and Pierce, 1981a; Pierce and Aune, 1981; Pierce and Kapp, 1976). Moreover, Mϕ-SF appears to

ISOLATION, CHARACTERIZATION, AND
UTILIZATION OF T LYMPHOCYTE CLONES

ISBN 0-12-249920-4

be modified SIRS; reaction of SIRS with Mϕ or low concentrations of peroxide yields Mϕ-SF (Aune and Pierce, 1981c). Mϕ-SF is an inhibitor of cell division by normal and neoplastic cells and of secretory processes (Aune and Pierce, 1981b; Pierce and Aune, 1981). Its action is not limited to cells of the immune system; Mϕ-SF also inhibits proliferation of normal and transformed fibroblasts. In an attempt to obtain sufficient material for purification and biochemical characterization of SIRS/Mϕ-SF, we have fused Con-A-activated murine spleen cells with the BW5147 cell line and cloned a cell line which produces SIRS constitutively. The cell line obtained from this fusion yields supernatant fluids with between 50- to 100-fold greater SIRS activity than can be obtained from Con-A-activated spleen cell cultures. Analysis to date shows that conventional SIRS and the product of the cloned hybrid T cell line (393.D2.6) are indistinguishable by the criteria tested. Supernatant fluids from cultures of BW5147 cells and other cloned hybrid cells from the same fusion are devoid of SIRS activity.

I. CHARACTERISTICS OF SIRS

The yield of SIRS from Con-A-activated spleen cells (Rich and Pierce, 1974), and from the SIRS-producing hybridoma T cell line (Aune and Pierce, 1981a,b,d) cultured in supplemented RPMI 1640 in the presence or absence of 10% horse serum are compared in Table I. Conventional sources of SIRS normally have between 50 and 150 units/ml when collected after a 48-hr incubation period. By contrast, hybridoma supernatant fluids contained between 2000 and 10,000 units/ml. Similar amounts were obtained from hybridoma cells cultured for 3 days in serum-supplemented and serum-free media. Production of these large quantities of SIRS in serum-free media will facilitate purification, since preliminary experiments suggest that 10–20 liters of SIRS-containing culture fluid will be necessary to obtain sufficient material for purification to homogeneity and initial biochemical characterization.

TABLE I

Yield of SIRS from Conventional and Hybridoma Sources

Source	SIRS (Units/ml)[a]
Con-A-activated spleen cells	50–150
T cell hybridoma (serum-supplemented medium)	2000–10,000
T cell hybridoma (serum-free medium)	2000–10,000

[a] One unit of SIRS is the amount necessary to suppress IgM PFC responses to SRBC 50%.

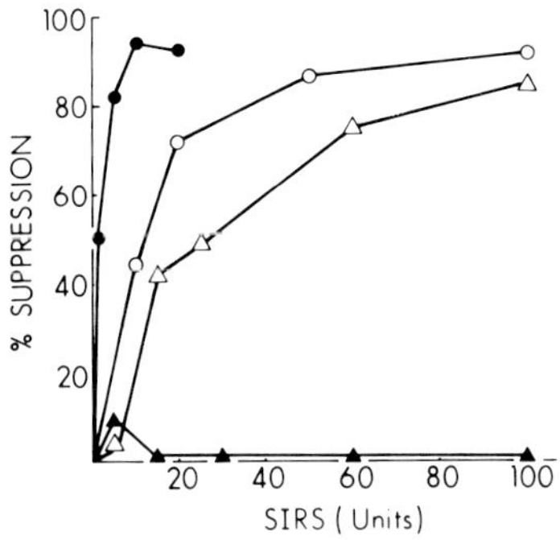

Fig. 1. Comparison of SIRS-mediated suppression of PFC responses by spleen cells or DNA synthetic responses by Mφ-like cell lines. The indicated quantities of SIRS were added to spleen cell cultures (●) or to Mφ-like cell lines, RAW 264.7 (○), P388D1 (△), J774.2 (▲) (3×10^5 cells/ml, 0.2 ml/well). PFC responses to SRBC were assayed on day 5. After 72 hr culture, Mφ were pulsed for 6 hr with 1 μCi ^{3}H-TdR, harvested, and radioactive incorporation determined by liquid scintillation spectrometry.

Figure 1 compares SIRS-mediated suppression of plaque-forming cell (PFC) responses to sheep red blood cells (SRBC) with SIRS-mediated inhibition of DNA synthesis in several Mφ-like cell lines. Two Mφ-like cell lines, RAW 264.7 and p388D_1 were relatively insensitive to inhibition by SIRS, compared to the PFC response, but could be completely inhibited upon addition of sufficient SIRS. By contrast, another Mφ-like cell line, J774.2 was not inhibited by SIRS even at the high concentrations. Other nonmacrophage cell lines, such as MOPC 315 and EL4, were not inhibited by SIRS under these conditions. The mechanism underlying SIRS-mediated inhibition of DNA synthesis by RAW 264.7 and p388D_1 cells is not completely clear at present. It is possible that both RAW 264.7 and p388D_1 cells convert SIRS to Mφ-SF and that Mφ-SF in turn inhibits division by these cells. This notion is supported by the fact that these cells are only inhibited after 48–72 hr of culture with SIRS; the time at which Mφ-SF activity is maximal (Aune and Pierce, 1981a). The RAW 264.7 cell line is routinely used to generate Mφ-SF from SIRS; p388D_1 cells has not generated detectable Mφ-SF (Aune and Pierce, 1981a). However, this cell line is known to produce Interleukin-1 (Mizel *et al.*, 1978), which may interfere with Mφ-SF-mediated suppression of PFC responses, the assay used to screen for Mφ-SF activity. Thus, in the present experiments p388D_1 may convert SIRS to Mφ-SF, which in turn inhibits DNA synthesis of p388D_1 cells. The Interleukin-1 present apparently does not interfere with inhibition under these circumstances. The effects of both Interleukin-1 and Interluekin-2 on SIRS/M -SF activity in a variety of assay systems are currently under active investigation. The failure of SIRS to inhibit DNA synthesis by the other cell lines quite possibly reflects the inability of these cells to produce sufficient H_2O_2 to convert SIRS to Mφ-SF

TABLE II

Conversion of SIRS to Mϕ-SF[a]

	Day 5 response (IgM PFC/culture)
Mϕ	5540 (0%)
SIRS (conventional)	5720 (0%)
SIRS (hybridoma)	6020 (0%)
SIRS (conventional) + Mϕ	840 (85%)
SIRS (hybridoma) + Mϕ	780 (86%)
10^{-8} *M* H_2O_2	5340 (3%)
SIRS (conventional) + 10^{-8} *M* H_2O_2	1100 (80%)
SIRS (hybridoma) + 10^{-8} *M* H_2O_2	990 (82%)

[a] SIRS (20 units) was added to RAW 264.7 Mϕ or reacted with 10^{-8} *M* H_2O_2. Mϕ supernatant fluids (100 μl) or SIRS–H_2O_2 reaction mixtures (equivalent to 10 SIRS units) were added to assay cultures on day 4. Control response was 5495 IgM PFC/culture. The numbers in parentheses represent percent suppression.

(Aune and Pierce, 1981c). Alternatively, SIRS may act directly to disrupt other cellular processes leading to inhibition of growth as measured by ^{3}H-TdR incorporation, and RAW 264.7 and p388D$_1$ may be sensitive to these effects.

Both conventional and hybridoma-derived SIRS yielded Mϕ-SF after culture with RAW 264.7 Mϕ or reaction with H_2O_2 (Table II). Mϕ-SF converted from conventional or hybridoma-derived SIRS and by Mϕ or reaction with H_2O_2 appear identical by all criteria tested to date (Aune and Pierce, 1981c). The most convenient quantitative assay for Mϕ-SF activity is to assay suppression of day 5 PFC responses to SRBC when Mϕ-SF is added on day 4. SIRS has no effect under these circumstances (Table II).

Our current working hypothesis of this suppressor T cell pathway is that SIRS, a product of concanavalin A-activated Lyt-2$^+$ T cells, is oxidized by peroxide to yield Mϕ-SF. Mϕ appears to serve only as a source of peroxide in this pathway. Mϕ-SF, in turn, reacts with target cell components (possibly a protein sulfhydryl) leading to rapid inhibition of cell division and secretory processes. SIRS/Mϕ-SF appears to have certain peroxidase-like properties. Not only does SIRS appear to react with peroxide to yield Mϕ-SF, but also Mϕ-SF is inactivated by certain peroxidase substrates (Aune and Pierce, 1981c). This is not to say that SIRS/Mϕ-SF acts catalytically, but rather that Mϕ-SF retains one or both oxidizing equivalents donated by peroxide similar to the classic oxidized forms of peroxidase (compound I or compound II) (Morrison and Schonbaum, 1976). Mϕ-SF appears to have greater stability than classic peroxidase derivatives and is able to react with or oxidize a substrate on or near the cell surface. The nature of the active site of SIRS is not known at present. The availability of the hybridoma T cell line producing SIRS should provide sufficient quantities of material for purification and biochemical analysis and will hopefully resolve several questions concerning the apparent oxidative basis of SIRS action.

II. SPECULATIONS

Characterization of lymphokines suffers from the imprecise nature of the biological assay used to identify them and the rather crude methods of characterization. Recently, we have found that murine fibroblast interferon (IFNβ) appears to derive its immunosuppressive properties through activation of suppressor T cells and the SIRS/Mϕ-SF pathway. By all criteria presently available to us IFNβ-activated and concanavalin A-activated suppressor T cells are identical, and the factor(s) derived from IFNβ-activated suppressor T cells appear identical to SIRS. However, this apparent identity is based largely on circumstantial evidence and suffers from the current state of the art of lymphokines. By preparing T cell hybridomas from IFNβ-activated suppressor T cells and comparing factors derived from these hybrid cell lines with hybridoma-derived SIRS on a biochemical basis, such as amino acid analysis and sequence, it will be possible to definitively compare these two factors.

The Con-A-activated suppressor T cell-SIRS/Mϕ-SF system has been a useful model to study mechanisms of nonspecific suppressor T cells and their products. The biological relevance, however, has been clouded by the manner in which these cells are activated. However, the finding that IFNβ activates this pathway and that SIRS/Mϕ-SF is produced by IFNβ-activated T cells changes this weather pattern and removes the clouds. This nonspecific suppressor pathway could have considerable significance for not only regulation of immune responses but more importantly for control of cell proliferation in general. Thus, the continuation of this line of investigation and the complete characterization of SIRS/Mϕ-SF have become very important.

ACKNOWLEDGMENTS

This investigation was supported by USPHS Research Grants AI-13915 and AI-15353. We thank Mr. John Mulkie of the Hybridoma Facility for assistance in generating hybridomas used in these studies. We thank Barbara Wollberg for expert and patient secretarial assistance.

REFERENCES

Aune, T. M., and Pierce, C. W. (1981a). Identification and initial characterization of a nonspecific suppressor factor (Mϕ-SF) produced by soluble immune response suppressor (SIRS)-treated macrophages. *J. Immunol.* **127,** 1828–1833.

Aune, T. M., and Pierce, C. W. (1981b). Mechanism of action of macrophage-derived suppressor factor produced by soluble immune response suppressor treated macrophages. *J. Immunol.* **127,** 368–372.

Aune, T. M., and Pierce, C. W. (1981c). Conversion of soluble immune response suppressor to macrophage-derived suppressor factor by peroxide. *Proc. Natl. Acad. Sci. U.S.A.* **78,** 5099–5103.

Aune, T. M., and Pierce, C. W. (1981d). Monoclonal soluble immune response suppressor (SIRS) derived from T cell hybridomas. *In* "Monoclonal Antibodies and T Cell Hybridomas" (G. J. Hammerling, U. Hammerling, and J. F. Kearney, eds.), pp. 516–522. Elsevier-North-Holland Biomedical Press, Amsterdam.

Cohen, S., Pick, E., and Oppenheim, J. J., eds. (1979). "The Biology of the Lymphokines." Academic Press, New York.

Mizel, S. B., Oppenheim, J. J., and Rosenstreich, D. L. (1978). Characterization of lymphocyte activating factor (LAF) produced by the macrophage cell line, P388D1. I. Enhancement of LAF production by activated T lymphocytes. *J. Immunol.* **120,** 1497–1503.

Morrison, M., and Schonbaum, G. R. (1976). Peroxidase-catalyzed halogenation. *Annu. Rev. Biochem.* **45,** 861–888.

Pierce, C. W., and Aune, T. M. (1981). Mechanism of action of soluble immune response suppressor (SIRS). *In* "Advances in Immunopharmacology" (J. Hadden, L., Chédid, P. Mullen, and F. Spreafico, eds.), pp. 397–404, Pergamon, Oxford.

Pierce, C. W., and Kapp, J. A. (1976). Regulation of immune responses by suppressor T cells. *Contemp. Top. Immunobiol.* **5,** 91–143.

Pierce, C. W., Tadakuma, T., and Kapp, J. A. (1979). Role of nonspecific and specific suppressor factors in immunity. *Ann. N.Y. Acad. Sci.* **332,** 336–344.

Rich, R. R., and Pierce, C. W. (1973). Biological expressions of lymphocyte activation. II. Generation of a population of thymus-derived suppressor lymphocytes. *J. Exp. Med.* **137,** 649–659.

Rich, R. R., and Pierce, C. W. (1974). Biological expression of lymphocyte activation. III. Suppression of plaque-forming cell responses *in vitro* by supernatant fluids from concanavalin A-activated spleen cell clultures. *J. Immunol.* **112,** 1360–1368.

Tadakuma, T., and Pierce, C. W. (1978). Mode of action of soluble immune response suppressor (SIRS) produced by concanavalin A-activated spleen cells. *J. Immunol.* **120,** 481–486.

Tadakuma, T., Kuhner, A. L., Rich, R. R., David, J. R., and Pierce, C. W. (1976). Biological expressions of lymphocyte activation. V. Characterization of a soluble immune response suppressor (SIRS) produced by concanavalin-A-activated spleen cells. *J. Immunol.* **117,** 323–330.

III

The Somatic Cell Genetic Analysis of Cytolytic T Lymphocyte Functions

14

An Overview

Markus Nabholz

I. CTL Lines . . . 166
II. Mutants . . . 170
A. *Vicia villosa*-resistant Mutants . . . 171
B. Antigen-Loss Variants . . . 172
III. Somatic Cell Hybrids . . . 173
IV. Outlook . . . 176
A. TCGF Dependence . . . 176
B. Specificity . . . 177
C. The Cytolytic Machinery . . . 178
References . . . 179

Cellular immunology is going through a phase of transition. The starting point is characterized by complex experimental systems which allow a description of immunological phenomena, the identification of the participating cell types and the measurement of their influences on immune responses, but not an analysis of the molecular basis of the phenomena observed. The transition is driven by the development of techniques for the isolation and maintenance of cloned cell lines which express immunological functions. An experimental approach combining somatic cell genetic techniques with biochemical and functional analysis of such cell lines could be the basis for an identification and characterization of the molecular components essential for the expression of the various lymphocyte specific activities.

A somatic cell genetic analysis of the functions characteristic of a particular differentiated cell type requires cell lines which express these functions with sufficient stability: the frequency with which inactive variants arise has to be low enough so as not to result in the rapid overgrowth of active lines by their nonfunctional derivatives. On the other hand, some source of stable inactive variants is required: their comparison with the active ("wild type") parental cells is the basis for discovering which cellular properties are essential for the specific activity analyzed. If the variants differ from the wild type genetically (i.e., if they are mutants) or by a stable chromosomally transmitted change in their state

ISOLATION, CHARACTERIZATION, AND
UTILIZATION OF T LYMPHOCYTE CLONES

ISBN 0-12-249920-4

of differentiation, then they can be used not only for the identification and characterization of the molecular differences between active and inactive cells but also for the localization and characterization of the genes controlling the expression of the molecules which confer upon the wild type cells their differentiated phenotype. The techniques of somatic cell hybridization (for a review, see Ringertz and Savage, 1976) allow a comparison of different variants by complementation tests and chromosome assignment of the genes controlling the differences between variants and wild type. Recombinant DNA technology will then permit isolation and definitive characterization of these genes.

The first T cell type with a definable function which became available in the form of established cell lines (in this chapter "established cell lines" are cloned cell populations with an apparently unlimited potential for proliferation) were mature cytolytic T lymphocytes (CTL). In this chapter we will discuss, on the basis of the experimental results available, to what extent and how these lines will be suitable for a somatic cell genetic analysis of CTL functions.

CTL-specific activities are perhaps the simplest of all T cell functions in terms of their measurements (for a review of CTL–target interaction, see Berke, 1980). The interaction of a single CTL with a target cell and the result—target cell lysis—can be observed under the microscope, and the activity of CTL populations can be measured within minutes to a few hours by a quantitative assay of isotope release from ^{51}Cr-labeled targets. Because of this relative simplicity and accessibility, much effort has been spent on the analysis of the CTL–target cell interaction, but we still know virtually nothing about its molecular basis. The repertoire of the determinant-specific recognition structures ("T cell receptors") which these cells must possess has been defined operationally in great detail (see Chapters 15–17 in this treatise), but none of the efforts to identify their molecular components have yielded any convincing results. The nature of the interaction(s) by which a CTL binds to its target cell and inflicts upon it an irreversible "lethal hit" which "programs" the target but not the killer cell for lysis is quite unclear. The use of metabolic inhibitors (see Martz, 1977) and antibodies (Hiserodt and Bonavida, 1981, and Section III,B) has allowed the definition of stages of the killer–target encounter but not provided any definitive clues about the components which give a CTL its capacity to induce target lysis or about the mechanism of lysis.

I. CTL LINES

Almost all of the murine CTL lines that have been derived until today have been established in one of two ways: (1) Either CTL precursors or CTL present in a mixed leukocyte culture are cloned directly by limiting dilution (Ryser and MacDonald, 1979) in microcultures containing irradiated spleen filler or stimulator cells and T cell growth factor [TCGF which is now called interleukin-2 (IL-2)]. When maintained in these conditions, many and, perhaps all CTL clones obtained from such cultures seem to have an infinite potential for proliferation (Glasebrook and Fitch, 1979). We call this type of line CTL-A line. (2) When whole MLC populations are cultured, without addition of further stimulator or filler cells in TCGF-containing medium, they will proliferate well for some time, then their growth rate often declines and some of the cultures are lost. In those populations which survive this "crisis," a rapidly growing TCGF-dependent cell population appears which expresses CTL activity and can easily be cloned in liquid cultures (Gillis and Smith, 1977). These cells do not depend on filler or stimulator cells. The first clone of established CTL lines were derived by this method (Nabholz *et al.*, 1978). We call them CTL-B lines.

Before comparing in greater detail the two types of lines, I will discuss briefly the history of the two different protocols. The second one was developed mainly to compare the cellular properties and physiology of normal lymphocytes with those of lymphoid tumor cells. The cultivation of normal lymphocytes had been given great impetus by the discovery that while such cells usually did not proliferate sufficiently in the tissue culture media to sustain growth of other types of cells, such as fibroblasts or many types of tumor cells, they could be stimulated to divide by certain plant lectins such as phytohemagglutinin. It became clear, however, that binding of such mitogens to lymphocytes was not sufficient to trigger their proliferation, which depended on the presence of more than one cell type in the cultures. It was probably the observations that supernatants of antigen- or mitogen-stimulated leukocyte cultures contained many different types of biologically active materials, such as colony stimulating factor, that suggested the experiments leading to the discovery that normal human T lymphocytes would initiate and maintain proliferation for many months when cultured in supernatants from PHA-stimulated leukocyte cultures (Morgan *et al.*, 1976; see Chapter 1 of this treatise). Finally Gillis and Smith (1977) demonstrated that murine CTL present in a mixed leukocyte–tumor cell culture could be kept growing for indefinite periods in a supernatant from concanavalin A (Con-A)-activated mouse spleen cells [Con-A supernatant (CS)], and cloned CTL lines were derived from such populations several months after the initiation of the *in vitro* culture (Nabholz *et al.*, 1978; Baker *et al.*, 1979).

After its discovery, the mixed leukocyte culture system was developed as a tool for an understanding of the genetic basis of graft rejection with the hope that it would serve as a predictor of the outcome of planned organ grafts in man. It contributed to a refined definition of the major histocompatibility complex (MHC) and a clearer appreciation of the complexity of T cell responses to tissue and other cell-bound antigens (for a review, see Nabholz and Miggiano, 1977). The demonstration that CTL directed against the stimulating cells did arise in MLC led to attempts to maintain these killer cells in culture by exposing them periodically to the same stimulator cells. The CTL activity of such populations can indeed be reactivated for a few cycles of restimulation, but then the peak activity of subsequent cycles almost always declines (Häyry, 1976; for an exception, see Dennert *et al.*, 1981), although the cells continue to respond by a wave of proliferation. At this time, it had become clear that at least two types of T lymphocytes participated in an MLC response (for a review, see Beverley, 1977): Some cells would proliferate but not become CTL. They had, on the other hand, an enhancing or "helping" effect on the maturation and/or proliferation of the other type of cell, the CTL precursors. The discovery that MLC supernatants, such as medium from T cell mitogen-activated leukocytes, contained lymphokines, including a factor "replacing" the requirement for T cell "help" in B lymphocyte responses (Dutton *et al.*, 1971), led to the suggestion that the "helper" activity for the CTL response could also be mediated by soluble factors. This hypothesis became even more attractive when it was demonstrated that supernatants from secondary MLC could induce rapid proliferation and reactivation of primed CTL precursors independent of reexposure to the priming stimulator cells (Ryser *et al.*, 1978).

Use of this type of supernatant allowed the cloning of the CTL present in MLC or their precursors in spleen with a much higher efficiency than in the previous attempts at limiting dilution analysis of CTL (Ryser and MacDonald, 1979); and Glasebrook and Fitch (1979) proceeded to show that at least some of the CTL clones obtained in this way could be propagated indefinitely in medium containing MLC or Con-A supernatant and irradiated spleen cells.

What are the differences between CTL-A lines obtained by immediate cloning of CTL precursors or MLC-activated CTL and the CTL-B lines derived from MLC populations maintained as mass cultures for several months in TCGF-containing medium? Proliferation of both types of lines continues to depend strictly on what is almost certainly the same T cell growth factor molecule present in both MLC and mitogen-activated culture supernatants. But while CTL-B lines grow in normal medium supplemented with a cell-free source of TCGF, CTL-A lines have additional requirements of unknown nature which are supplied by irradiated spleen "filler" cells (see also Glasebrook and Fitch, Chapter 23, for discussion). In the absence of TCGF, neither type of cell line can be induced to grow by exposure to stimulator cells carrying the determinants for which the lines are specific, although it appears that the growth of CTL-A clones can be enhanced by addition of appropriate allogeneic cells when TCGF is limiting (Lutz *et al.*, 1981). Both CTL-A and CTL-B cells are clearly of T cell origin. They express surface markers characteristic for normal T cells or CTL. CTL-A, as well as CTL-B, lines have been isolated which are stable in their lytic capacity and which express a clearly defined specificity which in the case of anti-viral, anti-tumor (Weiss *et al.*, 1981), anti-minor (von Boehmer *et al.*, 1979) histocompatibility antigen or anti-hapten (Haas *et al.*, 1980) activity is

MHC restricted. The level of cytolytic activity of either cell type does not depend on the stage of the cell cycle or the growth phase (exponential or stationary) of the cultures (Sekaly *et al.*, 1981).

Morphologically CTL-A cells are small, somewhat adherent cells with the features characteristic of those displayed by normal T lymphocytes activated in MLC. CTL-B cells, on the other hand, are much larger, and there is great variability in different lines between the predominant morphology and the tendency to adhere (Nabholz *et al.*, 1980a). Among a collection of half a dozen CTL-B lines, most can be distinguished simply on the basis of their morphological idiosyncrasies.

Analysis of the banding patterns of the chomosomes of CTL-A lines maintained for several years in culture has shown that almost all cells display a karyotype which is indistinguishable from that of normal cells. All of five independent CTL-B lines, on the other hand, showed at least some and often many and drastic deviations from the standard karyotype (see Johnson *et al.*, Chapter 5 in this treatise). (It should be noted that the source of TCGF was MLC supernatant for the CTL-A lines and crude CS for the CTL-B lines.) One plausible explanation for the differences between the two types of lines is that CTL-B lines, which are clearly less like normal CTL than CTL-A lines, are derived from CTL-A-like cells by a relatively rare ''transformation'' event which renders them independent of filler cells. The transformants would be the cells surviving the ''crisis'' observed in many early CTL-B cultures. That the postcrisis populations often consist of a single clone is, of course, consistent with this hypothesis (Engers *et al.*, 1980; Haas *et al.*, 1980). However, even if CTL-A seem indistinguishable from normal CTL, this does not mean that they have not undergone some changes, although more subtle, which have allowed them to escape the finite life spam characteristic for most, if not all, normal cells.

I want to consider briefly the relative usefulness of the two types of lines: CTL-A clones are easier to obtain in large numbers. This is their apparent normalcy, and the greater stability of their specificity establishes their advantage for the analysis of specificity repertoires. Once they are established, the maintenance of CTL-B lines is clearly less laborious. For biochemical or cell cycle analyses, the contamination of CTL-A populations with filler cell can be a nuisance. The presence of abnormal chromosomes of unidentifiable constitution is, on the other hand, a headache in the use of CTL-B cells for somatic cell genetics, but then again hybrid cells produced by fusion of CTL-B with thymomas much more stably express CTL-specific functions than comparable CTL-A hybrids (Nabholz *et al.*, 1981). Clearly, both types of CTL lines have their advantages and drawbacks, the relative importance of which will depend on the particular project envisaged. In time, we will probably learn how to produce ideal CTL lines combining all the advantages of both CTL-A and CTL-B lines without any of their disadvantages.

II. MUTANTS

A somatic cell genetic analysis of CTL lines depends on a source of stable heritable variants which are affected in one or other aspect of their CTL-specific functions. In many CTL-B lines, a quite large (intraclonal) quantitative variation in the cytolytic capacity is continuously generated, but completely inactive variants have rarely been found (Nabholz *et al.*, 1979). Whether such spontaneously arising quantitative variability is due to genetic differences or to multiple stable equilibria of the regulatory systems which control the cellular phenotype would be very hard to determine, particularly because the expression of CTL-specific functions—hereafter referred to as the CTL phenotype—is probably influenced by many properties of the cells which are not specific characteristics of CTL, e.g., cell mobility, size, or surface charge. Therefore this type of variation is not likely to be very useful for somatic cell genetic analysis of CTL.

What we are looking for is an experimental system which allows the selection of cytolytically completely inactive CTL line variants arising spontaneously with a low frequency, comparable to that of drug-resistant variants. If mutagen treatment could be shown to increase the frequency of such variants and their phenotype were stable, then one could reasonably assume that they are the consequence of genetic mutations. Unfortunately, a protocol for the efficient selection of cytolytically inactive cells has yet to be reported.

One characteristic of the CTL lines for which the selection of loss variants should be possible is their dependence on TCGF for growth and survival. So far attempts to select such mutants have been unsuccessful even after a mutagenesis protocol which increased the frequency of drug- and lectin-resistant variants by up to 1000-fold (Nabholz *et al.*, 1980a). An explanation for the apparently low frequency of TCGF-independent variants is suggested by the indication that TCGF dependence behaves like a dominant trait in hybrids between CTL and lymphoma lines (see below). These observations may mean that TCGF-dependence is imposed on CTL by a trans acting gene, both copies of which have to undergo a mutation for a cell to become TCGF independent.

In the absence of a technique allowing the selection of inactive mutants, the next best approach to the genetic analysis of the cytolytic function of CTL is the isolation of variants deficient in some property which might play a specific role in the CTL–target interaction. CTL-specific cell surface characteristics are obvious candidates, as it seems clear that specific target cell recognition and destruction must be processes mediated, at least in part, by cell surface interactions, and the search for CTL-specific monoclonal antibodies has become very popular. We should keep in mind, though, that this approach may be barking up the wrong tree, at least as far as the molecules mediating postrecognition steps go: We may just as plausibly surmise that successful delivery of the "lethal hit" depends on cell surface molecules which are expressed on many other cell types but which only in CTL are linked to a lytic machinery residing on the cytoplasmic side of the cell surface. If this is true, it may be profitable to screen not for CTL-specific antibodies but for antibodies which can inhibit target cell lysis by CTL.

The advantages of monoclonal antibodies over conventional antisera for this type of approach need hardly be stressed: Not only are they much more efficient reagents for the detection quantification, and characterization of tissue-specific antigens but their much better specificity should greatly facilitate the selection of antigen-loss variants. The isolation and characterization of such variants will be the critical test whether the affected antigenic molecule does indeed play a role in the expression of a specific cellular function.

A. *Vicia villosa*-Resistant Mutants

Several CTL line variants with specific alterations of the cell surface have been described. Conzelmann *et al.* (1980) isolated a number of independent mutants resistant to a lectin from *Vicia villosa* (VV) which is toxic for CTL-B lines but not for T lymphoma-derived lines. VV columns have been reported to retain specifically a subpopulation of activated T cells which include CTL, and the lectin binds specifically to a glycoprotein (gp) of normal T cells, T145, which appears upon activation concomittantly with cytolytic activity (Kimura *et al.*, 1979). CTL-B lines bind up to 10^7 molecules VV/cell, whereas T cell tumor lines show no detectable binding. CTL-B lines do indeed express T145, but VV absorbs not only this but many other gp's of these established cell lines.

Lectin-resistant CTL-B mutants were isolated in the hope of finding variants lacking T145 and in order to assess the importance of the high number of VV-binding sites for CTL activity. Isolation of variants depended on mutagenesis (with ethyl methane sulfonate). The levels of resistance of different mutants varied and correlated reasonably well with the reduction in the lectin-binding capacity. The resistant phenotypes were stable for several months of culture in the absence of VV. The most resistant variant grew well in concentrations of VV at least 100 times that toxic for the wild type and bound more than 1000-fold less lectin. The affinity of many of the gp for VV was greatly reduced, but all of five independent mutants still expressed a gp with a molecular weight and an isoelectric point close to that of wild type T145, and they killed target cells with approximately the same efficiency.

Thus these results did not furnish any evidence concerning the role of T145 in the cytolytic process, but they showed that variation over three orders of magnitude in the number of VV-binding sites did not affect cytolytic efficiency. The behavior of these variants is most easily explained by mutations affecting steps in a glycosylation pathway leading to the synthesis of VV-binding carbohydrate moieties on several different gp and possibly glycolipids

B. Antigen-Loss Variants

Most CTL lines express the T cell specific Thy-1 antigen as well as the Lyt-2 and Lyt-3 antigens which characterize a subset of T cells which includes CTL (see Beverley, 1977, for review). Lyt-2 and Lyt-3 were defined originally as alloantigens controlled by the same one or two genes, both closely linked to the Ig κ-chain locus (Gottlieb and Durda, 1977). Antibodies against either antigen can inhibit CTL activity (Shinohara and Sachs, 1979; Nakayama *et al.*, 1979; Sarmiento *et al.*, 1980), probably by preventing the binding of CTL to target cells. Until recently, they were the only defined antigens, antibodies against which could efficiently block lysis by CTL. These observations led to speculations that Lyt-2- and/or Lyt-3-bearing molecules might be part of the determinant-specific recognition structures ("T cell receptors") of CTL.

Dialynas *et al.* (1981) have described variants of a CTL-A line, L3, which were selected for loss of either Lyt-2 or Thy-1 expression on the cell surface using monoclonal antibodies and complement. All the variants described were isolated after mutagen treatment, but no effort was made to establish that the isolated variants had been induced by the mutagen. (To do so becomes very laborious in antibody–complement based selection systems, which require several cycles of treatment before variants are isolated.) Antigen expression by the variants was quantified using a cytofluorometry analysis, the lower limit of detection being probably around 1% of the amount of antigen expressed by the wild type cells.

The specificity and the cytolytic competence of the variants were analyzed by testing their cytolytic activity against an appropriate tumor target cell in the presence and absence of Con-A (addition of Con-A to a mixture of CTL and "inappropriate" targets is thought to overcome the requirement for specific target cell recognition and provoke nonspecific lysis of the latter).

The Thy-1 loss variant did not show any change in its lytic activity against the tumor target used. Of three Lyt-2 loss variants two (243/1, 243/2) were probably different isolates of the same variant which still carried detectable amounts (10% of the parental cells) of Lyt-2. Lyt-3 expression was reduced to the same level. The third variant, V4, expressed no detectable amounts of either Lyt-2 or Lyt-3. It showed less than 1% of the specific lytic activity of the parental cells, but its lytic competence was restored to that of L3 by the addition of Con-A. The other two variants showed a similar behavior, except that Con-A restores their cytolytic capacity only partially.

No genetic or biochemical characterization of these mutants has been reported. We do not know whether the extinction of Lyt-2 and Lyt-3 expression in V4 is due to a regulatory gene or whether both copies of the structural *Lyt-2* (and *Lyt-3*) gene presumably present in these cells carry mutations. Nor do we know what changes led to the large reduction but not complete extinction of *Lyt-2* and

Lyt-3 expression in the 243 variants. The results suggest interdependence of *Lyt-2* and *Lyt-3* expression.

The functional behavior of the variants reinforces the evidence suggesting a role of the molecules bearing the Lyt-2 and Lyt-3 determinants in an early phase of the CTL–target cell interaction, probably in the events leading to the formation of CTL–target conjugates, but they provide no further clues supporting the idea that these molecules determine the specificity of CTL.

III. SOMATIC CELL HYBRIDS

Somatic cells can be induced to fuse with each other with a high frequency by exposure to such agents as Sendai virus or polyethylene glycol. A small fraction of the resulting polykaryons subsequently undergoes nuclear fusion and gives rise to mononuclear proliferating hybrid cells. The major areas of application of this technique (see Ringertz and Savage, 1976, for review) have been in (1) the genetic analysis of somatic cells, (2) the study of the control of differentiation, and (3) the "immortalization" of a particular differentiated phenotype expressed by normal cells with a finite life span. The most popular application of this last possibility is undoubtedly the production of B cell hybridomas secreting antibodies of predetermined specificity.

In somatic cell genetics cell hybridization serves two purposes: (a) In complementation analysis, pairwise crosses of mutants with the same phenotype are used to distinguish between variants carrying different types of genetic lesions. (b) The other application, localization of genes on particular chromosomes, is possible because of the karyotypic changes occurring in somatic cell hybrids. Almost all somatic cell crosses involve at least one established (permanent) cell line with a heteroploid chromosome constitution, a property which it imparts on its hybrid derivatives. The latter are often karyotypically relatively unstable, and loss of parental chromosomes occurs with a frequency which depends on the combination of parental cells. In interspecies hybrids between human and rodent cells, there is almost always a strong preference for the loss of the human chromosomes. This has served as a substitute for the meiotic segregation in sexual genetics and has been the basis for the chromosomal assignment of more than 300 autosomal human genes. Intraspecies hybrids are often, but not always, karyotypically relatively stable and retain more or less the entire chromosome complements. If there is chromosome loss it may affect preferentially the complement of one parent, and in crosses between normal diploid cells and an established heteroploid cell line, the chromosomes of the normal parent are often lost more frequently. The usefulness of intraspecies hybrids for chromosome assignment studies is limited because it is impossible to distinguish homologous parental chromosomes. This limitation can be overcome by the use of cell lines or normal cells carrying chromosomal rearrangements of identifiable composition (for example, see Hengartner *et al.,* 1978).

After the possibility of producing somatic cell hybrids had been demonstrated, a large number of crosses between cells belonging to different histiotypes were made in the hope of gaining insight into the mechanisms controlling differentiation. The results of these experiments have, on the whole, been rather disappointing, and it is hard to summarize the findings obtained from the different types of crosses.

When cells or cell lines belonging to different cell lineages and expressing different differentiation programs are fused, the expression of any particular tissue-specific property can either continue or be extinguished. If expression of a particular differentiated product continues, the homologous gene of the nonexpressing parental cell may or may not be activated. Several of these situations may be observed in hybrids derived from the same cross, and in a cloned hybrid line an extinguished property may become reexpressed, e.g., as the result of the loss of a chromosome of the nonexpressing parent. Usually no properties characteristic for differentiation programs to which neither of the parental cells belongs become expressed. As one might expect, the more closely related the two parental cells are ontogentically, the less likely is extinction of their differentiated characteristics, and the most revealing and promising experiments in this field have perhaps been those involving cells representing different stages of differentiation of the same cell type. Good examples are the crosses between B cells and B cell tumor-derived lines representing different maturation stages of this cell lineage. Such hybrids have already provided considerable information on the genetic control of B cell development (Burrows *et al.,* 1979; Alt *et al..* 1980; Perry *et al.,* 1981; Raschke *et al.,* 1979).

Unless reexpression in negative hybrid clones is observed, it is difficult to decide whether extinction of a differentiated function is due to systematic loss of particular chromosomes of the differentiated cells or to negative control by the nonexpressing parent. When, in addition, normal differentiated cell populations are used, it can almost never be excluded that nonexpressing hybrids are derived from contaminating cells belonging to other histiotypes. A case in point is the early attempts to obtain established CTL lines from crosses between thymomas and a normal CTL-containing lymphocyte populations. Probably several hundred hybrids of this type have been tested in several laboratories and were found to be inactive (for a discussion of the recent report by Kaufmann *et al.,* 1981, see Chapter 17 in this treatise). This result could be attributed either to a selective outgrowth of hybrids derived from the contaminating non-CTL (one argument put forward was that fusion with a CTL was lethal), to extinction of CTL-specific functions by thymoma genes, or, finally, to consistent rapid loss of CTL chromosomes carrying genes whose expression was required for cytolytic competence. The finding that hybrids between cloned CTL-B lines and thymoma cells were also inactive

(M. Nabholz, unpublished observations) argued against, but did not exclude, the hypothesis that heterokaryons involving cytolytic cells were nonviable. The frequency of such hybrids was about 1 per 10^4 CTL in the fusion mixture, and it could not be excluded that all outgrowing lines were derived from rare inactive variants in the CTL-clone used.

Evidence that provides a clue as to which of the explanations for the extinction of CTL activity in CTL–thymoma hybrids is correct was provided by an experiment in which a polyethylene glycol-treated mixture of CTL-B and thymoma cells was plated out in selective medium, but Con-A supernatant was added to part of the cultures (Nabholz *et al.*, 1980b). Many hybrids grew out in both conditions, but their morphology was very different. The cells growing in normal medium resembled the parental thymoma cells: they were more or less round, undifferentiated, and formed colonies by piling up into regular pyramids. In most of the wells supplemented with Con-A supernatant a novel cell type appeared, which strongly adhered to plastic and had a very differentiated, sometimes almost fibroblast-like morphology. It turned out that almost all hybrids of this type had cytolytic activity and were dependent on TCGF for growth, while the thymoma-like hybrids were inactive and TCGF-independent. Further crosses between different AKR-thymomas and several CTL-B lines gave the same results, and most of the thymoma hybrids with CTL-A or CTL from secondary MLC were active when selected in TCGF, but they tended to lose cytolytic competence and TCGF-dependence much more rapidly than the CTL-B hybrids which maintained their CTL phenotype reasonably stably (Nabholz *et al.*, 1981).

We cannot yet exclude that the difference between the hybrids which express cytolytic activity (CTL^+) and are dependent on TCGF (CS^+) and those which are CTL^- CS^- is not genetic but depends on variables, such as the cell cycle stage of the fusion partners or a stochastic event occurring during or immediately after fusion. Some of our results do suggest that hybrids containing all the chromosomes contributed by the thymoma and the CTL parental cells are CS^+ CTL^+, and that CS^- CTL^- hybrids arise as the result of the loss of a CTL chromosome. The observations supporting this hypothesis are the following. (1) The frequency of hybrids isolated in normal medium is usually lower than the one of hybrids growing in TCGF-supplemented conditions. From a fusion between a tetraploid CTL-B and a diploid thymoma line only TCGF-dependent hybrids were obtained (Nabholz *et al.*, 1981). (2) In cloned TCGF-dependent hybrid populations, TCGF-independent variants arise which usually are cytolytically inactive and morphologically resemble the thymoma-like hybrids originally selected in normal medium (Conzelmann *et al.*, Chapter 17 in this treatise).

These findings suggest that extinction of differentiated functions observed in hybrid cells in other experimental situations may have been due to selection of hybrids in a medium lacking a constituent, the dependence on which is conferred by a chromosome required for the continued expression of the differentiated function. This possibility should be kept in mind in crosses where the growth requirements of the differentiated parental cells are not known, e.g., when normal nondividing cells are used.

IV. OUTLOOK

I think that the work discussed in this chapter shows that the analysis of CTL functions by somatic cell genetics is possible and that CTL lines provide an adequate source of material for such an approach. Some important technical problems still have to be solved before the arms for this type of attack is complete. Among these are the development of more efficient methods for the selection of antigen-loss variants; the production of stable active hybrids with CTL with a normal karyotype, the chromosomes of which are distinguishable from those of the noncytolytic parent (interspecies hybrids, or use of CTL derived from animals carrying translocation markers); and, most importantly, a system for the selection of cytolytically incompetent variants.

In this last section I want to consider briefly some of the ways in which somatic cell genetics can contribute to an elucidation of the molecular basis of the three most distinctive attributes of the CTL phenotype: specificity, cytolytic competence, and TCGF dependence.

A. TCGF Dependence

I will discuss this characteristic first because it is the one that seems most clearly and directly amenable to an analysis based on somatic cell genetics. While it may not be an exclusive property of CTL, it seems probably that most if not all CTL require TCGF for proliferation, at least *in vitro*. This dependence raises two questions: (1) What makes a cell TCGF-dependent? (2) How does the growth factor act?

As a first step in the analysis of the mechanism of action, we have studied the effect of TCGF removal on CTL-B lines and have found that it results in an accumulation and growth arrest of cells in the G_1 phase of the cell cycle (Sekaly *et al.*, Chapter 16 in this treatise). On reexposure to TCGF, arrested cells respond by a partially synchronized entry into the S phase, after a lag period of several hours (Sekaly *et al.*, 1982). The lytic activity per cell does not change appreciably even when they are cultured in the absence of TCGF for twice the cell cycle time, which suggests that TCGF or other CS components are not necessary for the expression of the lytic capacity. So far there is no evidence that TCGF is a signal which induces differentiation. On the other hand, the observation of an almost complete correlation between TCGF dependence and CTL activity in CTL–thymoma hybrids raises the question whether there is not only a genetic but also a functional linkage between these two manifestations of the CTL phenotype. In view of the morphological differences between CS^+ and CS^- hybrids, I wonder whether this correlation is not a reflection of differences in the cytoskeletal organization of the two cell types.

Be that as it may, the way to go seems fairly clear: Further characterization of the changes which occur in CTL lines after removal and after reexposure to TCGF should give us clues as to the mechanism of action of this molecule. Obvious changes to look for are those thought to play a role in the mitogenic activity of other growth factors or the cellular transformation by viruses, e.g., changes in the distribution of cytoskeletal proteins (Boschek *et al.*, 1981; Chinkers and Cohen, 1981; Sefton *et al.*, 1981).

If we do indeed find changes that are apparently controlled by TCGF, we should be able to learn something about the genetic basis of these responses and their relevance for the growth-promoting activity of this factor by looking for the same responses in CS^+ hybrids. Comparison of these hybrids with their CS^- variants or, even better, of CTL lines with their CS^- mutants, if they can be obtained, should, in turn, allow us to discern what molecular properties render a cell dependent on TCGF.

In this respect we have already found that CS^- variants can absorb about the same quantity of TCGF per cell as the CS^+ hybrids from which they were derived, i.e., 10 to 50 times more than the parental thymoma (Johnson *et al.*, Chapter 15 in this treatise). This suggests that TCGF dependence is not simply the consequence of the expression of a large concentration of TCGF receptors on the cell surface which have to be removed by internalization or shedding of TCGF–receptor complexes for the cell to be able to enter S phase.

B. Specificity

The question of the molecular and the genetic basis of T cell determinant-specific recognition structures ("T cell receptors") is at this time completely open. Technically, the problem is bogged down by the absence of an unambiguous and quantitative binding assay for T cell receptor molecules. None of the experiments pursuing the *idée fixe* that these receptors must have the same or similar molecular properties as antibodies has yielded any convincing evidence one way or the other. CTL-B lines have been used to search for somatic rearrangements involving immunoglobulin gene segments. The results (Forster *et al.*, 1980; Kronenberg *et al.*, 1980; Kurosawa *et al.*, 1981) were more intriguing than revealing, and it may well be time to go back to square one and to try to forget any preconceived ideas about the nature of the T cell receptor.

CTL lines should not only be useful to test rigorously some of these preconceived ideas, but may provide us with the means for an unbiased approach to the problem to T cell recognition. With regard to the first point they should permit us to determine, with considerable confidence, whether any particular chromosome does carry genes involved in specific T cell recognition by isolating, from CTL-thymoma hybrids which express the specificity of the parental CTL, segregants which have lost the CTL homologs of the chromosome in question. In some cases, such segregants can be selected out: selection of loss of expression of the H-2 antigens of the CTL parent should yield hybrids which have lost the chromosomes 17 of the CTL. In other cases, segregants may be frequent enough to be picked by random screening.

By screening hybrid subclones for the loss of cytolytic activity we may, in fact, be able to find segregants which have lost a chromosome carrying one of the genes controlling CTL specificity. Such variants would obviously be useful for the identification of these chromosomes, and the comparison of their cell surface molecules with those of the active parental hybrid might allow us to detect candidates for the molecular components of the T cell receptor. To distinguish receptor loss from variants which are not cytolytic because they have lost CTL genes which code for part of the cytolytic machinery, one could attempt to restore the activity by adding lectins to the CTL assay, which overcomes the requirement for specific target recognition for the lytic event. However, one must keep in mind that their effect may depend on the expression of a T cell receptor molecule on the CTL surface, i.e., they act by binding to a site on the receptor. One way to avoid this pitfall would be to isolate single specificity loss variants from hybrids expressing two independent specificities such as the ones described by Kappler *et al.* (1981).

C. The Cytolytic Machinery

This is the area where, I feel, the directions to take are least obvious, mainly because we have no good idea what to look for. Two technical breakthroughs could change this situation drastically: I already mentioned the need for a system allowing the selection of CTL line mutants deficient in a component essential for cytolytic activity. The other would be the development of an assay for the importance of molecular fractions of CTL for cytolytic activity, based on, e.g., the incorporation of such fractions into other cells or subcellular systems.

As it is, we do not know whether the only CTL-specific cell surface molecules that a CTL requires to be active are the T cell receptors themselves. Occupation of these by determinants on a target cell might trigger their interaction with other cell surface molecules which are not unique to CTL. The receptor may directly or indirectly transmit through the membrane signals whose transformation into cytolytic events depends on CTL-specific interactions with cytoplasmic molecules.

The genetic analysis of cytolytically incompetent segregants of CTL–thymoma hybrids should permit the chromosomal localization of CTL genes whose transcription is required for lytic competence and which are expressed on the thymoma homologs. But while it seems reasonable to look for T cell receptor gene products among the cell surface molecules, we do not know where the components of the lytic machinery should be located. It, therefore, may require a good dose of serendipity to detect which of the differences between the CTL^+ hybrids and their inactive variants are important for the cytolytic function.

ACKNOWLEDGMENTS

This work was supported by the Swiss National Science Foundation. I thank several of my collaborators for allowing me to cite their unpublished work. A. Conzelmann was a tireless and critical discussion partner.

REFERENCES

Alt, F. W., Bothwell, A. L. M., Knapp, M., Siden, E., Mather, E., Koshland, M., and Baltimore, D. (1980). Synthesis of secreted and membrane-bound immunoglobulin in Mu heavy chains is directed by mRNAs that differ at their 3′ ends. *Cell* **20,** 293.

Baker, P. E., Gillis, E., and Smith, K. A. (1979). Monoclonal cytolytic T-cell lines. *J. Exp. Med.* **149,** 273.

Berke, G. (1980). Interaction of cytotoxic T lymphocytes and target cells. *Prog. Allergy* **27,** 69.

Beverley, P. C. L. (1977). Lymphocyte heterogeneity. *In* "B and T Cells in Immune Recognition" (F. Loor and G. E. Roelants, eds.), pp. 35–57. Wiley, New York.

Boschek, C. B., Jockush, M., Friis, R. R., Back, R., Grundmann, E., and Bauer, H. (1981). Early changes in the distribution and organization of microfilament proteins during cell transformation. *Cell* **24,** 175.

Burrows, P. O., LeJeune, M., and Kearny, J. F. (1979). Evidence that murine pre-B cells synthesise a heavy chains but no light chains. *Nature (London)* **280,** 838.

Chinkers, M., and Cohen, S. (1981). Purified EGF receptor-kinase interacts specifically with antibodies to Rous sarcoma virus transforming protein. *Nature (London)* **290,** 514.

Conzelmann, A., Pink, R., Acuto, O., Mach, J.-P., Dolivo, S., and Nabholz, M. (1980). Presence of T145 on cytolytic T-cell lines and their lectin-resistant mutants. *Eur. J. Immunol.* **10,** 860

Dennert, G., Swain, S. L., Waterfield, J. D., Warner, J. F., and Dutton, R. W. (1981). Fine specificity mapping of 2 allospecific T cell lines: Recognition of private specificities in the *H-2 IA* subregion *Eur. J. Immunol.* **11,** 62.

Dialynas, D. P., Loken, M. R., Glasebrook, A. L., and Fitch, F. W. (1981). $Lyt\text{-}2^-/Lyt\text{-}3^-$ variants of a cloned cytolytic T cell line lack an antigen receptor functional in cytolysis. *J. Exp. Med.* **153,** 595.

Dutton, R. W., Falkoff, R., Hirst, J. A., Hoffmann, M., Kappler, J. W., Kettman, J. R., Lesley, J. F., and Vann, D. (1971). Is there evidence of a non-antigen specific diffusable chemical mediator from the thymus-derived cell in the initiation of the immune response. *In* "Progress in Immunology" (B. Amos ed.). pp. 355–368. Academic Press, New York.

Engers, H. D., Collavo, D., North, M., von Boehmer, H., Haas, W., Hengartner, H., and Nabholz, M. (1980). Characterization of cloned murine cytolytic T-cell lines. *J. Immunol.* **125,** 1481.

Forster, A., Hobart, M., Hengartner, H., and Rabbitts, T. H. (1980). An immunoglobuin heavy-chain gene is altered in two T-cell clones. *Nature (London)* **286,** 897.

Gillis, S., and Smith, K. A. (1977). Long term culture of tumor-specific cytotoxic T cells. *Nature (London)* **268,** 154.

Glasebrook, A. L., and Fitch, F. W. (1979). T cell lines which cooperate in generation of specific cytolytic activity. *Nature (London)* **278,** 171.

Gottlieb, P. O., and Durda, P. J. (1977). The I B-peptide marker and the Ly-3 surface alloantigen: Structural studies of a *Vk*-region polymorphism and a T-cell marker determined by linked genes. *Cold Spring Harbor Symp. Quant. Biol.* **41,** 805.

Haas, W., Mathur-Rochat, J., Pohlit, H., Nabholz, M., and von Boehmer, H. (1980). Cytotoxic T cell responses to haptenated cells. III. Isolation and specificity analysis of continuously growing clones. *Eur. J. Immunol.* **10,** 828.

Häyry, P. (1976). Anamnestic responses in mixed lymphocyte culture-induced cytolysis (MLC-CML) reaction. *Immunogenetics* **3,** 427.

Hengartner, H., Meo, T., and Muller, E. (1978). Assignment of genes for immunoglobulin K and heavy chains to chromosomes 6 and 12 in mouse. *Proc. Natl. Acad. Sci. U.S.A.* **75,** 4494.

Hiserodt, J. C., and Bonavida, B. (1981). Studies on the induction and expression of T cell-mediated immunity. XI. Inhibition of the "lethal hit" in T cell-mediated cytotoxicity by heterologous rat antiserum made against alloimmune cytotoxic T lymphocytes. *J. Immunol.* **126,** 256.

Kappler, J. W., Skidmore, B., White, J., and Marrack, P. (1981). Antigen-inducible, H-2-restricted, interleukin-2-producing T cell hybridomas. Lack of independent antigen and H-2 recognition. *J. Exp. Med.* **153,** 1198.

Kaufmann, V., Berke, G., and Eshhar, Z. (1981). Cytotoxic T lymphocyte hydridomas that mediate specific tumor-cell lysis *in vitro*. *Proc. Natl. Acad. Sci. U.S.A.* **78,** 2502.

Kimura, A., Wigzell, H., Holmquist, G., Ersson, B., and Carlsson, P. (1979). Selective affinity fractionation of murine cytotoxic T lymphocytes (CTL). Unique lectin specific binding of the CTL associated surface glycoprotein T145. *J. Exp. Med.* **149,** 473.

Kronenberg, M., Davis, M. M., Early, P. W., Hood, L. E., and Watson, J. D. (1980). Helper and killer T cells do not express B cell immunoglobulin joining and constant region gene segments. *J. Exp. Med.* **152,** 1745.

Kurosawa, Y., von Boehmer, H., Haas, W., Sakano, H., Trauneker, A., and Tonegawa, S. (1981). Identification of D segments of immunoglobulin heavy-chain genes and their rearrangement in T lymphocytes. *Nature (London)* **290,** 565.

Lutz, C. T., Glasebrook, A. L., and Fitch, F. W. (1981). Alloreactive cloned T cell lines. IV. Interaction of alloantigen and T cell growth factors (TCGF) to stimulate cloned cytolytic T lymphocytes. *J. Immunol.* **127,** 391.

Martz, E. (1977). Mechanism of specific tumor-cell lysis by alloimmune T lymphocytes: Resolution and characterization of discrete steps in the cellular interaction. *Contemp. Top. Immunobiol.* **7,** 301.

Morgan, D. A., Ruscetti, F. W., and Gallo, R. (1976). Selective *in vitro* growth of T lymphocytes from normal human bone marrow. *Science* **193,** 1007.

Nabholz, M., and Miggiano, V. (1977). The biological significance of the mixed leukocyte reaction. *In* "B and T Cells in Immune Recognition" (F. Loor and G. E. Roelants, ed.), Chapter 12, pp. 261–289. Wiley, New York.

Nabholz, M., Engers, H. D., Collavo, D., and North, M. (1978). Cloned T-cell lines with specific cytolytic activity. *Curr. Top. Microbiol. Immunol.* **81,** 176–187.

Nabholz, M., North, M., Engers, H. D., Collavo, D., von Boehmer, H., Haas, W., Hengartner, H., and McKenzie, I. F. C. (1979). Murine cytolytic T-cell lines: Stability of functional phenotype and expression of cell surface markers. *In* "T and B Lymphocytes: Recognition and Function" (F. H. Bach, B. Bonavida, E. Vitetta, and C. F. Fox, eds.), pp. 679–688. Academic Press, New York.

Nabholz, M., Conzelmann, A., Acuto, O., North, M., Haas, W., Pohlit, H., von Boehmer, H., Hengartner, H., Mach, J. P., Hengers, H. D., and Johnson, J. P. (1980a). Established murine cytolytic T-cell lines as tools for a somatic cell genetic analysis of T-cell functions. *Immunol. Rev.* **51,** 125.

Nabholz, M., Cianfriglia, M., Acuto, O., Conzelmann, A., Haas, W., von Boehmer, H., MacDonald, H. R., Pohlit, H., and Johnson, J. P. (1980b). Cytolytically active murine T-cell hybrids. *Nature (London)* **287,** 437.

Nabholz, M., Cianfriglia, M., Acuto, O., Conzelmann, A., Weiss, A., Haas, W., and von Boehmer, H. (1981). The production of murine cytolytic T cell hybrids. *In* "Monoclonal Antibodies and T cell Hybridomas" (G. H. Hammerling, U. Hammerling, and J. F. Kearney, eds.). Elsevier/North-Holland Biomed. Press, Amsterdam.

Nakayama, E., Hiroshi, S., Stockert, E., Oettgen, H. F., and Old, L. J. (1979). Cytotoxic T cells: Lyt phenotype and blocking of killing activity by Lyt antisera. *Proc. Natl. Acad. Sci. U.S.A.* **76,** 1977.

Perry, R. P., Kelley, D. E., Coleclough, C., and Kearney, J. F. (1981). Organization and expressions of immunoglobulin genes in fetal liver hybridomas. *Prod. Natl. Acad. Sci. U.S.A.* **78,** 247.

Raschke, W. C., Mather, E. L., and Koshland, M. E. (1979). The assembly and secretion of pentameric IgM in a fusion between a non-secreting B cell lymphoma and in IgG secreting plasmacytoma. *Proc. Natl. Acad. Sci. U.S.A.* **76,** 3469.

Ringertz, N. R., and Savage, R. E. (1976). "Cell Hybrids." Academic Press.

Ryser, J.-E., and MacDonald, H. R. (1979). Limiting dilution analysis of alloantigen-reactive T lymphocytes. I. Comparison of precursor frequencies for proliferative and cytolytic responses. *J. Immunol.* **122,** 1691.

Ryser, J.-E., Cerottini, J.-C., and Brunner, K. T. (1978). Generation of cytolytic T lymphocytes *in vitro.* IX. Induction of secondary CTL responses in primary longer-term MLC by supernatants from secondary MLC. *J. Immunol.* **120,** 370.

Sarmiento, M., Glasebrook, A. L., and Fitch, F. W. (1980). IgG of IgM monoclonal antibodies reactive with different determinants on the molecular complex bearing Lyt 2 antigen block T cell-mediated cytolysis in the absence of complement. *J. Immunol.* **125,** 2665.

Sefton, B. M., Hunter, T., Ball, E. H., and Singer, S. J. (1981). Vinculin: A cytoskeletal target of the transforming protein of Rous sarcoma virus. *Cell* **24,** 165.

Sekaly, R. P., MacDonald, H. R., Zaech, P., Glasebrook, A. L., and Cerottini, J.-C. (1981). T cell-mediated cytolysis is independent of growth phase and position in the mitotic cycle. *J. Exp. Med.* **154,** 575.

Sekaly, R. P., MacDonald, H. R., Zaech, P., and Nabholz, M. (1982). Cell cycle regulation of cloned cytolytic T cells by T cell growth factor: analysis by flow microfluorometry. Submitted for publication.

Shinkohara, N., and Sachs, D. H. (1979). Mouse alloantibodies capable of blocking cytotoxic T-cell function. I. Relationship between the antigen reactive with blocking antibodies and the Lyt-2 locus. *J. Exp. Med.* **150,** 432.

von Boehmer, H., Hengartner, H., Nabholz, M., Lernhardt, W., Schreier, M. H., and Haas, W. (1979). Fine specificity of a continuously growing killer cell clone specific for H-Y antigen. *Eur. J. Immunol.* **9,** 592.

Weiss, A., MacDonald, H. R., Cerottini, J.-C., and Brunner, K. T. (1981). Inhibition of cytolytic T lymphocyte clones reactive with Moloney leukemia virus-associated antigens by monoclonal antibodies: A direct approach to the study of H-2 restriction. *J. Immunol.* **126,** 482.

15

Karyotype Evolution of Cytolytic T Cell Lines

Judith P. Johnson/Maurizio Cianfriglia/
Andrew L. Glasebrook/Markus Nabholz

I. Karyotype Analysis of Functional T Cell Lines 183
A. Filler Cell-Independent CTL-B Lines 183
B. Murine T Cell Lines Maintained in the Presence of Stimulator or Filler Cells 188
C. Human T Cell Lines 189
II. Discussion 189
References 190

Since the original reports that human and murine T cells could be maintained in continuous culture by the addition of a T cell growth factor (TGGF, interleukin-2, IL-2) released by the lectin-stimulated lymphocytes, clones of cytolytic T cells (CTL), helper cells, and alloreactive proliferative cells have been isolated (see other chapters in this volume). The usefulness of these cell lines, particularly for somatic cell genetic and recombinant DNA studies, depends on the stability with which they maintain function, specificity, and a normal karyotype. We have examined the karyotypes of several murine CTL lines (see Table I), and our data show a high frequency of chromosomal rearrangements in some of these lines which make their use for cytogenetic studies problematical. The karyotypic evolution of such lines appears to be significantly affected by the procedures used to derive and establish them.

I. KARYOTYPE ANALYSIS OF FUNCTIONAL T CELL LINES

A. Filler Cell-Independent CTL-B Lines

The first cloned murine CTL lines that were established have now been maintained for 4 years in IL-2 without addition of filler or stimulator cells (Nabholz *et*

ISOLATION, CHARACTERIZATION, AND
UTILIZATION OF T LYMPHOCYTE CLONES

ISBN 0-12-249920-4

TABLE I

Origin and Characteristics of Murine T Cell Lines

Clone	Strain	Stimulator[a]	Maintained in	Established[b]	Activity	Specificity	Reference
B6.1	C57BL/6 ♀	C57B1/6 ♂	IL-2	3/78	Cytolytic	$H\text{-}2D^b$ ♂[c] $H\text{-}2D^d$	von Boehmer *et al.* (1979)
BD 2.118	(C57BL/6 × DBA/2)F_1	BALB/c	IL-2	11/78	Cytolytic	S194[e]	Nabholz *et al.* (1980)
DA 7	(AKR × DBA/2)F_1	C57BL/6	IL-2	11/77	Cytolytic	EL-4[d]	Nabholz *et al.* (1978)
HB.1	(AKR × DBA/2)F_1	C57BL/6	IL-2	9/77	Not cytolytic		Engers *et al.* (1980)
C.C3.11.75	BALB/c	C3H	Alloantigen[a]	11/75	Cytolytic, alloproliferative	I-A private[c]	Dennert *et al.* (1981)
B6.C.7.76	C57BL/6	BALB/c	Alloantigen[a]	7/76	Not cytolytic, alloproliferative	I-A private[c]	Dennert *et al.* (1981)
L3C5	C57BL/6	DBA/2	IL-2 + alloantigen[a]	1978	Cytolytic	$H\text{-}2D^d$[f]	Glasebrook and Fitch (1979)

[a] Stimulators and alloantigen are irradiated spleen cells.
[b] Beginning of *in vitro* culture (month and year).
[c] Lipopolysaccharide-induced lymphoblasts used as targets.
[d] C57BL/6-derived lymphoma.
[e] BALB/c-derived myeloma.
[f] Concanavalin A-induced lymphoblasts.

al., 1978; Baker *et al.*, 1979). IL-2 is usually provided in the form of supernatants of concanavalin A-stimulated mouse or rat spleen cells. These Thy-1^+ Lyt-2^+ CTL-B lines (Nabholz *et al.*, 1980) (for definition of CTL-A and CTL-B lines see Nabholz, Chapter 14 in this treatise) generally maintain their cytolytic activity and often also their specificity and are absolutely dependent on IL-2 for survival (reviewed in Nabholz *et al.*, 1980; Chapter 14 in this treatise; von Boehmer and Haas, 1981). The karyotypes of clones from four independently derived CTL-B lines (see Table I) have been analyzed in detail (Cianfriglia *et al.*, 1982), and their general karyotypic characteristics are presented in Table II.

None of the lines is karyotypically normal. However, the majority are cell populations with one discrete modal chromosomal number, and the same distinct structurally abnormal "marker" chromosomes are present in all metaphases. In addition, while each clone and subclone has unique characteristics, all lines tend to undergo similar kinds of karyotypic alterations, and some marker chromosomes were observed in independently derived lines. Structural aberrations are more frequent than numerical aberrations, in contrast to what is seen during the spontaneous evolution of murine fibroblast or epithelial cell cultures into permanent cell lines (Levan and Biesele, 1958; reviewed in Terzi, 1974).

TABLE II

Karyotypic Characteristics of Murine T Cell Lines

Cell	Age (months)	*N*[a]	NF[b]	Metacentrics	Remarks[c]
B6.1 subclones					
B6 1.1	25	42	43 (15)	1	
B6 1.2[d]	16	35	40 (12)	5	(*1.6*),(*2.6*),(7.8),(*9.10*),(*13.13*)
	25	35	41 (20)	6	(*1.6*),(*2.6*),(7.8),(*9.10*),(*13.13*)
B6 1.SF.1	25	42	43 (18)	1	
BD 2.118	25	31	40 (13)	9	(1.7),(*2.6*),(6.12),(*9.10*),(*13.13*),(19.10)
DA7 subclones					
DA 7.8	28	40	41 (18)	1	
DA 7.2.1	28	73	78 (17)	5	(*1.6*),(*13.13*),(11.11)
HB.1	10	39	40 (23)	1	
C.C3.11.75	31	40	40 (35)	0	translocation chr 1
B6.C.7.76	44	40	40 (28)	0	
L3C5	36	40	40 (41)	0[e]	

[a] Modal number of chromosomes.

[b] NF, fundamental number. In parentheses number of metaphases examined.

[c] (a.b) = Robertsonian fusions involving two whole recognizable mouse chromosomes (a and b). Italic are metacentrics which occur in more than one independent CTL-B line.

[d] The subclone B6 1.2 was analyzed twice in an interval of 9 months of continuous culture.

[e] Six out of 41 metaphases of L3C5 had 41 chromosomes. Of 14 completely analyzed Giemsa-banded metaphases, 11 appeared completely normal; of the remaining three each one was trisomic for a different chromosome (10, 14, 15).

The normal mouse karyotype consists of 20 pairs of acrocentric chromosomes each of which can be identified by its unique banding pattern (Nesbitt and Francke, 1973). All of the filler cell-independent lines carry at least one, and more often several, metacentric chromosomes. This common structural alteration of rodent chromosomes (Capanna *et al.*, 1976) presumably occurs by Robertsonian centric fusions (in which two acrocentric chromosomes fuse in the centrometric region to produce a single biarmed chromosome). This results in a reduced chromosome number but the number of chromosome arms (the fundamental number, *NF*) remains unchanged. All but one of the filler cell-independent CTL-B lines display a near diploid fundamental number. A more surprising observation is that a number of the chromosomes in these lines are structurally so different from any of the members of the mouse karyotype that their origin cannot be identified.

B6.1 and BD 2.118 are examples of lines which have extensive rearrangements producing unusual banding patterns (Fig. 1) and many metacentric chromosomes (Table II). An examination of several subclones of B6.1 demonstrates a broad range of variation, and the number of metacentric markers varies between 1 and 9 (Table II). Although they share many marker chromosomes consistent with their derivation from the same clone, subclones B6.1.1, 1.2, and 1.SF.1 are karyotypically distinct. Each carries unique metacentric and abnormal acrocentric chromosomes. This pattern can only be explained by a continual rapid evolution of the B6.1 karyotype, and this was directly observed when B6.1.2 was analyzed twice in an interval of 9 months (B6.1.2a,b). During this time the line underwent changes in the modal number of several normal chromosomes and acquired one new metacentric chromosome. Such instability is not characteristic of all CTL lines. When the uncloned H line was first examined (90 days after transfer to IL-2), all cells had a complement of 39 chromosomes which included one metacentric (Engers *et al.*, 1980). The same characteristics were seen in the clone HB.1 examined several months later. Thus, in this line a clone became predominant early during establishment of the line, and no further karyotypic changes occurred.

As fibroblast and epithelial cell cultures evolve into permanent lines, they often pass through a tetraploid stage and then slowly return to a hyperdiploid mode, although they then demonstrate great variation in the modal number of individual chromosomes (for reviews and interpretations, see Terzi, 1974; Harris, 1964, Chapter 4). The subclone DA 7.2.1 is the only example of a CTL line in which this process may be underway. It is subtetraploid ($N = 73$ but with a broad range) and carries variable numbers of individual chromosomes (e.g., five copies of chromosomes 5, 11 and 13, but only 2 recognizable copies of several other chromosomes). Four of the five copies of chromosome 13 are present as two 13/13 isochromosomes which suggests that tetraploidization occurred in a cell which had already undergone at least this rearrangement.

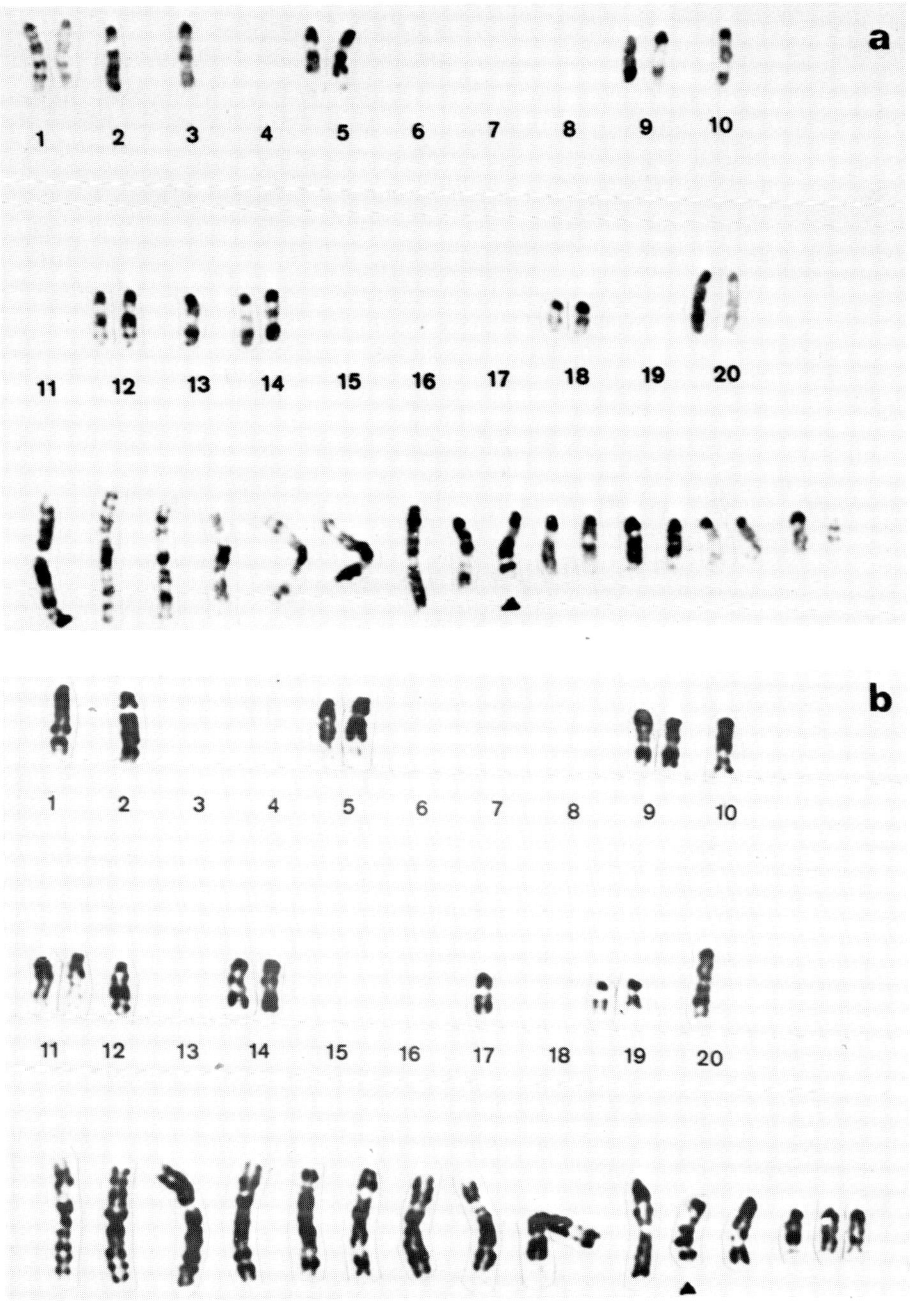

Fig. 1. Giemsa trypsin banded karyotypes of two independent CTL-B clones (a) B6.1.2. and (b) BD 2.118. Arrow denotes an acrocentric marker seen in both clones. Similar metacentric chromosomes are also found in both lines (see Table II).

When karyotypes of all clones are compared, it becomes clear that all chromosomes can be involved in numerical or structural alterations. Individual chromosomes can be trisomic, monosomic, or, in some cases, cannot be found at all. These numerical aberrations may be secondary to more fundamental structural rearrangements. For example, trisomies often occur when one copy of the affected chromosome is part of a metacentric. In the lines which carry unidentifiable marker chromosomes, it cannot be concluded that any chromosome is truly monosomic or absent. Metacentric chromosomes 1.6, 2.6, 9.10, and 13.13 have been found in several independently derived lines (see Table II), indicating that there is a nonrandom tendency to undergo centric fusion. However, no rearrangement is present in all lines. The same applies to acrocentric marker chromosomes: while the same markers have been identified in several independent lines (Fig. 1), no specific chromosomal alteration was found in all four filler cell-independent CTL-B lines.

B. Murine T Cell Lines Maintained in the Presence of Stimulator or Filler Cells

In addition to CTL-B lines we have examined one CTL-A line which requires both IL-2 and irradiated spleen filler or stimulator cells for growth (see Nabholz, Chapter 14 in this treatise for discussion), as well as two alloreactive T cell lines which apparently do not require IL-2 and are maintained by periodic restimulation with appropriate allogeneic spleen cells. The CTL-A clone was established in 1978 by cloning cells from a secondary mixed lymphocyte culture (MLC). The source of IL-2 used to maintain this line is secondary MLC supernatant (Glasebrook and Fitch, 1979). With regard to surface markers it is similar (Thy-1^+ Lyt-2^+) to the CTL-B lines described above, but the karyotype of most of the cells is completely normal (Table II), and the small fraction of cells with trisomies for different chromosomes probably arises continuously as the result of infrequent mitotic nondisjunction events.

Alloreactive T cells can be maintained in culture without addition of exogenous IL-2 if they are periodically restimulated with appropriate allogeneic leukocytes. Two lines have been described which have retained their antigenic specificity in culture for more than 5 years (Dennert *et al.*, 1981). Usually lines maintained in this way are noncytolytic (Häyry, 1976) and express Lyt-1 but not Lyt-2, and one of these two lines, B6.C.7.76, does fall into this group. It has an apparently completely normal karyotype (J. P. Johnson, S. L. Swain, and G. Dennert, unpublished). The other, C.C3.11.75, is unusual in that it is Lyt-1^+2^- but has retained specific cytolytic activity (Swain *et al.*, 1981). It carries a translocation involving one copy of chromosome 1 found in all metaphases examined, but all other chromosomes are apparently normal.

C. Human T Cell Lines

Human alloproliferative and CTL lines have been establishing by culturing cells from a primary or secondary MLC in the presence of IL-2, in the form of supernatants of phytohemagglutinin (PHA)-stimulated human leukocytes and irradiated allogeneic cells, either from peripheral blood or lymphoblastoid cell lines (see Chapters 35, 36, and 37). This protocol is similar to that used to derive the murine CTL-A clones. Like these cells, the human lines are dependent on both IL-2 and irradiated filler cells for growth. Thorough karyotypic studies have not yet been published, but preliminary observations from several laboratories suggest that major chromosomal abnormalities are frequent in these lines. One alloreactive clone maintained for 33 days in culture had a normal karyotype (J. P. Johnson and D. J. Schendel, unpublished observations) while a 6-month-old specific CTL clone was hyperdiploid with many rearranged chromosomes (C. Mawas, personal communication). Two HLA-A2 restricted clones with H-Y specificity were established and maintained in medium containing irradiated filler cells and PHA (Goulmy *et al.*, 1980). No IL-2 was added, but it is likely that the filler cells, in presence of the mitogen, produced sufficient growth factor to maintain the growth of the CTL. The lines were found to contain cells with extensive rearrangements when examined after 80 days of culture (E. Goulmy, personal communication). Human CTL lines pass through a period of poor growth, usually after about 2 months of culture, similar to the "crisis" observed during the establishment of CTL-B lines (Nabholz *et al.*, 1980).

II. DISCUSSION

The existence of CTL and alloproliferative lines which remain karyotypically normal and retain functional specificity although they have been in culture for as long as 5 years, demonstrates that it is possible to obtain the continuous growth of apparently normal T cells *in vitro*. These lines have been established and maintained in the presence of irradiated spleen cells. However, all filler cell-independent CTL lines that have been analyzed (including lines derived in Lausanne, Basel and by S. Gillis, personal communication) carry at least some and often many gross karyotypic abnormalities. There are many factors which can influence the frequency of chromosome aberrations (DeCarli and Lavizza, 1978; Sanford *et al.*, 1979) and filler cells may stabilize the karyotypes by counteracting some of these (Rothfels *et al.*, as discussed in Harris, 1964, p. 173). At the moment we cannot exclude that the difference between the karyotypes of CTL-A and CTL-B lines is due to the residual Concanavalian A in the IL-2 preparations used to maintain the CTL-B lines, or to hidden viral infections which occur in some laboratories but not in others. Mycoplasma infection would appear to be ruled out since CTL-B lines which are apparently not infected also have a high frequency of chromosomal aberrations.

Whereas one out of 5 cells of a 96 hr mixed leukocyte culture can give rise to a CTL-A clone, there are at least 100-fold less CTL in such populations which can grow in IL-2 alone (MacDonald *et al.*, 1980). Thus the precursors of CTL-B lines either belong to a very small fraction of normal CTL with different properties than CTL-A precursors, or, as we have suggested (see discussion by Nabholz, this volume) they are derived from CTL-A by a tranformation like event which renders them filler cell independent. It is tempting to speculate that the karyotype evolution of the CTL-B lines is causally related to this postulated transformation event, but this hypothesis will be difficult to prove, even if filler cell independent variants can be derived from CTL-A clones, and such variants do show a CTL-B like karyotype behavior.

We cannot yet make good guesses as to why human functional T cell lines seem to rapidly accumulate chromosomal abnormalities even if they are maintained in the presence of stimulator or filler cells. However, the IL-2 and filler cells used in the human system are different in many respects from those used to establish the CTL-A lines. In spite of the fact that it may be difficult to definitively identify the cause of the high frequency of karyotype abnormalities in CTL-B lines and human CTL lines, it is clearly important to learn how to control this frequency if such lines are to be useful for somatic cell genetic analyses.

ACKNOWLEDGMENTS

We thank D. J. Schendel for critical reading of the manuscript. This research was supported by the Deutsche Forschungsgemeinschaft Sonderforschungsbereich 37(B9) and by the Swiss National Science Foundation. M. Cianfriglia is the recipient of an EMBO fellowship.

REFERENCES

Baker, P. E., Gillis, S., and Smith, K. A. (1979). Monoclonal cytolytic T-cell lines. *J. Exp. Med.* **149,** 273.

Capanna, E., Gropp, A., Winking, H., Noak, G., and Civitelli, M. V. (1976). Robertsonian metacentrics in the mouse. *Chromosoma* **58,** 341.

Cianfriglia, M., Johnson, J. P., and Nabholz, M. (1982). In preparation.

DeCarli, L., and Lavizza, L. (1978). Induced chromosome variation in cultured cell populations. *In* "Origin and Natural History of Cell Lines" (C. Barigozzi, ed.), pp. 93–124. Alan R. Liss, Inc., New York.

Dennert, G., Swain, S. L., Waterfield, J. D., Warner, J. F., and Dutton, R. W. (1981). Fine specificity mapping of two allospecific T cell lines: Recognition of private specificities in the H-2 *IA* subregion. *Eur. J. Immunol.* **11,** 62.

Engers, H. D., Collavo, D., North, M., von Boehmer, H., Haas, W., Hengartner, H., and Nabholz, M. (1980). Characterization of cloned murine cytolytic T cell lines. *J. Immunol.* **125,** 1481.

Glasebrook, A. L., and Fitch, F. W. (1979). T cell lines which cooperate in generation of specific cytolytic activity. *Nature (London)* **278,** 171.

Goulmy, E., Blokland, E., van Rood, J., Charmot, D., Malissen, B., and Mawas, C. (1980) Production, expansion and clonal analysis of T cell with specific HLA-restricted male lysis. *J. Exp. Med.* **152,** 1825.

Harris, M. (1964) "Cell Culture and Somatic Variation." Holt, New York.

Häyry, P. (1976). Anamnestic responses in mixed lymphocyte culture-induced cytolytis (MLC-CML) reaction. *Immunogenetics* **3,** 417.

Levan, A., and Biesele, J. J. (1958). Role of chromosomes in carcinogenesis as studied in serial tissue culture of mammalian cells. *Ann. N.Y. Acad. Sci.* **71,** 1022.

MacDonald, H. R., Maryanski, J. L., and Cerottini, J.-C. (1980). Cloning of cytolytic T lymphocytes: Requirement for interleukin-2 and irradiated spleen cells. *Behring Inst. Mitt.* **67,** 182.

Nabholz, M., Engers, H. D., Collavo, D., and North, M. (1978). Cloned T cell lines with specific cytolytic activity. *Curr. Top. Microbiol. Immunol.* **81,** 176.

Nabholz, M., Conzelmann, A., Acuto, O., North, M., Haas, W., Pohlit, H., von Boehmer, H., Hengartner, H., Mach, J.-P., Engers, H., and Johnson, J. P. (1980). Established murine cytolytic T cell lines as tools for a somatic cell genetic analysis of T cell functions. *Immunol. Rev.* **51,** 125.

Nesbitt, M. N., and Francke, W. (1973). A system of nomenclature for band patterns of mouse chromosomes. *Chromosoma* **41,** 145.

Rothfels, K. H., Kupelwieser, E. B., and Parker, R. C. (1963). Effects of X-irradiated feeder layers on mitotic activity and development of aneuploidy in mouse embryo cells *in vitro*. *Proc. Can. Cancer Res. Conf.* **5,** 191–223.

Sanford, K. K., Parshad, R., Handleman, S. L., Price, F. M., Gantt, R. R., and Evans, U. J. (1979). Serum induced chromosome damage and neoplastic transformation of mouse cells *in vitro*. *In Vitro* **15,** 488.

Swain, S. L., Dennert, G., Wormsley, S., and Dutton, R. W. (1981). The Lyt phenotype of a long-term allospecific T cell line. Both helper and killer activities to IA are mediated by Ly-1 cells. *Eur. J. Immunol.* **11,** 175.

Terzi, M. (1974) "Genetics and the Animal Cells," pp. 27–41. Wiley, New York.

von Boehmer, H., and Haas, W. (1981). H-2 restricted cytolytic and noncytolytic T cell clones: Isolation, specificity and functional analysis. *Immunol. Rev.* **54,** 27.

von Boehmer, H., Hengartner, H., Nabholz, M., Lernhardt, W., Schreier, M. H., and Haas, W. (1979). Fine specificity of a continuously growing killer cell clone specific for H-Y antigen. *Eur. J. Immunol.* **9,** 592.

16

Growth Regulation of Cytolytic T Cell Lines by Interleukin-2

Rafick P. Sekaly/H. Robson MacDonald/Markus Nabholz

I. Mechanisms of Action of Growth Factors 194
II. Mechanisms of Action of TCGF on a Cloned CTL Line 196
A. Requirement for Continued Proliferation 196
B. Cell Cycle Kinetics 196
C. Cytolytic Activity 199
References 202

One of the central problems in cell biology is the elucidation of the factors and mechanisms which control cell reproduction or proliferation. As first defined by Howard and Pelc (1953), the mitotic cycle can be divided into four successive intervals, namely G_1, S, G_2, and MG_1 is the time gap between the completion of cell division and the beginning of DNA replication, S is the period of DNA replication, G_2 is the time gap between the end of DNA replication and the onset of cell division, and M is the time taken for cell division.

It has been known for many years that hormones, such as ACTH, growth hormone, and estrogen, are important for cell proliferation and differentiation *in vivo,* but these hormones do not stimulate the proliferation of their target cells *in vitro* (Masui and Garren, 1971). Among agents which stimulate both *in vitro* and *in vivo* proliferation of cells are the polypeptide growth factors (Rudland *et al.,* 1974; Gospodarowicz *et al.,* 1977, 1978), hormone-like substances that are released from many cell types and reach their destination by a variety of routes ranging from local diffusion to systemic transport. Present information suggests that many different polypeptide growth factors exist and that many remain unidentified and unpurified (Barnes and Sato, 1980). Serum and plasma appear to contain numerous different growth factors. Endocrine glands (Rudland *et al.,* 1974; Gospodarowicz *et al.,* 1978) (notably pituitary and submaxillary glands) and conditioned medium from tumor cells (sarcoma) (Todaro *et al.,* 1979) have also shown to be potent sources of growth factors. Many of these substances may

ISBN 0-12-249920-4

be related. Thus, nonsuppressible insulin-like activity, somatomedins in plasma, multiplication stimulating activity in serum, and nerve growth factors belong to a single family of genetically related proteins (Shields, 1978) with observed similarities in structure, while platelet growth factor, Antoniades human serum factor, and fibroblast growth factor are probably the same (Gospodarowicz and Moran, 1976).

The mechanisms of action of growth factors on cell proliferation have been extremely difficult to study in whole tissues. Most growth factor responsive tissues do not comprise a uniform cell population, and the control of cell proliferation in tissues involves the interaction of several hormones or growth factors and cells. Hence the isolation of clonal lines of growth factor responsive cells is of paramount importance for the study of the action of the growth factors.

In this chapter we shall review briefly the available information on the action of growth factors on the cell cycle of their relative target cells, which we will then compare with recent results obtained in the study of the cell cycle control of cytolytic T cell lines (CTL) by T cell growth factor (TCGF = interleukin = IL-2).

I. MECHANISMS OF ACTION OF GROWTH FACTORS

Growth factors act by binding to specific cell surface receptor sites (Gordon *et al.*, 1978). Whether a growth factor acts on a certain type of cell depends on the proportion of occupied receptor sites for the growth factor. The interaction of the growth factors with cells leads to a series of events inside the cell that culminates in the induction of DNA synthesis. Growth factors acting as mitogens have been grouped into two broad categories based on the stage of the cell cycle in which they appear to act (Stiles *et al.*, 1979). Agents such as epidermal growth factor (EGF) and fibroblast growth factor (FGF) prime a significant portion of a quiescent cell population to enter a state of competence, while other agents, notably the somatomedins, stimulate these competent cells to enter the S phase. In this chapter we shall restrict ourselves to the first category of growth factors with an emphasis on the mechanisms of action of EGF and FGF.

The usual method for studying kinetics of growth stimulation has been to take a quiescent culture, to add the stimulating agent (source of growth factor) to its medium, and to examine the modifications preceding DNA synthesis and mitosis. These transitions of cultures from the quiescent state into the growing state are characterized by several common kinetic features.

Normal untransformed quiescent cells are usually arrested in the G_1 phase of the cell cycle. Accordingly stimulated cells first enter the S phase and only later mitosis. Growth factor effects on DNA synthesis are noticed only after a certain lag period.

To activate DNA synthesis of cells, the stimulating agent is required during the whole latent period or at least during a large part thereof. Brooks (1976) has shown that the latent period preceding activation of DNA synthesis by resting cultures of 3T3 cells exposed to fresh serum as source of growth factor was 14 hr. In cultures of human glial cells, DNA synthesis stimulated by fresh serum or EGF started after a lag period of about 17 hr (Lindgren and Westermark, 1977). Transfer of chick fibroblasts into stimulator-free medium during any part of the latent period prevented activation of DNA synthesis (Rubin and Steiner, 1975).

The growth rate of normal cells is controlled by the concentration of the growth factors required for induction of DNA synthesis. In this context requirement of growth factor for cell proliferation can be studied by depriving cultured cells of the growth factor. Thus, the entry of chick fibroblasts into the S phase was reduced almost immediately after the removal of serum (Rubin and Steiner, 1975). Transfer of 3T3 cells from a medium enriched with growth factor a low serum medium led to a decrease in the rate of DNA synthesis after 5 hr (Brooks, 1976).

Kinetic characteristics of quiescent cultures stimulated to growth have been described above. To interpret these, several theoretical models of cell kinetics have been proposed (Rudland and Jimenez de Asua, 1979).

The first model assumed that the cell cycle of an individual cell is uniquely determined by its precise biochemical composition. Variation could arise because individual cells in the population differ in properties which determine their transit through the cycle. In a genetically homogeneous population such differences could occur because of unequal partition of cell constitutents at division or random fluctuation in cell cycle of important molecules present at low concentration. In this model, cells of resting cultures do not move through the cell cycle; instead they enter a special phase designated G_0. Stimulating agents activate cell reversion from G_0 to G_1 phase of the cycle.

The simplest transition probability model of the cell cycle suggests that the initiation of cell division depends on a single stochastic event or transition in G_1, which occurs at random. Each cell life is divided into two fundamentally different parts. After mitosis all cells enter a state (A) in which their activity is not directed toward replication. On leaving A state, cells enter the B phase in which their activities are directed toward replication in a deterministic fashion. Cell population growth rates are determined by the probability with which cells leave the A state, the duration of the B phase, and the rate of cell death. Growth factors, depending on their concentration, may change the rate of entry into the B phase.

In summary, growth stimulating agents to not immediately and irreversibly commit the exposed cells to DNA synthesis and division. The transition through the lag period is a lengthy and reversible process possibly requiring several external stimuli for its progress and completion.

II. MECHANISMS OF ACTION OF TCGF ON A CLONED CTL LINE

A. Requirement for Continued Proliferation

Several investigators have suggested that growth control in T lymphocytes under *in vitro* conditions is the result from the interaction of at least three distinct cell types (Möller, 1980). When antigen (Ag) is introduced into a mixed population, these cell types can respond in three ways: (1) release of lymphocyte activating factor (LAF) from monocytes/macrophage; (2) under the influence of LAF, some T cells release TCGF; (3) another subset of T cells expressed TCGF receptors and responds to TCGF by proliferation. It becomes apparent that functional T cell clonal expansion, although Ag initiated, is under the strict control by hormone-like soluble factors released by cells of the immune system.

Recent reports have demonstrated that cloned lines of T cells can be derived and maintained in medium containing TCGF (Nabholz *et al.*, 1980; MacDonald *et al.*, 1980; Glasebrook *et al.*, 1981). This provides an *in vitro* system in which T lymphocyte proliferation can be studied under constant environmental conditions, thus enabling analysis of the mode of action of this growth factor. Moreover, the fact that these T cell clones continue to express specific cytolytic activity makes it possible to study the control of functional activity by the growth factor. In this chapter, we describe the kinetics of action of TCGF on cytolytic T lymphocyte (CTL) line B6.1. obtained by multiple antigenic stimulation followed by a period of continuous culture in TCGF-containing medium (crude supernatant from rat spleen cells stimulated by concanavalin A) (von Boehmer *et al.*, 1979). Figure 1 indicates that in the presence of optimal TCGF concentrations, B6.1. cells have a doubling time of about 16.5 hr as calculated from the exponential phase of the growth curve. Complete removal of TCGF from the cell culture medium resulted in a leveling off of the growth curve which begins about 24 hr after removal of the factor.

B. Cell Cycle Kinetics

As we have mentioned on Section I most of the growth factor-dependent cells studied thus far accumulate in G_1 when they are transferred from a medium supplemented with growth factor to a growth factor free environment. It was thus of interest to look at the cell cycle distribution of exponentially growing B6.1.

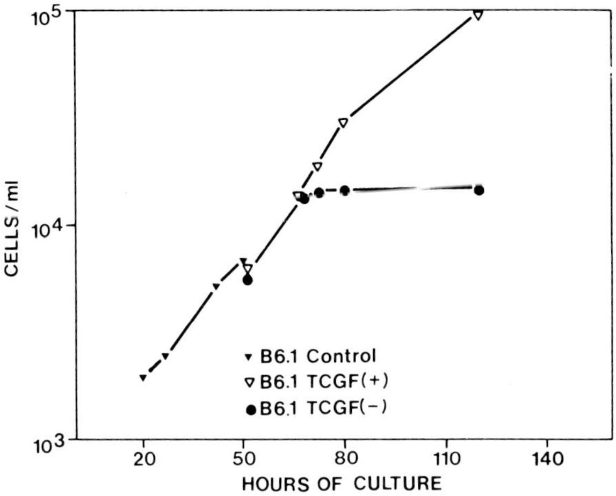

Fig. 1. Growth kinetics of B6.1. cells. 10^4 cells/well were plated in 1 ml of medium supplemented with 25% TCGF or in the absence of TCGF. The cell number per well was determined at various times using an electronic cell counter (Coulter Electronics). (▼) Growth of the control population. Growth of the population in the presence (▽) or in the absence (●) of TCGF.

cells deprived of TCGF. For this purpose, cells growing in TCGF-free medium for different time intervals were stained with the DNA binding dye propidium iodide (PI) after the cells had been treated with RNase, and the distribution of DNA content analyzed on a fluorescence activated cell sorter (Fig. 2). The proportion of cells in the S phase of the cell cycle was half that in control cultures after the cells had been deprived of TCGF for at least 6 hr. This fraction continued to decrease, and after 30 hr without TCGF about 91% of the cells were in the G_1 phase of the cell cycle, in comparison to 38% in an exponentially growing population. The number of DNA-synthesizing cells had fallen from 35% to 3%. These results suggest that cells stop in G_1 after removal of TCGF from the culture medium. It is unlikly that this accumulation of cells in G_1 is the result of a preferential death and disappearance of cells in the S, G_2, and M phases of the cell cycle because (1) cell number kept increasing for 24 hr after removal of TCGF (Fig. 1), and (2) the plating efficiency of B6.1. cells was not affected after the cells had been deprived of TCGF for intervals ranging up to 30 hr (data not shown).

It was thus of interest to confirm that cells completed at least one cycle after removal of TCGF. Therefore, we used a recently described technique (Böhmer, 1979) which is based on the quenching of fluorescence of the DNA-specific stain Hoechst 33342 by bromodeoxyuridine (BUdR) incorporated into DNA in place of thymidine. Preliminary experiments showed that presence of BUdR in the medium did not affect the proliferation and the cell cycle kinetics of B6.1.

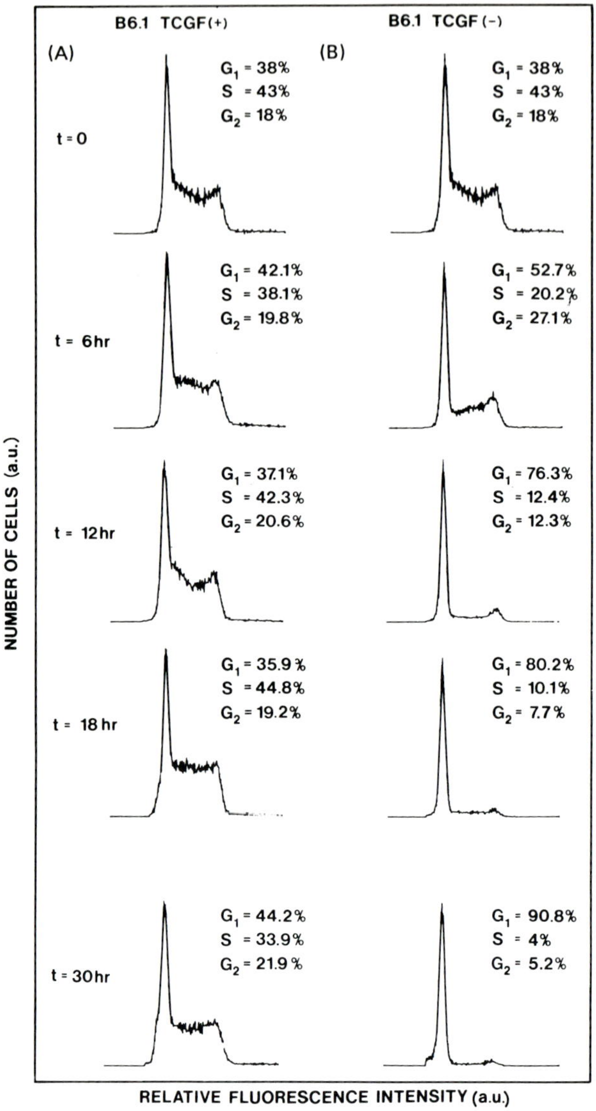

Fig. 2. Cell cycle distribution of B6.1. CTL line growing exponentially or at different times after removal of TCGF. Cells were harvested after they had been washed and maintained in medium without TCGF for different time intervals (0, 6, 12, 18, 30 hr). Following treatment with RNase (80 Kunitz units/ml), cells were stained with the DNA binding dye propidium iodide (50 μg/ml) in the presence of 0.05% NP40. The samples were then passed on a FACS II flow cytometer (Becton Dickinson, Mountainview, California) using the 488 nm excitation wavelength. A minimum of 50,000 cells were accumulated for each DNA histogram. A semiquantitative method was used to estimate the relative number of B6.1. cells in the different phases of the cell cycle, as described in detail elsewhere (Sekaly *et al.*, 1981).

Exponentially growing cultures of B6.1. cells were transferred from a TCGF-containing medium into a medium containing 10^{-5} *M* BUdR, harvested after different time intervals and stained with Hoechst in the presence of 0.05% NP 40 (Fig. 3). For each time point a culture maintained in TCGF was compared to one deprived of TCGF at the time of BUdR addition. The designation of the various peaks is explained in the legend of Fig. 3. Prior to addition to BUdR the fluorescence distribution corresponds to the real DNA distribution. When the cell progresses through the S phase, it will incorporate BUdR and thus will not increase its fluorescence intensity. After mitosis, the amount of detectable DNA will be half that present at the time of addition of BUdR. Figure 3 shows that by 3 hr, the G_2 + M peak had decreased, i.e., the cells in this phase at the time of BUdR addition have completed mitosis both in the exponentially growing population and in the population deprived of TCGF. After 8 hr the S′ compartment was empty. At 12 hr, we observe appearance of a new G_1'' peak with half the fluorescence intensity of the initial G_1 peak; it consists of cells which had been in G_1 at the moment of BUdR addition. After 20 hr most of the cells are in G_1''. It should be emphasized that the real DNA distributions as measured by PI have the shape of the zero time histograms in Fig. 2A, since the culture remains in the state of exponential growth, while the PI distribution of the cells in Fig. 2B indicates a progressive decrease of cells entering the S phase.

These results suggest that regulation of proliferation might occur at a random point during the G_1 phase of the cell cycle. Data obtained with the PI stain had indicated that cells accumulate in G_1 after removal of TCGF, while the results from the Hoechst–BUdR experiments confirmed that B6.1. cells complete at least one cycle before they accumulate in G_1. Preliminary experiments indicate that upon transfer of cells deprived of TCGF for 30 hr to a medium supplemented with the growth factor, the majority of the cells arrested in G_1 will enter the S phase. Many studies remain to be done to further clarify the influence of TCGF on the cell cycle kinetics of CTL. It is not clear from these data whether the block of cells in G_1 occurs at a single point. Alternatively, cells may arrest at any of several points in G_1 depending on their initial cell-associated TCGF association and on the location of the cell in the cell cycle at the moment of TCGF removal.

C. Cytolytic Activity

Quiescent cells probably undergo profound metabolic changes upon growth stimulation. In the case of TCGF stimulation of T cell proliferation it is not clear yet whether TCGF acts only as a growth promoting factor or whether it is also a differentiation inducing signal. We have compared the cytolytic activity of B6.1. growing exponentially or arrested after removal of TCGF for different time intervals. Cytolytic activity was measured in a short-term ^{51}Cr release assay

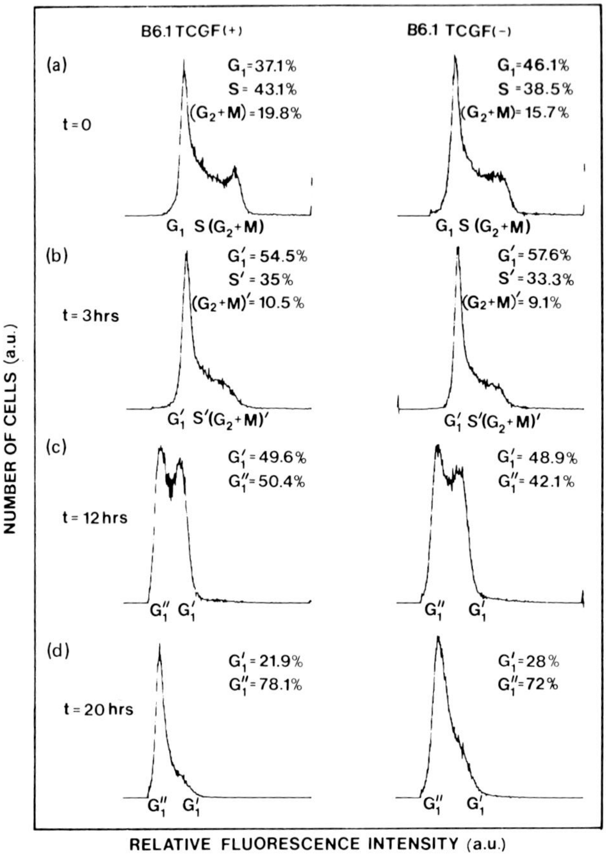

Fig. 3. Fluorescence distribution of Hoechst 33342 stained B6.1. cells maintained for various intervals in medium without TCGF but containing BUdR. Cells were plated in 25-ml culture flasks at a concentration of 10×10^4/ml and cultured in TCGF-containing medium until exponential growth was reestablished. Individual cultures were then harvested at various times after being washed and transferred to medium with or without TCGF and containing 2.0 mg/liter BUdR and 1.6 mg/liter deoxycytidine for (a) 0 hr, (b) 3 hr, (c) 12 hr, (d) 20 hr. Upon harvest cells were stained with the DNA binding dye Hoechst 33342 in presence of 0.05% NP40. The samples were passed on a FACS II Flow cytometer using the 351–364 nm excitation wavelength. G_1: cells in the G_1 phase of the cell cycle G_1': cells which had been in G_1 at the time of BUdR addition and have not passed yet through mitosis, G_1'': cells which had been in G_1 at the time of BUdR addition and have already passed through mitosis. Similar definitions are used for S and (G_2 + M) phase cells.

as described previously (Cerottini *et al.*, 1974). Data illustrated in Fig. 4 indicate that exponentially growing B6.1 lysed 50% of ^{51}Cr-labeled target cells at an effector: target cell ratio of 0.5 : 1. No significant decrease in the cytolytic activity was observed when the cells were deprived of TCGF for intervals ranging up to 30 hr (Fig. 4). These results are in agreement with prior observations (Sekaly *et al.*, 1981), indicating that the cytolytic activity of CTL obtained from noncycling or exponentially growing cultures was identical although in the latter report, resting cultures were obtained by letting the cells reach the plateau phase of growth, and it was not clear whether growth arrest was due to lack of TCGF or other media constituents. Thus while TCGF does control proliferation of B6.1. cells, expression of cytolytic competence *in vitro* is apparently not growth regulated.

In conclusion, this chapter brings new information on the mechanisms of action of TCGF and suggests that this molecule exerts its effects upon the control

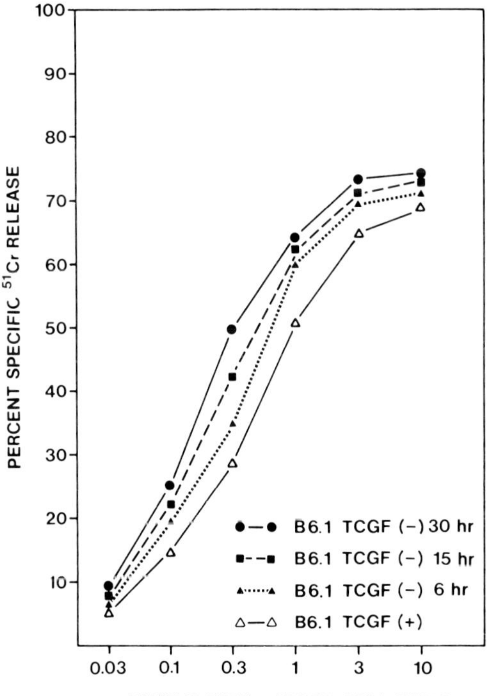

Fig. 4. Cytolytic activity of B6.1. CTL line deprived of TCGF for different periods. Exponentially growing B6.1. cells were transferred to medium without TCGF and later tested for lytic activity against 10^4 ^{51}Cr-labeled S194 target cells. Open symbols represent the cytolytic activity of exponentially growing control cultures. Closed symbols illustrate the cytolytic activity of B6.1. cells deprived of TCGF for 6 hr (▲), 15 hr (■), or 30 hr (●).

of proliferation of activated T cells in a manner similar to other polypeptide growth factors.

REFERENCES

Barnes, D., and Sato, G (1980). Serum free cell culture: A unifying approach. *Cell* **22,** 649.

Böhmer, R. M. (1979). Flow cytometric cell cycle analysis using the quenching of 33258 Hoechst fluorescence by bromodeoxyuridine incorporation. *Cell Tissue Kinet.* **12,** 101.

Brooks, R. F. (1976). Regulation of the fibroblast cell cycle by serum. *Nature* (*London*) **260,** 248.

Cerottini, J.-C., Engers, H. D., MacDonald, H. R., and Brunner, K. T. (1974). Generation of cytotoxic T lymphocytes *in vitro*. I. Response of normal and immune mouse spleen cells in mixed leukocyte cultures. *J. Exp. Med.* **140,** 703.

Glasebrook, A. L., Sarmiento, M., Loken, M. R., Dialynas, D. P., Quintans, J., Eisenberg, L., Lutz, C. T., Wilde, D., and Fitch, F. W. (1981). Murine T lymphocyte clones with distinct immunological function. *Immunol. Rev.* **54,** 225.

Gordon, P., Carpentier, J. L., Cohen, S., and Orci, L. (1978). Epidermal growth factor: Morphological demonstration of binding internalization and lysosomal association in human fibroblasts. *Proc. Natl. Acad. Sci. U.S.A.* **75,** 5025.

Gospodarowicz, D., and Moran, J. (1976). Growth factors in mammalian cell cultures. *Annu. Rev. Biochem.* **45,** 531.

Gospodarowicz, D., Mescher, A. L., Brown, K., and Birdwell, C. R. (1977). The role of fibroblast growth factor and epidermal growth factor in the proliferative response of the cornea and lens epithelium. *Exp. Eye Res.* **25,** 631.

Gospodarowicz, D., Greenberg, G., Bialecki, H., and Zettern, B. (1978). Factors involved in the modulation of cell proliferation *in vivo* and *in vitro*: The role of fibroblasts and epidermal growth factor in the proliferative response of mammalian cells. *In Vitro* **14,** 85.

Howard, A., and Pelc, S. R. (1953). Synthesis of deoxyribonucleic acid in normal and irradiated cells and its relation to chromosome breakage. *Heredity, Suppl.* **6,** 261.

Lindgren, A., and Westermark, B. (1977). Reset of the replicative phase of glial cells in culture. *Exp. Cell Res.* **106,** 89.

MacDonald, H. R., Cerottini, J.-C., Ryser, J.-E., Maryanski, J. L., Taswell, C., Widmer, M. B., and Brunner, K. T. (1980). Quantitation and cloning of cytolytic T lymphocytes and their precursors. *Immunol. Rev.* **51,** 93.

Masui, M., and Garren, L. D. (1971). On the mechanism of action of adrenocorticotropic hormone: The stimulation of thymidine kinase activity with altered properties and changed subcellular distribution. *J. Biol. Chem.* **246,** 5407.

Möller, G., ed. (1980). T cell stimulating growth factors. *Immunol. Rev.* **51,** 357.

Nabholz, M., Conzelmann, A., Acuto, O., North, M., Haas, W., Pohlit, H., von Boehmer, H., Hengartner, H., Mach, J.-P., Engers, H. D., and Johnson, J. P. (1980). Established murine cytolytic T-cell lines as tools for a somatic cell genetic analysis of T-cell functions. *Immunol. Rev.* **51,** 125.

Rubin, M., and Steiner, R. (1975). Reversible alteration in the mitotic cycle of chick embryo cells in various states of growth regulation. *J. Cell. Physiol.* **85,** 261.

Rudland, P. S., and Jimenez de Asua, L. (1979). Action of growth factors in the cell cycle. *Biochim. Biophys. Acta* **560,** 91.

Rudland, P. S., Seifert, N., and Gospodarowicz, A. (1974). Growth control in cultured human fibroblasts: Induction of the pleiotypic and mitogenic responses by a purified growth factor. *Proc. Natl. Acad. Sci. U.S.A.* **71,** 2600.

Sekaly, R. P., MacDonald, H. R., Zaech, P., Glasebrook, A. L., and Cerottini, J.-C. (1981). T. cell mediated cytolysis is independent of growth phase and position in the mitotic cycle. *J. Exp. Med.* **154,** 575.

Shields, R. (1978). Growth factors for tumours. *Nature* (*London*) **272,** 670.

Stiles, C. D., Capone, G. T., Scher, C. D., Antoniades, M. N., Van Wyk, J. J., and Pledger, W. J. (1979). Dual control of cell growth by somatomedins and platelet derived growth factor. *Proc. Natl. Acad. Sci. U.S.A.* **76,** 1279.

Todaro, G. J., DeLarco, J. E., Marquardt, H., Bryant, M. L., Sherwin, S. A., and Sliski, A. H. (1979). Polypeptide growth factors produced by tumor cells and virus transformed cells: A possible growth advantage for the producer cell. *Cold Spring Harbor Conf. Cell Proliferation* **6,** 113–127.

von Boehmer, H., Hengartner, H., Nabholz, M., Lernhardt, W., Schreier, M., and Haas, W. (1979). Fine specificity of a continuously growing killer cell clone specific for H-Y antigen. *Eur. J. Immunol.* **9,** 592.

17

Correlation between Cytolytic Activity, Growth Factor Dependence, and Lectin Resistance in Cytolytic T Cell Hybrids

Andreas Conzelmann/Patricia Corthesy/Markus Nabholz

I.	Introduction	205
II.	Origin in CTL Hybrids	206
III.	CTL Activity, VV Resistance, and CS Dependence of Hybrids	206
IV.	Selection of CS^- Variants from Cloned CS^+ Cytolytic Hybrids	210
V.	Conclusions	213
	References	214

I. INTRODUCTION

Recently it has been shown that fusion between murine cytolytic T cell lines and murine T lymphoma lines can yield hybrids which retain the specific cytolytic capacity of the CTL line parent (Nabholz *et al.*, 1980). The CTL lines used in these fusions are dependent on T cell growth factor (TCGF) without any additional requirements for feeder cells (CTL-B lines, see Nabholz *et al.*, 1981; Chapter 14 in this treatise). In the absence of TCGF the cells stop to grow and die within 2 to 3 days (Chapter 16 in this treatise). In the experiments reported here, we used supernatant from concanavalin A-stimulated rat spleen cells (CS) as a source of TCGF.

From crosses between such CTL-B lines and T lymphoma lines hybrids can be obtained with a high frequency. In our hands over a hundred such hybrids selected in the absence of CS were cytolytically inactive, whereas a large proportion of the hybrids selected in CS-containing medium displayed lytic activity. These can be cloned and maintain their activity with adequate stability (Nabholz *et al.*, 1981). The cytolytic hybrids continue to depend on CS for proliferation,

ISOLATION, CHARACTERIZATION, AND UTILIZATION OF T LYMPHOCYTE CLONES

ISBN 0-12-249920-4

while the hybrids selected in the absence of CS do not become cytolytic when cultured in CS. CS can be replaced by supernatant from secondary mixed leukocyte cultures or by partially purified TCGF of human origin (O. Acuto, unpublished observations). In certain crosses, the two types of hybrids can be distinguished by morphological criteria in that CS-dependent (CS^+) hybrids tend to adhere to plastic and assume a polygonal, fibroblast-like appearance, whereas CS-independent (CS^-) hybrids look like the thymoma parental cells (Nabholz *et al.*, 1980).

In this chapter we compare the two types of hybrids with regard to surface glycoproteins (gp's) and resistance to *Vicia villosa* lectin (VV). This lectin has been reported to specifically bind to cytolytic T lymphocytes (Kimura *et al.*, 1979). We have found that all CTL lines bind high amounts of VV and are very susceptible to its toxic effects, whereas thymomas bind 500- to 1000-fold less and are completely resistant (Conzelmann *et al.*, 1980).

II. ORIGIN OF CTL HYBRIDS

As described by Haas (1980), CSP.2.4 is a CTL line which displays specific, *H-2*-restricted cytolytic activity against 3-(sulfophenyldiazo)-4-hydroxyphenylacetic acid (SP)-coupled targets of $H\text{-}2^k$ haplotype. This line was fused with the AKR-thymoma line BW5147 ($HGPRT^-$, OUA^r) and hybrids were selected in HAT medium containing 10^{-3} M ouabain, either in the presence or in the absence of CS (Nabholz *et al.*, 1980). The hybrid nature of the selected cells was confirmed by analysis of cell surface markers and chromosome constitution. Four hybrid populations of each type were kept in culture in the presence or absence of CS according to the initial selection conditions. The hybrids are designated in the following way: The first number indicates the fusion from which they are derived, the second indicates the initial hybrid population. Thus, hybrids with a different second number are derived from independent fusion events. The third and further numbers designate clones and subclones derived from the initial hybrid population. Hybrids were cloned by limiting dilution on macrophage feeder layers.

III. CTL ACTIVITY, VV RESISTANCE, AND CS DEPENDENCE OF HYBRIDS

As summarized in Table I, the four CS-independent hybrid populations selected in the absence of CS (12.3, 12.4, 12.5, 12.21) neither show specific cytolytic activity nor do they lyse targets in the presence of 10 μg/ml concanavalin A (data not shown). They do not become cytolytic when they are grown in

TABLE I

Properties of Hybrid Populations Selected with or without CS

	CS[a] Day 0[b]	Cytolytic[c] activity Day 58	VV resistance[d] Day 65	VV resistance[d] Day 83	VV resistance[d,e] Day 84	VV resistance[d,e] Day 164	Cytolytic activity[c] Day 91
Hybrids							
12.3	−	0	105	>32	>100		N.T.
12.4	−	0	N.T.	>32	>100		N.T.
12.4.8	−	N.T.[f]	91	N.T.	N.T.		N.T.
12.5	−	0	>120	>32	>100		N.T.
12.21	−	0	>120	>32	>100		N.T.
12.7	+	15	N.T.	3		N.T.	12
12.9	+	26	6	1		N.T.	14
12.18	+	25	N.T.	2		N.T.	16
12.18.17	+	N.T.	2	N.T.		0.7	33
12.19	+	32	9	6		N.T.	50
12.19.2	+	N.T.	N.T.	N.T.		1.3	N.T.
Parental lines							
CSP.2.4		34	3.2	1.5	0.5		19
BW5147		0	>120	>32	>100		N.T.

[a] Selection of hybrids was done in the presence (+) or absence (−) of CS.

[b] Day 0 is the day of fusion.

[c] Chromium-51 release assay using haptenized (SP) LPS-blasts from CBA/J mice. Numbers indicate percent of specific ^{51}Cr-release during a 4-hr assay at a killer to target ratio of 1 : 1. (CS^- hybrids were grown in CS for several weeks before the assay.)

[d] 10^4 cells were plated out in variable concentrations of VV and growth was measured by cell counts after 3–4 days in culture. Numbers indicate the concentration of VV (in μg/ml) that reduces the cell counts to 50%. (100% = growth in the absence of VV.)

[e] CS^+ and CS^- hybrids were compared in the same experiment on day 164. However the CS^- hybrids had been frozen in between.

[f] N.T., not tested.

CS. These hybrids are resistant to the cytotoxic effect of high concentrations of VV (Fig. 1). On the other hand four independent populations of hybrids selected in the presence of CS (12.7, 12.9, 12.18, 12.19) were specifically cytolytic and their growth was inhibited by low concentrations of VV. The VV resistance of CS^+ and CS^- populations is close to the one shown by CSP.2.4 and BW5147 respectively. Growth curves of eight hybrid populations in the presence or absence of CS demonstrate that hybrids selected in CS grow only in the presence of CS, whereas hybrids selected without CS grow at the same rate with or without CS (data not shown). On day 89 after fusion, surface gp's of the hybrids were radiolabeled using galactose oxidase and neuraminidase, followed by reduction with tritiated borohydride, as described by Kimura and Wigzell

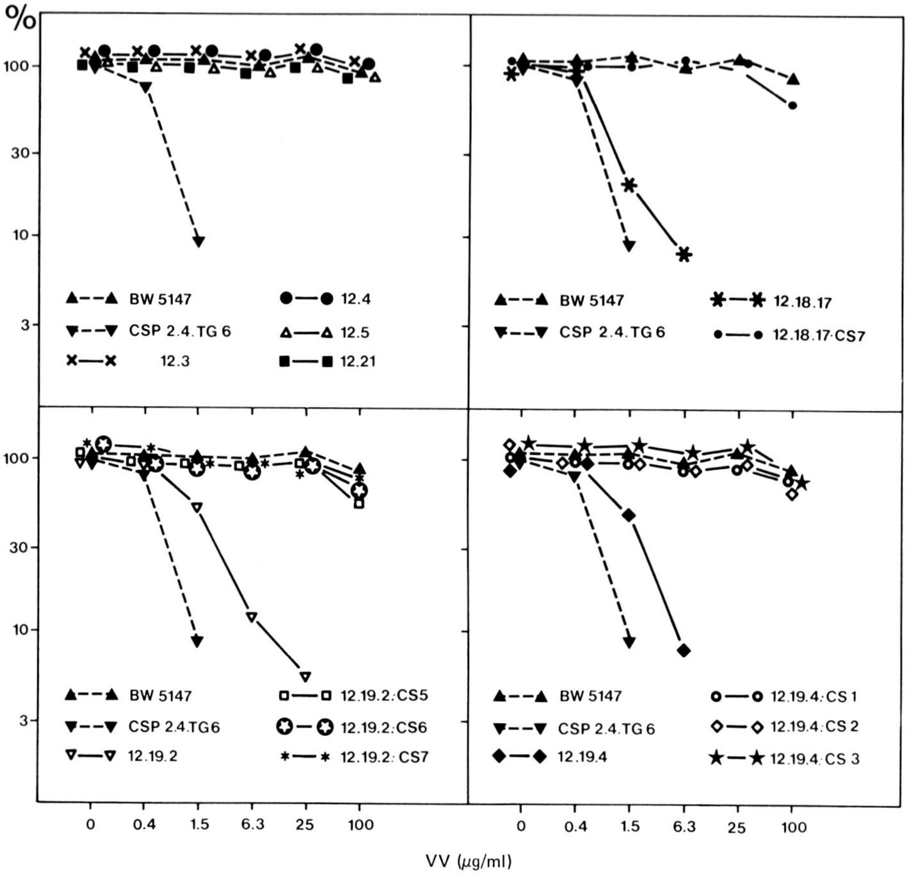

Fig. 1. VV resistance of the parental line BW5147 *TG^r OUA^r*, of a thioguanine-resistant mutant of the other parental line CSP.2.4, of hybrid populations selected without CS, and of clones from hybrids selected in the presence of CS as well as of CS^- variants. On day 164 after fusion, 10^4 cells were plated in 1 ml of medium containing CS and variable concentrations of VV. Growth was measured by cell counts after 4 days in culture at 37°C. Cell numbers in the control wells without VV are taken as 100%. Absolute cell numbers in the control wells varied from 2.8×10^5 (12.18.17) to 1.5×10^6 (12.5) according to the cell line.

(1978). The lysates of the cells were compared in the sodium dodecyl sulfate polyacrylamide gel electrophoresis (SDS-PAGE) system of Lämmli (Fig. 2). There is a clear difference in the surface gp pattern of hybrids selected in CS as compared to the ones selected without CS. The gp patterns of hybrids selected and maintained with or without CS resemble (but are not exactly identical with) the one of CSP.2.4 and BW5147, respectively.

From hybrid populations selected in CS, clones were isolated which stably

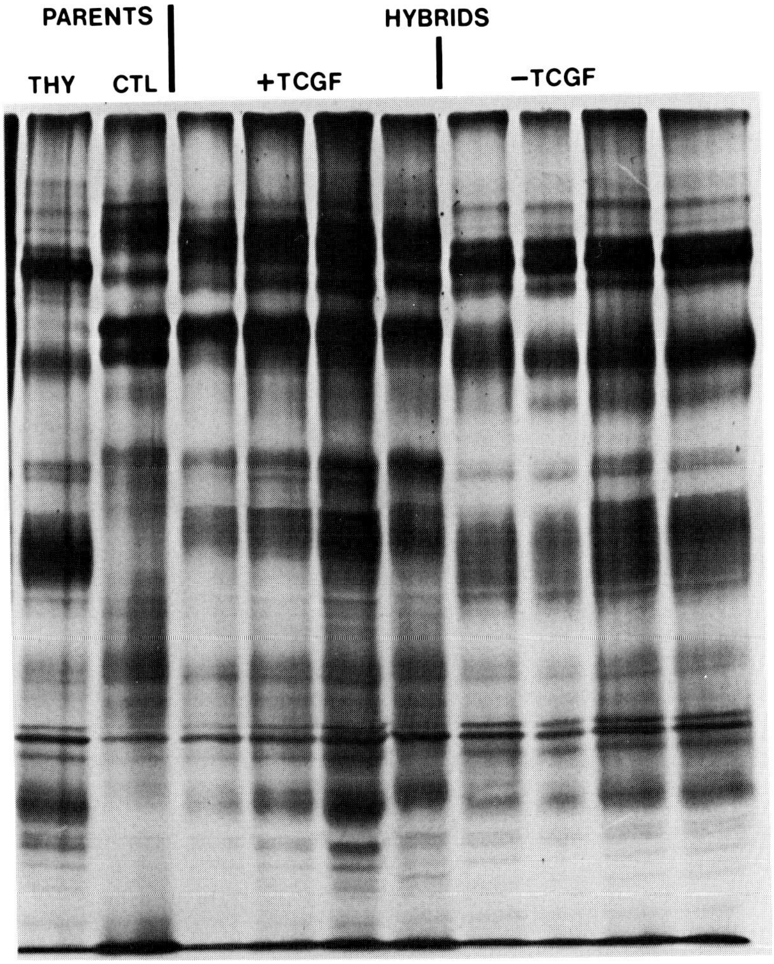

Fig. 2. Hybrid populations selected in CS [12.7, 12.9, 12.18, 12.19 (+ TCGF)] and without CS [12.3, 12.4, 12.5, 12.21 (− TCGF)] were harvested with EDTA, washed in α-methyl-D-mannoside, labeled with [^{3}H]borohydride using galactose oxidase and neuraminidase, and lysed in 0.5% NP40. After addition of SDS, the labeled surface gp's were separated in an 8% SDS-PAGE system under reducing conditions and developed by fluorography. Parental lines are THY, BW5147 thymoma, CTL, CSP.2.4. CTL line.

maintained the specific lytic activity and the other characteristics of the uncloned hybrids, i.e., which were VV sensitive and dependent on CS for growth and survival.

IV. SELECTION OF CS^- VARIANTS FROM CLONED CS^+ CYTOLYTIC HYBRIDS

The experiments described so far indicate that the cytolytic hybrids of fusion 12 are CS^+, VV-sensitive, and possess a distinct surface gp pattern, whereas CS^- hybrids from this fusion are relatively resistant to VV, have a different surface gp pattern, and do not possess any cytolytic activity.

We had proposed (Nabholz *et al.*, 1980) that the two types of hybrids differed in their chromosomal constitution, and that one type was derived from the other by segregation of one or several parental chromosomes. There were some indications that CS^- were derived from CS^+ hybrids: (1) if selection of hybrids was done in CS-containing medium, the frequency of hybrids was higher than if selection was done without CS (Nabholz *et al.*, 1981); (2) in a fusion involving a tetraploid CTL line, many hybrids were obtained in the plates containing CS but no hybrids in the ones without CS. Clearly if transition from CS^+ to CS^- is due to the segregational loss of genes contributed by the CS^+ parental line, the frequency of CS^- hybrids is expected to be much lower in fusions involving a tetraploid CS^+ parental line. Therefore, we decided to test whether CS^- variants could be selected from CS^+ clones.

Cells from three CS^+ clones (derived from two independent hybrid populations) were plated at concentrations of 10^4 to 6×10^2 cells/well/100 μl in flat bottom 96-well microtiter plates in medium without CS. Selection of CS^- variants started 50 days after cloning. CS^- variants were obtained from all three clones, but their frequency within the CS^+ clones can be estimated only roughly, since we have not tested the cloning efficiency of CS^- variants under these conditions. At the lowest cell concentration (600 cells/well) growth was observed in 4 out of 8 wells with clone 12.18.17, 6 out of 8 wells with 12.19.2, and 8 out of 8 wells with 12.19.4. The CS^- isolates are designated by adding CS and a number to the name of the clone from which they are derived. In the case of 12.19.2 and 12.19.4, several CS^- isolates were kept, but there is no evidence that these variants are independent, i.e., that they are not derived from the same variant subclone.

CS^- variants were tested for cytolytic activity, CS dependence, and VV resistance without further cloning, and the data are summarized in Table II. It is clear that the variants grow as fast in the absence of CS as the CS^+ parents in presence of CS. The parents have remained CS dependent. (The 3-fold increase in cell number of 12.19.2 in the absence of CS might indicate that at the time of assay the CS^- variants have become a sizable fraction of the 12.19.2 clone.) The CS^-

TABLE II

Properties of CS^+ and CS^- Variants

	CS dependence[a] Day 142		Cytolytic activity[b] Day 155	VV resistance Day 164
	+CS	−CS		
Hybrids				
12.18.17	26	1.0	47	0.7
12.18.17.CS7	29	21	2	>100
12.19.2	43	3	41	1.3
12.19.2.CS5	34	39	0	>100
12.19.2.CS6	68	78	5	>100
12.19.2.CS7	60	57	0	>100
12.19.4	50	0.9	61	1.5
12.19.4.CS1	15[c]	11[c]	0	>100
12.19.4.CS2	21[c]	19[c]	0	>100
12.19.4.CS3	52	56	0	>100
Parental lines				
CSP.2.4	N.T.[d]	N.T.		0.5
BW5147	N.T.	N.T.		>100

[a] 10^4 cells are put into culture with (+CS) or without (−CS) CS added to the medium. Figures indicate cell counts multiplied by 10^{-4} obtained after 4 days of culture.

[b] ^{51}Cr-release assay using S194 myeloma cells as targets, Numbers indicate percent of specific ^{51}Cr-release during a 4-hr assay at a killer to target ratio of 1 : 1 in the presence of 10 μg/ml of concanavalin A.

[c] Values were obtained after 3 days of culture.

[d] N.T., not tested.

variants show no or only marginal cytolytic activity, whereas the parental hybrid lines remained strongly cytolytic. The variants are very resistant to VV, whereas the VV sensitivity of the parental hybrids has not changed significantly (Fig. 1). On day 155, the surface gp's of the variants and parental hybrids were labeled with neuraminidase/galactose oxidase and tritiated borohydride. Figure 3 shows the SDS-PAGE fluorogram of this experiment. All CS^- variants show a similar gp pattern that is different from the gp pattern of the parental hybrids. Moreover, the gp's of the variants are not very different from the gp's of CS^- hybrid populations shown in Fig. 2.

These experiments have been repeated with CS^+ subclones 12.18.17.4, 12.19.4.16, and 12.19.4.20, which were isolated 169 days after fusion. Selection of CS^- variants was started on day 257 and from each subclone one variant was isolated. These variants were highly resistant to VV and showed no significant cytolytic activity except for one, 12.19.4.16 CS8.4, which gave 15% specific ^{51}Cr release on S194 myeloma targets at a 10:1 killer to target ratio in a 4-hr assay.

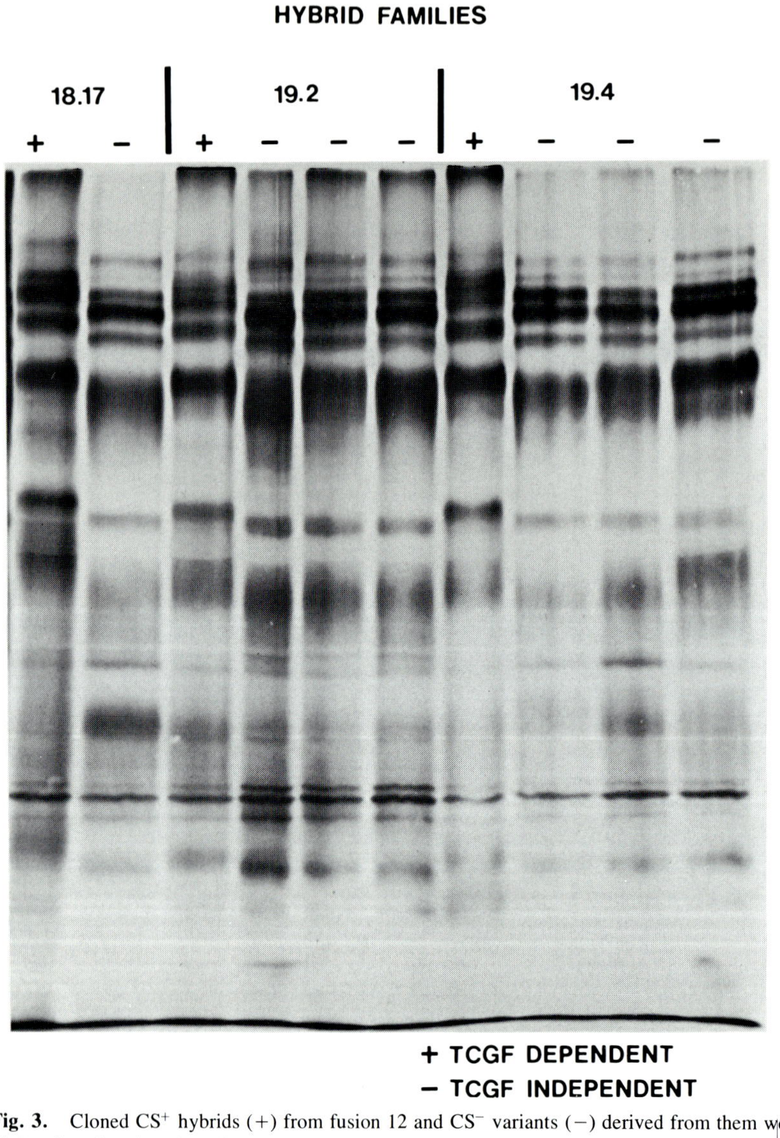

Fig. 3. Cloned CS^+ hybrids (+) from fusion 12 and CS^- variants (−) derived from them were labeled and analyzed as described in legend to Fig. 2. The hybrids are the ones listed in Table II.

V. CONCLUSIONS

The finding that somatic crosses between CTL-B lines and thymomas yield hybrids with two different stable phenotypes has confronted us with two questions: (1) What determines the phenotype of these hybrids? (2) Why is cytolytic activity associated with dependence on CS and susceptibility to the toxic effects of VV?

We discussed above the observations that led us to believe that the hybrids selected in the absence of CS are early arising variants derived from CS^+ hybrids. It may be difficult to prove this hypothesis, but we have shown that it is indeed possible to select CS^- variants from cloned CS^+ hybrids and that such variants resemble the hybrids originally isolated in the absence of CS in their resistance to VV and their gp pattern. However, while most of them also have lost detectable cytolytic activity, two out of eight variants still show some cytolytic competence, although much less than their CS^+ parents.

Our results seem to be in contradiction with those of Kaufmann *et al.* (1981). Fusing BW5147 thymoma cells with activated normal CTL these authors obtained cytolytic hybrids which grow in normal medium without addition of TCGF. We have screened over 100 hybrids selected in the absence of CS, including 20 derived from normal CTL (Nabholz *et al.*, 1981), all of which were inactive. It is possible, as suggested by Kaufmann *et al.* (1981), that their hybrids are derived from infrequent normal CTL which do not depend on external TCGF for growth (Chaper 22 in the treatise). Alternatively their hybrids may be similar to those cytolytically active CS^- variants we describe here.

Earlier we suggested that CS^- variants may originate from CS^+ hybrids through segregation of one or several CTL chromosomes carrying genes which in their active state impose TCGF dependence on a cell. In addition to the observations mentioned in Section IV this hypothesis is supported by the fact that no such variants could be obtained from CTL-B lines even after treatment with ethylmethane sulfonate. To further support this hypothesis we will have to show that the transition from CS^+ to CS^- is correlated with the loss of particular CTL chromosomes.

At present we cannot rule out other explanations, but at least we have some evidence which argues against the conjecture that CS^- variants are induced by the withdrawal of CS during the selection: (1) CS^- hybrids, which are *Vicia villosa* resistant, do arise among the hybrids selected in presence of CS. (2) The frequency of cells growing in the absence of CS in cloned CS^+ hybrids increases with time of culture after cloning (data not shown).

What is the significance of the observation that (1) all CS^+ hybrids are sensitive and all CS^- hybrids or variants are resistant to growth inhibition by *Vicia villosa* lectin, and (2) All CS^- hybrids display no or much less cytolytic activity than CS^+ hybrids?

The hypothesis that these traits are controlled by a gene or genes active in CTL but not in thymomas and located on a single CTL chromosome awaits confirmation by karyotype analysis. At present we cannot exclude that while CS^+ hybrids retain at least one copy of all CTL chromosomes, selection in medium without CS results in the isolation of cells which have lost not one but several CTL chromosomes. If there are genes on many different chromosomes which are expressed in CTL but not thymomas and which control VV sensitivity or CTL activity then even random loss of several CTL chromosomes might result most of the time in extinction of these traits. Alternatively, it might be that the correlations observed turn out to be a peculiarity of the hybrids described here, which are all derived from the same CTL-B line carrying several chromosomal translocations (M. Cianfriglia, unpublished observations; see Chapter 15 in this treatise for a description of CTL line karyotypes).

Analysis of VV resistant mutants (Conzelmann *et al.*, 1980) has already shown that CTL-B lines can lose their sensitivity to VV without becoming CS independent or losing their cytolytic capacity, and we have found that while all CS^- hybrids are VV resistant, the reverse is not true. Selection for VV resistance does yield CS^- but also CS^+ cytolytically active hybrid variants (A. Conzelmann, unpublished observations). This suggests, not unexpectedly, that VV sensitivity depends on the expression of more than one unlinked genes active in CTL but not in thymomas.

Our results clearly raise a number of intriguing questions concerning the genetic control of the CTL phenotype. Fortunately they also indicate that CTL lines and hybrids provide appropriate tools for answering them.

ACKNOWLEDGMENTS

We thank Dr. J.-P. Mach for the generous gift of purified VV lectin. This work was supported by the Swiss National Science Foundation, the Schweizerische Krebsliga, and the Thurgauische Krebsliga.

REFERENCES

Conzelmann, A., Pink, R., Acuto, O., Mach, J.-P., Dolivo, S., and Nabholz, M. (1980). Presence of T145 on cytolytic T-cell lines and their lectin-resistant mutants. *Eur. J. Immunol.* **10,** 860.

Haas, W., Mathur-Rochat, J., Pohlit, H., Nabholz, M., and von Boehmer, H. (1980). Cytotoxic T cell responses to haptenated cells. III. Isolation and specificity analysis of continuously growing clones. *Eur. J. Immunol.* **10,** 828.

Kaufmann, Y., Berke, G., and Eshhar, Z. (1981). Cytotoxic T lymphocyte hybridomas that mediate specific tumor-cell lysis *in vitro*. *Proc. Natl. Acad. Sci. U.S.A.* **78,** 2502.

Kimura, A. K., and Wigzell, H. (1978). Cell surface glycoproteins of murine cytotoxic T lymphocytes. I. T145, a new cell surface glycoprotein selectively expressed on $LY1^{-}2^{+}$ cytotoxic T lymphocytes. *J. Exp. Med.* **147,** 1418.

Kimura, A. K., Wigzell, H., Holmquist, G., Ersson, B., and Carlsson, P. (1979). Selective affinity fractionation of murine cytotoxic T lymphocytes (CTL). Unique lectin specific binding of the CTL associated surface glycoprotein T145. *J. Exp. Med.* **149,** 473.

Nabholz, M., Cianfriglia, M., Acuto, O., Conzelmann, A., Haas, W., von Boehmer, H., MacDonald, H. R., Pohlit, H., and Johnson, J. P. (1980). Cytolytically active murine T-cell hybrids. *Nature (London)* **287,** 437.

Nabholz, M., Cianfriglia, M., Acuto, O., Conzelmann, A., Weiss, A., Haas, W., and von Boehmer, H. (1981). The production of murine cytolytic T cell hybrids. *In* "Monoclonal Antibodies and T cell Hybridomas" (G. H. Hämmerling, U. Hämmerling, and J. F. Kearney, eds.), pp. 537–547. Elsevier/North-Holland Biomedical Press, Amsterdam.

IV

Clonal Analysis by Limiting Dilution

18

An Overview

R. G. Miller

I. Theory of Limiting Dilution 220
II. Experimental Conditions Required for Limiting Dilution Analysis of CTL-P Frequencies 224
III. The CTL-P Frequency Problem 228
References 230

Limiting dilution assays in cell biology (and cellular immunology) form a special subclass of all cell transfer assays in which the particular objective is to measure the frequency of the cells giving rise to a response. In all cell transfer assays, one transfers cells into an animal or a culture tube and sometime later measures the response produced by those cells. Limiting dilution assays treat the special case in which the assay is sufficiently sensitive that the difference between obtaining a significant response and no response at all is determined by the presence or absence of a single cell transferred into the assay vessel.

Porter and Berry (1963) were interested in measuring the frequency of cells in a transplantable leukemia capable of actually transplanting the disease. They transplanted mice with varying numbers of leukemia cells and found a range of cell doses in which some of the mice developed leukemia and others did not. The proportion of responding mice as a function of cell dose fit the zero-order term of the Poisson distribution (Section II). This enabled them to conclude that the presence or absence of a single cell in the transferred cell suspension was determining whether or not the leukemia grew. From the measured distribution of responding and nonresponding mice they were then able to calculate the frequency of this critical cell and found that essentially every cell of the leukemia could transfer the disease.

Similar limiting dilution techniques have been extensively used to study the cells responsible for antibody production. The interpretation of these experiments tends to be more ambiguous than the transplantable leukemia experiments of Porter and Berry (1963) because the cell (or cells) determining the ability to

ISBN 0-12-249920-4

respond are a very small fraction of all the cells transferred. Before the distinction between B and T cells had been made, Kennedy *et al.* (1966) measured the minimum number of spleen cells that must be transferred into an irradiated mouse to enable the mouse to mount an immune response against sheep red blood cells. Again, the proportion of responding mice as a function of cell dose followed the zero-order term of the Poisson distribution, and they were able to measure the frequency of what they referred to as the "antigen sensitive cell" as about 1 in 10^6 spleen cells transferred. They did not know whether the antibody-producing cell precursor or some accessory cell with which it must interact was limiting the response. The mathematical analysis only tells one that some single cell (or cell interaction) is determining the presence or absence of a response. If this cell were the precursor of the antibody-producing cell, one would expect the number of antibody-producing cells obtained to increase linearly with the number of antigen-sensitive cells transferred. However, Gregory and Lajtha (1968) showed that the number of antibody-producing cells obtained increased quadratically with the number of antigen-sensitive cells transferred, suggesting that it was something other than the presence or absence of an antibody-producing cell precursor (B cell) which was limiting the response. The fact that it is the least frequent cell, and not necessarily the precursor of the cell ultimately detected, which determines whether or not there is a response should always be kept in mind when interpreting limiting dilution assays. More recently, Andersson *et al.* (1977) have developed a limiting dilution assay which clearly measures B cell frequency *in vitro*: The fraction of responding cell cultures as a fraction of cell dose fits the zero-order term of the Poisson distribution, and the number of antibody-producing cells obtained is a linear function of the number of cells transferred.

It is only recently that limiting dilution technology has been applied to T cells, particularly to the measurement of the frequency of the precursor of the cytotoxic T lymphocyte. Three groups [Skinner and Marbrook (1976), Fischer-Lindahl and Wilson (1977), and Teh *et al.* (1977)] independently developed assays for measuring this frequency *in vitro*. This chapter will be primarily concerned with reviewing these procedures plus some subsequent developments. It should be mentioned that this frequency can also be measured *in vivo* (Skinner *et al.*, 1978).

I. THEORY OF LIMITING DILUTION

Limiting dilution analysis can, in principle, be applied to any cell transfer assay system which is sufficiently sensitive to detect the response from a single transferred responsive cell. However, this chapter is concerned with the measurement of cytotoxic T lymphocyte precursor (CTL-P) frequency in the mixed lymphocyte reaction (MLR) so the theory will be developed in the context of this particular application. In a typical MLR, lymphoid cells from one inbred mouse strain (responder cells) are cultured with inactivated (e.g., by irradiation) lymphoid cells from a second inbred mouse strain. When the two strains differ at the major histocompatibility complex (*H-2* in the mouse), cytotoxic T lymphocytes (CTL) capable of recognizing and destroying cells sharing H-2 with the stimulating cell population develop from their precursors (CTL-P) in the responder cell population. We wish to measure the frequency of these precursors.

Let ν be the frequency of CTL-P in a suspension of responder cells and assume for the present (but see section III) that all other cells required for CTL-P activation are present in the suspension at much higher frequency. Set up large numbers of replicate cultures containing varying number N of responding cells and a fixed number of stimulating cells. Cultures for which $N\nu >> 1$ contain, on average, many CTL-P and all such cultures are likely to develop CTL. Cultures for which $N\nu << 1$ are unlikely to contain any CTL-P and few will develop CTL. At intermediate concentrations of responder cells ($N\nu \sim 1$), some cultures will contain 1 or more CTL-P and others will contain none at all. The Poisson distribution allows one to predict the probability $P_n(N, \nu)$ of any number n of CTL-P in a culture as a function of N and ν. Thus

$$P_n\ (N,\ \nu) = (N\nu)^n e^{-N\nu}/n! \qquad (1)$$

Experimentally, it is simplest to distinguish between those cultures that respond or fail to respond, corresponding to cultures which contain at least one CTL-P or no CTL-P. One then measures the fraction f of nonresponding cultures as a function of N. The fraction f is then an experimental estimate of the probability of a culture containing N responder cells failing to respond. This probability is given by the first term of Eq. (1):

$$P_0\ (N,\ \nu) = e^{-N\nu} \qquad (2)$$

When this equation is plotted semilogarithmically, as shown by the solid line in Fig. 1 (with $\nu = 0.01$) the frequency ν can be read directly as the slope of the line or, more simply, as the inverse of that value of N for which the probability of no response is $1/e$ (0.37).

What is the best procedure for analyzing experimental data obtained in a limiting dilution experiment? The analysis procedure adopted should do two things: (1) Provide an estimate of CTL-P frequency and the standard error of this estimate. (2) Test how well the experimental data do, in fact, fit the limiting dilution model. The first step in any analysis procedure is to assume that the experimentally determined values of f (fraction of nonresponding cultures) are valid estimates of $P_0\ (N,\ \nu)$. One can then plot the data. Figure 2 is an example of such data. The data points appear to fall on a straight line which intersects the origin approximately at 1. By this subjective criterion, condition (2) stated above

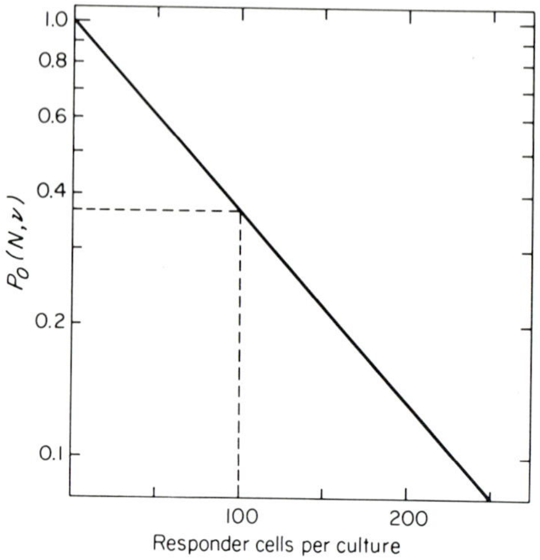

Fig. 1. Plot of the zero-order term of the Poisson equation for $\nu = 0.01$ [Eq. (2) in the text].

appears to be met. One can then use Eq. (1) to estimate the frequency either from the slope of the line or from the inverse of that value of N for which 37% of the cultures do not respond. The fitting procedure can be made somewhat more rigorous by making a least-squares fit of a straight line to the data points. However, a few moments thought will convince one that any such line fitting procedure is of dubious statistical validity. In an actual experiment, one counts responding cultures, and one expects statistical variations in the number of cultures that respond. Clearly, the larger the number of cultures that respond in a group, the smaller the percentage error in the number of responding cultures. Thus, assuming all groups contain the same number of cultures, a group in which 90% ($f = 0.10$) of the cultures responded should be given more weight in estimating ν than a group in which only 10% ($f = 0.90$) of the cultures responded. This is difficult to do with direct least-squares analysis. However, Porter and Berry (1963) have worked out a statistically valid procedure for determining frequencies from limiting dilustion data. Their procedure has the additional advantage that it allows the computation of a value of χ^2 for testing the fit of the data to the limiting dilution model. Although somewhat complex, it is easily programmed. We have programmed it for both computer and programmable calculator (HP67) and use it for all limiting dilution calculations. Taswell (1981) has recently reexamined the whole problem of how to analyze limiting dilution data and also came to the conclusion that the Porter and Berry procedure was the best method. It should be pointed out that different methods of analyzing the same set of data can give different frequencies because of the varying statisti-

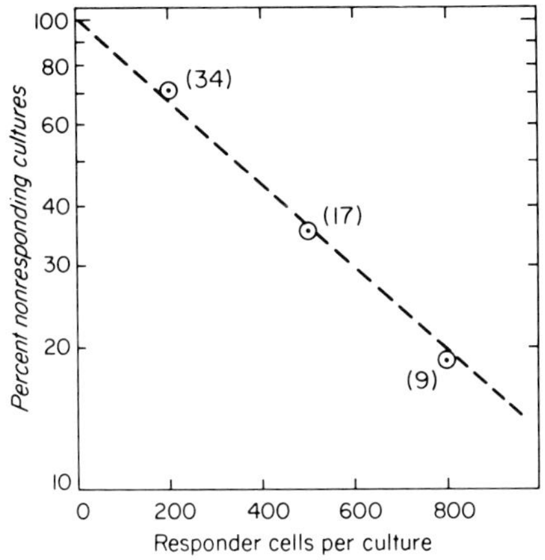

Fig. 2. Plot of percent nonresponding cultures versus number of responder cells per culture for RNC lymph node cells in an RNC anti-DBA/2 response. The number of nonresponding cultures (out of 48 tested) is indicated beside each data point. The data were fit using the Porter and Berry procedure which gave a frequency of 2005 per 10^6 LN cells, 95% confidence limits of 1598 to 2516, and a χ^2 value of 0.414. The fit is indicated by the dotted line.

cal weights assigned to the data points. Thus, it is critical that the method of analysis used be explicitly stated.

In bulk MLR cultures, the CTL produced come from many different precursors. This makes studies of the fine specificity of CTL difficult. For example, when CTL from a bulk culture can lyse target cells unrelated to the stimulator cells, is this due to a small subpopulation of CTL originating from only a few precursors or a property of all CTL in the culture? In contrast, in MLR cultures set up near limiting dilution, there is a large probability that all the CTL in a responding culture are derived from a single precursor. Assuming that all members of such a clone have the same specificity, and there is as yet no experimental evidence counter to this assumption, such cultures should have all the advantages for studying CTL specificity as do monoclonal antibodies in comparison with conventional antibodies in studies of antibody specificity. Figure 3 is a graph of the probability of a responder culture being clonal versus the probability of the culture responding at all calculated using Poisson statistics. From the graph, if 1/10 of a group of identical cultures respond, then the probability is about 0.95 that a particular responding culture is clonal. Such clonal cultures can easily be established as cell lines using the techniques described elsewhere in this treatise. This general approach has been successfully used by several investigators for studying CTL fine specificity (see, for example, Teh *et al.*, 1978a; Brunner *et al.*, 1980).

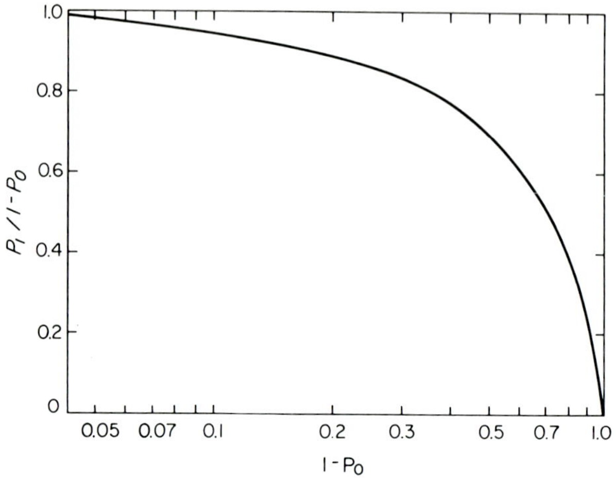

Fig. 3. Probability of a responding culture in a group of identical cultures being clonal $P_1(1-P_0)$ versus the probability of a culture in the same group responding at all $(1-P_0)$ calculated using Eq. (1) in the text.

II. EXPERIMENTAL CONDITIONS REQUIRED FOR LIMITING DILUTION ANALYSIS OF CTL-P FREQUENCIES

To achieve satisfactory results in a limiting dilution experiment, the following conditions must be met: (1) The culture conditions must be such that a single CTL-P can survive and produce normal progeny after activation. (2) The assay for CTL must be sufficiently sensitive to detect the progeny of a single CTL-P, i.e., the assay must clearly distinguish cultures containing a single clone of CTL from nonresponding cultures. (3) All cells and/or factors other than CTL-P which are required for CTL production must be present in excess, i.e., the presence or absence of CTL-P must be the only factor determining whether a culture will respond.

Three groups [Skinner and Marbrook (1976), Fischer-Lindahl and Wilson (1977), and Teh *et al.* (1977a,b)] independently established experimental conditions for successful limiting dilution assays, and since then many other groups have also reported success. No group has had problems meeting the first two conditions stated above using standard tissue culture conditions routinely used for MLR cultures and the ^{51}Cr-release assay for CTL activity as originally described by Brunner *et al.* (1968). The third condition is somewhat harder to meet and several different procedures, which may not be completely equivalent, have been devised. As shown clearly in other chapters in this treatise, IL-2 must be present for an activated CTL-P to expand into a clone of CTL. It appears that one or more of the cells required for production of IL-2 can be diluted out by limiting dilution before the cultures become limiting for CTL-P. This deficiency can be overcome by adding conditioned medium (Fischer-Lindahl and Wilson, 1977), by adding cells (Teh *et al.*, 1977a,b), or by choice of a special tissue culture vessel (Skinner and Marbrook, 1976).

Table I is a compilation of CTL-P frequency results obtained by various investigators using various procedures for attempting to ensure that CTL-P are the only limiting cell. Whenever possible, the frequencies are for C57BL/6 (B6) lymph node or spleen cells responding against DBA/2 (D2) spleen cells, but to include the whole range of methodologies, a few other strain combinations have been included. It has been generally found that the CTL-P frequency in a B6 anti-D2 response is particularly high. The frequency of CTL-P in spleen has been found to be about three times lower than in lymph node (Fischer-Lindahl and Wilson, 1977; Teh *et al.*, 1977a; MacDonald *et al.*, 1980). The frequencies listed do not include error estimates for two reasons. First, some authors have not made error estimates and do not give sufficient information for an independent estimate to be made. Second, different and not directly comparable procedures (see Section II) have been used to extract the frequency from the limiting dilution curve. Nevertheless, I conclude that the 95% confidence limits for all the table entries are no more than twofold above and below the entries independent of the analysis method used. On this basis, there would appear to be significant differences between the different procedures. These are discussed below.

Fischer-Lindahl and Wilson (1977) achieved limiting dilution conditions by supplementing their cultures with 50% conditioned medium from a 48-hr primary MLR. It appears that much more active conditioned medium can be obtained by stimulating mouse or rat spleen cells with Con-A for 24–48 hr and that the required factor or factors are identical to or copurify with IL-2 (Wagner *et al.*, 1980; Teh and Teh, 1980; Miller *et al.*, 1980). The most active conditioned medium of all can be obtained from the supernatant of a secondary MLR (Ryser and MacDonald, 1979; MacDonald *et al.*, 1980). This conditioned medium gives frequencies two to five times higher than those obtained using Con-A-induced supernatants. The reasons for these differences are not clear at the present time, but there are two likely explanations. There is always a problem in distinguishing responding from nonresponding cultures. The more active supernatants produce larger clones of CTL which are more easily distinguished from nonresponding cultures. Thus, with the less active supernatants, one might merely be losing a substantial fraction of responding cultures below the detection threshold. One should keep in mind that the limiting dilution approach will always give one a lower limit to the true frequency. The second possibility is that the CTL-P of a given specificity are heterogeneous in their activation and/or growth properties. One could then say that secondary MLR supernatant contains some factor(s) in addition to IL-2 which allow detection of additional classes of CTL-P of a given specificity. Goronzy *et al.* (1981) have identified two popula-

TABLE I

Comparison of CTL-P Frequencies Measured in Different Systems

Responder cells	Strain combinations	Special culture additions	CTL-P per 10^6 responder cells	References
LN	B6 αD2	Primary MLR SN	1220	Fischer-Lindahl and Wilson (1977)
LN	B6 αB6D2F_1	B6.nu spleen	1130	Teh *et al.* (1977a)
LN	B6 αD2	B6.nu spleen	1642	Teh and Teh (1980)
LN	B6 αD2	Con-A SN	2844	Teh and Teh (1980)
LN	B6 αD2	Secondary MLR SN	14710	MacDonald *et al.* (1980)
Spleen	B6 αBALB/c	Con-A SN	2200	Wagner *et al.* (1980)
Spleen	B6 αD2	Con-A SN	1930	Goronzy *et al.* (1981)
Spleen	B6 αBALB/c.nu	None	330	Ceredig (1980)
Spleen	CBA α (CBA $\times$ DBA)F_1	(Special culture vessel)	770	Skinner and Marbrook (1976)

tions of CTL-P, a low-frequency subset detected following activation with allogeneic cells in the presence of a Con-A-induced conditioned medium (see Table I entry) and a high-frequency subset which can be detected following activation with Con-A in bulk cultures and reculture under limiting dilution conditions. The frequency of this second subset is comparable to that seen by MacDonald *et al.* (1980) using secondary MLR supernatant.

Teh *et al.* (1977a,b) achieved limiting dilution conditions by supplementing their cultures with nude spleen cells syngeneic to the responder cells. The nude spleen cells do not themselves contribute CTL-P and appear to replace some other cell which has been lost through dilution (Miller *et al.,* 1977). The requirement for nude spleen can be replaced with a conditioned medium enriched in IL-2 (Teh and Teh, 1980; Miller *et al.,* 1980). The frequencies obtained are directly comparable to those of Fischer-Lindahl and Wilson (1977) using primary MLR supernatant. Extensive analysis (Miller *et al.,* 1977) suggested that all or most CTL-P activated under the culture conditions used were detected as clones of CTL. However, different frequencies could be obtained using different types and concentrations of stimulator cells, and, in some cases, using very large numbers of spleen cells as stimulator cells, frequencies as high as 10,000 per 10^6 were obtained (Miller *et al.,* 1977). It was concluded that there might be a broad spectrum of CTL-P of a given specificity differing in their activation requirements.

Ceredig (1979, 1980) was able to achieve limiting dilution conditions by using nude spleen cells as stimulator cells and not making any other culture additions. Presumably, limiting dilution conditions are being met in the same way as by Teh *et al.* (1977a,b), although Miller (1980) has presented evidence that the Ceredig protocol should lead to a reduced CTL-P frequency as a result of inactivation of some of the CTL-P by a population of suppressor cells in the nude spleen capable of suppressing a response against their own (but not other) H-2 antigens.

There have been several recent reports (Gillis *et al.,* 1979; Hünig and Bevan 1980; Ando and Hurme, 1981; Gillis and Watson, 1981) that nude spleen cells can generate CTL *in vitro* if the cultures are supplemented with IL-2. However, we (R. G. Miller and H. Derry, unpublished) cannot obtain CTL from nude mouse spleen cells on adding IL-2 unless the nude mice are at least 11 weeks old, and even then, the responses are orders of magnitude lower than from normal mice. Nevertheless, if nude spleen cells are used, controls should be included to ensure that they are not responsive.

In all of the above studies, the MLR cultures were set up in plastic microtiter trays such that each culture was totally separate from all the others. Special additions, either cells or factors, had to be added to achieve limiting dilution. Skinner and Marbrook (1976), however, made no special additions to their cultures to achieve limiting dilution. In their system, the cells settle into 64 microwells within a polyacrylamide raft containing 3.8 ml of culture medium and fetal calf serum. The porous matrix on which the cells grow was devised to prevent any nutritional limitations. Although cells cannot move between microwells, it seems probable that soluble factors can and that this explains the success of the system. It may be, however, that even under these improved culture conditions, sufficient factor is produced only when there are strong antigenic differences capable of producing large quantities of such factor(s).

III. THE CTL-P FREQUENCY PROBLEM

In the MLR, the major histocompatibility complex stimulates a disproportionately large number of T lymphocytes, as many as 1–2% of the total number of lymphocytes in the responding population (Wilson *et al.*, 1968). The responding cells, however, appear to constitute several different subclasses only one of which gives rise to CTL, the apparent end-product effector cell of the response (Cantor and Boyse, 1975). This has spurred several groups to attempt to measure frequencies of CTL precursors (CTL-P) to see if they are also high. The results in Table I, primarily for B6 anti-D2 (H-2^b anti-H-2^d) range from $330/10^6$ to $14710/10^6$, i.e., from 0.03 to 1.5% of all responder cells. Analysis of the above numbers (Fischer-Lindahl and Wilson, 1977; Miller *et al.*, 1977; Teh *et al.*, 1978a) shows that the initial enigma of finding an explanation for the high frequency of responding cells in an MLR still remains; the total CTL-P pool constitutes only a few percent of the responding cell pool so that one finds again that up to several percent of the total CTL-P pool are being activated to make CTL specific for the sensitizing alloantigen. Whether the wide variation in percent of cells responding in different assay systems results from variations in sensitivity of cells recruited from a CTL-P pool of fixed size or whether the different assay systems are recruiting CTL-P from pools of different sizes is not clear at the present time. As argued in the preceding section, I prefer the latter explanation. In any case, the enigma of extremely high responsiveness to MHC antigens remains. The CTL-P frequency remains high even in an MLR between H-2 congenic strains of mice (Table II) or, in an even more extreme case, in an MLR between two strains of mice differing only by a single mutation in *H-2K* or *H-2D* (Widmer and Macdonald, 1980).

The very high frequency of CTL-P reactive to MHC antigens imply that either CTL-P are not initially specificity restricted but become so during a response, or that there is extensive cross-reaction between different *H-2* haplotypes. The latter appears to be the case as shown by the studies of Teh *et al.* (1978a,b; Teh, 1979) and confirmed by Taswell *et al.* (1980). Clearly the role of the MHC will remain a central question in studies of T cells.

TABLE II

Comparison of CTL-P Frequencies Measured in MLR between Congenic or H-2 Mutant Mice

Responder cells	Strain combinations	Special culture additions	CTL-P per 10^6 responder cells	References
Spleen	B6 αB6.H-2^k	Secondary MLR SN	860	MacDonald *et al.* (1980)
LN	B6 αB6.H-2^k	B6.nu spleen	1220	R. G. Miller (unpublished)
LN	B6 αC3H	B6.nu spleen	1179	R. G. Miller (unpublished)
LN	B6 αB6.H-2^k	Con-A SN	8700	Langhorne and Fischer-Lindahl (1981)
LN	B6 αBALB/c	Con-A SN	8600	Langhorne and Fischer-Lindahl (1981)
Spleen	B6 αB6-H-2^{ba}	Secondary MLR SN	1300	Widmer and MacDonald (1980)

REFERENCES

Andersson, J., Coutinho, A., Lernhardt, W., and Melchers, F. (1977). Clonal growth and maturation to immunoglobulin secretion "*in vitro*" of every growth-inducible B-lymphocyte. *Cell* **10,** 27.

Ando, I., and Hurme, M. (1981). Self-MHC-restricted cytotoxic T-cell response without thymic influence. *Nature* (*London*) **289,** 494.

Brunner, K. T., Mauel, J., Cerottini, J.-C., and Chapuis, B. (1968). Quantitative assay of the lytic action of immune lymphoid cells on ^{51}Cr-labelled allogeneic target cells *in vitro;* inhibition by isoantibody and by drugs. *Immunology* **14,** 181.

Brunner, K. T., MacDonald, H. R., and Cerottini, J.-C. (1980). Antigenic specificity of the cytolytic T lymphocyte (CTL) response to murine sarcoma virus-induced tumors. II. Analysis of the clonal progeny of CTL precursors stimulated *in vitro* with syngeneic tumor cells. *J. Immunol.* **124,** 1627.

Cantor, H., and Boyse, E. A. (1975). Functional subclasses of T lymphocytes bearing different Ly antigens. II. Co-operation between subclasses of Ly^{+} cells in the generation of killer activity. *J. Exp. Med.* **141,** 1390.

Ceredig, R. (1979). Frequency of alloreactive cytotoxic T cell precursors in the mouse thymus and spleen during ontogeny. *Transplantation* **28,** 377.

Ceredig, R. (1980). Frequencies of alloreactive cytotoxic T-lymphocyte precursors responding to H-2 antigens alone. *Immunology* **40,** 163.

Fischer-Lindahl, K., and Wilson, D. B. (1977). Histocompatibility antigen-activated cytotoxic T lymphocytes. II. Estimates of the frequency and specificity of precursors. *J. Exp. Med.* **145,** 508.

Gillis, S., and Watson, J. (1981). Interleukin-2 induction of hapten-specific cytolytic T cells in nude mice. *J. Immunol.* **126,** 1245.

Gillis, S., Union, N. A., Baker, P. E., and Smith, K. A. (1979). The *in vitro* generation and sustained culture of nude mouse cytolytic T-lymphocytes. *J. Exp. Med.* **149,** 1460.

Goronzy, J., Schaefer, U., Eichmann, K., and Simon, M. M. (1981). Quantitative studies on T cell diversity. II. Determination of the frequencies and Lyt phenotypes of two types of precursor cells for alloreactive cytotoxic T cells in polyclonally and specifically activated splenic T cells. *J. Exp. Med.* **153,** 857.

Gregory, C. J., and Lajtha, L. G. (1968). Kinetic study of the production of Ab-forming cells from their precursors. *Nature* (*London*) **218,** 1079.

Hünig, T., and Bevan, M. J. (1980). Specificity of cytotoxic T cells from athymic mice. *J. Exp. Med.* **152,** 688.

Kennedy, J. C., Till, J. E., Siminovitch, L., and McCulloch, E. A. (1966). The proliferative capacity of antigen-sensitive precursors of hemolytic plaque-forming cells. *J. Immunol.* **96,** 973.

Langhorne, J., and Fischer-Lindahl, K. (1981). Role of non-H-2 antigens in the cytotoxic T cell response to allogeneic H-2. (Submitted for publication.)

MacDonald, H. R., Cerottini, J.-C., Ryser, J.-E., Maryanski, J. L., Taswell, C., Widmer, M. B., and Brunner, K. T. (1980). Quantitation and cloning of cytolytic T lymphocytes and their precursors. *Immunol. Rev.* **51,** 93.

Miller, R. G. (1980). An immunological suppressor cell which inactivates cytotoxic T lymphocyte precursor cells recognizing it. *Nature* (*London*) **287,** 544.

Miller, R. G., Teh, H.-S., Harley, E., and Phillips, R. A. (1977). Quantitative studies of the activation of cytotoxic lymphocyte precursor cells. *Immunol. Rev.* **35,** 38.

Miller, R. G., Lalande, M. E., Derry, H., and Paetkau, V. (1980). Second signal requirements of cytotoxic T lymphocyte precursors. *Behring Inst. Mitt.* **67,** 41.

Porter, E. H., and Berry, R. J. (1963). The efficient design of transplantable tumor assays. *Br. J. Cancer* **17,** 583.

Ryser, J.-E., and MacDonald, H. R. (1979). Limiting dilution analysis of alloantigen-reactive T lymphocytes. I. Comparison of precursor frequencies for proliferative and cytolytic responses. *J. Immunol.* **122,** 1691.

Skinner, M. A., and Marbrook, J. (1976). An estimation of the frequency of precursor cells which generate cytotoxic lymphocytes. *J. Exp. Med.* **143,** 1562.

Skinner, M. A., Marbrook, J., and Baguley, B. C. (1978). Splenic foci of cytotoxic lymphocytes in a graft-versus-host reaction. *Int. Arch. Allergy Appl. Immunol.* **56,** 334.

Taswell, C. (1981). Limiting dilution assays for the determination of immunocompetent cell frequencies. I. Data analysis. *J. Immunol.* **126,** 1614.

Taswell, C., MacDonald, H. R., and Cerottini, J.-C. (1980). Clonal analysis of cytolytic T lymphocyte specificity. I. Phenotypically distinct sets of clones as the cellular basis of cross-reactivity to alloantigens. *J. Exp. Med.* **151,** 1372.

Teh, H.-S. (1979). Frequency estimations of cytotoxic precursors to trinitrophenyl-modified alloantigens and determination of the degree of cross-reactivity between allodeterminants and trinitrophenyl-modified self determinants. *Immunogenetics* **8,** 99.

Teh, H.-S., and Teh, S.-J. (1980). Direct evidence for a two-signal mechanism of cytotoxic T-lymphocyte activation. *Nature (London)* **285,** 163.

Teh, H.-S., Harley, E., Phillips, R. A., and Miller, R. F. (1977a). Quantitative studies on the precursors of cytotoxic lymphocytes. I. Characterization of a clonal assay and determination of the size of clones derived from single precursors. *J. Immunol.* **118,** 1049.

Teh, H.-S., Phillips, R. A., and Miller, R. G. (1977b). Quantitative studies on the precursors of cytotoxic lymphocytes. II. Specificity of precursors responsive to allo-antigens and to Concanavalin A. *J. Immunol.* **118,** 1057.

Teh, H.-S., Phillips, R. A., and Miller, R. G. (1978a). Quantitative studies on the precursors of cytotoxic lymphocytes. IV. Specificity and cross-reactivity of cytotoxic clones. *J. Immunol.* **120,** 425.

Teh, H.-S., Phillips, R. A., and Miller, R. G. (1978b). Quantitative studies on the precursors of cytotoxic lymphocytes. V. The cullular basis for the cross-reactivity of TNP-specific clones. *J. Immunol.* **121,** 1711.

Wagner, H., Hardt, C., Heeg, K., Pfizenmaier, K., Solbach, W., Bartlett, R., Stockinger, H., and Rollinghoff, M. (1980). T–T cell interactions during cytotoxic T lymphocyte (CTL) responses: T cell derived helper factor (interleukin 2) as a probe to analyze CTL responsiveness and thymic maturation of CTL progenitors. *Immunol. Rev.* **51,** 215.

Widmer, M. B., and MacDonald, H. R. (1980). Cytolytic T lymphocyte precursors reactive against mutant K^b alloantigens are as frequent as those reactive against a whole foreign haplotype. *J. Immunol.* **124,** 48.

Wilson, D. B., Blyth, J. L., and Nowell, P. C. (1968). Quantitative studies on the mixed lymphocyte interaction in rats. III. Kinetics of response. *J. Exp. Med.* **128,** 1157.

19

Clonal Analysis of Helper and Cytolytic T Cells: Multiple, Independently Regulated Precursor Sets at Frequencies Suggesting a Limited Repertoire

Klaus Eichmann/Jörg Goronzy/Ute Hamann/ Peter H. Krammer/Rudolf C. Kuppers/Inga Melchers/ Markus M. Simon/Gabriele Zahn

I. The Assay 234
II. Multiple Populations of T Precursor Cells 236
III. Independent Regulation of Each Precursor Population 238
IV. Lyt-Phenotypic Differences between T Precursor Populations 241
V. Conclusions 241
A. Size of the T Cell Repertoire for Foreign Antigens 241
B. Specificity and Cross-Reactivity of T Cells 241
C. Regulation of T Cell Specificity 242
References 243

T cells are a heterogeneous mixture of functionally and physically distinct cell types. The function of each T cell is not autonomous but is regulated by other T lymphocytes, both *in vivo* and in unseparated T lymphocyte populations *in vitro*. Therefore, the functional analysis of T cells as a pool, be it *in vivo* or in mass tissue culture, is of limited value. Initial attempts to limit the experimental complexity of systems used to study T cell functions have therefore used a variety of approaches to fractionation, including purification or depletion of T cells with certain antigen specificities (Haas and von Boehmer, 1978), or positive and negative selection procedures based on the expression of alloantigens such as the Lyt and Qat series (Cantor and Boyse, 1977; Hämmerling *et al.*, 1979; Eardley *et al.*, 1978; Simon and Eichmann, 1980; Zahn *et al.*, 1981).

As a further step in this direction, T cells are currently being analyzed at the

ISOLATION, CHARACTERIZATION, AND
UTILIZATION OF T LYMPHOCYTE CLONES

ISBN 0-12-249920-4

clonal level. Two different approaches have been used, one based on long-term tissue culture of functional T cell clones or hybridomas and the other based on short-term limiting dilution analysis (reviewed in Haas and von Boehmer ,1978). Both approaches give incomplete information and are complementary to each other; whereas the latter can yield information on the T cell repertoire, the former allows repeated analysis of the same clone and supplies large numbers of cells for analysis.

Clonal analyses of T cells by limiting dilution have been performed by many laboratories (reviewed in von Boehmer *et al.*, 1980). Comparisons of the results, however, have been difficult because the types of assays used were designed for the particular T cell being analyzed. In addition, the vast majority of clonal assays have been directed toward the analysis of only one T cell type, namely, the precursors of cytotoxic T cells specific for major histocompatibility antigens. The study of long-term T cell lines, although including both helper and cytotoxic functions, has been of limited information because of the uncertainty about how representative such T cells are for the normal T cell population.

In view of this situation, our laboratory has developed an assay which combines elements of the two approaches mentioned above: namely, limiting dilution of T cells together with an activation protocol that ensures differentiation and/or expansion of functional T cells. This method can serve as a general limiting dilution protocol for the characterization of the precursors for any T cell whose function can be determined *in vitro* (Eichmann *et al.*, 1980; Goronzy *et al.*, 1981). Results from this assay allow the comparison of precursor frequencies and clonal properties of various functionally distinct T cells specific for a variety of antigens. In addition, the assay allows the characterization of effector and regulatory T cells in the same experiment.

I. THE ASSAY

Since our aim was to study all T cell types, we use polyclonal activation rather than specific antigen activation and include several experimental steps that ensured differentiation and/or expansion of as many different T cell types as possible. Nylon wool-purified T cells are activated for a period of 2 days with concanavalin A (Con-A) in bulk culture. Thereafter, activated T cell blasts are recovered and subjected to limiting dilution, using I1-2-containing conditioned medium (TCGF) and irradiated filler cells. After 1 week of culture under these conditions, individual cultures are assayed for T cell functions by appropriate assays (Eichmann *et al.*, 1980; Goronzy *et al.*, 1981), and the results are analyzed according to Poisson distribution (Documenta Geigy, 1960).

The exact details of this method are given in the Appendix. Here, we discuss some important reservations regarding the validity of such an assay for making statements on the composition of the normal T cell repertoire. These reservations concern the use of certain steps which may be selective for or against certain T cell populations.

The first selection step in our procedure is the use of nylon wool to purify T cells. We, as well as others (Tada *et al.*, 1978), have obtained results that suggest some degree of selectivity of nylon wool fractionation within the T cell pool. However, we also found that precursor frequencies for various T cell types are not significantly different when nylon wool-purified T cells were compared with whole spleen cells (Goronzy *et al.*, 1981; Melchers and Eichmann, 1981a,b). Therefore, we consider the possible selectivity of nylon wool fractionation a minor problem.

A more serious problem is posed by the step in our procedure involving Con-A activation. For example, a large body of literature suggests that Con-A may selectively activate suppressor cells (Möller, 1972). We have analyzed carefully two aspects of Con-A activation: the proportion of T cells going into division and the question of whether these activated cells differ functionally from the total T cell pool. Depending on the strain of mice, between 15 and 40% of T cells are induced to proliferate (Watanabe *et al.*, 1977; I. Melchers and R. Kuppers, unpublished). The frequencies of sheep red blood cell reactive helper cells (Melchers and Eichmann, 1981a,b) and the frequencies of alloreactive cytotoxic cells (Goronzy *et al.*, 1981) were compared before and after Con-A activation. Since the frequencies differed less than twofold, it appears that little if any selection among T cells occurs upon Con-A activation. Thus, Con-A-activated T cells can be used for quantitative studies on T cell diversity and repertoire.

The subsequent expansion and differentiation in TCGF certainly represents another possible selection step in our procedure. This has been minimized by choosing an optimal way to prepare Il-2-containing supernatant which allows the growth of up to 50% of all Con-A-activated T cells. Figure 1 shows experiments comparing the frequencies of Con-A blasts grown in secondary MLC supernatant (Mls activation only), in mouse spleen Con-A supernatant, and in rat spleen Con-A supernatant. It is evident that secondary MLC supernatant only allows the growth of 1/18 Con-A blasts. Whereas mouse Con-A supernatant is superior to MLC supernatant, rat Con-A supernatant promotes the growth of 1/3.5 Con-A blast, and, in many experiments, growth frequencies of 1/2 are reached (Eichmann *et al.*, 1980).

The growth frequencies and kinetics in selected *Lyt-1*$^+$ and *Lyt-2*$^+$ T cells are similar and are not significantly different from nonselected T cells (Kuppers *et al.*, 1981). However, the growth period and colony size are better for *Lyt-2*$^+$ cells than for *Lyt-1*$^+$ cells. Furthermore, we find that T helper cells do not necessarily have to divide to be detected in our assay (Melchers and Eichmann, 1981b). Thus, we feel that we analyze the repertoire of the majority of the T cell population, since we can detect activity of at least some nondividing cells in addition to the dividing cells which constitute about 50% of the cells.

We have also used limiting dilution of normal T cells with subsequent activa-

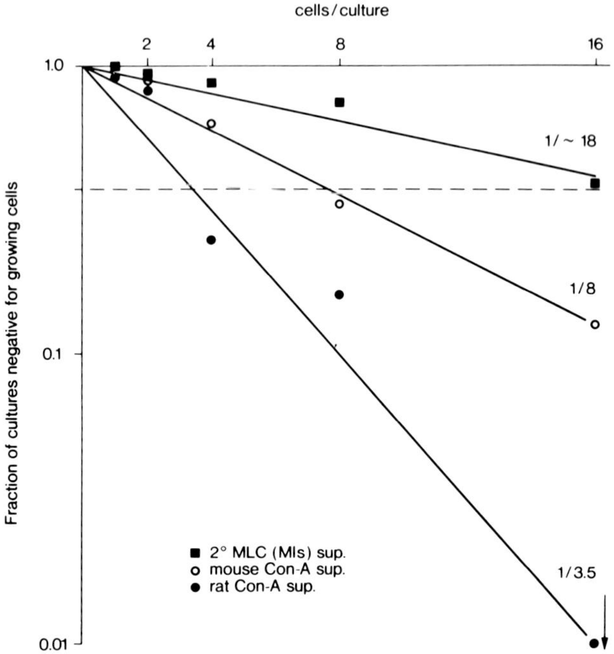

Fig. 1. Precursor frequency determinations for Con-A activated cells induced to grow in various conditioned media. 2° MLC (Mls) Sup, supernatant from BALB/c spleen cells (*H-2^d*, *Mls^b*) restimulated with DBA/2 (*H-2^d*, *Mls^a*) stimulator cells. Mouse Con-A sup, Supernatant from C57BL/6 spleen cells cultured for 24 hr with 5 μg/ml Con-A. Rat Con-A sup., supernatant from Spraque Dawley rat spleen cells cultured for 24 hr with 5 μg/ml Con-A. All supernatants were used at 20% final concentration. Cultures with growing cells were determined by visual examination using an inverted microscope.

tion by alloantigens to determine the frequency of several T cell types. In contrast to Con-A activation prior to limiting dilution, these methods select only those cells that can react to the particular antigen under the limiting dilution conditions. As will be discussed below, both types of methods have revealed similar frequencies for certain T cell precursor sets, suggesting to us that our frequency determinations closely reflect those of the normal T cell repertoire.

II. MULTIPLE POPULATIONS OF T PRECURSOR CELLS

When a single cell type is limiting, there is a linear relationship between the number of cells per culture and the logarithm of the fraction of non-responding cultures. Thus, as shown in Fig. 1, only one type of T cell is limiting for growth of T cells in Il-2 containing media. In contrast, at different cell concentrations, there are several limiting T cell types for the expression of T cell functions. This is exemplified by the data in Fig. 2 which represent the determinations in three inbred mouse strains of T helper (Th) precursor frequencies for the antibody response to trinitrophenylated *Streptococcus* A (Strep A) bacteria. The relationships between the numbers of T cells per culture and the fraction of nonresponding cultures show two linear positive slopes and an intermediate, nonlinear, negative slope. We have interpreted this as indicating two distinct types of Th cells of high (1/1500–1/6000) and low (1/50,000–1/30,000) frequency, the more frequent of which is sensitive to suppression (see below) (Eichmann *et al.*, 1980). In a study of Th precursor cells reactive to sheep red blood cells (SRBC), we find a similar situation; however, three types of precursors are seen, two of which are suppressible (Melchers and Eichmann, 1981a,b). Indeed we have found multiple populations for the majority of Th precursors and cytotoxic T lymphocyte (CTL) precursors analyzed. A survey of these results is represented

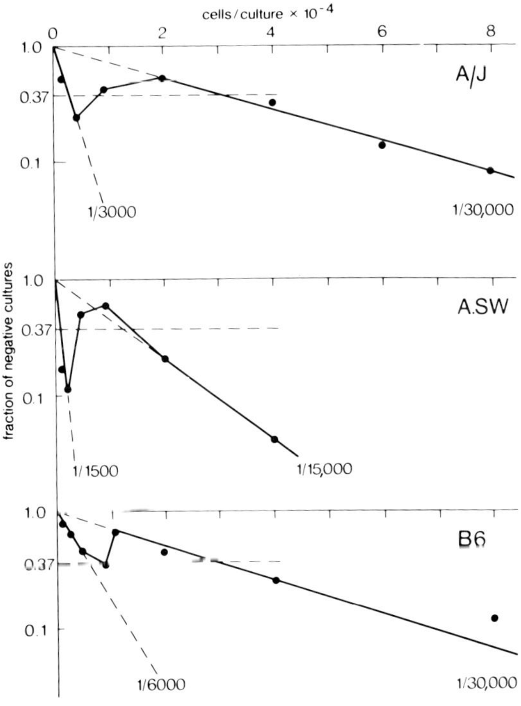

Fig. 2. Precursor frequencies for T helper cells from three inbred strains specific for antibody response to trinitrophenylated group A streptococci (TNP-Strep A). T cells were activated with Con-A in 2 day bulk culture, then placed in limiting dilution together with syngeneic PEC and Con-A supernatant for 7 days. Thereafter, each culture was assayed for helper activity by adding B cells and TNP-Strep A and testing for TNP-specific plaque-forming cells on day 4.

in Table I. From this summary it appears that there are three frequency ranges for T precursor cells. For most T cell functions analyzed, we find precursors in either two or three of these ranges and rarely only in one.

Table I also compares the precursor frequencies for a number of different T cell types and specificities. What is most surprising is that the high frequency range (1/50–1/700) is not restricted to alloreactive cells but is also seen for SRBC-specific Th and trinitrophenyl-specific CTL. Furthermore, alloreactive cells are also found in the intermediate set. Thus, the often quoted "high frequency" of alloreactive cells may have to be redisputed.

III. INDEPENDENT REGULATION OF EACH PRECURSOR POPULATION

As stated above (Fig. 2), at certain cell concentrations we find the fraction of positive cultures decreasing with increasing numbers of cells per culture, a phenomenon which represents some form of suppression (Eichmann *et al.*, 1980; Goronzy *et al.*, 1981; Melchers and Eichmann, 1981b). Suppression is in each

TABLE I

Precursor Frequencies for Helper and Cytotoxic T Cells of Various Specificities

T cell function	Antigen	Frequency: Frequent set	Intermediate set	Rare set
Th	Strep A[a]		1/900–1/10,000	1/10,000–1/100,000
	SRBC[b]	1/50–1/250	1/1,500–1/9,000	1/12,000–1/70,000
	CRBC[b]	1/50–1/250	1/1,500–1/9,000	1/12,000–1/70,000
	T15 Id[c]		1/5,000–1/20,000	1/50,000–1/500,000
	H-2[d,h]		1/2,200–1/4,000	
	H-2 + Mls[d,h]	1/150–1/500	1/2,200–1/4,000	
CTL	H-2[e]	1/150–1/600	1/2,000–1/8,000	
	TNP + H-2[f]	1/100–1/700	1/1,500–1/9,000	1/12,000–1/10,000
	HY + H-2[g,h]		1/5,000–1/13,000	

[a] Data from Eichmann *et al.*, 1980.
[b] Data from Melchers and Eichmann, 1981a,b.
[c] J. Cerny, G. Hämmerling, W. Kuon, and K. Eichmann, unpublished observation.
[d] Data from Simon *et al.*, 1981a,b.
[e] Data from Goronzy *et al.*, 1981.
[f] Data from Hamann *et al.*, 1981a,b.
[g] Data from Zahn *et al.*, 1981.
[h] Frequencies determined in normal T cells activated by antigen in limiting dilution, rather than in Con-A blasts.

case specific for only one of the multiple populations, because with further increase of the cell input positive cultures increase again in number. These findings indicate the existence of another, less frequent cell population which is insensitive to the suppression mechanism that inactivates the more frequent population.

Several experiments have been performed to investigate this situation. Figure 3 shows results from an experiment in which alloreactive CTL precursors are determined in Con-A-activated T cells and, for comparison, by limiting dilution of normal T cells with subsequent activation by allogeneic stimulating cells (Goronzy *et al.*, 1981). It is evident that the frequent CTL precursor is revealed by both assays. However, it is not suppressed in alloantigen-activated cells so that infrequent CTL precursors are not revealed. Thus, in contrast to Con-A activation, exposure to alloantigen either does not activate the suppressive mechanism or converts the frequent precursor cell to a nonsuppressable state.

Further information on the nature of the suppression comes from experiments using T cells selected for their Lyt phenotypes assayed in a different limiting dilution protocol. This protocol, designed to determine the precursor frequency of alloreactive Th cells for CTL, involves the activation of T cells by allogeneic stimulator cells with and without TCGF and their subsequent assay for help in a detection system consisting of thymocytes and the same stimulator cells (Simon *et al.*, 1981a,b). As shown in Table II using a number of experimental variations,

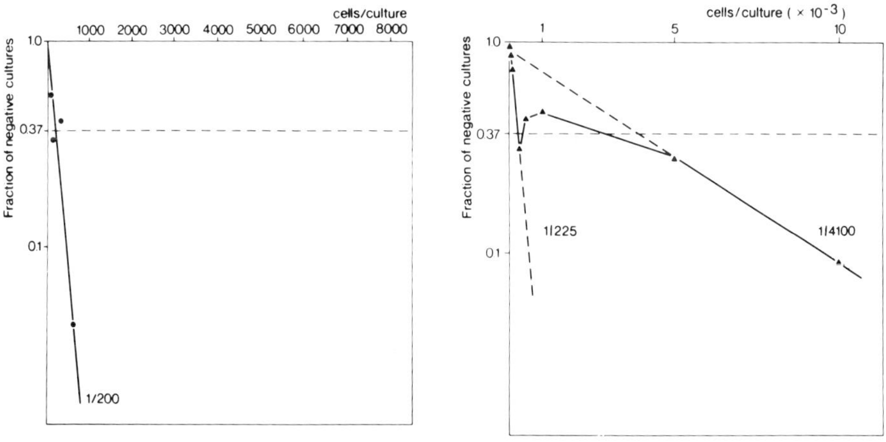

Fig. 3. Precursor frequencies for C57BL/6 cytotoxic T cells with specificity for DBA/2 target cells. Left: Normal T cells were placed in limiting dilution together with irradiated allogeneic stimulator cells and Con-A supernatant for 7 days and thereafter analyzed for cytotoxic activity. Right: T cells were first activated with Con-A in 2 day bulk culture, then placed in limiting dilution together with syngeneic PEC and Con-A supernatant for 7 days. Thereafter, all cultures were assayed DBA/2 (P815) target cells by a ^{51}Cr release assay.

TABLE II

Precursor Frequency and Regulation of Alloreactive T Helper Cells, Dependence on Experimental Conditions[a]

			Frequency			
Cells	Antigen[b]	Con-A Sup.[c]	Frequent set	(Suppr.)	Intermediate set	(Suppr.)
T	H-2	–	–	?[d]	1/1920	++[d]
T	H-2 + Mls	–	–	?	1/2390	++
Lyt-1	H-2	–	–	?	1/3790	(+)
Lyt-1	H-2 + Mls	–	–	?	1/4760	(+)
T	H-2 + Mls	+	–	+++	—	+++
Lyt-1	H-2 + Mls	+	1/150	++	1/2690	–

[a] Data from Simon *et al.*, 1981a,b.

[b] Antigen present during limiting dilution period and in detection system, consisting of thymocytes and allogeneic stimulator cells. H-2, activation by H-2 congenic cells; H-2 + Mls, activation by totally allogeneic cells including Mls difference.

[c] Rat Con-A supernatant present during limiting dilution period.

[d] ?, precursor set possibly suppressed and therefore not detected; +++, strong suppression so that precursor set is not detected; ++, suppression of precursor set at increasing cell concentrations; (+), suppression only at very high cell concentrations; –, no suppression detected.

we find one type of Th precursors corresponding in frequency to the intermediate set in Table I. Using nonselected T cells, this Th precursor is suppressed at increasing cell concentrations. Using purified Lyt-1^+ cells, suppression is largely abrogated. This suggests that the suppression of the intermediate set may be due to a typical Lyt-1^-2^+ suppressor T (Ts) cell.

In addition, Lyt-1^+ cells reveal under appropriate experimental conditions an additional, more frequent set of Th precursors which is suppressed at cell concentrations between the frequent and intermediate sets. Thus, this suppression must be due to a Lyt-1^+2^- cell and may therefore act indirectly through an inducer cell (Eardley *et al.*, 1978). Further work on the nature of suppression in this system is needed.

It can also be seen from Table II that multiple sets of T precursor cells may be difficult to demonstrate using antigen activation. Only under a very defined set of conditions do we detect the frequent set of alloreactive Th. Since these conditions include the use of Lyt-1^+ cells which are presumably devoid of Ts cells, it is appropriate to assume that the reason for the failure to detect the frequent Th set under most experimental conditions is suppression. Indeed, we think that in all experimental situations which do not reveal a frequent precursor set, this set is suppressed rather than absent.

IV. Lyt-PHENOTYPIC DIFFERENCES BETWEEN T PRECURSOR POPULATIONS

In our attempts to find functional differences between the multiple precursor populations, we have determined their Lyt phenotypes. For Strep A reactive Th we have found that the intermediate set is Lyt-1^+2^+, whereas the rare set is Lyt-1^+2^- (Eichmann *et al.*, 1980). For alloreactive CTL we found that the frequent set consists predominantly but not entirely of Lyt-1^+2^+ cells, whereas the intermediate set consists predominantly of Lyt-1^-2^+ cells (Goronzy *et al.*, 1981). These observations may indicate that, with decreasing frequency, T cell precursor sets represent sequential maturation steps on the way from a virgin to the memory status.

V. CONCLUSIONS

A. Size of the T Cell Repertoire for Foreign Antigens

For most complex antigens, such as allogeneic H-2 and xenogeneic red blood cells, we find frequencies for the most frequent precursor set that center around 1/200 splenic or lymph node T cells. On the basis of our Lyt data and because they represent the most frequent T cell population in nonimmune mice, we think that this figure characterizes the virgin T cell repertoire. Thus, if we conceded between 10 and 50 different antigenic determinants or reactive T cell clones for each complex antigen, the T cell repertoire would consist of between 2000 and 10,000 different combing sites. We would like to stress that this is a maximal estimate because arguments such as cross-reactivity or degeneracy would only diminish this figure. It should also be pointed out that if T cell combining sites were indeed made of V_H regions (Rajewsky and Eichmann, 1977), this would be an expected size for the repertoire. If the T cell repertoire were indeed of this limited size, it must be highly cross-reactive in order to accommodate the much larger repertoire of antigens.

B. Specificity and Cross-Reactivity of T Cells

Although many conflicting results on T cell specificity have been published, a general consensus has been reached on a rather fine discriminatory capacity of T cells. This consensus is based primarily on experiments performed with mixed populations of T cells using the restimulation approach, i.e., asking the question of whether T cells primed with antigen A can or cannot be restimulated with antigen B.

In contrast, using the clonal approach, T cell cross-reactivity seems to be more frequently observed (reviewed in von Boehmer *et al.*, 1980). The most prominent recent example is the high frequency of alloreactive T cell clones that cross-react with Mls determinants (Molnar-Kimber *et al.*, 1980; Simon *et al.*, 1981b). As can be seen from Table II, although H-2 as well as Mls determinants are strongly stimulatory for T cells, only insignificant differences are observed between Th frequencies for II-2, and for H-2 + Mls. Thus, on the clonal level, T cell cross-reactivity appears to be greater than was expected from the restimulation approach using mixed T cell populations. Furthermore, the old observations on T helper cell monogamy (Waldman *et al.*, 1976; Sullman and Feinstein, 1977) have been neglected in this discussion, being compatible with a complete lack of antigen specificity of T helper cells.

It should be pointed out that these statements concern specificity for foreign antigens and not restriction specificity, which has not been studied extensively by limiting dilution. For specificity to foreign antigens, however, it seems that the high degree of specificity seen with mixed T cell populations may in part be regulatory in nature.

C. Regulation of T Cell Specificity

We have presented evidence previously that, in nonselected T cells, secondary, Lyt-1^-2^+ CTL precursors only respond to the homologous alloantigen used for priming and do not respond to a cross-reacting alloantigen, although they are able to respond to this alloantigen when tested as isolated Lyt-1^-2^+ cell population (Simon and Abenhardt, 1980; Simon and Eichmann, 1980). The prevention of a cross-reacting secondary response was clearly due to suppression. This undoubtedly represents an example for the regulation of T cell restimulation toward a greater degree of specificity.

In conjunction with the independent regulation of virgin and memory precursor populations, this can be used to construct a T cell system that gets by with a limited repertoire and yet appears highly specific. The functional principle of this system may be suppression of cross-reactivity. Although at present there is no clear idea on the mechanism of this suppression, it seems likely that it should be based on binding affinity and some form of competition between suppression and activation by antigen. Taken together, we think that the understanding of the suppressive regulation of multiple T presursor sets may be a key to the understanding of T cell specificity.

ACKNOWLEDGMENTS

We like to thank Ms. I. Falk, U. Schaefer, A. Michnay, C. Löschmann, A. Moll, S. Leidig, and Mr. W. Muller for able technical assistance.

REFERENCES

Cantor, H., and Boyse, E. A. (1977). Regulation of the immune response by T cell subclasses. *Contemp. Top. Immunobiol.* **7,** 27.

Documenta Geigy (1960). "Wissenschaftliche Tabellen," 6th ed., p. 170. Geigy.

Eardley, D. D., Hugenberger, J., McVay-Bourdeau, L., She, F. W., Gershon, R. K., and Cantor, H. (1978). Immunoregulatory circuits among T cell sets. I. T helper cells induce other T cell sets to exert feedback inhibition. *J. Exp. Med.* **147,** 1106.

Eichmann, K., Falk, I., Melchers, I., and Simon, M. M. (1980). Quantitative studies on T cell diversity. I. Determination of the precursor frequencies for two types of streptococcus A specific helper cells in non-immune, polyclonally activated splenic T cells. *J. Exp. Med.* **152,** 477.

Goronzy, J., Schaefer, U., Eichmann, K., and Simon, M. M. (1981). Quantitative studies on T cell diversity. II. Deptermination of the frequencies and Lyt phenotypes of two types of precursor cells for alloreactive cytotoxic T cells in polyclonally and specifically activated splenic T cells. *J. Exp. Med.* **153,** 857.

Haas, W., and von Boehmer, H. (1978). Techniques for separation and selection of antigen-specific lymphocytes. *Curr. Top. Microbiol. Immunol.* **84,** 1.

Hamann, U., Rehberger, R., Eichmann, K., and Krammer, P. H. (1981a). Receptors and regulation of major histocompatibility restricted cytotoxic T lymphocytes. *In* "Immunoglobulin Idiotypes and their Expression" (C. Janeway, E. Sercarz, and H. Wigzell, eds.), p. 441. Academic Press, New York.

Hamann, U., Eichmann, K., and Krammer, P. H. (1981b). Regulation and precursor frequencies of MHC-restricted TNP-specific cytotoxic T lymphocytes. *Immunobiology* (abstr.) **160,** 33.

Hämmerling, G. J., Hämmerling, U., and Flaherty, L. (1979). Qat-4 and Qat-5, new murine T cell antigens governed by the *Tla* region and identified by monoclonal antibodies. *J. Exp. Med.* **150,** 108.

Kuppers, R., Simon, M. M., and Eichmann, K. (1981). Single cell analysis of the growth of Lyt phenotype subsets in IL-2 supernatants. *Immunobiology* (abstr.) **160,** 63.

Melchers, I., and Eichmann, K. (1981a). Frequency estimates of precursor helper T cells in non-immune mice after polyclonal activation and differentiation *in vitro*. *Immunobiology* (abstr.) **160,** 72.

Melchers, I., and Eichmann, K. (1981b). Quantitative studies on T cell diversity. III. Frequencies of precursor cells for T helper cells reactive to sheep red blood cells: Differentiation, clone size and specificity. (Submitted for publication.)

Möller, G., ed. (1972). Lymphocyte activation by mitogens. *Transplant. Rev.* **11.**

Molnar-Kimber, K. L., Webb, S. R., Sprent, J., and Wilson, D. B. (1980). T cell lines with dual specificity for strong Mls and H-2 determinants. *J. Immunol.* **125,** 2643.

Rajewski, K., and Eichmann, K. (1977). Antigen receptors on T helper cells. *Contemp. Top. Immunobiol.* **7,** 69.

Simon, M. M., and Abenhardt, B. (1980). Generation of effector cells from T cell subsets. II. Lyt-123 T cells contain the precursors for all primary cytotoxic effector cells and for cells involved in the regulation of cytotoxic responses. *Eur. J. Immunol.* **10,** 334.

Simon, M. M., and Eichmann, K. (1980). T cell subsets participating in the generation of cytotoxic T cells. *Springer Semin. Immunopathol.* **3,** 39.

Simon, M. M., Goronzy, J., and Eichmann, K. (1981a). Comparison of the frequencies of alloantigen-specific T helper cell precursors in unselected and in selected T cell subpopulations after specific activation. *Immunobiology* **159,** 19 (abstr.).

Simon, M. M., Goronzy, J., Schaefer, U., and Eichmann, K. (1981b). Frequency analysis of alloantigen-specific T helper cell precursors in unselected T cells and in selected Lyt-1 T cell subpopulations after specific activation. *In* "Mechanisms of Lymphocyte Activation" (H. Kirchner and K. Resch, eds.), p. 270. Elsevier/North-Holland Biomedical Press, Amsterdam.

Sullman, S. F., and Feinstein, A. (1977). The relative distribution of foci forming antibodies to two different haptens in repopulated mouse spleens. *Eur. J. Immunol.* **7,** 421.

Tada, T., Tahemori, T., Okumura, K., Nonaka, M., and Tokuhisa, T. (1978). Two distinct types of helper T cells involved in the secondary antibody response: independent and synergistic effects of Ia^- and Ia^+ helper T cells. *J. Exp. Med.* **147,** 446.

von Boehmer, H., and Haas, W. (1981). H-2 restricted cytolytic and non-cytolytic T cells clones: Isolation, specificity and functional analysis. *Immunol. Rev.* **54,** 27.

von Boehmer, H., Haas, W., Pohlit, H., Hengartner, H., and Nabholz, M. (1980). T cell clones, their use for the study of specificity, induction and effector-function of T cells. *Springer Semin. Immunopathol.* **3,** 1.

Waldman, H., Levkovits, I., and Feinstein, A. (1976). Restriction in the functions of single T cells. *Immunology* **3,** 533.

Watanabe, T., Fathman, G., and Coutinho, A. (1977). Clonal growth of T cells in vitro: Preliminary attempts to a quantitative approach. *Immunol. Rev.* **35,** 3.

Zahn, G., Hämmerling, G. J., Eichmann, K., and Simon, M. M. (1981). Expression of Qat-4 and Qat-5 alloantigens on cytotoxic precursor and effector cells: Different surface phenotypes of alloreactive and H-2 restricted cytotoxic T cells. *Eur. J. Immunol.* **12,** 43.

20

Frequency, Regulation, and H-2 Epitope Specificity of Alloreactive and *H-2*-Restricted CTL Clones

Günter J. Hämmerling/Cornelia Weyand/Jörg Goronzy

I. Topographic Arrangement of Alloantigenic Determinants on the H-2K^k Molecule 245
II. Distinct CTL Subpopulations with Different Precursor Frequencies Detected by Limiting Dilution Analysis 246
III. Target Inhibition by mc Anti-H-2 of CTL Clones Generated in the Limiting Dilution System 247
IV. Target Inhibition of *H-2K^k*-Restricted, TNP-Specific CTL Clones . . 248
V. Conclusions 249
References 251

H-2 antigens are known to be the primary target structures for murine cytotoxic T lymphocytes (CTL). However, it is not clear if alloreactive CTL recognize the same determinants or domains on the H-2 molecule which are characterized by alloantibodies, and if the same determinants serve also as restriction sites for recognition by *H-2*-restricted CTL. In the present chapter we will summarize our findings on the frequency of alloreactive and *H-2*-restricted CTL clonotypes, regulatory mechanisms controlling their generation, and their epitope specificity as assessed by target inhibition with a panel of monoclonal anti-H-2 antibodies (mcAb).

I. TOPOGRAPHIC ARRANGEMENT OF ALLOANTIGENIC DETERMINANTS ON THE H-2K^k MOLECULE

Using competitive antibody binding assays with six different monoclonal (mc) anti-H-2 (Lemke *et al.*, 1979), we have observed previously that alloantigenic determinants are concentrated in two spatially separated clusters on the H-2K^k

ISOLATION, CHARACTERIZATION, AND
UTILIZATION OF T LYMPHOCYTE CLONES

ISBN 0-12-249920-4

molecule (Lemke and Hämmerling, 1981). Thus, binding of any given mc anti-H-2 was only blocked by mcAb within one cluster, while mcAb belonging to the other cluster did not interfere with binding. These findings are schematically illustrated in Fig. 1.

II. DISTINCT CTL SUBPOPULATIONS WITH DIFFERENT PRECURSOR FREQUENCIES DETECTED BY LIMITING DILUTION ANALYSIS

For analysis of the fine specificity of individual CTL clones, a limiting dilution system was established (Weyand *et al.*, 1981b). Increasing numbers of DBA/2 responder spleen cells (from 50 to 10^4 cells/well) were stimulated in microtiter plates with 10^6 irradiated A/J stimulator spleen cells for 7 days in the presence of 5% crude T cell growth factor (TCGF) from concanavalin (Con-A)-stimulated rat spleens. Cytotoxicity was assayed against ^{51}Cr-labeled L929 ($H\text{-}2^k$) tumor cells. In a large set of limiting dilution experiments, we observed consistently multiphasic Poisson distributions. A representative triphasic Poisson plot is depicted in Fig. 2 which shows three sets of experimental values each fitting to a straight line. All lines cross the ordinate at about 1.0, indicating that only one cell type is limiting.

With increasing numbers of responding cells, there is a linear increase in the number of wells with cytolytic activity; these data yield a precursor frequency estimate of about 1/400 for this first CTL population. However, a further increase in the number of responding cells results in a decrease in number of wells with CTL activity, suggesting the action of suppressive mechanisms on the most frequent CTL population. Then, with higher cell numbers, a second CTL population becomes apparent (*f* about 1/1200 to 1/3000, depending on the experiment), which also becomes suppressed. This allows a third CTL population to become visible (*f* about 1/3000 to 1/4000). It should be noted that on many occasions we observed only biphasic curves with populations CTL_I and CTL_{II} or with CTL_{II} and CTL_{III}. The reasons for these variations are not clear, but the batch of TCGF,

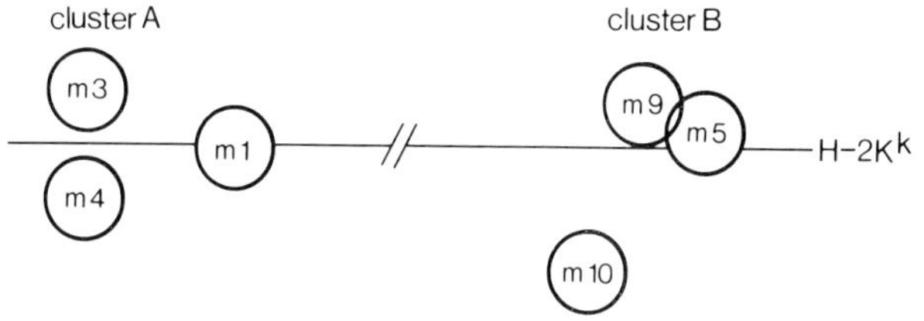

Fig. 1. Schematic topographic arrangement of allodeterminants on the H-2K^k molecule (Lemke and Hämmerling, 1981).

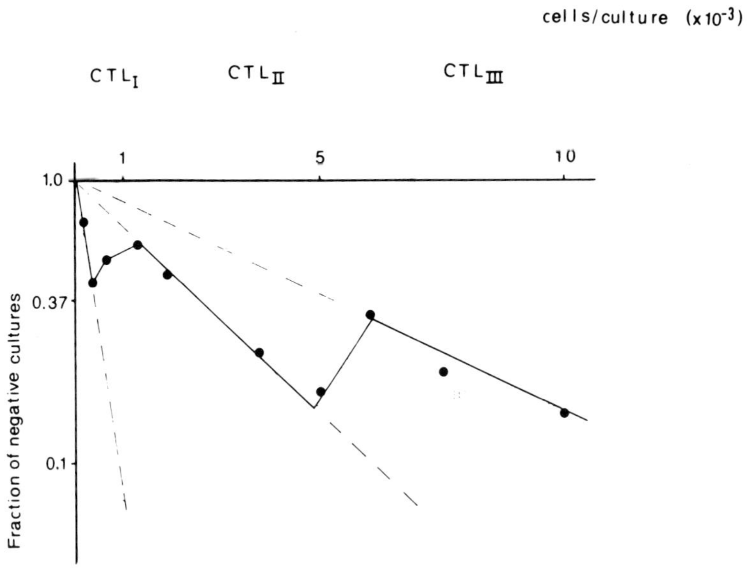

Fig. 2. Three H-2K^k specific CTL populations with different precursor frequencies demonstrated by limiting dilution analysis.

the origin of mice, etc., could play a role. In cases where in the Poisson plot only CTL_I and CTL_{II} could be demonstrated, the presence of the third population was also obvious from a decrease and subsequent increase of ^{51}Cr release values at higher responder cell doses.

III. TARGET INHIBITION BY mc ANTI-H-2 OF CTL CLONES GENERATED IN THE LIMITING DILUTION SYSTEM

The H-2 epitope specificity of CTL clones within each subpopulation was determined by target inhibition with mc anti-H-2. Each limiting dilution well was split into two equal aliquots, and cytolytic activity was assayed without and in the presence of an optimal concentration (mcAb (Weyand *et al.*, 1981b). The results of these blocking studies revealed a surprising pattern as summarized in Table I.

As expected, each individual antibody blocked only a fraction of CTL clones, suggesting that CTL are heterogenous and specific for different H-2 epitopes. However, clones within the different subpopulations display distinct receptor repertoires. Thus, clones from CTL_I were only blocked by mcAb to cluster A, while CTL_{II} clones were blocked to about the same percentage by both mcAb's to clusters A and B. In contrast CTL_{III} were predominantly blocked by mcAb to cluster B. Altogether the results suggest the presence of an high frequency

TABLE I

Target Inhibition by mc Anti-H-2 of Alloreactive Clones in Different CTL Populations[a]

Specificity of mcAB	Percent H-2K^k-specific CTL clones blocked by mc anti-H-2K^k		
	CTL_I (*f* 1/400)	CTL_{II} (*f* 1/1500)	CTL_{III} (*f* 1/4000)
Cluster A	48, 52, 72	10, 41, 53	8, 24, 28
Cluster B	0, 0, 0	52, 55, 59	65, 68, 72
Mixed mcAB	85	90	95
Ratio A : B	1 : 0	1 : 1.6	1 : 3.6

[a] Three mcAb to cluster A (m1, m3, m4) and three to cluster B (m5, m9, m10) were used. In this order for each mcAb the percentage of inhibited clones is shown. The ratio A : B gives a rough estimate of the total fraction of clones blocked by cluster A antibodies compared to cluster B antibodies. The mcAb are described in Lemke *et al.* (1979), the clusters are illustrated in Fig. 1, and CTL subpopulations are shown in Fig. 2.

alloreactive CTL population with predominant specificity for cluster A determinants. This population is suppressed at higher cell doses and allows other populations to become visible with preferential activity toward cluster B. In recent studies (Weyand *et al.*, 1981a), we have observed that CTL generated under bulk culture conditions are also predominantly blocked by cluster B antibodies, namely, three times more efficiently than with cluster A antibodies. Thus bulk culture CTL appear to consist mainly of populations identical or similar to CTL_{III}, while the high frequency and cluster A-specific populations appear to be suppressed.

IV. TARGET INHIBITION OF *H-2K*^{k}-RESTRICTED, TNP-SPECIFIC CTL CLONES

Next, we approached the question whether or not an individual H-2 molecule would contain more than one restriction site which is recognized in conjunction with the hapten trinitrophenyl (TNP) by *H-2*-restricted CTL. *H-2K*^{k}-restricted TNP-specific CTL clones were generated in an analogous limiting dilution system with CBA responders stimulated in the presence of TCGF by 10^6 TNP conjugated A/J splenocytes. After 7 days, wells were split and cytotoxicity assayed with and without mc anti-H-2K^k against TNP modified L929 targets. Again triphasic Poisson curves were frequently found similar to Fig. 2 with the following average frequencies: TNP-CTL_I 1/700, TNP-CTL_{II} 1/1800, and TNP-CTL_{III} 1/3500 (data not shown).

Target inhibition by the six mc anti-H-2K^k showed again that only a fraction of

H-2-restricted CTL clones could be blocked by each individual antibody, while a mixture of all Ab inhibited the vast majority of clones (see Table II). These data provide evidence that an H-2 molecule contains various epitopes or domains which can serve as restriction sites for different *H-2*-restricted clones. As shown in Table II, in the *H-2*-restricted system all three CTL populations were inhibited to a large degree by mcAb to cluster B. However, again the less frequent population, CTL_{III}, was more efficiently blocked by cluster B antibodies than the high frequency population CTL_{I}, but the effects are less striking than in the allosystem (see Table I). Thus twofold more clones of the CTL_{I} population are blocked by Ab against cluster B as compared to cluster A antibodies. In the CTL_{II} population, the ratio of clones specific for cluster B compared to clones specific for cluster A is about 3:1, and in CTL_{III} it is roughly 4:1. Again, these data suggest a shift in the expressed repertoire of CTL populations depending on the responder cell doses. It should be mentioned in this context that our previous studies on target inhibition of TNP-specific CTL generated in bulk culture also demonstrated a preponderance of cluster B restricted CTL (Weyand *et al.*, 1981a).

V. CONCLUSIONS

The data presented here demonstrate that under limiting dilution conditions in the allosystem ($H\text{-}2^d$ anti-$H\text{-}2K^k$), a high frequency population can be found with preferential specificity for $H\text{-}2K^k$ epitopes within cluster A. This population is subject to a suppressive mechanism which after emergence and suppression of another population with intermediate frequency allows a low frequency population to become visible with predominant reactivity to cluster B determinants. Similar observations were also made in the TNP system in which more clones of

TABLE II

Target Inhibition by mc Anti-H-2K^k of TNP-Specific Clones in Different CTL Subpopulations[a]

Specificity of mcAb	Percent TNP-specific CTL clones blocked by mc anti-H-2K^k		
	CTL_{I} (f 1/700)	CTL_{II} (f 1/1800)	CTL_{III} (f 1/3500)
Cluster A	19, 36, 39	9, 20, 31	8, 23, 19
Cluster B	61, 51, 62	71, 53, 70	78, 61, 85
Mixed mcAb	93	90	96
Ratio of A : B	1 : 1.8	1 : 3.2	1 : 4.4

[a] For target inhibition of limiting dilution clones (CBA anti-CBA TNP), three mcAb to cluster A (m1, m3, m4) and three to cluster B (m5, m9, m10) were used. The percentage of inhibited clones is shown in this order for each mcAb. The ratio A : B gives a rough estimate of the total fraction of clones blocked by cluster A antibodies compared to cluster B antibodies.

the low frequency population were restricted by cluster B epitopes than clones of the high frequency population. The results indicate that the multiphasic Poisson curves observed by us are not laboratory artifacts but do indeed reflect the existence of different CTL populations with distinct receptor repertoire.

The nature of the suppressive mechanism is still unknown, but it may be a suppressor cell. The putative suppressor cell could havc idiotype, antigen (H-2 epitope), or perhaps other specificity. In any case, the suppressor cell must be of high precursor frequency because onset of suppression is often observed at input doses of only 500 cells per well. So far multiphasic Poisson curves for CTL precursors have been reported by only a few other investigators (Goronzy *et al.*, 1981; also see Eichmann *et al.* Chapter 19 in this treatise), while in general limiting dilution analysis of CTL precursors has resulted in single straight regression lines (e.g., Fischer-Lindahl and Wilson, 1977; Teh *et al.*, 1977; MacDonald *et al.*, 1980). The reasons for this apparent discrepancy are still unresolved, but source and quality of the TCGF-containing supernatant as well as strain combinations, etc., may be of relevance.

Altogether, our data suggest that H-2 molecules contain several distinct determinants or restriction sites which serve as target structures for different CTL clones. Heterogeneity of target specificities also was described by Sherman (1980). Our data allow the additional conclusion that the target specificities on the H-2K^k molecule are clustered in two major domains, and that alloreactive CTL recognize basically the same polymorphic determinants or domains which are defined by alloantibodies. Furthermore, the same domains also harbor the restriction sites for TNP-specific CTL. At first sight, the results appear to support the dual recognition models of *H-2* restriction with one binding site specific for TNP and the other one specific for allodeterminants. However, they also satisfy altered self models if one assumes that for steric reasons T cells can recognize only two major modified domains on the H-2 molecule, namely, cluster A and B. In this context, the fact that in both alloreactive and anti-TNP systems a comparable shift of the expressed repertoire from cluster A- to cluster B-specific populations is observed could be coincidental. Other *H-2*-restricted systems need to be investigated to determine whether this is a general phenomenon. Finally, the regulatory effects demonstrated in the limiting dilution system emphasize strongly that the spectrum of specificities observed under particular experimental conditions (e.g., in bulk culture) does not necessarily reflect the potential repertoire of the T cells.

ACKNOWLEDGMENTS

This work was in part supported by DFG. We thank Mrs. S. Muller for preparation of this manuscript.

REFERENCES

Fischer-Lindahl, K., and Wilson, D. B. (1977). Histocompatibility antigen-activated cytotoxic T lymphocytes. II. Estimates of the frequency and specificity of precursors. *J. Exp. Med.* **145,** 503.

Goronzy, J., Schaefer, U., Eichmann, K., and Simon, M. M. (1981). Quantitative studies on T cell diversity. II. Determination of the frequencies and Lyt phenotypes of two sets of precursor cells for alloreactive cytotoxic T cells in polyclonally and specifically activated splenic T cells. *J. Exp. Med.* **153,** 857.

Lemke, H., and Hämmerling, G. J. (1981). Topographic arrangement of H-2 determinants defined by monoclonal hybridoma antibodies. *In* "Monoclonal Antibodies and T Cell Hybridomas" G. J. Hämmerling, U. Hämmerling, and J. F. Kearney, eds.), p. 102. Elsevier/North-Holland Biomedical Press, Amsterdam.

Lemke, H., Hämmerling, G. J., and Hämmerling, U. (1979). Fine specificity analysis with monoclonal antibodies of antigens controlled by the major histocompatibility complex and by the *Qa/TL* region in mice. *Immunol. Rev.* **47,** 175.

McDonald, H. R., Cerottini, J. C., Ryser, J. E., Maryanski, J. L., Taswell, C., Widmer, M. B., and Brunner, K. T. (1980). Quantitation and cloning of cytolytic T lymphocytes and their precursors. *Immunol. Rev.* **51,** 93.

Sherman, L. A. (1980). Dissection of the B10.D2 anti-H-2K^b cytolytic T lymphocyte receptor repertoire. *J. Exp. Med.* **151,** 1397.

Teh, H. S., Harley, E., Phillips, R. A., and Miller, R. G. (1977). Quantitative studies on the precursors of cytotoxic lymphocytes. I. Characterization of a clonal assay and determination of the size of clones derived from single precursors. *J. Immunol.* **118,** 1049.

Weyand, C., Hämmerling, G. J., and Goronzy, J. (1981a). Recognition of H-2 domains by cytotoxic T lymphocytes. *Nature (London)* **292,** 627.

Weyand, C., Goronzy, J., and Hämmerling, G. J. (1981b). Recognition of polymorphic H-2 domains by T lymphocytes. I. Functional role of different H-2 domains for the generation of alloreactive cytotoxic T lymphocytes and determination of precursor frequencies. *J. Exp. Med.* **154,** 1717.

21

Production of Lymphokines by Murine T Cells Grown in Limiting Dilution and Long-Term Cultures

Peter H. Krammer/Michael Dy/Lothar Hultner/
Peter Isakson/Ursula Kees/Marie-Luise Lohmann-Matthes/
Fabrizio Marcucci/Andrea Michnay/
Ellen Puré/Anneliese Schimpl/Fritz Staber/
Ellen S. Vitetta/Michael Waller

I. Introduction 253
II. Analysis of Lymphokine Release in Limiting Dilution Microcultures 254
III. Analysis of Lymphokine Production from Long-Term T Cell Clones and Lines 258
IV. Conclusions 261
References 261

I. INTRODUCTION

T lymphocytes regulate the immune response by interacting with other T cells or with cells from other compartments of the immune system. Such interactions are accompanied by release of soluble T cell factors. The effector functions of these factors may be antigen specific or nonspecific. The nonspecific lymphokines are potent soluble mediators which act on other lymphocytes, macrophages, or on cells which are unrelated to the immune system. It is obvious that such a system must use complex regulatory mechanisms to assure physiological homeostasis. No unifying hypothesis can yet relate the specific and nonspecific pathways of the response or explain the operation of the entire system. This is in part due to the fact that the molecular nature of the antigen-specific or -nonspecific molecules by which T cells exert their regulatory role is unknown. In addition, although many lymphokines are produced during immune reactions

ISOLATION, CHARACTERIZATION, AND
UTILIZATION OF T LYMPHOCYTE CLONES

ISBN 0-12-249920-4

in which T cells are primarily involved, we have not defined the signals which stimulate the release of such lymphokines from a particular cell type. Since many lymphokines released during an immune response act on a variety of target cells, it is important to know whether a particular cell can release several lymphokines and what mechanisms control their activity.

In order to analyze some of these questions in detail, we have used two systems. In the first system, mitogen-activated T cells from nonimmune mice are plated in limiting dilution cultures (Eichmann *et al.*, 1980), and the mitogen-induced release of lymphokines from the clonal progeny of a limited number of precursor T cells is analyzed. These experiments allow us to test directly the reactivity of such T cells in the microcultures and to determine whether a single T cell releases several lymphokines into the culture supernatant. This analysis gives a frequency estimate for lymphokine-producing T cells and describes their activity. The data derived from such experiments provide evidence for the simultaneous production of several lymphokines by a single T cell alone. In the second system, we have studied the mitogen-induced release of lymphokines from TCGF-dependent T cell clones grown in long-term culture. Results obtained with several long-term T cell clones and lines releasing different lymphokines imply that lymphokine activity is exerted by at least several different molecules.

II. ANALYSIS OF LYMPHOKINE RELEASE IN LIMITING DILUTION MICROCULTURES

To analyze the lymphokines released from T cells and to define the activity of these lymphokines, an optimal experimental situation should allow us to test the activity of the clonal progeny of every T cell. In order to minimize selection of T cell subsets, selective growth, and induction we used the following experimental procedure (the details of the methods are described in the Appendix).

Murine spleen cells are activated in bulk culture by stimulation with concanavalin A (Con-A) for 2 days. Dead cells and debris are removed by separation over Ficoll. Ficoll-enriched cells are plated in limiting dilution microcultures at 1, 2, 4, etc., cells per well in the presence of irradiated allogeneic peritoneal exudate cells in culture medium supplemented with T cell growth factor (TCGF) (from rat spleen cells induced with Con-A for 24 hr). The cells are allowed to grow for 7–12 days during which time they are fed twice with TCGF-containing medium. The cells in each microwell are then thoroughly washed, pulsed with Con-A for 3 hr, washed again in fresh culture medium, and allowed to release lymphokines into the supernatant for 24 hr. Individual supernatants are then tested for the presence of a variety of lymphokines as shown in Table I: immune interferon (IFN-γ), macrophage activating factor (MAF), colony stimulating factor (CSF) [CSF for neutrophilic granulocytes and macrophages (GM-CSF),

TABLE I

Test Systems for Lymphokines

Lymphokines	Test systems for analysis
Immune interferon (IFN-γ)	Virus plaque reduction assay (Campbell *et al.*, 1975)
Macrophage activating factor (MAF)	Induction of cytotoxicity of purified bone marrow macrophages on P815 tumor cells (Lohmann-Matthes *et al.*, 1979)
Colony stimulating factors (CSF) for neutrophilic granulocytes and macrophages (GM-CSF), for megakaryocytes (Meg-CSF), for eosinophilic granulocytes (Eo-CSF), for erythrocytes (E-CSF)	Formation of colonies of hematopoietic cells in semisolid agar cultures of bone marrow cells (Staber and Johnson, 1980)
Histamine-producing cell-stimulating factor (HCSF)	Induction of an increase in histamine production by bone marrow cells (Dy *et al.*, 1981)
T cell growth factor (TCGF)	Growth support of a TCGF-dependent T cell clone in long-term culture (Krammer and Michnay, 1981)
T cell replacing factor (TRF)	Induction of anti-sheep red blood cell (SRBC) plaque forming cells in spleen cells from Nu/Nu mice immunized with SRBC (Schimpl and Wecker, 1972)
B cell differentiation factors (BCDF)	Induction of IgM secretion and switch to IgG secretion by purified B cells (Isakson *et al.*, 1982)

megakaryocytes (Meg-CSF), eosinophilic granulocytes (Eo-CSF), and erythrocytes (E-CSF)], histamine-producing cell-stimulating factor (HCSF), T cell growth factor (TCGF), T cell replacing factor (TRF), and B cell differentiation factors (BCDF). The assay systems for lymphokine activities are listed in Table I. Although we have tested only a limited number of lymphokines under these conditions, this methodology can be applied to all lymphokines whose release can be triggered by mitogens. Furthermore, with sensitive microassays, it is possible to test each supernatant simultaneously for the presence of several lymphokines.

It should be noted that it is essential to wash the cells in medium lacking TCGF prior to Con-A induction, since TCGF preparations themselves contain lymphokines. For various purposes it is important that the cells in microculture wells reach suitable clone sizes. This allows the determination of cell-mediated activities in aliquots of cells (T cell help, suppression, or cytotoxicity) as well as an assessment of lymphokine production by these cells. It should also be noted that the induction of IFN-γ can occur in serum-free medium without a significant loss in activity. This may be true of other lymphokines as well.

The frequency of cultures with growing cells is determined after 7–12 days of culture by visual examination, and the results are analyzed according to Poisson distribution. To estimate the frequencies of lymphokine-producing T cells determined according to Poisson distribution, supernatants from individual cultures of cells grown in limiting dilution are scored as positive when the lymphokine titer is equal to or higher than one or several (predetermined for each assay) standard deviations above the arithmetic mean of the controls from wells negative for T cell growth. For frequency estimates, the relationship between the number of responder cells added per microculture and the fraction of nonresponding cultures per group is analyzed by the least-squares method and fit to the zero-order term of the Poisson equation. Estimates of precursor frequencies are determined by the slope of the regression line.

In the above experimental system between 20 and 50% of the Con-A-activated murine spleen cells from bulk cultures grow and in limiting dilution microcultures a growth frequency as high as $f = 1/2$ can be obtained. Furthermore, the activity of T helper (Th), T suppressor (Ts), and cytotoxic T lymphocytes (CTL), and the frequency of T cells releasing a variety of lymphokines can be determined. This suggests that our data reflect a random determination of the T cell repertoire from nonimmune mice (see the discussion by Eichmann *et al.*, Chapter 19 in this treatise). There are, however, several experimental steps during this procedure which might favor selection of certain T cell subpopulations. These steps include Con-A activation, Ficoll purification, growth in limiting dilution microcultures, and induction of lymphokines by Con-A. Even if we assume that our system reflects the expression of a random T cell repertoire, this hypothesis remains to be proved by a single cell assay for T cells.

The release of IFN-γ, CSF, and MAF in limiting dilution microcultures is not constitutive but can be induced by mitogens. A similar situation might apply to other lymphokines, but this possibility has not been extensively tested. In addition, under limiting dilution culture conditions, normal regulation and growth control might be bypassed such that very high titers of lymphokines can be obtained. For example, individual selected microcultures containing 10^4–10^5 cells yield titers of IFN-γ higher than 10^4 international units (Krammer *et al.*, 1982). Furthermore, we observed that IFN-γ is produced by both cytotoxic and noncytotoxic T cells, but that the cultures with the most potent cytolytic activity give the highest IFN-γ titers (Krammer *et al.*, 1982). The activity of different microculture supernatants varies considerably, and this might be due to cellular heterogeneity rather than to variation in clone size.

Similar considerations apply to the production of CSF. The number of colonies in semisolid agar cultures generated from bone marrow cells stimulated by CSF-containing T cell supernatants shows considerable variation. GM-CSF can be demonstrated in all CSF positive supernatants. Moreover, supernatants with high GM-CSF activity also contain rare CSF subtypes, such as (with decreasing frequency) Meg-CSF, Eo-CSF, and E-CSF. The production of these rare CSF subtypes is usually associated with the production of GM-CSF. Thus, from an initial plating of cell numbers which give a high statistical chance of one precursor cell per well, supernatants with unique mixtures of GM-CSF and one or more of the rare CSF subtypes can be obtained. In only a few supernatants with high GM-CSF activity, however, can GM-CSF alone be detected. This suggests that the mitogen-induced release of particular lymphokines is related to the presence of particular T cells at a certain stage of growth or to the presence of different T cell subsets.

The frequency estimates we determined for T cells releasing IFN-γ, CSF, MAF, and TCGF, are shown in Table II. It is evident that at a growth frequency of between $f = 1/3$ and 1/28 the frequencies of IFN-γ ($f = 1/10$), CSF (1/6), and TCGF (1/15) producing T cells are rather high. In addition, in preliminary experiments designed to determine the frequencies for TRF and BCDF-producing T cells (data not shown), the frequencies were lower than those described above the IFN-γ and TCGF. In all cases, the regression lines from data plotted according to Poisson statistics were essentially linear and showed single hit kinetics. This indicates that T cells are limiting with respect to lymphokine release and hence suggests that they are the producer cells. Since the frequency estimates for cells producing IFN-γ and CSF are high, we could speculate that a large portion of the T cells produce these lymphokines and that the subpopulations of such T cells are overlapping, i.e., one T cell might release several lymphokines. This remains to be definitely established, however, by splitting supernatants from T cells initially plated in limiting dilution microcultures at a very low cell density to obtain an even higher statistical chance that the cells are derived from one precursor T lymphocyte.

TABLE II

Frequency of Lymphokine-Producing Cells in Con-A-Activated B6 Spleen Cells

Lymphokine	Frequency[a]
IFN-γ	1/10
CSF	1/6
MAF	1/91
TCGF	1/15

[a] The growth frequencies in these experiments were $f = 1/4$ (IFN-γ), $f = 1/3$ (CSF), $f = 1/28$ (MAF), and $f = 1/5$ (TCGF) Krammer and Michnay (1981).

III. ANALYSIS OF LYMPHOKINE PRODUCTION FROM LONG-TERM T CELL CLONES AND LINES

The majority of T cell clones obtained from primary limiting dilution microcultures in medium supplemented with TCGF alone cannot be propagated in culture beyond a period of 3 weeks. However, a few clones are capable of long-term growth in medium and TCGF. We obtained such homogeneous T cells as clones from a 4 day culture prepared with cells from the draining axillary and inguineal lymph nodes of AKR/J mice sensitized on the abdominal skin by 2,4,6-trinitrophenyl chloride [picryl chloride (PC)] 5 days earlier (Krammer *et al.*, 1980). These clones have been passaged in tissue culture for more than 18 months with a doubling time of 15 to 20 hr. Their growth is strictly dependent on the presence of TCGF in the medium. Cells from these clones are stimulated with Con-A or phytohemagglutinin (PHA) and tested for lymphokine production using various culture conditions (Marcucci *et al.*, 1981). A second type of long-term T cell line, maintained *in vitro* for approximately 2 years, was derived from secondary alloreactive AKR-anti-C57BL/6 (B6) cells regularly restimulated by irradiated B6 stimulator cells and maintained in culture medium supplemented with TCGF. Proliferation of these I-A^b-specific lines is dependent upon the presence of stimulator cells and TCGF in the medium, and lymphokine release from these lines is either induced by stimulation with Con-A or irradiated allogeneic stimulator cells.

Although T cell clones and lines provide a useful source of cells for biochemical purposes and for genetic engineering, it has to be kept in mind that the conclusions derived from studies with these cells must be verified using normal cell populations. Growth of TCGF-dependent T cells in a long-term cultures occurs rarely and only with cells on which a strong selective pressure has been applied over a long period of culture. T cells in long-term culture are more easily established and established at a higher frequency in medium with TCGF and the stimulating antigen. However, if these cells are not cloned at an early stage they might undergo selective pressure during a prolonged culture period. Therefore, the information provided by these clones and lines may also not be representative of the T cell repertoire. In addition, T cells from long-term TCGF-supplemented cultures, might be aberrant with respect to karyotype, gene expression, and regulation of their gene products (Nabholz *et al.*, 1980; Johnson, *et al.*, Chapter 15 in this treatise).

The conclusions drawn from the limiting dilution analysis, that single T cells are responsible for the production of several lymphokines, are supported by the analysis of T cell clones and lines maintained in long-term culture. As is the case for the induction of lymphokine release from T cells in short-term limiting dilution microcultures, TCGF-dependent T cell clones grown in long-term culture can be triggered by mitogen or antigen to release lymphokines. Table III

TABLE III

Lymphokine Release from Long-Term T Cell Lines and Clones

Long-term cultured cells	Growth dependent on		Lymphokines									
				CSF								
	Antigen	TCGF	IFN-γ	GM	Meg	Eo	E	MAF	HCSF	TCGF	TRF	BCDF
PC-AKR-Clone 29	−	+	+	+	+	−	−	+	−	−	−	−
PC-AKR-Clone 96	−	+	+	−	−	−	−	+	−	−	−	−
AKR-anti-B6 line 7.1.1a	+	+	−	+	+	+	+	NT[a]	+	−	−	+
AKR-anti-B6 line 7.1.2	+	+	−	+	+	+	+	NT	+	−	−	+

[a] NT, not tested.

shows two representative examples, PC-AKR-CL29 and PC-AKR-CL96. Both clones could be grown to large cell numbers in the presence of TCGF alone and produce IFN-γ, GM-CSF, Meg-CSF, MAF, and IFN-γ and MAF, respectively. In particular, PC-AKR-CL29 released quantities of IFN-γ and MAF which have never been observed using bulk culture conditions. In addition, by generating subclones of PC-AKR-CL29 by single cell isolation, we could demonstrate formally that the clonal progeny of one precursor cell is capable of releasing several lymphokines (IFN-γ, CSF, and MAF).

AKR-anti-B6 lines 7.1.1a and 7.1.2 are two representative examples of alloreactive T cell lines with antigen specificity. The growth of these lines is dependent on the presence of antigen and TCGF. These lines were tested for production of various lymphokines. Neither line produced IFN-γ, TCGF (as tested on a cytotoxic and a noncytotoxic, TCGF-dependent T cell clone), or TRF, but both released high quantities of CSF and the various CSF subtypes as well as HCSF and BCDF.

Assuming that one lymphokine does not have pleiotropic, concentration-dependent effects, we can deduce from the pattern of lymphokine release from these clones and lines, as well as from the activity pattern of IFN-γ, CSF , and MAF from PC-AKR-CL29 subclones (data not shown) that the lymphokines listed in Table I are not identical in molecular nature. This conclusion must remain open for HCSF and BCDF, since we do not have clones which discriminate between the two. Most importantly, however, BCDF is not identical to TRF. For practical purposes of biochemical isolation and gene cloning, it is important to note that the quantities of lymphokines released from these clones and lines sometimes exceed the quantities obtained from bulk cultures by several hundredfold. Furthermore, it is noteworthy that in the case of the alloreactive AKR-anti-B6 T cell lines, lymphokines can be released by incubation with the appropriate antigen, i.e., B6 stimulator cells.

These observations lead to the following questions: (a) which T cell is the lymphokine-producing T cell under physiological conditions? (b) What is the signal which triggers lymphokine release? (c) Is this signal identical for all lymphokines? In principal, an antigen-specific signal, either the antigen as such or anti-idiotypic reagents stimulating the antigen-specific receptor might be sufficient. Alternatively, a polyclonal signal stimulating a variety of T cells could be delivered either by other lymphocytes, or by macrophages in a manner similar to that postulated for TCGF release by *Lyt-1*$^+$ T cells.

Our data suggest that one producer cell can release several lymphokines. This is especially intriguing since such lymphokines seem to act on different target cells. Several possibilities for regulating this system might be envisaged. Lymphokine production could be regulated on the level of the producer cell, i.e., by altering the rate of lymphokine production or by stimulating or inhibiting the clonal expansion of the lymphokine-producing cells. Alternatively, the lymphokine activity could be regulated at the target cell level, i.e., by a competitive mechanism. These possibilities might not be mutually exclusive. The several lymphokines may belong to a family of structurally related molecules which have evolved from a common precursor, and the genes encoding some of the lymphokines may be arranged in tandem so that a common inductive signal may trigger the transcription of several genes simultaneously. While these issues remain to be explored, further insight into the complex biological mechanisms linking specific immunity to the release of nonspecific factors will be obtained by studying the physiological role of molecules which have been purified to homogeneity.

IV. CONCLUSIONS

In this chapter we describe a new method for determining the frequency and activity of lymphokine-producing splenic T cells from adult mice. Concanavalin A-activated T cells were grown for 7 to 12 days in limiting dilution microcultures in the presence of T cell growth factors (TCGF) and allogeneic peritoneal exudate filler cells. The cells were then washed and plated in microcultures in Con-A-containing medium in order to induce the release of lymphokines into the supernatant. The T cells produced immune interferon, colony stimulating factors, macrophage activating factors, and TCGF. The high frequency of producer T cells suggests that single T cells might release several lymphokines. This assumption was supported by the analysis of T cell clones and lines in long-term culture. For future biochemical characterization of the lymphokines it is important to notc that some of the clones and lines produce very high quantities of lymphokines. In addition, since single T cells are capable of simultaneously releasing several lymphokines which act on a variety of target cells, the entire system must be highly regulated *in vivo*.

REFERENCES

Campbell, J. B., Grunberger, T., Kochman, M. A., and White, S. L. (1975). Microplaque reduction assay for human and mouse interferon. *Can. J. Microbiol.* **3,** 1247.

Dy, M., Lebel, B., Kamoun, P., and Hamburger, J. (1981). Histamine production during the anti-allograft response. Demonstration of a new lymphokine enhancing histamine synthesis. *J. Exp. Med.* **153,** 293.

Eichmann, K., Falk, I., Melchers, I., and Simon, M. M. (1980). Quantitative studies on T cell diversity. I. Determination of the precursor frequencies for two types of streptococcus A-specific helper cells in non-immune, polyclonally activated splenic T cells. *J. Exp. Med.* **152,** 477.

Isakson, P., Puré, E., Vitetta, E. S., and Krammer, P. H. (1982). T cell-derived B cell differentiation factor(s) (BCDF): Effect on the isotope switch of murine B cells. *J. Exp. Med.* **155,** 734.

Krammer, P. H., and Michnay, A. (1981). Frequency of T cell growth factor producing murine spleen cells. *In* "Mechanisms of Lymphocyte Activation" (K. Resch and H. Kirchner, eds.) p. 357. Elsevier/North-Holland Biomedical Press, Amsterdam.

Krammer, P. H., Rehberger, R., and Eichmann, K. (1980). Antigen receptors on major histocompatibility complex-restricted T lymphocytes. I. Preparation and characterization of syngeneic antisera against trinitrophenyl-activated T cell blasts and demonstration of their specificity for idiotypes on cytotoxic T lymphocytes. *J. Exp. Med.* **151,** 1166.

Krammer, P. H., Marcucci, F., Waller, M., and Kirchner, H. (1982). Heterogeneity of soluble T cell products. I. Frequency and correlation analysis of cytotoxic and immune interferon (IFN-γ) producing spleen cells in the mouse. *Eur. J. Immunol.* (in press).

Lohmann-Matthes, M.-L., Domzig, W., and Taskov, H. (1979). Antibody-dependent cellular cytotoxicity against tumor cells. I. Cultivated bone marrow-derived macrophages kill tumor targets. *Eur. J. Immonol.* **9,** 261.

Marcucci, F., Waller, M., Kirchner, H., and Krammer, P. H. (1981). Production of immune interferon (IFN-γ) by murine T cell clones from long-term cultures. *Nature* (*London*) **291,** 79.

Nabholz, M., Conzelmann, A., Aurto, O., North, M., Haas, W., Polith, H., von Boehmer, H., Hengartner, H., Mach, J.-P., Engers, H., and Johnson, J. P. (1980). Established murine cytolytic T-cell lines as tools for a somatic cell genetic analysis of T-cell functions. *Transplant. Rev.* **51,** 125.

Schimpl, A., and Wecker, E. (1972). Replacement of T cell function by a T cell product. *Nature* (*London*) *New Biol.* **273,** 15.

Staber, F. G., and Johnson, G. R. (1980). The responses of hematopoietic precursor cells in mice to bacterial cell-wall components. *J. Cell. Physiol.* **105,** 143.

V

Murine T Cell Clones Reactive with Alloantigens

22

An Overview

Andrew L. Glasebrook/Frank W. Fitch

I. Conditions for Deriving T Cell Clones 266
A. Strategies for Cloning T Cells 266
B. Cloning Methods 268
II. Cytolytic T Cell Clones 269
III. Noncytolytic T Cell Clones 273
IV. Factors Produced by Alloreactive T Cell Clones 276
V. Conclusions 278
References 280

Cell-mediated immune responses are initiated by T cell subpopulations with diverse and highly specialized functions. These include T cells which exhibit specific and/or nonspecific cytolytic, helper, or suppressor functions. However, definitive analysis of cell-mediated immune responses has been hampered by the heterogeneity of cell populations. Although the development of monoclonal antibodies toward specific differentiation antigens has helped partially to distinguish T cell subsets, the enrichment of functional T cell populations using positive or negative selection methods still yield heterogeneous mixtures of cells. Delineation of the cellular and molecular events in cell-mediated immune responses has now become possible with the availability of cloned, monospecific, functional T cell lines.

This chapter will discuss primarily the derivation and analysis of functional murine T cell clones which are specific for viral or alloantigens. Cell populations for cloning have been obtained routinely after restimulation *in vitro* with antigen in mixed leukocyte culture (MLC) or mixed leukocyte–tumor cell culture (MLTC). Such systems are characterized by T cell proliferation which may result in the generation of CTL. Functional analysis of the T cell clones isolated has reflected the heterogeneity of responding T cells. These include T cell clones which are either cytolytic or noncytolytic and which are specific for major histocompatibility complex (MHC), non-MHC, or viral antigens. Some of these clones secrete biologically active lymphokines; others do not. The significance of

ISOLATION, CHARACTERIZATION, AND
UTILIZATION OF T LYMPHOCYTE CLONES

ISBN 0-12-249920-4

the ability to derive stable, functional T cell clones can not be overstated. It has now become possible to dissect the immune response and delineate the reactivities, specificity repertoire, and regulatory functions of T cells. The following sections summarize clonal analysis of various T cell functions. The findings demonstrate considerable heterogeneity and cross-reactivity in T cell responses.

I. CONDITIONS FOR DERIVING T CELL CLONES

A. Strategies for Cloning T Cells

The derivation of T cell clones has been approached in basically two different ways which may influence the heterogeneity of functional clones isolated. The first method involves cloning T cells from long-term cultures which have adapted to continuous growth in interleukin-2 (IL-2) containing medium (Nabholz *et al.*, 1978; Baker *et al.*, 1979; von Boehmer *et al.*, 1979; Watson, 1979; Schreier and Tees, 1980; Fresno *et al.*, 1981; Snodgrass *et al.*, 1981). Often, cell populations have been repeatedly stimulated *in vitro* followed by repetitive culture in medium supplemented with IL-2. Cells were then cloned and maintained in IL-2 in the absence of antigen and feeder cells. Although cells obtained after antigen stimulation could be cloned in IL-2 with a high plating efficiency (Haas *et al.*, 1980; Rosenberg *et al.*, 1980), the frequency of continuously growing T cell clones isolated was usually (von Boehmer *et al.*, 1979; Haas *et al.*, 1980; Nabholz *et al.*, 1980) though not always (Rosenberg *et al.*, 1980; Schawaller *et al.*, 1980), very low. The presence of irradiated syngeneic feeder cells during cloning did not appreciably increase the plating efficiency nor the frequency with which T cell clones could be established. However, propagation of cells in IL-2 for 4 to 10 weeks prior to cloning could increase the frequency almost 100% (Haas *et al.*, 1980). This suggests that the derivation of T cell clones which grow continuously in IL-2 in the absence of antigen and feeder cells is an adaptive event requiring the generation and/or selection of variants in long-term cultures (Watson, 1979; Nabholz *et al.*, 1980). The adaptation of T cells for continuous growth in IL-2 is most likely a rare event, since long-term cultures of cells maintained in only IL-2-containing medium tend to "clone themselves" (Haas *et al.*, 1980; Nabholz *et al.*, 1980). Derivation of functional T cell clones by this method then may not be representative of the T cell repertoire.

An alternative approach involves cloning T cells from short-term cultures in the presence of antigen, irradiated feeder cells, and IL-2-containing medium (Glasebrook and Fitch, 1979; Hengartner and Fathman, 1980; Sredni and Schwartz, 1980; Weiss *et al.*, 1980; MacDonald *et al.*, 1980a; Kimoto and Fathman, 1980; Braciale *et al.*, 1981; von Boehmer and Haas, 1981). In the majority of cases, cells obtained after primary or secondary stimulation *in vitro* have been cloned immediately in the presence of the original stimulating antigen, irradiated feeder cells, and IL-2-containing medium. Similar culture conditions have then been used to maintain the continuous growth of derived clones *in vitro*. Irradiated spleen cells have been used most often as feeder cells, although cells from other sources may be used but with a reduction in plating efficiency (Nabel *et al.*, 1981a). In cloning T cells which respond to soluble antigens, irradiated syngeneic spleen cells can function as antigen-presenting cells and feeder cells. In deriving T cell clones reactive to viral or alloantigens, irradiated spleen cells can provide both antigen and feeder cells. The cell which provides the "feeder effect" appears to be an adherent, non-T cell (Lutz *et al.*, 1981a). In contrast to the approach for deriving clones from long-term cultures, conditions for cloning T cells from short-term cultures are optimal when both antigen and feeder cells are present in addition to IL-2 (MacDonald *et al.*, 1980b). It would appear that "variant" clones are not necessarily selected by this approach (see below). The high frequency with which continuously growing T cell clones can be established after short-term culture (25 to 90%, A. L. Glasebrook, unpublished observations) would favor such an interpretation. As such, this approach may be more suited toward analysis of heterogeneity in cellular responses.

Cell populations have often been enriched for antigen-specific cells by stimulation with antigen one or more times *in vivo* and/or *in vitro* prior to cloning. However, it has been possible to establish functional T cell clones from naive or immature T cell populations (Rosenberg *et al.*, 1980; Nabel *et al.*, 1981a; Hapel *et al.*, 1981). Cells obtained from normal animals either have been cloned immediately (Rosenberg *et al.*, 1980; Nabel *et al.*, 1981a) or after varying periods of culture in media containing IL-2 (Nabel *et al.*, 1981a) or IL-3 (Hapel *et al.*, 1981). The use of feeder cells and/or preincubation of cells in IL-2-containing medium prior to cloning increased the plating efficiency (Nabel *et al.*, 1981a). However, the frequency of clones obtained was much lower compared to that observed for cells previously stimulated with antigen (Rosenberg *et al.*, 1980; Braciale *et al.*, 1981). It is unclear from these studies whether undifferentiated T cells can be cloned and maintained in continuous culture *in vitro*. Several studies would indicate that the expression of T cell receptors for IL-2 is dependent on antigenic or mitogenic stimulation (Robb *et al.*, 1981). Although partially purified IL-3 was used in one study (Hapel *et al.*, 1981), residual mitogen in conditioned medium may have stimulated the T cells which were eventually cloned (Rosenberg *et al.*, 1980; Nabel *et al.*, 1981a). Alternatively, medium components may have stimulated the expression of T cell receptors of growth-promoting factors.

It is unclear to what extent T cell clones isolated by the two approaches outlined above are different. Cloned T cells derived from long-term cultures most probably represent variants which have been selected on the basis of growth in IL-2. They appear "abnormal" in that growth is independent of feeder cells and antigen, and they often have chromosomal abnormalities (Engers *et al.*, 1980; Chapter 15 in this treatise). Fluctuations in function have also been observed

(Nabholz *et al.*, 1979; Rosenberg *et al.*, 1980; Engers *et al.*, 1980); these may be attributable to serum components (Schreier *et al.*, 1980) and to the rapid generation/selection of new variants. In contrast, T cell clones derived from short-term cultures in the presence of feeder cells, antigen, and IL-2, appear "normal"; they possess normal karyotype (Chapter 15 in this treatise), and the majority have been functionally stable for long periods in culture (Glasebrook and Fitch, 1980; Sredni *et al.*, 1980; Weiss *et al.*, 1980; Braciale *et al.*, 1981). While the rate at which new variants are generated and/or selected in cultures containing feeder cells and antigen would appear to be low, variants can arise (Ely *et al.*, 1981). Although cell proliferation is optimal in the presence of feeder cells, antigen, and IL-2, nearly all such clones can be grown continuously in IL-2 alone after an indeterminate period of culture (A. L. Glasebrook, unpublished observations). However, chromosomal alterations may develop as soon as 1 week after cells are cultured only in IL-2-containing medium from different sources (R.-P. Sekaly, personal communication). The use of crude preparations of IL-2-containing medium may contribute to the "crisis" (lengthening of doubling time and refractoriness to IL-2 stimulation) often observed for T cell clones maintained in IL-2 alone (Smith and Ruscetti, 1981). Although it is unclear what function feeder cells and antigen fulfill, physical and biological properties of T cell clones are maintained best when feeder cells and antigen are present in addition to conditioned medium. Frequent subcloning may be necessary, however, to ensure homogeneity of particular T cell clones.

B. Cloning Methods

The majority of strategies employed for cloning T cells have involved the use of conditioned medium containing IL-2. Culture fluids obtained from mitogen- or alloantigen-stimulated spleen cells (Morgan *et al.*, 1976; Gillis and Smith, 1977), MLC cells (Ryser *et al.*, 1978), tumor cells (Gillis *et al.*, 1980; Shimizu *et al.*, 1980; Farrar *et al.*, 1980), and T cell hybridomas (Harwell *et al.*, 1980; Stull and Gills, 1981) have been found to be convenient sources of conditioned medium. All contain IL-2 and all would appear to be equally effective at promoting the *in vitro* growth of T cells when used at optimal concentrations.

Although cell populations may "clone themselves" when maintained in long-term culture only with IL-2, it is necessary to use one of several cloning methods in order to be certain that cells obtained from short-term and long-term cultures in fact represent clones. Three methods have been used for cloning T cells. The majority of clones reported have been derived by techniques of limiting dilution (Chapters 18–21). In this approach, cells are cloned in liquid culture by aliquoting a known limiting number of cells per microwell. Depending on the culture conditions, proliferating cells become visible after 6 to 14 days. The probability that cells within individual microwells represent clones can be estimated using Poisson statistics. The advantages of limiting dilution are that it is rapid and allows for the derivation and functional screening of a large number of clones prior to expansion.

Another approach to deriving T cell clones in liquid culture is micromanipulation (Zagury *et al.*, 1975). Individual cells are picked either mechanically or by hand using a capillary and repeatedly expelled or pipetted to ensure there is only a single cell present before transfer to a microwell. The advantage of this method is that it provides reasonable certainty that "clones" arising are true clones, making it particularly useful for subcloning. However, the procedure is time consuming. The use of the fluorescence activated cell sorter (FACS) to clone *Thy-1*$^+$ T cells achieves similar results (A. Nordin, personal communication) and may be the method of choice when large numbers of short-term clones are desired.

The third method for cloning T cells involves the use of semisolid agar (Nabholz *et al.*, 1978; von Boehmer *et al.*, 1979; Rosenberg *et al.*, 1980; Hengartner and Fathman, 1980; Sredni and Schwartz, 1981). T cells are suspended in 0.2–0.5% soft agar and seeded over an agar layer which may contain feeder cells. When colonies develop, they are extracted with a fine capillary and transferred to liquid culture. T cells can be cloned in semisolid agar in the presence (von Boehmer *et al.*, 1979; Rosenberg *et al.*, 1980; Braciale *et al.*, 1981) or absence (Fathman and Hengartner, 1978; Sredni *et al.*, 1980) of IL-2. If IL-2 is not included, antigen and feeder cells must be provided, and colonies have been found to contain a mixture of cells (Hengartner and Fathman, 1980; Sredni and Schwartz, 1980; Braciale *et al.*, 1981). A disadvantage of agar cloning is that it is difficult to assess the clonality of colonies which grow initially in agar. A serious consideration is the possible recruitment of nearby cells into the colony, since large numbers of cells must be seeded, and T cells can migrate within the agar.

Cloning T cells in liquid culture by limiting dilution or micromanipulation with a high plating efficiency is dependent on the presence of IL-2 (MacDonald *et al.*, 1980b). The plating efficiency is often greater than 25% and may approach 100% (Baker *et al.*, 1979; Rosenberg *et al.*, 1980; Glasebrook and Fitch, 1980; Haas *et al.*, 1980). However, a maximum plating efficiency of 1% has been observed in agar (Hengartner and Fathman, 1980; Sredni *et al.*, 1980; Rosenberg *et al.*, 1980) which may approach 100% during subcloning (Sredni and Schwartz, 1980). The low plating efficiency for T cells in agar may indicate that growth in agar is selective for subpopulations of T cells or colony forming units (Sredni and Schwartz, 1981).

II. CYTOLYTIC T CELL CLONES

The generation of cytolytic activity in MLC is greatest 4 to 6 days after initiation of culture, after which time the level of cytolytic activity per cell declines. In contrast to MLC cell populations, CTL clones express a constant level of cytolytic activity per cell. Upon subculture of cloned CTL, lytic activity per culture reaches a peak and then declines with continued culture, but lytic activity per cell remains constant (Glasebrook *et al.*, 1981a). The magnitude of cytolytic activity expressed per culture is, therefore, directly proportional to the extent of cell proliferation. As would be expected from these results, there is no association between lytic activity of cloned cells and the stage of the cell cycle. Cloned CTL collected in exponential growth and separated by FACS into populations of cells in G_1, S, or G_2 phases of the cell cycle were equally lytic (Sekaly *et al.*, 1981). Depending on the initial cell input, cloned cells may go through four to seven doublings before reaching a saturation density, typically about 10^6 cells/ml.

Populations of CTL generated by antigenic stimulation are specific in that they predominantly lyse target cells bearing the original stimulating antigens. Often, however, low levels of lytic activity for target cells which do not bear stimulating antigens can be detected. This has been observed for both alloreactive CTL (Peck *et al.*, 1976; Fischer-Lindahl and Wilson, 1977) and CTL specific for viral or hapten determinants (Bevan, 1977; Finberg *et al.*, 1978), in which case antigen recognition is restricted by the MHC of the antigen-presenting cells. The ability of CTL populations to express a range of reactivities suggests that individual CTL receptors may recognize determinants shared (cross-reactive) with those of the stimulator antigens. In this regard, cloned T cells have provided much information detailing the reactivity of receptor(s) on individual T cells.

We have observed previously that CTL clones derived from allogeneic MLC are quite heterogeneous in their expression of cytolytic activity (Glasebrook and Fitch, 1980). While the majority of CTL clones isolated from secondary MLC lysed target cells bearing the original stimulating alloantigens, more complex patterns of reactivity were observed as the panel of target cells was expanded. At least seven different patterns of lysis were observed for nine CTL clones tested against eleven different target cells. Some clones were specific for the H-2K or H-2D alloantigens of the original stimulating cells, while other clones exhibited cross-reactive or heteroclitic lysis of target cells. Schawaller *et al.* (1980) observed that CTL clones derived from tertiary MLC were either specific for the immunizing antigen or cross-reactive with syngeneic or unrelated allogeneic target cells. Taswell *et al.* (1980) have analyzed the cross-reactivity of alloreactive CTL using a quantitative approach involving the generation of a large number of short-term clones from primary MLC. They observed that for 211 CTL clones isolated, 81% could be characterized as specific, 9% as heteroclitic, and 9% as cross-reactive. Unfortunately, only two target cells were used to evaluate cytolytic activity, so these data must be considered to provide an underestimation of cross-reactive T cell clones. Collectively, however, these data indicate that alloantigen-stimulated CTL may be reactive for unique or shared haplotype determinants. A more definitive quantification of cross-reactive antigenic recognition by CTL requires an expanded panel of target cells to test large numbers of clones derived by limiting dilution or micromanipulation. An alternative approach is to study the blocking of target cell antigens by monoclonal antibodies directed toward MHC determinants (Weiss *et al.*, 1981).

Lysis of allogeneic target cells can be observed with self-MHC-restricted CTL, suggesting that there are overlapping populations of MHC-restricted and alloreactive CTL. Results obtained at the clonal level indicate that individual MHC-restricted CTL may show a specific pattern of cross-reactivity with allogeneic target cells. Gillis and Smith (1977) observed that MLTC prepared with allogeneic Friend leukemia virus (FLV)-induced cells lysed both syngeneic and allogeneic FLV-induced tumor cells. Analysis of 20 CTL clones derived from a long-term CTL line revealed at least three patterns of cytolytic reactivity (Baker *et al.*, 1979). Similar findings by Weiss *et al.* (1980) also confirmed the heterogeneity of T cell reactivities in MHC-restricted immune responses (Chapter 24 in this treatise). Some clones lysed only syngeneic Moloney murine leukemia virus (MoLV)-infected target cells. Other clones were capable of lysing both syngeneic and allogeneic MoLV-infected target cells. The majority of clones within this latter group, however, were also capable of lysing uninfected allogeneic target cells.

MHC-restricted CTL clones specific for type A influenza virus have been established by Braciale and co-workers (1981; Chapter 23 in this treatise). The CTL clones isolated were of F_1 origin stimulated by infected parental cells. In this study, only one of thirteen F_1 CTL clones analyzed caused significant lysis of uninfected or infected allogeneic target cells. The cytotoxicity of all clones was restricted by one or the other but not both parental haplotypes, although lysis of both infected parental target cells was readily observed with primary cultures of cells. The inability of the clones to lyse allogeneic cells may be explained by their F_1 origin (Haas *et al.*, 1980). Alternatively, differences in the stimulation (virus preparations versus infected cells) and/or time after which cells are cloned may influence the percentage of cross-reactive CTL clones observed.

Another example of dual specificity by cloned CTL is the response toward male-specific antigen. Von Boehmer *et al.* (1979) have shown that cloned CTL from female C57BL/6 mice which were reactive with C57BL/6 male target cells also lysed both male and female target cells expressing H-2D^d alloantigens. For all clones analyzed, CTL recognition of non-MHC antigens appears to be restricted by the *H-2K* or *H-2D* locus of the antigen-presenting cells. This has been observed for CTL clones reactive toward MoLV antigens, type A influenza virus, and haptens. Collectively, the results obtained with MHC-restricted cloned CTL would indicate that the restriction is often not as stringent as observed with bulk populations. Cloned CTL frequently show unexpectedly strong reactivity for apparently unrelated antigens with which the bulk populations react poorly.

Caution, however, must be exercised in interpreting the "apparent" cross-reactivities of CTL clones, especially when using tumor target cells. CTL clones may demonstrate quantitative fluctuations in cytolytic activity toward mitogen-induced blast or tumor target cells not bearing the original stimulating antigens when assayed over a period of several weeks (von Boehmer and Haas, 1981). It cannot be excluded that variation in the cytolytic activity of clones is a result of alteration in nonspecific surface properties rather than changes in affinity or density of antigen-specific receptors. Also, it cannot be assumed that tumor cells, or even mitogen-induced blasts, express all the "proper" antigens of their respective haplotype. In this regard, some tumor cells have been found to express allogeneic MHC determinants inconsistent with their haplotype of origin (Garrido *et al.*, 1976), even when detected using monoclonal antibodies (H. R. MacDonald, personal communication). Also, an IL-2-secreting subline of EL-4 (Farrar *et al.*, 1980) was found to express cell surface antigens not found on other "EL-4" tumor lines (H. R. MacDonald, personal communication). We can conclude from these observations that tumor cells may express additional or aberrant forms of MHC antigens, and this altered antigenic expression may vary with tumor cell lines maintained in different labs.

The reactivity patterns of isolated CTL clones suggests considerable heterogeneity in T cell immune responses. Most studies, however, were not initiated with the purpose of defining the T cell repertoire, and the relatively small number of clones provide only suggestive evidence that the CTL repertoire is large. The most detailed analysis of CTL repertoire has been carried out by Sherman (1980; Chapter 25 in this treatise). The response of B10.D2 T cells to H-2K^b antigens was studied since inbred strains of H-2K^b mutant mice were available which expressed different antigenic determinants resulting from point mutations. Short-term CTL clones were assayed for lytic activity against mitogen-induced normal or seven different mutant *H-2K^b* blast cells. A total of 128 reactivity patterns were possible. Forty-three CTL clones from seven different donor mice expressed 23 different reactivity patterns, indicating that at least 23 different determinants are present on the H-2K^b molecule. All CTL clones were lytic for normal H-2K^b target cells.

Braciale *et al.* (1981; Chapter 23 in this treatise) have analyzed the fine specificity of CTL clones specific for type A influenza viruses using a panel of target cells infected with serologically related or distinct type A viruses. Three major types of recognition patterns were apparent for twelve CTL clones. Some clones reacted exclusively to the immunizing virus strain. Other clones were subtype specific, being directed toward determinants shared by viruses of the same subtype as the immunizing virus. A third group of clones exhibited cross-reactive recognition of determinants shared by all subtypes of type A influenza viruses. Further analysis of the T cell repertoire will be dependent on the availability of serologically distinct forms of the stimulating antigen.

Definitive analysis of the T cell receptor has remained elusive. Use of T cell clones may prove useful in such studies. In particular, analysis of CTL clones using techniques of somatic cell genetics appears promising (Chapters 14–17 in this treatise). Dialynas *et al.* (1981) have derived variant clones from a highly cytolytic, anti-H-2D^d CTL clone by selection with antibody and complement after treatment of the cells with the mutagen ethyl methanesulfonate. A variant clone lacking the cell surface marker Thy 1.2 expressed the same level and specificity of cytolytic activity as that of the parent clone. Variant clones lacking Lyt-2, however, expressed markedly reduced levels of specific cytolytic activity. In the presence of lectin the level of cytolytic activity increased and, for one variant clone, was indistinguishable from that of the parent clone. These results suggest that Lyt-2 is not required for cytolytic activity but appears to enhance the establishment of specific effector cell–target cell interactions. Lyt-2 may function to stabilize low affinity receptors since not all CTL clones are inhibitable by anti-Lyt-2. The expression of cytolytic activity by *in vivo* primed CTL populations is much more difficult to inhibit with anti-Lyt-2 (MacDonald *et al.*, 1981), and CTL clones obtained by priming *in vivo* are not inhibitable even by microgram quantities of anti-Lyt-2 (H. R. MacDonald, personal communication).

All of the CTL clones reported in the literature are strictly dependent on the presence of IL-2 for continued growth *in vitro*. It has become apparent, however, that a few CTL clones can proliferate upon antigen stimulation independently of exogenously added IL-2. Such CTL clones were first observed by Widmer and Bach (1981) and by Glasebrook *et al.* (1982a). Such "bifunctional" CTL clones were derived after short-term culture and cloning in the presence of filler cells, antigen, and IL-2. Such a strategy is probably crucial to the derivation of these clones as their frequency in primary MLC is approximately 1/6 (Glasebrook *et al.*, 1982a). CTL clones isolated from C57BL/6 anti-H-2^d MLC proliferate when stimulated with *H-2^d* cells, specifically lyse H-2^d target cells, and also produce IL-2, immune interferon, and macrophage activating factor (Glasebrook *et al.*, 1982b; Widmer and Bach, 1981; Chapter 28 in this treatise). Such clones were *Lyt-1*$^+$*2*$^+$ or *Lyt-1*$^-$*2*$^+$, and all functions could be inhibited by monoclonal anti-Lyt-2 antibody (Glasebrook *et al.*, 1982b). Although the frequency of such cells in fully allogeneic MLC combinations is low, it is tempting to speculate that in MLC combinations involving only H-2K and H-2D differences the frequency may be much higher. This would explain the observations that IL-2 production in response to H-2K stimulation is dependent on *Lyt-2*$^+$ cells (Okada and Henney, 1980).

III. NONCYTOLYTIC T CELL CLONES

The other major type of cloned T cell is noncytolytic and proliferates when stimulated by specific antigen in the absence of IL-2. These clones do not express Lyt-2 and may or may not express Lyt-1 (Glasebrook and Fitch, 1980). In certain strain combinations, proliferating alloreactive T cell clones may express nonspecific cytolytic activity when assayed in the presence of lectin (A. L. Glasebrook, unpublished observations). Although such clones do not express specific cytolytic activity, this may be due to the failure to provide appropriate target cells.

Noncytolytic clones can be maintained by repetitive stimulation with antigen/feeder cells, although the addition of conditioned medium containing IL-2 often results in optimal cell proliferation (Glasebrook and Fitch, 1979; Hengartner and Fathman, 1980). Clones maintained in conditioned medium alone retain their original antigenic specificity (Schreier *et al.*, 1980). Cells removed from IL-2-containing culture then proliferate in the absence of IL-2 when stimulated with the appropriate antigens, but this may require culturing the cloned cells at a relatively high cell density. Recent reports suggest that a lymphokine which has been called IL-3 and which is found in conditioned medium may be responsible for the continued growth of these clones *in vitro* (Hapel *et al.*, 1981). All T cells maintained or cloned in IL-3 were found to be *Lyt-2*$^-$. IL-3 does not support the continuous growth of *Lyt-2*$^+$ CTL clones *in vitro*. Naive T cells cloned in the presence of IL-3 may proliferate in culture medium alone. All clones analyzed secreted detectable quantities of IL-3 but not IL-2. Stimulation of cells with phorbol myristate acetate, however, induced IL-2 secretion. While proliferating T cell clones have been widely used for analysis of immune responses, it is clear that analysis of the requirements for continued growth of these cells *in vitro* has lagged behind.

Proliferating alloreactive T cell clones have been useful in studying the nature of antigens which stimulate in MLC. While stimulation with MHC antigens causes T cell proliferation, certain non-MHC antigens may also induce T cells to proliferate. In particular, strong *Mls* locus determinants in MHC-compatible strain combinations stimulate high levels of T cell proliferation *in vitro* (Festenstein, 1973). The precursor frequency of T cells reactive to *Mls* locus determinants appears to be equivalent to or higher than that for MHC antigens (Janeway *et al.*, 1980; Lutz *et al.*, 1981b). It is controversial as to whether recognition of *Mls* locus determinants is MHC-restricted due to the inherent restraints in using MHC-compatible strain combinations, the source of responding T cells, and the poorly defined nature of the *Mls* locus antigens themselves. It would appear, however, that responses to *Mls* locus antigens in primary MLC are MHC-restricted (Peck *et al.*, 1977; Janeway *et al.*, 1980), while responses to strong *Mls* locus antigens in secondary MLC are not (Molnar-Kimber and Sprent, 1980; Janeway *et al.*, 1980).

We were surprised to observe that of three noncytolytic proliferating T cell clones independently derived from secondary C57BL/6 anti-DBA/2 MLC, all were reactive toward non-MHC antigens. DBA/2 spleen cells express the strongly stimulating Mls^a alloantigen. We concluded that the reactivity of the clones was most likely for Mls^a based on (1) the specificity of proliferation observed using a panel of stimulating cells, (2) the ability of DBA/2 B cells but not DBA/2 T cells plus syngeneic adherent cells to stimulate clone cell proliferation, and (3) the lack of reactivity towards F_1 progeny from a cross of DBA/2 with CBA/N, which possess an X-linked immune B cell defect involving nonexpression of Mls determinants (Glasebrook *et al.*, 1981a). Recognition of Mls^a by these clones (comparable to that observed with cells from secondary MLC) was not MHC-restricted, since Mls^a presented in association with $H\text{-}2^k$ or $H\text{-}2^d$ were equally effective in stimulating clone cell proliferation. It cannot be excluded, however, that these clones were restricted by a determinant shared between $H\text{-}2^{d,k}$ or among all *H-2* haplotypes. It is interesting that all *Mls* locus reactive T cell clones produced IL-2, and some defined strongly stimulating determinants on strains expressing supposedly weakly stimulating determinants (Glasebrook and Fitch, 1980).

Sprent and co-workers (Molnar-Kimber *et al.*, 1980) have observed that long-term T cell lines exhibit dual specificity for MHC and strong *Mls* locus determinants. BALB/c lymph node cells were repeatedly stimulated *in vitro* with MHC-compatible but Mls-different DBA/2 spleen cells. After the fifth stimulation, high proliferative responses were obtained against stimulator cells bearing the original priming Mls alloantigens which were not MHC restricted. However, significant proliferative responses were also observed against Mls-compatible cells expressing foreign MHC determinants. Repeated stimulation of the T cell line with Mls-compatible but MHC-different cells did not reduce responses to the original priming Mls determinants. The cell lines could be stimulated either by Mls determinants or by MHC determinants alone. Clones derived from such T cell lines retained the ability to recognize *Mls* locus and MHC determinants (Chapter 27 in this treatise). However, a significant proportion of clones recognized only *Mls* locus antigens, which may explain why we failed to derive MHC, *Mls* locus reactive T cell clones. Similar results have been reported by Braciale *et al.* (Chapter 23 in this treatise) for an influenza virus-specific cytolytic T cell clone. Optimal growth of the clone was observed only when cells were cultured with specific antigen (infected spleen cells) and IL-2, conditions which we had previously found to be optimal for CTL clones (Glasebrook and Fitch, 1979). Cells proliferated poorly when cultured with uninfected spleen cells and IL-2. However, optimal proliferation was obtained when clone cells were cultured with IL-2 and uninfected spleen cells expressing strongly stimulating *Mls* locus determinants.

T cells may possess receptors for *Mls* locus determinants which are different from those which recognize MHC antigens. Alternatively, *Mls* locus determinants may be cross-reactive with particular MHC determinants. Also, it should be stressed that ascribing T cell reactivities in MHC-compatible strain combinations to *Mls* locus differences may not always be justified. The strain distribution of *Mls* locus determinants has been defined operationally by the ability to stimulate T cell responses in MHC-compatible strain combinations, but other minor histocompatibility differences also are included. Coutinho *et al.* (1981) originally attributed the primary MLR between C3H/HeJ and C3H/Tif to *Mls* locus differences. Analysis of progeny of backcrosses between F_1 hybrids and C3H/HeJ indicated that the MLR stimulating determinants segregated from antigens (LyM-1) which are closely linked to the *Mls* locus (Coutinho *et al.,* 1981). Although proliferative T cell responses in MHC-compatible strain combinations may be directed toward background antigens not associated with the *Mls* locus, such responses still represent stimulation by *non*-MHC antigens. As such, they are useful for comparing T cell recognition and function of different alloantigens.

Cloned T cells reactive with "conventional" soluble antigens also may have dual reactivity for antigen and MHC determinants. A cloned T cell which proliferated when cultured with DNP-ovalbumin and cells bearing I-A^k antigens also proliferated when stimulated with cells bearing I-A^s alone (Sredni and Schwartz, 1980; Chapter 31 in this treatise). Other haplotypes tested were nonstimulatory.

Although (A × B) F_1 cells stimulated the proliferation of either A or B parental T cells, results obtained with parental lymph node cells suggested the existence of unique F_1 hybrid MLC-stimulating determinants (Fathman and Nabholz, 1977). Definitive proof for the existence of unique hybrid stimulating determinants was provided by clones of noncytolytic proliferating T cells which were stimulated to proliferate only with F_1 alloantigens (Fathman and Hengartner, 1978). Clones were derived from cultures of responder A strain lymph node cells stimulated repeatedly with C57BL/6 or (C57BL/ × A) F_1 hybrid spleen cells. Analysis of proliferative specificity using congenic or recombinant congenic F_1 stimulating cells indicated that the unique F_1 hybrid stimulating determinants were encoded within the *I-A* region of the MHC (Kimoto and Fathman, 1980; Chapter 30 in this treatise). This would indicate that free combinatorial association of the parental *I-A* α and β chains in the F_1 hybrid would generate new antigenic determinants. For clones reactive to unique F_1 hybrid antigens, the stimulating determinant seemed to be derived from trans complementation between the $I\text{-}A^k$ and $I\text{-}A^b$ region gene products. For clones reactive with both parental and F_1 cells, the stimulating determinant resulted from a cis complementation of $I\text{-}A^b$ region gene products. These results demonstrate that F_1 hybrid *I* region antigens may be recognized by T cells as alloantigens. Other studies utilizing T cell clones have indicated that recognition of soluble antigens can be restricted by different combinatorial associations of *I-A* and *I-E* region gene products (Kimoto and Fathman, 1981; Chapter 30 in this treatise).

IV. FACTORS PRODUCED BY ALLOREACTIVE T CELL CLONES

Appropriate stimulation of some cloned T cells may induce the secretion of soluble "factors" which mediate a variety of activities. Supernatant fluids obtained from allogeneic secondary MLC contain practically every factor for which an assay exists (MacDonald *et al.*, 1980a). More restricted genetic combinations may result in fewer activities detected in MLC supernatant fluids, suggesting that stimulation with certain antigens may induce secretion of particular factor activities and not others. Results from the work of Cantor and Boyse (1975) and Bach *et al.* (1976) indicated that the proliferation and differentiation of *Lyt-2,3*$^+$ CTL precursor cells in MLC was enhanced or induced by a population of "amplifier" T cells. These were characterized as *Lyt-1*$^+$, *2, 3*$^-$ cells which appear to be stimulated by specific alloantigens, perhaps encoded by the *I* region.

The emergence of technology for cloning functional T cells has enabled analysis of these cellular interactions using a reductionist approach. The minimal requirements for reconstituting an immune response can now be determined using T cell clones. It was found early that a synergistic expression of specific cytolytic activity was observed when noncytolytic proliferating T cell clones reactive toward non-MHC (Mls) antigens were cultured together with CTL clones and stimulating alloantigen in the absence of IL-2 (Glasebrook and Fitch, 1979). Similar results were observed when the interacting T cell clones were separated by a Millipore membrane, indicating that the interactions were mediated by soluble factors (Glasebrook and Fitch, 1980). Similar results were also obtained with cell populations (Wagner *et al.*, 1980). Further analysis indicated that the factors were neither antigen specific nor MHC restricted, although antigenic-specific stimulation of the proliferating T cell clones was required (Schreier and Tees, 1980; Schreier *et al.*, 1980; Glasebrook and Fitch, 1980; Glasebrook *et al.*, 1981c). An exception are the T cell clones described by Nabel *et al.* (1981b) which are antigen nonresponsive and produce several biologically active factors constitutively. A wide range of factor activities could be detected in supernatant fluids collected from cultures of a proliferating T cell clone (L2) stimulated with non-MHC alloantigens (Ely *et al.*, 1981). These included IL-2, factors promoting polyclonal stimulation of B cells, colony stimulating factor (CSF), interferon (IFN-γ), induction of Ia antigen expression by macrophages *in vitro*, and stimulation of production of complement components by guinea pig macrophages.

Since T cell clones had been stimulated with T cell-depleted alloantigens, the possibility remained that some of the factor activities could be of macrophage origin. This possibility was excluded by demonstrating that T cell clones, even after having been maintained in IL-2 for 4 weeks to deplete residual stimulator cells, secreted the same range of factor activities on stimulation with the mitogen concanavalin A alone (Ely *et al.*, 1981; Marcucci *et al.*, 1981; Glasebrook *et al.*, 1982c; Chapters 21 and 28 in this treatise). Similar results have been reported for T cell clones reactive to male-specific antigens (O. Kanagawa, personal communication) and T cell clones derived in the presence of IL-3 (Hapel *et al.*, 1981). Mitogenic stimulation of IL-2 production by lymphomas (Gillis *et al.*, 1980; Farrar *et al.*, 1980; Shimizu *et al.*, 1980) and T cell hybridomas

(Harwell *et al.*, 1980) also has been reported. These observations should lead to a definitive analysis of T cell-derived soluble products.

While one clone (L2) appears to secrete every factor imaginable, this is clearly not the case for all T cell clones. When four factor activities were measured, various clones could produce none, some, or all of the factors (Glasebrook *et al.*, 1982c). IL-2-dependent CTL clones as well as noncytolytic proliferating T cell clones also can secrete numerous biologically active factors. When grouped according to function, phenotype, and factors secreted, at least 11 different patterns could be observed for T cell clones isolated from MLC (Glasebrook *et al.*, 1981b). Dissociations of factor activities have been observed in T cell clones, suggesting that several different molecules account for these activities. IL-2 activity has been separable from macrophage activation factor MAF, CSF, IFN-γ, and factors which induce antigen-specific B cell responses (BCGF). This has been determined by differences in the time course of production (Ely *et al.*, 1981; Schrier *et al.*, 1980), heterogeneous T cell clones (Glasebrook *et al.*, 1982c; Marcucci *et al.*, 1981), variant T cell clones (Ely *et al.*, 1981), and physical and chemical separation of the molecules (Nabel *et al.*, 1981b; Hubner *et al.*, 1981; Watson and Mochizuki, 1980). Analysis of culture supernatants from cloned T cells has also indicated dissociation between CSF and MAF/IFN-γ (A. Kelso, personal communication). Numerous different alloantigens would appear capable of inducing secretion of multiple factor activities. However, the numbers of established T cell clones analyzed so far for factor production have been few, and results obtained may not indicate the full range of functional heterogeneity. In most instances, analysis for production has been incidental since T cell clones have been derived for other purposes.

V. CONCLUSIONS

The ability to maintain continuously growing clones of functional T cells *in vitro* has prompted a reexamination of immune responses at the clonal level. This has included analysis of the responding cells involved, the soluble factors which are produced, and the stimulating antigens which are recognized. While T cell clones have provided much information relating observations for cell populations to individual cells, T cell clones may not be useful in all instances. For example, cloned CTL appear not to revert to "memory" cells but express full cytolytic activity regardless of cell or culture cycle. This complicates analysis of the molecular events required for induction of CTL. T cell clones in which expression of specific cytolytic activity can be modulated would be useful for such purposes. In contrast, proliferation and/or lymphokine production by noncytolytic T cell clones is not constitutive but is modulated by antigenic stimulation. These cells provide a simple model system for study of T cell recognition and lymphokine release. Culture conditions influence the ease with which T cell clones can be obtained as well as the properties of the resulting clones. A better understanding of the effects of culture conditions would facilitate isolation of T cell clones having particular functions.

Although many cytolytic and noncytolytic T cell clones appear to be specific for the immunizing antigens, there may be cross-reactive lysis or recognition of unrelated antigens. MHC-restricted T cells often can be shown to cross-react with alloantigens if the panel of stimulating or target cells is sufficiently large. While MHC-restricted T cells reactive with alloantigens occur with some frequency, it has been difficult to show that alloreactive cells also react with conventional antigens. Alloreactive T cells do, however, cross-react with antigens not involved in the original stimulation. The exact nature of the determinants involved in cross-reactions is unclear. Monoclonal antibodies reactive with MHC antigens should allow a more precise characterization of the cross-reacting antigens and provide a better understanding of T cell specificity.

The observations that alloreactive or MHC-restricted T cells can also recognize non-MHC (*Mls* locus) antigens (this chapter and Chapters 23 and 27 in this treatise) have been interpreted as providing evidence for either cross-reactivity between or independent recognition of *Mls* locus and MHC and/or viral antigens. However, it is unclear what such T cells actually recognize. *Mls* locus antigens remain poorly defined due to the lack of congenic strains and specific antisera. There is an alternative explanation for the above results: *Mls* locus antigens may be composed of several different determinants which together constitute the strongly stimulating $Mls^{a,d}$ loci. Weakly or nonstimulating strains ($Mls^{b,c}$) may express only one or two determinants which, by themselves, would not be strongly stimulatory in bulk cell cultures but which could be recognized by individual Mls reactive T cell clones. Thus, reactivity of a T cell clone with cells from two strains differing at *H-2*, one expressing "strongly" stimulating Mls antigens and the other expressing "weakly" stimulating Mls antigens, may not be the result of dual recognition of MHC and Mls but rather recognition by individual T cells of a specific "minor" Mls determinant shared between the two strains. We have suggested previously such an explanation based on the analysis of Mls reactive T cell clones (Glasebrook and Fitch, 1980). Experiments testing the effect on the Mls response of antibodies which block the allogeneic or MHC-restricted response should be particularly informative. It may be possible to map the strain distribution of *Mls* locus antigens using Mls reactive T cell clones and thus provide an unambiguous description of their expression.

The studies discussed above have been performed with T cell clones *in vitro*. However, the biological functions of cloned T cells *in vivo* is of both theoretical and practical interest. Cloned helper T cells can function effectively *in vivo* (Schreier and Tees, 1980; Tees and Schreier, 1980; Schreier *et al.*, 1980), but the results obtained with cloned CTL generally have been disappointing (Engers *et al.*, 1981; Gillis and Watson, 1981; Giorgi and Warner, 1980). Although protection has been observed when cloned CTL were mixed with tumor cells and injected together, protection was not found if cloned CTL were injected intravenously and the tumor was given intraperitoneally (Engers *et al.*, 1981). This may relate to the dependence of CTL on IL-2. Intravenously injected CTL may die quickly due to a lack of IL-2. Gillis and Watson (1981) reported that administration of IL-2 together with cloned T cells resulted in an enhanced protective effect. In addition, the recirculation pattern of cloned CTL may be abnormal, since the majority of intravenously injected CTL were trapped in the lungs and liver. Perhaps trapping of cloned cells in the lung accounted for the observation that influenza-specific cloned CTL could protect mice after intranasal challenge with virus (Lin and Askonas, 1980).

In any case, it should be possible to determine the role of CTL and other cell types in allograft rejection and in tumor immunity *in vivo* using T cell cloning techniques. T cell clones have been derived from cells infiltrating tumors (Brunner *et al.*, 1981). Such approaches together with development of methods for retaining function of cloned cells *in vivo* should enable practical application of T cell clones.

REFERENCES

Bach, F. H., Bach, M. L., and Sondel, P. M. (1976). Differential function of major histocompatibility complex antigens in T-lymphocyte activation. *Nature (London)* **259,** 273.

Baker, P. E., Gillis, S., and Smith, K. A. (1979). Monoclonal cytolytic T-cell lines. *J. Exp. Med.* **149,** 273.

Bevan, M. J. (1977). Killer cells reactive to altered self antigens can also be alloreactive. *Proc. Natl. Acad. Sci. U.S.A.* **74,** 2094.

Bianchi, A. J. J., Hooijkaas, H., Benner, R., Tees, R., Nordin, A. A., and Schreier, M. H. (1981). Clones of helper T cells mediate antigen-specific, H-2-restricted DTH. *Nature (London)* **290,** 62.

Braciale, T. J., Andrew, M. E., and Braciale, V. L. (1981). Heterogeneity and specificity of cloned lines of influenza-virus-specific cytotoxic T lymphocytes. *J. Exp. Med.* **153,** 910.

Brunner, K. T., MacDonald, H. R., and Cerottini, J.-C. (1981). Quantitation and clonal isolation of cytolytic T lymphocyte precursors selectively infiltrating murine sarcoma virus-induced tumors. *J. Exp. Med.* **154,** 362.

Cantor, H., and Boyse, E. A. (1975). Functional subclasses of T lymphocytes bearing different Ly antigens. II. Cooperation between subclasses of ly^+ cells in the generation of killer activity. *J. Exp. Med.* **141,** 1390.

Coutinho, A., Augustin, A. A., Forni, L., and Fischer-Lindahl, K. (1981). Genetics of a non-H-2 antigen that stimulates "unrestricted" helper T cells and MLR. *J. Immunol.* **127,** 21.

Dialynas, D. P., Loken, M. R., Glasebrook, A. L., and Fitch, F. W. (1981). Lyt-2^-/Lyt-3^- variants of a cloned cytolytic T cell line lack an antigen receptor functional in cytolysis. *J. Exp. Med.* **153,** 595.

Ely, J. M., Prystowsky, M. B., Eisenberg, L., Quintans, J., Goldwasser, E., and Fitch, F. W. (1981). Alloreactive cloned T cell lines. V. Differential kinetics of IL-2, CSF, and BCSF release by a cloned T amplifier cell and its variant. *J. Immunol.* **127,** 2345.

Engers, H. D., Collavo, D., North, M., von Boehmer, H., Haas, W., Hengartner, H., and Nabholz, M. (1980). Characterization of cloned murine cytolytic T cell lines. *J. Immunol.* **125,** 1481.

Engers, H. D., Sorenson, G. D., Terres, G., Glasebrook, A. L., Horvath, C., and Brunner, K. T. (1981). Functional *in vivo* of cytolytic T lymphocytes generated *in vitro*. *In* "Mechanisms of Lymphocyte Activation" (K. Resch and H. Kirchner, eds.). Elsevier/North-Holland Biomedical Press, Amsterdam (in press).

Farrar, J. J., Fuller-Farrar, J., Simon, P. L., Hilfiker, M. L., Stadler, G. M., and Farrar, W. L. (1980). Thymoma production of T cell growth factor (interleukin 2). *J. Immunol.* **125,** 2555.

Fathman, C. G., and Hengartner, H. (1978). Clones of alloreactive T cells. *Nature (London)* **272,** 617.

Fathman, C. G., and Nabholz, M. (1977). *In vitro* secondary MLR. II. Detection of semi-allogeneic (F1) MLR stimulating determinants. *Eur. J. Immunol.* **7,** 370.

Festenstein, H. (1973). Immunogenetic and biological aspects of *in vitro* lymphocyte allotransformation (MLR) in the mouse. *Transplant. Rev.* **15,** 62.

Finberg, R., Burakoff, S. J., Cantor, H., and Benacerraf, B. (1978). The biologic significance of alloreactivity. II. T cells stimulated by Sendai virus coated syngeneic cells specifically lyse allogeneic target cells. *Proc. Natl. Acad. Sci. U.S.A.* **75,** 5145.

Fischer-Lindahl, K., and Wilson, D. B. (1977). Histocompatibility antigen-activated cytotoxic T lymphocytes. II. Estimates of the frequency and specificity of precursors. *J. Exp. Med.* **145,** 508.

Fresno, M., Nabel, G., McVay-Boudreau, L., Furthmayer, H., and Cantor, H. (1981). Antigen-specific T lymphocyte clones. I. Characterization of a T lymphocyte clone expressing antigen-specific suppressive activity. *J. Exp. Med.* **153,** 1246.

Garrido, F., Schirrmacher, V., and Festenstein, H. (1976). H-2 like specificities of foreign haplotypes appearing on a mouse sarcoma after vaccinia virus infection. *Nature (London)* **259,** 225.

Gillis, S., and Smith, K. A. (1977). Long term culture of tumor-specific cytotoxic T cells. *Nature (London)* **268,** 154.

Gillis, S., and Watson, J. (1981). Interleukin-2 dependent culture of cytolytic T cell lines. *Immunol. Rev.* **54,** 81.

Gillis, S., Scheid, M., and Watson, J. (1980). Biochemical and biologic characterization of lymphocyte regulatory molecules. III. The isolation and phenotypic characterization of interleukin-2 producing T cell lymphomas. *J. Immunol.* **125,** 2570.

Giorgi, J. V., and Warner, M. (1981). Continuous cytotoxic T cell lines reactive against murine plasmacytoma tumor-associated antigens. *J. Immunol.* **126,** 322.

Glasebrook, A. L., and Fitch, F. W. (1979). T-cell lines which cooperate in generation of specific cytolytic activity. *Nature (London)* **278,** 171.

Glasebrook, A. L., and Fitch, F. W. (1980). Alloreactive cloned T cell lines. I. Interactions between cloned amplifier and cytolytic T cell lines. *J. Exp. Med.* **151,** 876.

Glasebrook, A. L., Sarmiento, M., Loken, M. R., Dialynas, D. P., Quintans, J., Eisenberg, L., Lutz, C. T., Wilde, D., and Fitch, F. W. (1981a). Murine T lymphocyte clones with distinct immunological functions. *Immunol. Rev.* **54,** 225.

Glasebrook, A. L., MacDonald, H. R., Kelso, A., and Brunner, K. T. (1982a). IL-2-independent proliferating cytolytic T cell clones. I. Frequency, specificity, and phenotype. (Submitted for publication.)

Glasebrook, A. L., MacDonald, H. R., and Brunner, K. T. (1982b). IL-2-independent proliferating cytolytic T cell clones. II. Inhibition of cytolytic activity, proliferation, and soluble factor production by monoclonal anti-Lyt-2. (Submitted for publication.)

Glasebrook, A. L., Kelso, A., Zubler, R. H., MacDonald, H. R., Engers, H. D., and Brunner, K. T. (1982c). Heterogeneity of soluble factor production by cytolytic and non-cytolytic alloreactive T cell clones. (Submitted for publication.)

Glasebrook, A. L., Kelso, A., MacDonald, H. R., and Engers, H. D. (1981b). Heterogeneity of T cell clones. *Transpl. Clin. Immunol.* **13,** 63.

Glasebrook, A. L., Quintans, J., Eisenberg, L., and Fitch, F. W. (1981c). Alloreactive cloned T cell lines. II. Polyclonal stimulation of B cells by a cloned helper T cell line. *J. Immunol.* **126,** 240.

Haas, W., Mathur-Rochat, J., Pohlit, H., Nabholz, M., and von Boehmer, H. (1980). Cytotoxic T cell responses to haptenated cells. III. Isolation and specificity analysis of continuously growing clones. *Eur. J. Immunol.* **10,** 828.

Hapel, A. J., Lee, J. C., Farrar, W. L., and Ihle, J. N. (1981). Establishment of continuous cultures of Thy 1.2^+, Lyt 1^+, 2^- T cells with purified Interleukin 3. *Cell* **25,** 179.

Harwell, L., Skidmore, B., Marrack, P., and Kappler, J. (1980). A concanavalin A inducible, interleukin 2 producing T cell hybridoma. *J. Exp. Med.* **152,** 893.

Hengartner, H., and Fathman, C. G. (1980). Clones of alloreactive T cells. I. A unique homozygous MLR-stimulating determinant present on B6 stimulators. *Immunogenetics* **10,** 175.

Hubner, L., Kniep, E. M., Laukel, H., Song, C., Fischer, H., Gassel, W. D., Havemann, K., Kickhofen, B., Lohmann-Matthes, M. L., Schimpl, A., and Wecker, E. (1981). Chemical characterization of macrophage cytotoxicity factor, macrophage migration inhibiting factor, T-helper cell replacing factor and colony-stimulating murine spleen cells *Immunobiology* **157,** 169.

Janeway, C. A., Lerner, E. A., Jason, J. M., and Jones, B. (1980). T lymphocytes responding to *Mls*-locus antigens are *Lyt-1*$^+$, *2*$^-$ and *I-A* restricted. *Immunogenetics* **10,** 481.

Kimoto, M., and Fathman, G. (1980). Antigen-reactive T cell clones. II. Transcomplementing hybrid *I-A*-region gene products function effectively in antigen presentation. *J. Exp. Med.* **152,** 759.

Kimoto, M., and Fathman, C. G. (1981). Antigen-reactive T cell clones. II. Unique homozygous and (high responder × low responder) F_1 hybrid antigen-presenting determinants detected using poly(Tyr, Glu)-poly(D,L-Ala)—poly(Lys)-reactive T cell clones. *J. Exp. Med.* **153,** 375.

Lin, Y.-L., and Askonas, B. A. (1981). Biological properties of an influenza A virus-specific killer T cell clone. Inhibition of virus replication *in vivo* and induction of delayed-type hypersensitivity reactions. *J. Exp. Med.* **154,** 225.

Lutz, C. T., Glasebrook, A. L., and Fitch, F. W. (1981a). Alloreactive cloned T cell lines. III. Accessory cell requirements for the growth of cloned cytolytic T lymphocytes. *J. Immunol.* **126,** 1404.

Lutz, C. T., Glasebrook, A. L., and Fitch, F. W. (1981b). Enumeration of alloreactive helper T lymphocytes which cooperate with cytolytic T lymphocytes. *Eur. J. Immunol.* **11,** 726.

MacDonald, H. R., Cerottini, J.-C., Ryser, J.-E., Maryanski, J. L., Taswell, C., Widmer, M. B., and Brunner, K. T. (1980a). Quantitation and cloning of cytolytic T lymphocytes and their precursors. *Immunol. Rev.* **51,** 93.

MacDonald, H. R., Maryanski, J. L., and Cerottini, J.-C. (1980b). Cloning of cytolytic T lymphocytes: Requirement for interleukin-2 and irradiated spleen cells. *Behring Inst. Mitt.* **67,** 182.

MacDonald, H. R., Thiernesse, N., and Cerottini, J.-C. (1981). Inhibition of T cell-mediated cytolysis by monoclonal antibodies directed against Lyt-2: Heterogeneity of inhibition at the clonal level. *J. Immunol.* **126,** 1671.

Marcucci, F., Walter, M., Kirchner, H., and Krammer, P. (1981). Production of immune interferon by murine T-cell clones from long-term cultures. *Nature (London)* **291,** 79.

Molnar-Kimber, K. L., and Sprent, J. (1980). Absence of H-2 restriction in primary and secondary mixed-lymphocyte reactions to strong Mls determinants. *J. Exp. Med.* **151,** 407.

Molnar-Kimber, K. L., Webb, S. R., Sprent, J., and Wilson, D. B. (1980). T cell lines with dual specificity for strong Mls and H-2 determinants. *J. Immunol.* **125,** 2643.

Morgan, D. A., Ruscetti, F. W., and Gallo, R. (1976). Selective *in vitro* growth of T lymphocytes from normal human bone marrows. *Science* **193,** 1007.

Nabel, G., Fresno, M., Chessman, A., and Cantor, H. (1981a). Use of cloned populations of mouse lymphocytes to analyze cellular differentiation. *Cell* **23,** 19.

Nabel, G., Greenberger, J. S., Sakakeeny, M. A., and Cantor, H. (1981b). Multiple biologic activities of a cloned inducer T-cell population. *Proc. Natl. Sci. U.S.A.* **78,** 1157.

Nabholz, M., Engers, H. D., Collavo, D., and North, M. (1978). Cloned T-cell lines with specific cytolytic activity. *Curr. Top. Microbiol. Immunol.* **81,** 176.

Nabholz, M., North, M., Engers, H., Collavo, D., von Boehmer, H., Haas, W., Hengartner, H., and McKenzie, I. F. C. (1979). Murine cytolytic T-cell lines: Stability of functional phenotype and expression of cell surface markers. *In* "T and B Lymphocytes: Recognition and Function" (F. H. Bach, B. Bonavida, E. S. Vitetta, and C. F. Fox, eds.), pp. 679–688. Academic Press, New York.

Nabholz, M., Conzelmann, A., Acuto, O., North, M., Haas, W., Pohlit, H., von Boehmer, H., Hengartner, H., Mach, J.-P., Engers, H., and Johnson, J. P. (1980). Established murine cytolytic T-cell lines as tools for a somatic cell genetic analysis of T-cell functions. *Immunol. Rev.* **51,** 125.

Okada, M., and Henney, C. S. (1980). The differentiation of cytotoxic T cells *in vitro*. II. Amplifying factor(s) produced in primary mixed lymphocyte cultures against K/D stimuli require the presence of Lyt-2^+ cells but not Lyt-1^+ cells. *J. Immunol.* **125,** 300.

Peck, A. B., Alter, B. J., and Fischer-Lindahl, K. (1976). Specificity in T cell mediated lympholysis: Identical genetic control of the proliferative and effector phases of allogeneic and xenogeneic reactions. *Transplant. Rev.* **29,** 189.

Peck, A. B., Janeway, C. A., and Wigzell, H. (1977). T lymphocyte responses to *Mls* locus antigens involve recognition of *H-2 I*-region gene products. *Nature (London)* **266,** 840.

Robb, R. J., Munck, A., and Smith, K. A. (1981). T-cell growth factor receptor: Quantitation, specificity and biological relevance. *J. Exp. Med.* **154,** 1455.

Rosenberg, S. A., Spiess, P. J., and Schwartz, S. (1980). *In vitro* growth of murine T cells. IV. Use of T-cell growth factor to clone lymphoid cells. *Cell. Immunol.* **54,** 293.

Ryser, J.-E., Cerottini, J.-C., and Brunner, K. T. (1978). Generation of cytolytic T lymphocytes *in vitro*. IX. Induction of secondary CTL responses in primary long-term MCL by supernatants from secondary MLC. *J. Immunol.* **120,** 370.

Schreier, M. H., and Tees, R. (1980). Clonal induction of helper T cells. Conversion of specific signals into non-specific signals. *Int. Arch. Allergy Appl. Immunol.* **61,** 227.

Schreier, M. H., Iscove, N. N., Tees, R., Aarden, L., and von Boehmer, H. (1980). Clones of killer and helper T cells: Growth requirements, specificity and retention of function in long-term culture. *Immunol. Rev.* **51,** 315.

Schawaller, R., Röllinghoff, M., and Wagner, H. (1980). Fine specificity and cytolytic activity of continuously growing alloreactive cytoltoxic T lymphocyte clones. *Scand. J. Immunol.* **11,** 449.

Sekaly, R.-P., MacDonald, H. R., Zaech, P., Glasebrook, A. L., and Cerottini, J.-C. (1981). Cytolytic T lymphocyte function is independent of growth phase and position in the mitotic cycle. *J. Exp. Med.* **154,** 575.

Sherman, L. A. (1980). Dissection of the B10.D2 anti-H-2K^b cytolytic T lymphocyte receptor repertoire. *J. Exp. Med.* **151,** 1386.

Shimizu, S., Kanaka, Y., and Smith, R. (1980). Mitogen-initiated synthesis and secretion of T cell growth factors by a T lymphoma cell line. *J. Exp. Med.* **152,** 1436.

Smith, K. A., and Ruscetti, F. W. (1981). T-cell growth factor and the culture of cloned functional T-cells. *Adv. Immunol.* **31,** 137.

Snodgrass, H. R., Bosma, M. J., and Wilson, D. B. (1981). T lymphocytes specific for immunoglobulin allotype. II. Cloned *Igh-1^b* specific cytotoxic T cells. *J. Exp. Med.* **154,** 491.

Sredni, B., and Schwartz, R. H. (1980). Alloreactivity of an antigen-specific T-cell clone. *Nature* (*London*) **287,** 855.

Sredni, B., and Schwartz, R. H. (1981). Antigen-specific, proliferating T lymphocyte clones. Methodology, specificity, MHC restriction and alloreactivity. *Immunol. Rev.* **54,** 187.

Sredni, B., Tse, H. Y., and Schwartz, R. H. (1980). Direct cloning and extended culture of antigen-specific MHC-restricted, proliferating T lymphocytes. *Nature* (*London*) **283,** 581.

Stull, D., and Gillis, S. (1981). Constitutive production of interleukin-2 activity by a T cell hybridoma. *J. Immunol.* **126,** 1680.

Taswell, C., MacDonald, H. R., and Cerottini, J.-C. (1980). Clonal analysis of cytolytic T lymphocyte specificity. I. Phenotypically distinct sets of clones as the cellular basis of cross-reactivity to alloantigens. *J. Exp. Med.* **151,** 1372.

Tees, R., and Schreier, M. H. (1980). Selective reconstitution of nude mice with long-term cultured and cloned specific helper T cells *Nature* (*London*) **283,** 780.

von Boehmer, H., and Haas, W. (1981). H-2 restricted cytolytic and noncytolytic T cell clones: Isolation, specificity and functional analysis. *Immunol. Rev.* **54,** 27.

von Boehmer, H., Hengartner, H., Nabholz, M., Lernhardt, W., Schreier, M. H., and Haas, W. (1979). Fine specificity of a continuously growing killer cell clone specific for H-Y antigen. *Eur. J. Immunol.* **9,** 592.

Wagner, H., Hardt, C., Hecg, K., Pfizenmaler, K., Solbach, W., Bartlett, R., Stockinger, H., and Rollinghoff, M. (1980). T-T cell interactions during cytotoxic T lymphocyte (CTL) responses: T cell derived helper factor (interleukin 2) as a probe to analyze CTL responsiveness and thymic maturation of CTL progenitors. *Immunol. Rev.* **51,** 215.

Watson, J. (1979). Continuous proliferation of murine antigen-specific helper T lymphocytes in culture. *J. Exp. Med.* **150,** 1510.

Watson, J., and Mochizuki, D. (1980). Interleukin 2: A class of T cell growth factors. *Immunol. Rev.* **51,** 257.

Weiss, A., Brunner, K. T., MacDonald, H. R., and Cerottini, J.-C. (1980). Antigenic specificity of the cytolytic T lymphocyte response to murine sarcoma virus-induced tumors. III. Characterization of cytolytic T lymphocyte clones specific for Maloney leukemia virus associated cell surface antigens. *J. Exp. Med.* **152,** 1225.

Weiss, A., MacDonald, H. R., Cerottini, J.-C., and Brunner, K. T. (1981). Inhibition of cytolytic T lymphocyte clones reactive with Moloney leukemia virus-associated antigens by monoclonal antibodies: A direct approach to the study of H-2 restriction. *J. Immunol.* **126,** 482.

Widmer, M. B., and Bach, F. H. (1981). Antigen driven helper cell-independent cloned cytolytic T lymphocytes. *Nature* (*London*) **294,** 750.

Zagury, D., Bernard, J., Thiemesse, N., Foldman, M., and Berke, G. (1975). Isolation and characterization of individual functionally reactive cytotoxic T lymphocytes. Conjugation, killing, and recycling at the single cell level. *Eur. J. Immunol.* **5,** 818.

23

Cloned Continuous Lines of *H-2*-Restricted Influenza Virus-Specific CTL: Probes of T Lymphocyte Specificity and Heterogeneity

T. J. Braciale/V. L. Braciale/M. E. Andrew

I. Properties of Influenza-Specific CTL Clones 286
A. Patterns of *H-2* Restriction 286
B. Specificity of Viral Antigen Recognition 287
C. Proliferative Response of CTL Clones 288
D. Simultaneous Expression of Alloreactive and *H-2* Restricted Recognition by CTL Clones 290
E. Strong *Mls* Locus Recognition by Cloned *H-2* Restricted CTL . . 291
II. Conclusions 293
References 294

Since the initial realization that T cells represent a distinct lymphocyte set, one of the central issues in cellular immunology has been the nature of the foreign antigen receptor on T lymphocytes and the relationship of this receptor to the immunoglobulin receptor on the B lymphocyte. The hallmark of the B lymphocyte response to foreign antigens is its high degree of specificity and remarkable degree of diversity. In considering the T lymphocyte response to a particular foreign antigen, an analysis of the specificity and extent of repertoire diversity of the responding T lymphocytes should at least provide correlative information on the relationship of the T and B lymphocyte antigen recognition structures. Although numerous attempts have been made to carry out such analyses in a variety of model systems, a major difficulty in evaluating T lymphocyte specificity and diversity has been the necessity of employing heterogeneous populations of T lymphocytes in these studies.

This chapter will deal with recent work from this laboratory on the characteri-

ISOLATION, CHARACTERIZATION, AND
UTILIZATION OF T LYMPHOCYTE CLONES

ISBN 0-12-249920-4

zation of continuous cloned lines of *H-2* restricted cytolytic T lymphocytes (CTL) directed to the type A influenza viruses. In addition to stimulating a potent CTL response *in vivo* and *in vitro* (Braciale, 1977), the type A influenza viruses have been extremely well characterized both biochemically and antigenically (Kilbourne, 1975). More importantly, nature has provided a large series of variant virus strains with readily demonstrable antigenic (serologic) differences associated with distinct virion polypeptides (Webster and Laver, 1975). These features of the type A influenza viruses make them an extremely useful probe for analyzing CTL recognition at the clonal level.

I. PROPERTIES OF INFLUENZA-SPECIFIC CTL CLONES

A. Patterns of *H-2* Restriction

In analyzing the properties of *H-2* restricted CTL lines ostensibly derived from individual CTL precursors (Braciale *et al.*, 1981a), perhaps the major consideration is whether these lines are indeed of clonal origin. Based on the extensive evidence obtained with heterogeneous populations of *H-2* restricted CTL (Zinkernagel and Doherty, 1979) certain predictions can be made concerning the properties of *H-2* restricted CTL clones. Specifically, in addition to possessing specificity for the stimulating foreign antigen, cloned CTL populations should be restricted in target cell recognition by either the *H-2K* or the *H-2D* locus product of the donor *H-2* haplotype. In our studies influenza-specific CTL clones have been established from BALB/c ($H\text{-}2^d$), C57BL/6 ($H\text{-}2^b$), and (BALB/c × C57BL/6) CB6F_1 ($H\text{-}2^{d/b}$) mice. We included the CB6F_1 mice in our studies because previous work with heterogeneous populations of virus-specific CTL in F_1 mice indicated the existence of two subpopulations of CTL, i.e., CTL restricted to virus in association with *H-2* products of either of the two parental haplotypes but not both (Doherty *et al.*, 1976). Therefore at the clonal level influenza-specific CTL lines of $H\text{-}2^{b/d}$ origin should exhibit only one of four possible patterns of *H-2* restriction, i.e., recognition of virus-infected cells expressing either K^d, D^d, K^b, or D^b. Table I shows the results of such an analysis on a series of CB6F_1 clones directed to influenza A/JAPAN/305/57. Individual F_1 CTL lines lyse infected target cells of the $H\text{-}2^d$ haplotype (P815 cells) or the $H\text{-}2^b$ haplotype (MC57G) but not both. In addition, when tested on a fibroblast cell line derived from an *H-2* recombinant mouse strain ($H\text{-}2K^dD^b$) (Table I) lysis of infected recombinant HTGSV target cells by individual $H\text{-}2^d$ or $H\text{-}2^b$ restricted clones is selective. Since this recombinant target cell should be susceptible to lysis by CTL clones restricted to the *K* end of $H\text{-}2^d$ or the *D* end of $H\text{-}2^b$, this result indicates restriction of individual CTL clones by one end of the appropriate parental haplotype. As expected, a heterogeneous population of

TABLE I

H-2 Restriction of Cytotoxicity by Influenza Virus-Specific CTL Clones[a]

CTL clone	Percent specific ^{51}Cr release from target cells					
	P815 ($H\text{-}2K^d,D^d$)		MC57G ($H\text{-}2K^b,D^b$)		HTGSV ($H\text{-}2K^d,D^b$)	
	Uninfected	Infected	Uninfected	Infected	Uninfected	Infected
11-1	1	88	3	2	0	31
13-1	1	5	11	53	0	7
14-1	11	88	3	4	2	68
14-17	0	85	1	1	1	0
20-15	0	0	0	39	0	37
$CB6F_1$[b]	2	85	2	29	5	67

[a] Clones are all of $CB6F_1$ ($H\text{-}2^{d/b}$) origin. The effector cell–target cell ratio is 5 : 1. The assay time is 6 hr. Values are the mean of quadruplicate assays with standard errors (always less than 5% of mean values) omitted. Adapted from Braciale *et al.* (1981a).

[b] Indicates heterogeneous population of secondary CTL generated *in vitro*.

influenza-specific CTL of $CB6F_1$ origin lyses all three infected target cell types (Table I). A more extensive analysis of *H-2* restricted recognition by CTL clones is presented elsewhere (Braciale *et al.*, 1981a).

B. Specificity of Viral Antigen Recognition

Previous studies on the viral antigen specificity of heterogeneous populations of CTL directed to the type A influenza viruses suggested considerable heterogeneity in the response to this antigen (Braciale, 1977, 1979; Effros *et al.*, 1977; Zweerink *et al.*, 1977). In particular, several studies demonstrated the simultaneous induction of two distinct CTL subpopulations (Braciale, 1977; Effros *et al.*, 1977). One subpopulation recognized target cells infected with serologically related type A influenza strains of the same subtype as the immunizing influenza strain, i.e., subtype specific, while the other subpopulation recognized target cells infected with any type A influenza virus, independent of subtype, i.e., type specific. Since both CTL subpopulations were generated simultaneously upon immunization with a given influenza strain, the two subpopulations were not physically separable and their presence could only be established using cold target inhibition protocols (Braciale, 1977; Effros *et al.*, 1977). CTL with subtype-specific or type-specific patterns of virus recognition should, however, be readily separable at the clonal level. Therefore, another useful criterion for clonality in this system was the demonstration of CTL lines with either subtype or type specific recognition.

Table II shows the results of such an analysis with three representative $H\text{-}2^d$ restricted CTL clones selected for recognition of influenza A/JAP/57 (H_2N_2). Included in this analysis are $H\text{-}2^d$ target cells infected with the selecting A/JAP/57 strain, target cells infected with the serologically related A/AA/67 virus also of the H_2N_2 subtype, target cells infected with two serologically distinct type A strains of different subtypes A/PR/8 (H_1N_1) and A/PC/75 (H_3N_2), as well as target cells infected with the unrelated type B strain LEE. One clone, 14–13, shows the typical type-specific recognition with lysis of type A virus-infected targets irrespective of subtype. Subtype-specific recognition is exhibited by a second clone, 14–7 with selective lysis of target cells infected with either the immunizing A/JAP/57 (H_2N_2) virus or the serologically related A/AA/67 (H_2N_2) virus. Thus the two patterns of viral antigen recognition are separable at the clonal level, thereby further substantiating the clonal origin of the CTL lines. Unexpectedly a third pattern of viral antigen recognition also emerged which was heretofore not demonstrable in a heterogeneous CTL response. As exemplified by clone 14–1, CTL clones were isolated which exclusively recognized the immunizing A/JAP/57 virus strain.

These observations directly support the concept the *H-2* restricted CTL can exhibit both considerable heterogeneity and specificity in antigen recognition. Results of Sherman (1980) also indicate considerable heterogeneity among alloreactive CTL when assessed at the clonal level. Using recombinant influenza virus strains it has been possible to determine directly the influenza virion surface glycoprotein (hemagglutinin or neuraminidase) to which particular unique or subtype specific CTL clones are directed (Braciale *et al.*, 1981a).

C. Proliferative Response of CTL Clones

These *H-2* restricted CTL clones were isolated, expanded, and maintained in the presence of both viral antigen and T cell growth factor (TCGF)-containing concanavalin A (Con-A) supernatant. This fact probably accounts for a striking

TABLE II

Influenza Virus Specificity of CTL Clones[a]

	Percent specific ^{51}Cr release from P815 ($H\text{-}2^d$) target cells					
CTL clone	Uninfected	A/JAP/57 (H_2N_2)	A/AA/67 (H_2N_2)	A/PR/8 (H_1N_1)	A/PC/75 (H_3N_2)	B/Lee
14-13	0	68	70	78	76	2
14-7	0	75	64	1	2	2
14-1	2	57	4	5	7	6

[a] As in Table I except that effector cell–target cell ratio is 1 : 1

property of these CTL lines which is that both exogeneous TCGF and specific antigenic stimulation (in the form of virus-infected antigen presenting cells) are required for the continued *in vitro* proliferation of these CTL clones. Data in Table III demonstrate this requirement for antigen and TCGF for stimulation of a representative $H\text{-}2^d$ restricted $CB6F_1$ CTL clone using [^{3}H]thymidine incorporation as a measure of cellular proliferation. Both virus-infected F_1 spleen cells and exogenous TCGF are required for optimal proliferation of this line. Significant proliferation is also observed upon stimulation with virus-infected BALB/c ($H\text{-}2^d$) spleen cells but not in the presence of infected C57B1/6 ($H\text{-}2^b$) spleen cells. This requirement for both TCGF and antigen appears to be a general property of the influenza-specific CTL clones. To date, at least ten lines have been extensively analyzed. All require specific antigenic stimulation as well as an exogenous source of TCGF for continued *in vitro* propagation.

Because of the requirement for specific antigenic stimulation in cloned CTL propagation, it has been possible to demonstrate that the antigenic requirements for proliferation of the CTL clones directly parallels their patterns of *H-2* restricted viral antigen recognition. Table IV shows the proliferative response of four $CB6F_1$ clones which exhibit either unique, subtype-, or type-specific patterns of lysis of influenza-infected target cells. Clones 11-1 and 14-1, which lyse A/JAP/57-infected target cells exclusively, proliferate only in response to F_1 spleen cells infected with this virus, whereas the subtype-specific clone 14-7 proliferates in response to both A/JAP/57 virus and the serologically related A/AA/67 virus. The type-specific clone, 14-13, in addition, proliferates in response to the serologically distinct A/PR/8 virus.

TABLE III

Requirement for Antigen and TCGF in the Proliferative Response of Influenza-Specific CTL Clones[a]

Stimulating spleen cells	Virus (A/JAP/57)	TCGF	^{3}H-TdR incorporation by CTL clone 11-1 (cpm)
$CB6F_1$ ($H\text{-}2^{d/b}$)	+	−	339 ± 79
None	−	+	2,174 ± 209
$CB6F_1$	−	+	1,553 ± 198
$CB6F_1$	+	+	23,878 ± 2,406
BALB/c ($H\text{-}2^d$)	−	+	501 ± 137
BALB/c	+	+	32,887 ± 1,326
C57BL/6 ($H\text{-}2^b$)	+	+	1,087 ± 174

[a] Quadruplicate cultures of 10^4 viable cells from CTL clone 11-1 were examined for proliferation by ^{3}H-TdR incorporation. Values are the mean ± SEM of ^{3}H-TdR incorporation at the peak of the response (day 4 of culture). Spleen cells received 2000 R of irradiation prior to use as stimulator cells in proliferation assays. Adapted from Andrew and Braciale (1981).

TABLE IV

Virus Specificity of Proliferation by Cloned CTL[a]

Stimulating virus strain	^{3}H-TdR incorporation (cpm) 11-1	14-1	14-7	14-13
A/JAP/57	27,732 ± 1254	41,660 ± 1268	22,539 ± 828	31,610 ± 1960
A/AA/67	1,178 ± 222	1,733 ± 242	24,310 ± 2149	61,228 ± 5284
A/PR/8	1,713 ± 84	1,173 ± 138	490 ± 59	30,616 ± 2802
B/LEE	2,887 ± 240	3,109 ± 650	430 ± 76	1,171 ± 475
None	2,683 ± 279	2,323 ± 527	989 ± 197	—

[a] Four CB6F$_1$ CTL clones were examined for their proliferative response to syngeneic (F$_1$) spleen cells infected with the indicated type A influenza strain [in the presence of medium supplemented with 10% (v/v) TCGF]. The cytolytic specificities of these clones are: 11-1, A/JAP/57 only; 14-1, A/JAP/57 only; 14-7, A/JAP/57 and A/AA/67; 14-3, A/JAP/57, A/AA/67, and A/PR/8. Adapted from Andrew and Braciale (1981).

D. Simultaneous Expression of Alloreactive and *H-2* Restricted Recognition by CTL Clones

During the initial screening of a panel of CTL clones for *H-2* restricted recognition, an unexpected pattern of lysis was observed. One clone of CB6F$_1$ origin which exhibited unique recognition of the immunizing (selecting) virus strain, A/JAP/305/57, in association with $H\text{-}2K^d$, simultaneously expressed cytotoxic activity on uninfected target cells of the $H\text{-}2^k$ haplotype. Data in Table V documents the simultaneous expression of *H-2* restricted virus-specific cytotoxicity and alloreactivity by this CB6F$_1$ clone, 14–2. Data on two other A/JAP/305/57 specific $H\text{-}2K^d$ restricted CB6F$_1$ clones, 11–1 and 14–13, which

TABLE V

Expression of Virus-Specific and Alloreactive Cytotoxicity by CTL Clone 14-2[a]

	Percent specific ^{51}Cr release from target cells P815 ($H\text{-}2^d$)					L929 ($H\text{-}2^k$)
CTL clone	Uninfected	A/PR/8 (H_1N_1)	A/JAP/57 (H_2N_2)	A/AA/67 (H_2N_2)	B/Lee	Uninfected
14-2	0	0.6	54	2	0	27
11-1	8	9	50	10	11	0
14-13	1	65	47	53	4	0.3

[a] Three CB6F$_1$ CTL clones (all restricted to $H\text{-}2^d$) were tested for cytotoxicity on the indicated target cells at an effector–target cell ratio of 2.5 : 1. Adapted from Braciale *et al.* (1981b).

lacked cytotoxicity for $H\text{-}2^k$ targets, is also included. Further analysis of this alloreactive recognition using uninfected target cells from *H-2* recombinant mouse strains indicates that clone 14–2 is cytotoxic for cells expressing the $H\text{-}2K^k$ locus product (Braciale *et al.*, 1981b). In addition, because of the requirement for specific antigenic stimulation in clonal proliferation it was possible to demonstrate that proliferation of clone 14–2 could be stimulated either by virus-infected spleen cells expresssing $H\text{-}2K^d$ or uninfected spleen cells of the $H\text{-}2K^k$ haplotype (Table VI).

It should be emphasized that this dual specificity CTL line was isolated and expanded under totally syngeneic conditions, i.e., in the presence of infected $CB6F_1$ spleen cells. As discussed in detail elsewhere (Braciale *et al.*, 1981b) several other lines of evidence, including cold target inhibition experiments and subcloning of this line, directly support the notion that line 14–2 is derived from a single virus-specific CTL precursor and therefore that a given homogeneous CTL population can simultaneously exhibit *H-2* restricted and alloreactive recognition. This observation is consistent with recent results of other investigators (von Boehmer *et al.*, 1979; Sredni and Schwartz, 1980) who have demonstrated such dual specificity T cells at the clonal level.

E. Strong *Mls* Locus Recognition by Cloned *H-2* Restricted CTL

A hallmark of T lymphocytes is their vigorous proliferative response to foreign major histocompatibility locus products of the species in the mixed leukocyte culture. In the mouse, a strong proliferative response by T lymphocytes has also been observed in response to a difference at a gene locus, (the *Mls* or *M* locus) which maps outside of the *H-2* gene complex (Festenstein, 1973). *Mls* locus reactive T lymphocytes, like alloreactive T lymphocytes, appear to be represented in high frequency among mature peripheral T lymphocytes (Janeway *et al.*, 1980). In contrast to the response to alloantigen, however, T lymphocytes

TABLE VI

Proliferative Response of Dual Specificity CTL Clone 14-2

Stimulator spleen cell	^{3}H-TdR incorporation (cpm)
$CB6F_1$ ($H\text{-}2^{d/b}$)	362 ± 204
$CB6F_1$ + A/JAP/57 virus	33,500 ± 1,991
BALB/c ($H\text{-}2^d$) + A/JAP/57 virus	33,844 ± 999
C57BL/6 ($H\text{-}2^b$) + A/JAP/57 virus	647 ± 52
CBA/J ($H\text{-}2^k$)	38,044 ± 951
B10.BAR4 ($H\text{-}2K^kD^b$)	48,004 ± 951
B10.OH ($H\text{-}2K^dD^k$)	653 ± 138

responding to an *Mls* locus difference appear to exhibit little or no cytotoxicity for the appropriate *Mls* locus incompatible target cells (Festenstein, 1973; von Boehmer and Sprent, 1974).

Our interest in the *Mls* locus was an outgrowth of a fortuitous observation made during an analysis of the proliferative response of our virus-specific CTL clones (Table VII). We observed that one of the virus-specific $CB6F_1$ clones, 14–13, proliferated in response to allogeneic CBA/J ($H\text{-}2^k$; Mls^d) spleen cells. As demonstrated above (Table VI) the dual specific clone, 14–2, also responded to the $H\text{-}2K^k$ bearing CBA/J stimulator cells. In contrast to clone 14–2, however, clone 14–13 failed to respond to two other stimulator cell types of the $H\text{-}2^k$ haplotype, B10.BR ($H\text{-}2^k$, Mls^b) and CBA/CaJ ($H\text{-}2^k$; Mls^b) spleen cells (Table VII). This lack of responsiveness to B10.BR and in particular to CBA/CaJ suggested that clone 14–13 was responding to a gene product which mapped outside of $H\text{-}2^k$. The fact that CBA/J expresses the Mls^d allele, whereas CBA/CAJ expresses the Mls^b allele raised the possibility that clone 14–13 ($H\text{-}2^{b/d}$; Mls^b) was proliferating in response to the Mls^d locus expressed on the CBA/J spleen cells. Since CBA/J is the only mouse strain expressing the Mls^d allele, it was not possible to directly demonstrate Mls^d recognition using appropriate Mls^d compatible stimulator cells. However since the Mls^d allele is highly cross-reactive with (and perhaps identical to) the Mls^a allele, we could demonstrate that uninfected histocompatible stimulator cells expressing the Mls^a allele, i.e., DBA/2($H\text{-}2^d$; Mls^a) and NZB($H\text{-}2^d$; Mls^a) could specifically stimulate proliferation of clone 14–13 (Table VII). It is also of note that CTL clone 14–13 failed to lyse T lymphoblast target cells from the CBA/J, DBA/2, or NZB strains. A more detailed discussion of this phenomenon is presented elsewhere (Braciale and Braciale, 1981).

TABLE VII

Strong *Mls* Locus Recognition by Influenza Virus-Specific CTL Clone 14-13[a]

Stimulator spleen cells	*H-2;Mls* genotype	^{3}H-TdR incorporation by CTL clone (cpm)		
		14-13	14-2	14-7
$CB6F_1$	*bxd;b*	2,936 ± 103	1,706 ± 543	1,388 ± 116
$CB6F_1$ + A/JAP/57	*bxd;b*	45,660 ± 3081	42,504 ± 4929	56,131 ± 1623
CBA/J	*k;d*	37,293 ± 1336	48,876 ± 1582	572 ± 119
B10.BR	*k;b*	2,237 ± 676	38,970 ± 3912	430 ± 159
CBA/CaJ	*k;b*	327 ± 98	—	—
DBA/2	*d;a*	12,079 ± 1096	2,151 ± 235	1,790 ± 465
NZB	*d;a*	8,471 ± 418	1,797 ± 247	2509 ± 425
SJL	*s;c*	2,566 ± 310	2,764 ± 413	851 ± 354

[a] Adapted from Braciale and Braciale (1981).

To date we have examined a total of eight virus-specific CTL clones (all of the *Mls*^{b} type) and have found three clones which apparently proliferate in response to a strong *Mls* locus difference, i.e., *Mls*^{d} and/or *Mls*^{a}. Five other clones, all of which exhibit a *H-2* restricted proliferative response to influenza virus, failed to proliferate in response to either an *Mls*^{d}, *Mls*^{a}, or *Mls*^{c} locus difference, e.g., clone 14–7 in Table VII.

II. CONCLUSIONS

In this chapter we have attempted to summarize briefly recent work with *H-2* restricted, influenza virus-specific CTL clones which touches upon several aspects of T lymphocyte function. Perhaps the central theme which has emerged from this analysis is the degree of heterogeneity among CTL at the clonal level. This heterogeneity is evident both in the immunologic specificity of these clones and in their expression of cell surface markers. Our limited analysis of the fine specificity of viral antigen recognition by these cloned CTL lines already suggests considerable diversity in the CTL response to a given antigenic moiety. Obviously the extent of this diversity can best be dissected at the clonal level with an antigen such as the type A influenza hemagglutinin where a variety of antigenic variants of this moiety are available (Gerhard *et al.*, 1981). Clearly, information on the fine specificity and degree of repertoire diversity of CTL will be necessary for a complete understanding of the structure of the antigen receptor on CTL. This information can best be obtained at the clonal level.

Our observation that specific antigenic stimulation as well as TCGF is required for proliferation of the influenza-specific CTL clones is at variance with early reports on the proliferative requirements for CTL clones maintained in the presence of TCGF (von Boehmer *et al.*, 1979), and probably reflects the fact that our clones were selected and maintained in the presence of both antigen and TCGF (Andrew and Braciale, 1981; Weiss *et al.*, 1980). The availability of cloned CTL lines which are dependent on antigen and TCGF for proliferation will allow us to examine the requirements for antigen presentation and accessory cells in CTL activation and to assess the regulatory effect of the various factors in the crude TCGF preparations. This type of analysis should begin to shed light on the more complex issue of CTL induction *in vivo* and *in vitro*.

The demonstration of a CTL clone with simultaneous expression of *H-2* restricted virus recognition and alloreactivity for a specific unrelated *H-2* haplotype is perhaps not surprising in light of the considerable body of evidence indicating overlap between the MHC-restricted and alloreactive T cells (e.g., Lemonnier *et al.*, 1977; Bevan, 1977). A major question that remains unanswered is the extent of the overlap between MHC restricted and alloreactive T cells.

Perhaps the most surprising result to emerge from our analysis was the demonstration of apparent reactivity to a strong *Mls* locus difference by a *H-2* restricted virus-specific CTL clone. One possible explanation for the existence of such *H-2* restricted CTL clones with reactivity toward strong *Mls* difference is that this reactivity is a reflection of a separate recognition system for T lymphocyte activation which is independent of foreign antigen-induced T lymphocyte activation (Braciale and Braciale, 1981). Recent results of Sprent and collaborators (Molnar-Kimber *et al.*, 1980) are pertinent to the issue of *Mls* locus recognition by T lymphocytes and are described in detail elsewhere in this treatise.

Many of the major questions regarding the mechanism of antigen recognition by T lymphocytes and the processes of T lymphocyte activation and regulation can only be fully answered by characterization of the relevant cell surface structures on the T lymphocyte. Whether this analysis is carried out at the level of the genes coding for these structures or by direct biochemical analysis of the molecules, homogeneous populations of functional T lymphocytes provide an obvious and most appropriate source of material for this analysis. Of equal, if not greater, importance is the potential for therapeutic application of functional cloned T lymphocyte lines. In the case of the system described herein, it should now be possible to assess unambiguously the role of various T lymphocyte subsets on the outcome of experimental influenza infection in mice by adoptive transfer of functional homogeneous T lymphocyte populations representative of the various subsets. Application of this technology for immunotherapy and reconstitution in man may also soon be a reality.

ACKNOWLEDGMENTS

This work is supported by Grant AI-15608 from the United States Public Health Service and by research support from Brown and Williamson Tobacco Corporation; Philip Morris, Inc.; R. J. Reynolds Tobacco Company, and the United States Tobacco Company.

REFERENCES

Andrew, M. E., and Braciale, T. J. (1981). Antigen-dependent proliferation of cloned continuous lines of H-2 restricted influenza virus-specific cytotoxic T lymphocytes. *J. Immunol.* **127,** 1201.

Bevan, M. J. (1977). Killer cells reactive to altered self antigens can also be alloreactive. *Proc. Natl. Acad. Sci. U.S.A.* **74,** 2094.

Braciale, T. J. (1977). Immunologic recognition of influenza virus-infected cells. I. Generation of a virus-strain specific and a cross-reactive subpopulation of cytotoxic T cells in the response to type A influenza viruses of different subtypes. *Cell Immunol.* **33,** 423.

Braciale, T. J. (1979). Specificity of cytotoxic T cells directed to influenza virus hemagglutinin. *J. Exp. Med.* **149,** 856.

Braciale, T. J., Andrew, M. E., and Braciale, V. L. (1981a). Heterogeneity and specificity of cloned lines of influenza virus-specific cytotoxic T lymphocytes. *J. Exp. Med.* **153,** 910.

Braciale, T. J., Andrew, M. E., and Braciale, V. L. (1981b). Simultaneous expression of H-2-restricted and alloreactive recognition by a cloned line of influenza virus-specific cytotoxic T lymphocytes. *J. Exp. Med.* **153,** 1371.

Braciale, V. L., and Braciale, T. J. (1981). *Mls* locus recognition by a cloned line of H-2 restricted influenza virus-specific cytotoxic T lymphocytes. *J. Immunol.* **127,** 859.

Doherty, P. C., Blanden, R. V., and Zinkernagel, R. M. (1976). Specificity of virus immune effector T cells for H-2K or H-2D compatability interactions. Implications for H-antigen diversity. *Transplant. Rev.* **29,** 89.

Effros, R. B., Doherty, P. C., Gerhard, W., and Bennink, J. (1977). Generation of both cross-reactive and virus-specific T cell populations after immunization with serologically distinct influenza A viruses. *J. Exp. Med.* **145,** 557.

Festenstein, H. (1973). Immunogenetic and biological aspects of *in vitro* lymphocyte allotransformation (MLR) in the mouse. *Transplant. Rev.* **15,** 62.

Gerhard, W., Yewdell, J., Frankel, M. E., and Webster, R. (1981). Antigenic structure of influenza virus hemagglutinin defined by hybridoma antibodies. *Nature* (*London*) **290,** 713.

Janeway, C. A., Lerner, E. A., Jason, J. M., and Jones, B. (1980). T lymphocytes responding to *Mls*-locus antigens are Lyt-$1^{+}2^{-}$ and *I-A* restricted. *Immunogenetics* **10,** 481.

Kilbourne, E. D., ed. (1975). "The Influenza Viruses and Influenza." Academic Press, New York.

Lemonnier, F., Burakoff, S. J., Germain, R. N., and Benacerraf, B. (1977). Cytolytic thymus-derived lymphocytes for allogeneic stimulator cells crossreact with chemically modified syngeneic cells *Proc. Natl. Acad. Sci. U.S.A.* **74,** 1229.

Molnar-Kimber, K. L., Webb, S. R., Sprent, J., and Wilson, D. B. (1980). Cell lines with dual specificity for strong Mls and H-2 determinants. *J. Immunol.* **125,** 2643.

Sherman, L. A. (1980). Dissection of the B10.D2 anti-H-$2K^{b}$ cytolytic T lymphocyte repertoire. *J. Exp. Med.* **157,** 1386.

Sredni, B., and Schwartz, R. H. (1980). Alloreactivity of an antigen-specific T cell clone. *Nature* (*London*) **287,** 855.

von Boehmer, H., and Sprent, J. (1974). Expression of *M* locus differences by B cells but not T cells. *Nature* (*London*) **249,** 363.

von Boehmer, H., Hengartner, H., Nabholz, M., Lenhardt, W., Schreier, M., and Haas, W. (1979). Fine specificity of a continuously growing killer cell clone specific for H-Y antigen. *Eur. J. Immunol.* **9,** 592.

Webster, R. G., and Laver, W. G. (1975). Antigenic variation of influenza virus. *In* "The Influenza Viruses and Influenza" (E. D. Kilbourne, ed.), p. 269. Academic Press, New York.

Weiss, A., Brunner, K. T., McDonald, H. R., and Cerrotini, J.-C. (1980). Antigenic specificity of the cytolytic T lymphocyte response to murine sarcoma virus-induced tumors. III. Characterization of cytolytic T lymphocyte clones specific for Moloney leukemia virus-associated cell surface antigens. *J. Exp. Med.* **152,** 1210.

Zinkernagel, R. M., and Doherty, P. C. (1979). MHC-restricted cytotoxic T cells: Studies on the biological role of polymorphic major transplantation antigens determining T cell restriction specificity, function and responsiveness. *Adv. Immunol.* **27,** 51.

Zweerink, H. J., Askonas, B. A., Millican, D., Courtneidge, S. A., and Skehel, J. J. (1977). Cytotoxic T cells to type A influenza viruses: Viral hemagglutinin induces A-strain specificity while infected cells confer cross-reactive cytotoxicity. *Eur. J. Immunol.* **7,** 630.

24

Cytolytic T Lymphocyte Clones Recognizing Murine Sarcoma Virus-Induced Tumor Antigens

K. Theodor Brunner/Arthur Weiss/
H. Robson MacDonald/Jean-Charles Cerottini

I. Optimal Microculture Conditions for the Generation of MoLV-Specific CTL Clones . . . 298
II. Frequency Determination of MoLV-Specific CTL Precursors . . . 300
III. Isolation and Maintenance of MoLV-Specific CTL Clones . . . 301
IV. Specificity of MoLV-Specific CTL Clones . . . 302
V. Surface Phenotype of MoLV-Specific CTL Clones . . . 309
VI. Conclusions . . . 309
References . . . 310

The present chapter summarizes and extends recent studies from our laboratory describing the generation *in vitro* and characterization of Moloney leukemia virus (MoLV)-specific cytolytic T lymphocyte (CTL) clones. The results demonstrate that under appropriate culture conditions, MoLV-specific CTL clones can be generated from CTL precursors (CTL-P) by directly plating small (limiting) numbers of normal or primed lymphoid cells (or single primed cells obtained by micromanipulation) into micro-mixed leukocyte–tumor cell cultures (micro-MLTC). The frequency of CTL-P contained in various lymphoid cell populations was studied by applying limiting dilution analysis, and cytolytic activity and specificity of clonal CTL populations were assayed using a panel of target cells and inhibition by antibody. Most of the clones studied so far showed high cytolytic activity and stability, and all were restricted to syngeneic MoLV-derived tumor cells.

Previous studies of the murine sarcoma virus (MSV) tumor model had shown that CTL restricted to MoLV-derived tumor cells are generated *in vivo* during the growth and subsequent rejection of MSV-MoLV induced sarcomas (Levy and

ISOLATION, CHARACTERIZATION, AND
UTILIZATION OF T LYMPHOCYTE CLONES

ISBN 0-12-249920-4

Leclerc, 1977). In addition, lymphoid cells collected at the time of and up to several months after tumor regression showed secondary type CTL responses when stimulated *in vitro* with syngeneic MoLV-derived tumor cells (Plata *et al.*, 1975). This indicated the presence of increased frequencies of CTL-P in the immune cell populations.

Specificity studies further showed that cytolytic activity was preferentially directed against MoLV-derived tumor cells syngeneic with the effector cells (Plata *et al.*, 1976). More specifically, lysis of $H\text{-}2^b$ MoLV-derived target cells required identity at the $H\text{-}2D^b$ locus, whereas lysis of $H\text{-}2^d$ MoLV-derived targets required identity at $H\text{-}2K^d$ (Gomard *et al.*, 1977). This restriction appeared, however, not to be complete, since a minor degree of cross-reactivity with allogeneic MoLV-derived tumor cells was noted.

CTL responses measured at the population level could only provide indirect evidence concerning frequency and specificity of CTL and their precursors. With the recent introduction of interleukin-2 (IL-2) as a nonspecific stimulant able to induce and/or maintain *in vitro* proliferation of antigen-activated T cells (Smith, 1980), it has become possible to define microculture conditions allowing the clonal expansion of small (limiting) numbers of CTL-P, to obtain minimal estimates of their frequency in various cell populations, and to characterize the progeny derived, at least theoretically, from single CTL-P. Evidence was also provided demonstrating that CTL-P as well at CTL responded by clonal expansion, i.e., that mature CTL behaved operationally as CTL-P (Maryanski *et al.*, 1980). The present studies confirm the applicability of limiting dilution microculture techniques to the clonal analysis of MSV tumor-reactive CTL.

I. OPTIMAL MICROCULTURE CONDITIONS FOR THE GENERATION OF MoLV-SPECIFIC CTL CLONES

Results obtained in allogeneic systems had shown that secondary MLC supernate(s) (SN) as a source of IL-2 facilitated the response of small numbers of alloreactive CTL-P in micro-MLC (MacDonald *et al.*, 1978; Ryser and MacDonald, 1979). Optimal CTL responses in MLC also require the presence of accessory cells (including macrophages) which are usually provided for by the stimulating spleen cells. To define optimal microculture conditions in the syngeneic tumor system under investigation, it was therefore considered important to add, in addition to irradiated MoLV-derived tumor (stimulator) cells and secondary MLC SN, a source of accessory cells in the form of irradiated syngeneic spleen cells. When the requirement for these various supplements was tested in experiments in which micro-MLTC contained a standard number (6000/culture) of C57BL/6 regressor (responder) spleen cells, a requirement for all three supplements (stimulator cells, accessory cells, and secondary MLC SN) in the generation of optimal numbers of cytolytic microcultures was demonstrated (Brunner *et al.*, 1980). In a similar experiment presented in Fig. 1, a secondary MLTC population (obtained following restimulation *in vitro* of C57BL/6 regressor spleen cells) was chosen as a source of responder cells, and 2, 10, and 50 of these cells were cultured in the presence of irradiated syngeneic MB1-2 tumor (stimulator) cells, irradiated syngeneic spleen (accessory) cells, and/or secondary MLC SN. On day 7 of culture, each of 24 replicate microcultures was assayed for cytolytic activity against 2×10^3 ^{51}Cr-labeled MB1-2 target cells. Results show that optimal culture conditions again depended on the presence of all three supplements (stimulating cells, accessory cells, and secondary MLC SN). Generation of cytolytically active microcultures was dependent upon both antigenic stimulation and presence of secondary MLC SN, since no significant responses were seen when responder cells were either cultured with secondary MLC SN and irradiated syngeneic spleen cells or with stimulator cells and spleen cells.

On the other hand, a considerable although suboptimal number of positive microcultures was observed in the presence of stimulating cells and sedondary MLC SN, but absence of syngeneic spleen cells. This suggests a relative but not absolute requirement for accessory cells. However, since stimulating tumor cells were obtained from ascites fluid, suboptimal numbers of accessory cells contaminating the tumor cells may have been introduced into the cultures.

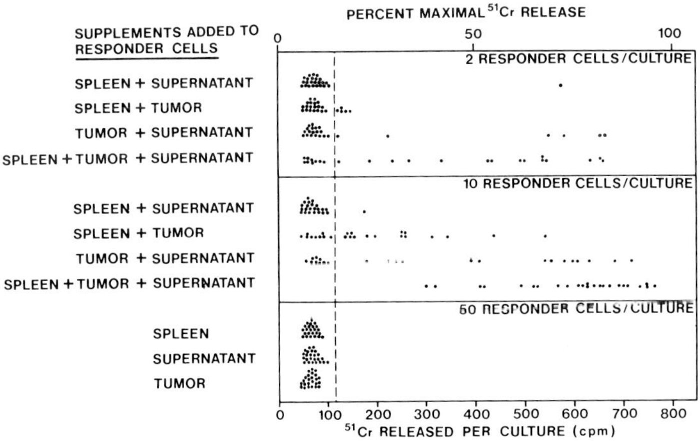

Fig. 1. Optimal microculture conditions for induction of MoLV-specific CTL. Groups of 24 microwells containing 2, 10, or 50 C57BL/6 secondary MLTC (responder) cells were supplemented with secondary MLC SN and/or irradiated MoLV-derived syngeneic (MB1-2) lymphoma cells (tumor) and/or irradiated syngeneic spleen cells (spleen) as indicated. After 7 days, microwells were assessed for cytotoxicity against ^{51}Cr-labeled MB1-2 target cells. The dotted line represent 3 S.D. above the mean ^{51}Cr release value in a group of 24 control microwells containing cell supplements but no responder cells.

II. FREQUENCY DETERMINATION OF MoLV-SPECIFIC CTL PRECURSORS

Since CTL responses could be detected with small numbers of primed responder cells in micro-MLTC supplemented with syngeneic MoLV-derived tumor (stimulator) cells, normal syngeneic spleen cells, and secondary MLC SN, it was also possible to estimate the frequency of MoLV-specific CTL-P contained in various lymphoid cell populations by applying limiting dilution analysis. As described in detail in previous communications (Brunner *et al.*, 1980; Weiss *et al.*, 1980), various (limiting) numbers of responder cells were placed in micro-MLTC and the cultures assayed on day 7–8 for cytolytic activity. Positive cultures were defined as those in which ^{51}Cr-release exceeded spontaneous release values by three standard deviations (determined in a group of parallel wells which contained irradiated stimulating cells and secondary MLC SN but no responder cells). Minimal estimates of CTL-P frequencies were calculated by analysis of the Poisson distribution relationship between the number of responding cells per microculture and the percentage of nonresponding cultures. Experimental values were fitted to the zero-order term Poisson equation by the minimum χ^2 method (Taswell, 1981). Figure 2 shows an example of such a determination. The experiment from which the data are derived was one of a series designed to answer the question of a possible selective accumulation of MoLV-specific CTL-P in tumor tissue at the time of tumor rejection. To this end, limiting numbers of lymphoid cells obtained from tumors, blood, or spleen of C57BL/6 mice injected 10 days previously with MSV–MoLV complex were cultured in micro-MLTC with 3×10^4 irradiated syngeneic MB1–2 lymphoma cells, 10^6 irradiated syngeneic spleen cells, and 25% (v/v) secondary MLC SN (Brunner *et al.*, 1981). After 7 days incubation, sets of 24 replicate microcultures were assayed for cytolytic activity against 2000 ^{51}Cr-labeled MB1–2 target cells in a 3.5 hr test, and CTL-P frequencies determined as described. Results presented in Fig. 2 show frequencies of 1/87, 1/468, and 1/936 for tumors, PBL, and spleens, respectively, i.e., 5- to 11-fold higher in the tumors as compared to blood and spleen. These results strongly suggested selective accumulation of MoLV-specific CTL-P in tumor tissue at the time of onset of tumor regression.

Limiting dilution analysis was further applied to the evaluation of the effect of *in vivo* and *in vitro* immunization on the frequency of MoLV-specific CTL-P in various lymphoid cell populations. Table I summarizes results obtained in six (or more) experiments for each of the populations tested. It can be seen that spleens obtained 15 days after immunization with MSV–MoLV complex contained CTL-P at an almost 10-fold higher frequency than normal spleens, while secondary stimulation *in vitro* with syngeneic MoLV-derived lymphoma cells resulted in a further 100-fold increase. These results (including those presented in Fig. 1) also illustrate the high plating efficiency of CTL-P contained in secondary MLTC populations, reaching at a CTL-P frequency of 1/3, at least 50%.

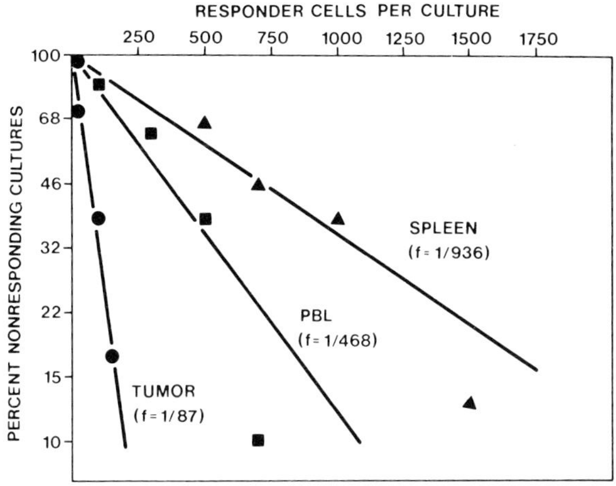

Fig. 2. Frequency determination of MoLV-specific CTL-P in lymphoid cells from tumors, blood, and spleen of C57BL/6 mice injected 10 days previously with MSV–MoLV complex. Frequencies were calculated by fitting experimental values to the zero-order term Poisson equation by the minimum χ^2 method. The nonresponding cultures are those which were negative for cytolytic activity against MB1-2 target cells.

III. ISOLATION AND MAINTENANCE OF MoLV-SPECIFIC CTL CLONES

The dramatic increase in frequency of MoLV-specific CTL-P (from 1/500 up to 1/2) after *in vitro* restimulation of C57BL/6 regressor spleen cells suggested the use of secondary MLTC cells as a source of responder cells in attempts to generate directly large numbers of MoLV-specific CTL clones. Very small

TABLE I

Effect of Immunization on the Frequency of MoLV-Specific CTL-P in C57BL/6 Mice[a]

Immunization	Lymphoid cell population	Mean frequency (reciprocal)
None	Spleen	7400
In vivo	Spleen (day 10)	806
	PBL (day 10)	430
	Tumor (day 10)	83
	Spleen (day 15)	480
In vivo–in vitro	Secondary MLTC (day 7)	4

[a] Normal or regressor lymphoid cells or secondary MLTC cells from C57BL/6 mice were stimulated with irradiated MoLV-derived syngeneic MB1-2 lymphoma cells under limiting dilution micro-MLTC conditions described in Fig. 1. Microcultures were assayed for cytotoxicity against ^{51}Cr-labeled MB1-2 target cells, and CTL-P frequencies calculated as described in Fig. 2.

(limiting) number of secondary MLTC responder cells (1–3 per well) could be used (see results with 2 responder cells per well, Fig. 1), thus assuring a relatively high probability that the CTL populations generated in individual microcultures were indeed derived from single precursors (i.e., were monoclonal), even at a relatively high percentage of positive cultures. In addition, individual secondary MLTC cells could be isolated by micromanipulation and directly plated. This latter technique is now currently used in our laboratory to reclone CTL populations obtained by limiting dilution (See Section IV).

Since positive micro-MLTC were typically found to contain from 1 to 5 × 10^4 CTL, it was possible to split the content of individual microwells for direct assay on a panel of up to five target cell types. For further analysis, selected populations were expanded and maintained by serial restimulation as described elsewhere (Weiss *et al.*, 1980). Many of the clones could be maintained for extended periods of time, i.e., from several months to over 1 year, without loss of activity or specificity, and without development of gross chromosomal abnormalities (Weiss *et al.*, 1980). However, considerable variations in growth potential of individual isolates were observed, some of the clones being lost after one or several expansions. Cytolytic activity against the stimulating lymphoma cells was high for most of the clones assayed, leading to 50% target cell lysis in a 3.5 hr ^{51}Cr release assay at lymphocyte to target cell ratios of 0.3:1 to 3:1 (Fig. 5 and Weiss *et al.*, 1980; Brunner *et al.*, 1981).

IV. SPECIFICITY OF MoLV-SPECIFIC CTL CLONES

The studies so far described have shown that it was possible to study the frequency of MoLV-specific CTL-P, and as a direct corollary, to approach cloning by first enriching for MoLV-specific CTL in secondary mass cultures (secondary MLTC) followed by the application of limiting dilution or micromanipulation techniques. In using this approach, we have generated large numbers of clones and assayed them directly (or after recloning and/or expansion) for specificity by two methods, one involving the use of a panel of target cells and the other inhibition of lytic activity with monoclonal antibodies.

In a first study in C57BL/6 mice, large numbers of CTL clones were generated with limiting numbers (1–3/well) of secondary MLTC (responder) cells and syngeneic MB1–2 lymphoma (stimulator) cells in micro-MLTC. After 7 days of incubation, the cultures were split and tested for cytolytic activity on four target cell types, i.e., syngeneic MB1–2 (*H-2*^{b}) and allogeneic LSTRA (*H-2*^{d}) MoLV-derived lymphoma cells, and unrelated P815 and E1–4 tumor cells of the same haplotypes. A series of selected clones (14) were subcloned by limiting dilution, expanded in 1 ml cultures and assessed using the four tumor targets employed in the initial screening procedure. Results revealed three distinct specificity patterns (Weiss *et al.*, 1980). The majority of the clones lysed only syngeneic MoLV-derived target cells. A subpopulation, however, lysed allogeneic ($H\text{-}2^d$) target cells, either MoLV-derived or not, in addition to syngeneic MoLV-derived target cells. The third pattern, which was quite rare, involved lysis of both types of MoLV-derived but no detectable lysis of the unrelated target cells. All specificity phenotypes were found to be stable by recloning experiments.

More recently, we have attempted to select for MoLV-specific $H\text{-}2^b$ CTL clones which also react with $H\text{-}2^d$ alloantigens (or $H\text{-}2^d$ restricted MoLV-specific antigens) by making conjugates between cells from C57BL/6 secondary MLTC populations and either P815 ($H\text{-}2^d$) tumor or LSTRA ($H\text{-}2^d$) MoLV-associated tumor cells. These conjugates were then micromanipulated into microwells and grown up in the presence of syngeneic MB1–2 stimulator cells, syngeneic spleen cells, and secondary MLC SN. Clones so derived were then tested for cytolytic activity against syngeneic (MB1–2) or allogeneic (LSTRA) MoLV-derived target cells. In addition, concanavalin A (Con-A) blasts from the congeneic strains B10.D2 ($H\text{-}2K^dD^d$), B10A.5R ($H\text{-}2K^bD^d$), and B10.HTG ($H\text{-}2K^dD^b$) were included as target cells in an effort to more precisely define the specificity which is cross-reactive with $H\text{-}2^d$.

Figure 3 shows the specificity patterns of two clones showing clearly defined cross-reactivity with $H\text{-}2K^d$ or $H\text{-}2D^d$, respectively, confirming that CTL clones with cross-reactivity between MoLV-associated H-2 determinants and allogeneic unmodified H-2 determinants exist (Weiss *et al.*, 1980; MacDonald *et al.*,

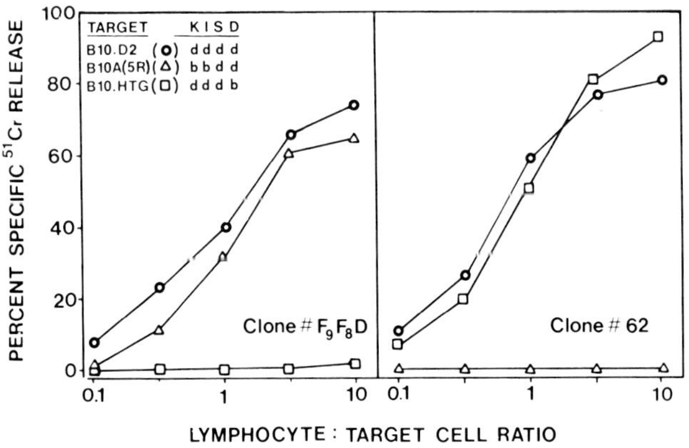

Fig. 3. Cross-reactivity of MoLV-specific C57BL/6 CTL clones. Two clones selected on the basis of cross-reactivity with allogeneic ($H\text{-}2^d$) tumor cells were expanded and assayed for cytotoxicity against ^{51}Cr-labeled Con-A blasts from B10.D2, B10.A (5R), and B10.HTG mice. Both clones also lysed MoLV-derived $H\text{-}2^b$ and $H\text{-}2^d$ tumor cells (not shown). (Reprinted from MacDonald *et al.*, 1982.)

1982). Figure 4 presents results of an experiment in which 88 conjugates between secondary MLTC cells and allogeneic LSTRA tumor cells were micromanipulated into microwells and grown up in the presence of MB1-2 stimulator cells. When the cultures (of which 66 showed visible growth upon microscopic examination) were tested for cytolytic activity against the syngeneic MB1-2 and the allogeneic LSTRA targets, 70 were found to be positive on MB1-2 and 28 (40%) of these were also positive on LSTRA, while none were cytolytic for LSTRA cells only. Of the 28 cultures cytolytic for both targets, 14 (20%) appeared clearly to be "double reactors," lysing both the syngeneic and the allogeneic tumor cells to a similar degree.

The results of this experiment demonstrate the power of micromanipulation as a tool for direct cloning from lymphoid cell populations strongly enriched in CTL-P, and suggest its potential application in selective cloning of CTL-P form-

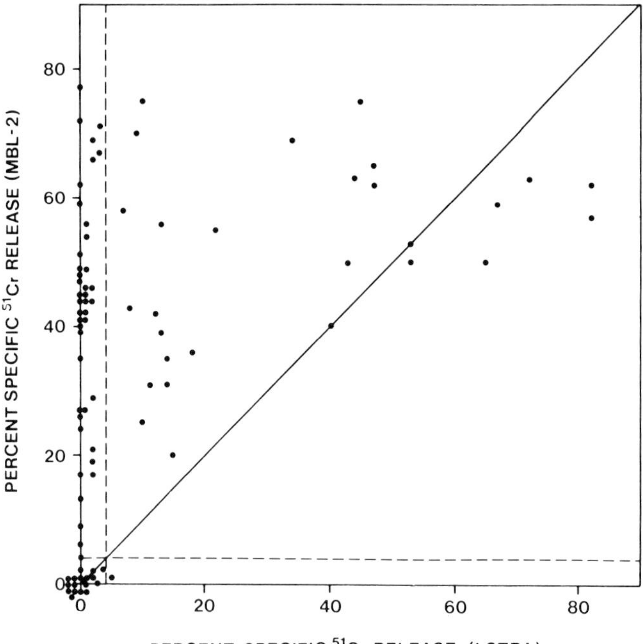

Fig. 4. Cross-reactivity of MoLV-specific C57BL/6 CTL clones. Eighty-eight conjugates between C57BL/6 secondary MLTC cells and allogeneic MoLV-derived LSTRA tumor cells were micromanipulated into wells of a 96-well microplate and stimulated with 3×10^4 irradiated (5000 rad) syngeneic MB1-2 tumor cells in the presence of 10^6 irradiated (2000 rad) syngeneic spleen cells and 25% (v/v) secondary MLC SN. After 7 days, the wells were assessed microscopically for cell growth, and the content of each microculture split and tested for cytotoxicity against ^{51}Cr-labeled MB1-2 and LSTRA target cells. Each point represents the activity of a single clone tested against the two targets.

ing antigen-specific conjugates. The fact that 70 of the 88 conjugates plated gave rise to cytolytic microcultures shows the high plating efficiency (80%) of the system, allowing the isolation of large numbers of unambiguous clones in one step. Similarly high plating efficiencies are encountered when individual secondary MLTC cells rather than conjugates are micromanipulated into micro-MLTC (results not shown). On the other hand, further studies are needed to demonstrate clearly that antigen-specific CTL can be enriched by this conjugate method. The fact that about 20% of the conjugate-forming clones were clearly "double reactors" (as compared to less than 3% of clones derived from secondary MLTC and 7% from regressor cell populations) (Weiss *et al.*, 1980; Brunner *et al.*, 1980) suggests enrichment in such clones, but also demonstrates that many of the conjugates must have been nonspecific. On the other hand, the fact that all the microcultures which were microscopically positive for growth were cytolytic shows that all conjugates giving rise to growth were formed with CTL-P.

The panel of target cells used to study the specificity of clones reactive with MoLV-associated antigens was further extended to include tumor target cell lines induced by Friend, Gross, or radiation-leukemia viruses. Studies of CTL activity at the population level had shown cross-reactivity between Friend, Moloney, and Rauscher (FMR) leukemia virus-associated antigens and lack of cross-reactivity with Gross virus associated antigens suggesting the main reactive antigen to be an "FMR-like" substance (Gomard *et al.*, 1978; Plata and Lilly, 1979). In an experiment presented in Fig. 5, four CTL clones directly derived by limiting dilution from MSV–MoLV-induced tumors in C57BL/6 mice (Brunner *et al.*, 1981) were expanded and subsequently tested in parallel for cytolytic activity against 6 target cell lines: MB1–2, the stimulating C57BL/6 MoLV-derived lymphoma, RB1–5, a C57BL/6 Rauscher leukemia virus-derived lymphoma line which may in fact be superinfected with MoLV (Taniyama and Holden, 1979); B.GV, a BALB.B ($H\text{-}2^b$) Gross-virus induced lymphoma; HF1/B, a BALB.B ($H\text{-}2^b$) Friend virus-induced lymphoma; TC-96, a (C57BL/6 × A)F_1 ($H\text{-}2^b \times H\text{-}2K^kD^d$)$F_1$ Friend virus-induced lymphoma, and RLV 136.5, a C57BL/6 radiation-leukemia virus-induced tumor line. As shown by the results in Figure 5, both Moloney and Rauscher virus induced lines (MB1–2 and RB1–5), as well as one of the two Friend virus-induced lines (HF1/B) were lysed by all four clones, whereas the three other lines (TC-96, B.GV, RLV 136.5) were resistant. All four clones showed approximately the same (low) reactivity against the HF1/B line and the same (strong) reactivity against the MB1–2 line, whereas two clones showed a considerably higher reactivity against RB1–5 than against MB1–2 cells, pointing to considerable heterogeneity at the clonal level of MoLV-specific CTL. Lysis of the HF1/B line appears to confirm, and lack of lysis of TC-96 to contradict, cross-reactivity between Moloney and Friend virus-associated antigens. However, definite conclusions cannot be drawn without further studies demonstrating the presence (or absence) of relevant viral and

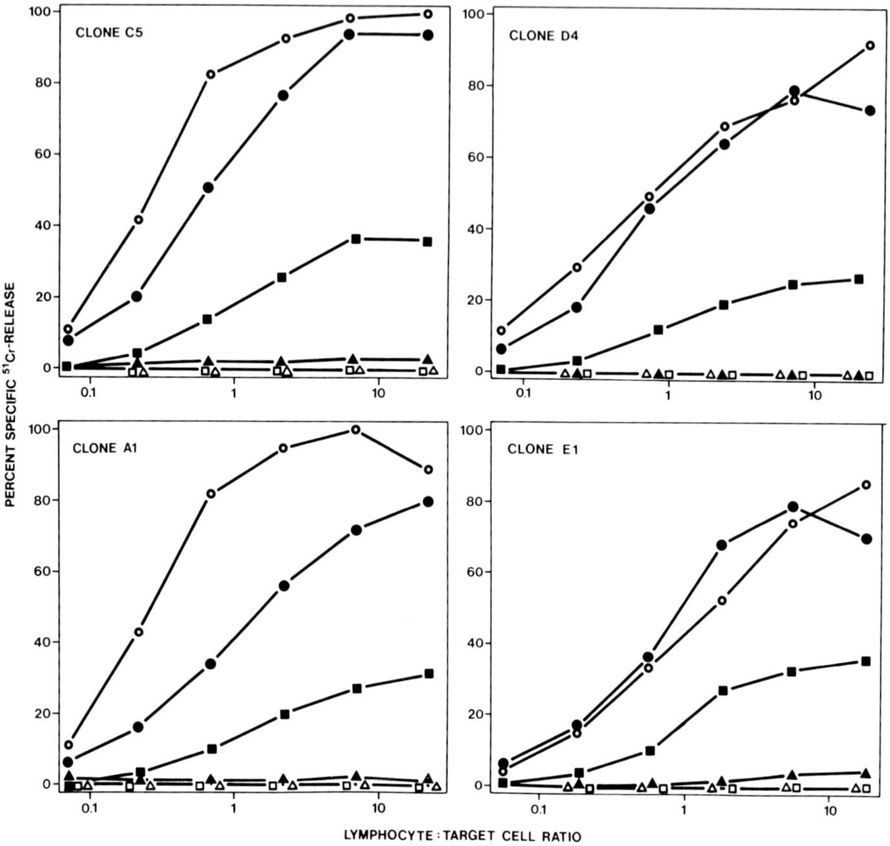

Fig. 5. Specificity of MoLV-specific C57BL/6 CTL clones. Four clones (C5, D4, A1, and E1) isolated by limiting dilution micro-MLTC from lymphoid cells infiltrating MSV–MoLV-induced tumors were expanded and assayed for cytolytic activity against six ^{51}Cr-labeled target cell types: MB1–2 and RB1–5, two C57BL/6 MoLV-derived lymphomas (●, ○); HF1/B (BALB.B) and TC-96 (B10 × A.BY)F_1, two Friend virus-induced erythroleukemia cell lines (■, ▲); B.GV, a BALB.B Gross virus-induced lymphoma (△); and RLV 136.5, a C57BL/6 radiation leukemia virus-induced lymphoma (□).

H-2 antigens at the respective target cell surfaces. Lack of lysis of B.GV cells agrees with results showing lack of cross-reactivity between the FMR group viruses and the Gross virus, and lack of lysis of the RLV 1365 (radiation leukemia) line confirms lack of reactivity with a line induced in C57BL/6 mice with an unrelated virus. Studies with large numbers of clones and better defined target cells, preferably freshly infected lymphoid cells (Gomard *et al.*, 1980; Collavo *et al.*, 1981; Stukart *et al.*, 1981), are needed to answer the question of cross-reactivity between cells infected with different serologically defined murine RNA leukemia viruses at the clonal level.

An alternative approach to the analysis of clonal specificity of MoLV-specific CTL was based on the use of monoclonal antibodies directed against H-2 determinants on the target cells to inhibit lysis. As shown previously at the population level, MoLV-specific CTL preferentially lyse syngeneic MoLV-derived tumor target cells, and (monoclonal) antibodies directed against appropriate H-2 (restriction) determinants inhibit target cell lysis (Lindahl and Lemke, 1979). In extending these studies to the clonal level, we have evaluated the inhibitory effect of three monoclonal antibodies, two directed against H-2D^b determinants and one against H-2K^b, on the lytic interaction between CTL clones and MoLV-derived syngeneic target cells. The analysis was performed on six established cloned CTL lines (Weiss *et al.*, 1980) as well as on a series of 51 short-term putative clones (Weiss *et al.*, 1981) in the C57BL/6 anti-MSV–MoLV system. In the experiment involving the six CTL lines, MB1–2 (C57BL/6) target cells were pretreated with varying concentrations of the monoclonal antibodies prior to the exposure to cloned CTL. Results showed that cytolysis was inhibited in a dose-dependent fashion by anti-H-2D^b antibodies but not by anti-H-2K^b antibodies in every case. The same result was obtained in experiments with short-term CTL clones. Figure 6 illustrates the results of such an experiment in which 96 microcultures were prepared. Of these, 20 were cytolytic for MB1–2 cells. In cultures tested in the presence of the anti-H-2^b alloantiserum (Fig. 6a), significant inhibition of cytolysis by all 20 putative clones was observed. Similarly, both the anti-H-2D^b monoclonal antibodies inhibited the activity of 19 out of 20 clones to a comparable degree (Fig. 6b and d). It should be noted that the clone that could not be inhibited by either of the two anti-H-2D^b antibodies was the same one, and this clone was inhibited by the anti-whole haplotype antiserum. As shown in Fig. 6c, none of the clones was significantly inhibited by a concentration of the anti-H-2K^b monoclonal antibody which resulted in 90% inhibition of lysis of the same target cells by alloreactive effector cells. In fact, all three monoclonal antibodies had previously been characterized in terms of their ability to inhibit specifically the lytic activity of alloreactive CTL populations directed against the relevant determinants H-2D^b and H-2K^b.

In this experiment and others, a total of 51 independent C57BL/6 clones were assessed for restriction to the *H-2D^b* and *H-2K^b* regions by using these monoclonal reagents. Restriction to the *H-2D^b* region was observed in 44 of these 51 clones. Of the remaining 7 clones, none was inhibited by the anti-H-2K^b antibody, and 3 were inhibited by anti-whole *H-2^b* haplotype antiserum. It is thus evident that the recognition of MoLV-associated antigens by the majority of CTL clones was restricted to the *H-2D^b* region as defined by the monoclonal antibodies used, and that there exists limited heterogeneity in the *H-2* restriction of such clones.

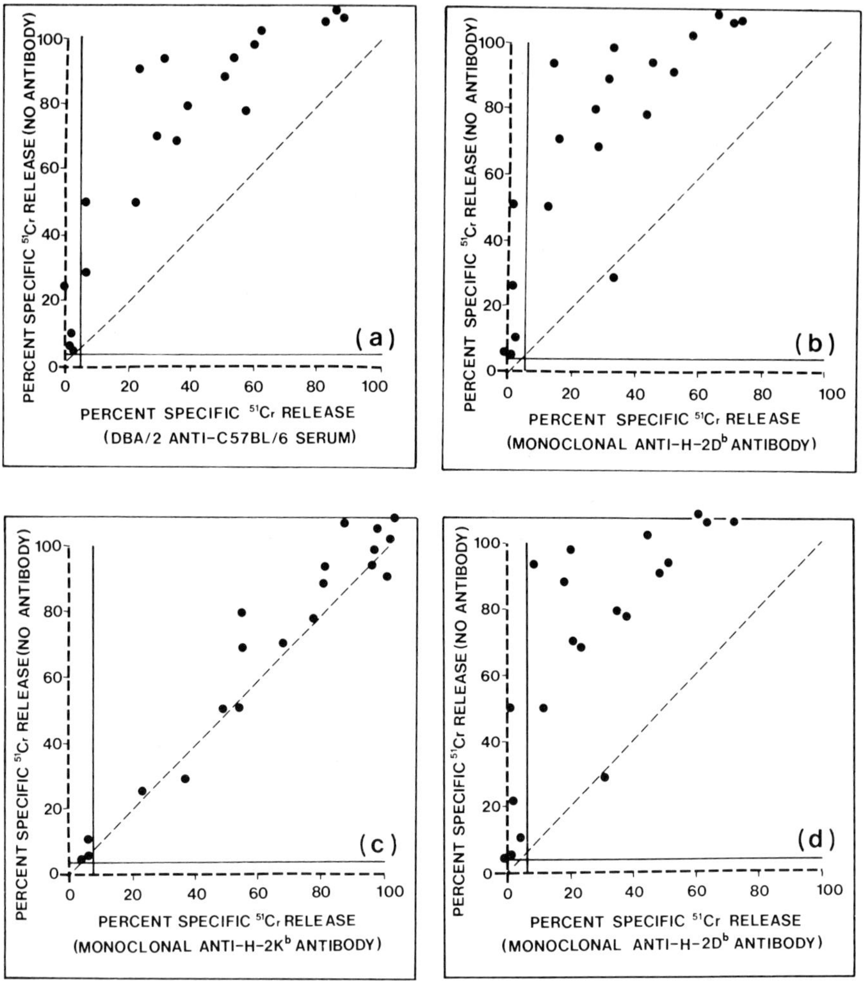

Fig. 6. Ability of monoclonal antibodies to inhibit the lytic activity of MoLV-specific CTL clones. Micro-MLTC prepared under limiting dilution conditions with C57BL/6 regressor spleen cells were assessed for cell growth microscopically, and positive microcultures (20 of 96) were split into 5 aliquots. Each aliquot was assessed for cytolytic activity against 2000 ^{51}Cr-labeled MB1-2 target cells which had been incubated with or without antibody. The cytolytic activity observed in the absence of antibody was compared to that obtained with 1:40 dilution of DBA-2 anti-C57BL/6 alloantiserum, anti-H-2^{b} (a); 1:100 dilution of B-22-249-RI, anti-H-2D^{b} antibody (b); 1:100 dilution of B8-24-1, anti-H-2K^{b} antibody (c); or H141-40, anti-H-2D^{b} antibody (d). (Reprinted from Weiss *et al.*, 1981).

V. SURFACE PHENOTYPE OF MoLV-SPECIFIC CTL CLONES

The surface phenotype of a number of MoLV-specific CTL clones has been investigated using monoclonal antibodies and the fluorescence activated cell sorter (FACS). All clones tested thus far expressed readily detectable amounts of Thy-1 and Lyt-2 alloantigens. When the Lyt phenotype of three MoLV-specific C57BL/6 clones was compared to that of normal thymocytes (Weiss *et al.*, 1980), it was found that both Lyt-1 and Lyt-2 antigens were expressed on the surface of the cells of all three clones, that the Lyt-1 density of the clones was at least equivalent to that on thymocytes, and that Lyt-2 appeared even more abundant. However, there was heterogeneity in the density of Lyt-1 among the clones, the quantity of Lyt-1 on one clone being twice that seen on the two others. Since it has been observed by Glasebrook and Fitch (1980) that a significant number of CTL clones do not stain above background levels for Lyt-1, and since most (if not all) CTL precursors are of the Lyt-1^+2^+ phenotype (Teh and Teh, 1980; Cerottini and MacDonald, 1981) it would seem possible that loss of expression of Lyt-1 may occur during propagation of certain CTL clones. Such a loss was not, however, observed with the three MoLV-specific clones described above, since the stability of the difference in Lyt-1 expression in time was confirmed in determinations 2 months apart.

VI. CONCLUSIONS

In the present chapter, we have summarized recent results from our laboratory describing the generation and the properties of MoLV-specific CTL clones. The results demonstrate that the techniques developed in allogeneic systems were directly applicable to a syngeneic system, i.e., that it was possible to approach cloning as a direct corollary of studies examining the frequency of specific CTL-P by first enriching for antigen-specific cells of the CTL lineage by a short culture period (typically 6–7 days) and directly to clone CTL from these enriched populations by limiting dilution or micromanipulation techniques. Most of the clones thus obtained were found to have high cytolytic activity (50% lysis of lymphocyte–target cell ratios ranging from 0.3 : 1 to 3 : 1) and many could be maintained *in vitro* apparently indefinitely in the presence of IL-2 and specific antigen. Such clones were stable in terms of activity and specificity, had apparently normal DNA content, and expressed Thy-1, Lyt-1, and Lyt-2 surface antigens. Specificity analysis indicated restriction of the majority of C57BL/6 MoLV-specific clones to H-$2D^b$ determinants, and a relatively high degree of cross-reactivity with unmodified allogeneic target cells, suggesting considerable overlap between populations reactive with modified syngeneic and allogeneic MHC determinants.

ACKNOWLEDGMENTS

We thank Dr. U. Hämmerling, Deutsches Krebsforschungzentrum, Heidelberg, GFR, and Dr. G. Köhler, Basel Institute for Immunology, Switzerland, for the generous gifts of monoclonal antibodies; Dr. F. Plata, Pasteur Institute, Paris, France, for the HF1/B cells; Dr. B. Chesebro, Rocky Mountain Laboratory, Hamilton, Montana, for the TC-96 cells; and Dr. E. Kedar, The Lautenberg Center for General and Tumor Immunology, the Hebrew University-Hadassah Medical School, Jerusalem, Israel, for the RLV 136.5 cells. We also wish to thank C. Contat and C. Horvath for expert technical assistance.

REFERENCES

Brunner, K. T., MacDonald, H. R., and Cerottini, J.-C. (1980). Antigenic specificity of the cytolytic T lymphocyte (CTL) response to murine sarcoma virus-induced tumors. II. Analysis of the clonal progeny of CTL precursors stimulated *in vitro* with syngeneic tumor cells. *J. Immunol.* **124,** 1627.

Brunner, K. T., MacDonald, H. R., and Cerottini, J.-C. (1981). Quantitation and clonal isolation of cytolytic T lymphocyte precursors selectively infiltrating murine sarcoma virus-induced tumors. *J. Exp. Med.* **154,** 362.

Cerottini, J.-C., and MacDonald, H. R. (1981). Limiting dilution analysis of alloantigen-reactive T lymphocytes. V. Lyt phenotype of cytolytic T lymphocyte precursors reactive against normal and mutant H-2 antigens. *J. Immunol.* **126,** 490.

Collavo, D., Zanovello, P., Biasi, G., and Chieco-Bianci, L. (1981). T lymphocyte tolerance and early appearance of virus-induced cell surface antigens in Moloney-murine leukemia virus neonatally injected mice. *J. Immunol.* **126,** 187.

Glasebrook, A. L., and Fitch, F. W. (1980). Alloreactive cloned T cell lines. I. Interactions between cloned amplifier and cytolytic T cell clones. *J. Exp. Med.* **151,** 876.

Gomard, E., Duprez, V., Reme, T., Colombani, M. J., and Levy, J. P. (1977). Exclusive involvement of $H\text{-}2D^b$ or $H\text{-}2K^b$ product in the interaction between T-killer lymphocytes and syngeneic $H\text{-}2^b$ and $H\text{-}2^d$ viral lymphomas. *J. Exp. Med.* **146,** 909.

Gomard, E., Levy, J. P., Plata, F., Henin, Y., Duprez, V., Bismuth, A., and Reme, T. (1978). Studies on the nature of the cell surface antigen reacting with cytolytic T lymphocytes in murine oncornavirus-induced tumors. *Eur. J. Immunol.* **8,** 228.

Gomard, E., Henin, Y., Colombani, M. J., and Levy, J. P. (1980). Immune response genes control T killer cell response against Moloney tumor antigen cytolysis regulating reactions against the best available H-2 + viral antigen association. *J. Exp. Med.* **151,** 1468.

Levy, J. P., and Leclerc, J. C. (1977). The murine sarcoma virus-induced tumor: Exceptions or general model in tumor immunology? *Adv. Cancer Res.* **24,** 1.

Lindahl, K. F., and Lemke, H. (1979). Inhibition of killer-target cell interaction by monoclonal anti-H-2 antibodies. *Eur. J. Immunol.* **9,** 526.

MacDonald H. R., Ryser, J.-E., Engers, H. D., Brunner, K. T., and Cerottini, J.-C. (1978). Differentiation pathway of murine cytolytic T lymphocytes: Analysis by limiting dilution. *In* "Human Lymphocyte Differentiation: Its Application to Cancer" (B. Serrou and C. Rosenfeld, eds.), pp. 23–28. Elsevier/North-Holland Biomedical Press, Amsterdam.

MacDonald, H. R., Sekaly, R. P., Kanagawa, O., Thiernesse, N., Taswell, C., Cerottini, J.-C., Weiss, A., Glasebrook, A. L., Engers, H. D., Kelso, A., Brunner, K. T., and Bron, C. (1982). Cytolytic T lymphocyte clones. *Immunobiol.* **161,** 84–106.

Maryanski, J. L., MacDonald, H. R., and Cerottini, J.-C. (1980). Limiting dilution analysis of alloantigen-reactive T lymphocytes. IV. High frequency of cytolytic T lymphocyte precursor cells in MLC blasts separated by velocity sedimentation. *J. Immunol.* **124,** 42.

Plata, F., and Lilly, F. (1979). Viral specificity of H-2 restricted T killer cells directed against syngeneic tumors induced by Gross, Friend, or Rauscher leukemia virus. *J. Exp. Med.* **150,** 1174.

Plata, F., Cerottini, J.-C., and Brunner, K. T. (1975). Primary and secondary *in vitro* generation of cytolytic T lymphocytes in the murine sarcoma virus system. *Eur. J. Immunol.* **5,** 227.

Plata, F., Jongeneel, V., Cerottini, J.-C., and Brunner, K. T. (1976). Antigenic specificity of the cytolytic T lymphocyte (CTL) response to murine sarcoma virus generated secondary CTL with syngeneic tumor cells. *Eur. J. Immunol.* **6,** 823.

Ryser, J.-E., and MacDonald, H. R. (1979). Limiting dilution analysis of alloantigen-reactive T lymphocytes. I. Comparison of precursor frequencies for proliferative and cytolytic responses. *J. Immunol.* **122,** 1691.

Smith, K. A. (1980). T cell growth factor. *Immunol. Rev.* **51,** 337.

Stukart, M. J., Vos, A., and Melief, C. J. M. (1981). Cytotoxic T cell response against lymphoblasts infected with Moloney (Abelson) murine leukemia virus. Methodological aspects and H-2 requirements. *Eur. J. Immunol.* **11,** 251.

Taniyama, T., and Holden, H. T. (1979). *In vitro* induction of T-lymphocyte-mediated cytotoxicity by infectious murine type C oncornaviruses. *J. Exp. Med.* **150,** 1367.

Taswell, C. (1981). Limiting dilution assays for the determination of immunocompetent cell frequencies. I. Data analysis. *J. Immunol.* **126,** 1614.

Teh, H.-S., and Teh, S.-J. (1980). The use of a clonal assay for cytotoxic T lymphocytes to determine the Ly phenotypes of the cytotoxic precursors and effector cells to alloantigens and trinitrophenyl-modified self antigens. *J. Immunol.* **125,** 1977.

Weiss, A., Brunner, K. T., MacDonald, H. R., and Cerottini, J.-C. (1980). Antigenic specificity of the cytolytic T lymphocyte response to murine sarcoma virus-induced tumors. III. Characterization of cytolytic T lymphocyte clones specific for Moloney leukemia virus-associated cell surface antigens. *J. Exp. Med.* **152,** 1210.

Weiss, A., MacDonald, H. R., Cerottini, J.-C., and Brunner, K. T. (1981). Inhibition of cytolytic T lymphocyte clones reactive with Moloney leukemia virus-associated antigens by monoclonal antibodies: A direct approach to the study of H-2 restriction. *J. Immunol.* **126,** 482.

25

The Specificity Repertoire of Cytolytic T Lymphocytes

Linda A. Sherman

I.	Analysis of Receptor Specificity	314
II.	CTL Receptor Repertoire of the B10.D2 Anti-H-$2K^b$ Response	315
III.	Specificity Repertoire of the bm11 Anti-H-$2K^b$ Response	317
IV.	The C57BL/6 Anti-bm11 CTL Response: A Model for Determinant Recognition	319
V.	The Influence of MHC on Receptor Repertoire	320
	References	322

Perhaps the most unique feature of the immune system is the diversity of lymphocyte receptors. Recent advances in understanding of the organization and expression of structural genes for the immunoglobulin variable region have begun to provide an appreciation of how the organism may effect such extensive diversity (Johnson *et al.*, 1981). Indeed, it would appear that molecular mechanisms are sufficiently diverse and sophisticated that the challenge to the immune system may not necessarily be the ability to construct a particular antigen-specific receptor but rather selectively to recruit receptors which are most valuable to both the organism and the species. In order to probe mechanisms responsible for repertoire selection, it is necessary to develop methods for describing the receptor repertoire. It should then be possible to assess the influence of a variety of environmental and genetic variables on repertoire selection.

This laboratory has developed an experimental system which permits analysis of the receptor repertoire of cytolytic T lymphocytes (CTL) (Sherman, 1980). As described below, these analyses have provided new information concerning both the receptor repertoire of T cells and the antigenic determinants which are recognized. The results suggest a novel view of determinant recognition. In addition, this experimental approach permits genetic analysis of repertoire as demonstrated by comparison of inbred murine strains which differ in their major histocompatibility complex (MHC).

ISOLATION, CHARACTERIZATION, AND UTILIZATION OF T LYMPHOCYTE CLONES

ISBN 0-12-249920-4

I. ANALYSIS OF RECEPTOR SPECIFICITY

The strategy currently used in our laboratory to identify receptor specificity is based on analysis of alloantigen-specific monoclonal CTL using a panel of closely related antigens. The alloantigen used in these studies is the H-2K^b molecule, and the panel consists of seven different K^b mutants each of which differ from the standard (wild type) H-2K^b molecule by only one or two amino acid substitutions (Nairn *et al.,* 1980). The distribution of the particular determinant recognized by a receptor among the members of the panel serves to describe receptor specificity. This approach was based on the observation that a population of K^b-specific CTL contained CTL clones which could be fractionated on the basis of monolayer adsorption using a K^b mutant (Klein, 1978).

The main advantage of this method is that it provides a description of all antigen-stimulated receptor specificities. Therefore, assuming minimum selective pressure is involved in the method used in obtaining antigen-specific CTL clones, the results should provide a representative profile of the repertoire under consideration. Of the methods currently available for obtaining CTL clones, the techniques involved in stimulation of CTL precursors under limiting dilution culture conditions are most suitable for obtaining large numbers of antigen-specific CTL clones with minimum danger of skewing the repertoire, and is, therefore, most suitable for repertoire studies. However, clones obtained in limiting dilution cultures must first be expanded before they are of sufficient size to test on all members of the panel. Such expansion has been achieved by further incubation of each clone in media containing T cell growth factor(s). After 6 days in culture, successfully expanded clones are tested for lytic activity on 9 different targets. These include the wild type (Kh), 7 different K^b mutants, and D2.GD (H-2K^d, D^b) which serves as a negative control and also indicates if lysis involves recognition of the D^b molecule which is present on all members of the panel.

For this analysis, it is of critical importance that the specificity observed is the result of a single CTL clone. Several precautions are taken to assure a high probability of monoclonality. First, clones are initially obtained from limiting dilution cultures in which the CTL precursor is the limiting entity as determined on the basis of the correlation with statistical predictions for a single hit phenomenon (Miller *et al.,* 1977). Second, the number of responder cells placed in each microculture well is such that 20% or less of all wells contain an H-2K^b-specific CTL precursor. The probability that each positive well is monoclonal is then 90% or more. Finally, after panel analysis is performed, clones are only considered if lysis on all members of the panel either falls above 60% (positive) or below 25% (negative) of the value on the homologous target. This attempts to avoid wells containing two or more clones, since the admixture of clones with nonidentical specificity would be expected to result in lysis which is highest on the homologous target. It has been found that a higher proportion of cultures than is statistically predicted (10%) result in such "partial" reactivities. To further investigate the basis of such specificity, presumptive clones were recloned and the specificity was investigated. As indicated in Table I, the reactivity pattern (RP) obtained for the subclones is identical to that of the original clones. This would indicate that (1) the fine specificity of a clone is stable and (2) a single clone can give rise to partial reactivity on one or more mutants (Table I, clone B). Nevertheless, in order to avoid ambiguity in the assignment of reactivity patterns, such clones have not been included in repertoire analysis.

II. CTL RECEPTOR REPERTOIRE OF THE B10.D2 ANTI-H-2K^b RESPONSE

An example of the results obtained from panel analysis of the specificity of 78 CTL clones obtained from studies of 20 individual B10.D2 mice is presented in Table II. These clones identify 33 different receptor specificities. In addition, since a determinant is defined on the basis of differential receptor recognition, these 33 different RP define 33 different determinants present on a single alloantigen. One RP which recurs at a comparatively high frequency includes recognition of all the H-2 mutants. These clones may represent H-2K^b-specific receptors which recognize region(s) of the molecule not altered in any of the mutants. However, since it is also possible that a receptor which does not discriminate between the H-2K^b mutants may not be specific for the H-2K^b molecule, this specificity pattern is excluded from further consideration in repertoire analyses.

TABLE I

Stability of Clonal Specificity

	Percent ^{125}I-labeled UdR release from indicated target cells[a]					
	Kh	bm8	bm3	bm4	bm9	bm10
Clone A[b]	*60*	*57*	9	2	*62*	0
subclone	*17*	*19*	0	0	22	1
Clone B[b]	*62*	*48*	33	*47*	*51*	*48*
subclone	*57*	*54*	29	*61*	*50*	*53*

[a] Italic values represent positive recognition of that particular strain.

[b] Expanded CTL clones were subcloned by limiting dilution. Clones obtained from dilutions which yielded <20% positive wells were reexpanded and tested on the indicated targets. Results demonstrated the stability and reproductivity of the phenotypic expression of a single clone. This is true even when partial reactivities are observed as the reactivity on bm3 of clone B and its subclone. Methods involved in obtaining CTL clones by limiting dilution, expanding such clones, and assaying for reactivity on the indicated panel of target cells are as described previously (Sherman, 1980).

TABLE II

The B10.D2 Anti-K^b CTL Repertoire

				bm9	+	+	+	+	−	−	−	−
				bm10	+	+	−	−	+	+	−	−
				bm11	+	−	−	+	+	−	−	+
bm8	bm1	bm3	bm4									
+	+	+	+		9[a]	·	·	·	·	·	·	·
+	+	−	+		·	1	·	·	·	·	·	·
+	−	−	+		·	·	·	1	·	1	1	·
+	−	+	+		4	·	·	2	·	·	·	·
−	+	+	+		3	·	·	·	·	·	·	·
−	+	−	+		·	·	1	·	·	·	·	·
−	−	−	+		·	1	1	·	·	3	3	·
−	−	+	+		1	·	1	·	·	·	·	·
+	+	+	−		2	·	·	·	·	·	·	·
+	+	−	−		·	·	2	·	·	·	·	·
+	−	−	−		·	2	·	·	·	1	·	·
+	−	+	−		1	·	·	1	·	·	·	2
−	+	+	−		·	·	·	1	·	·	·	·
−	+	−	−		·	·	·	1	·	·	·	·
−	−	−	−		·	·	14	·	·	2	4	·
−	−	+	−		3	·	2	4	·	·	1	1

[a] Numbers represent the total number of clones observed with a particular reactivity pattern. Data represents 78 clones obtained from 20 individual mice (Sherman, 1982).

Another relatively recurrent RP is characterized by recognition of only bm9 among the mutants. This particular RP is shared by 20% of all anti-H-2K^b clones considered in these analyses. Although one possible explanation for such frequent recurrence is the existence of a predominant clonotype within the B10.D2 anti-H2K^b response (analogous to public idiotypes in antibody responses), it is also possible that a recurrent RP represents recognition of one or more determinants by multiple and idiotypically distinct receptors as discussed below. Immunochemical analysis is necessary to distinguish between these possibilities.

With the exception of the two comparatively frequent RP discussed above, the B10.D2 anti-H-2K^b repertoire is consistent with the predicted results of a random distribution among 47 different receptor specificities as calculated using the Poisson distribution. This estimate permits a calculation of the minimum size of the total CTL receptor repertoire. For example, based on the frequency of H-2K^b-specific CTL precursors [one in 12,000 spleen cells (Sherman, 1980)], and estimates on the frequency of spleen cells which are CTL precursors as determined using (concanavalin A) Con-A stimulation and lysis in the presence of mitogen [~3% (Goronozy *et al.*, 1981)], the frequency of cells with a particular RP is calculated to be ~1/20,000 CTL precursors. This suggests a minimum size of the repertoire of 20,000 specificities.

This technique resolves only those specificities which recognize determinants expressed differently on the panel of mutant cells and certainly does not permit the conclusion that two receptors with the same RP are idiotypically identical or even that they react with the same determinant. The fact that any single RP may include many distinct clonotypes is shown by the data presented in Table III. Here, several pairs of clones derived from B10.BR responders display identical RP against the mutant panel yet can be distinguished on the basis of reactivity on a third party alloantigen (K^d). Approximately 4% of all B10.BR anti-K^b-specific CTL clones were found to cross-react with K^d. This is similar to previous estimates of the frequency of alloreactive CTL clones which demonstrate third-party reactivity (MacDonald *et al.*, 1980). Therefore, the assumption that a particular RP defined by the K^b mutants represents only one specificity results in underestimation of the actual diversity of the T cell repertoire. Thus, this assay provides only an estimate of the minimum number of antigen-specific receptors and antigenic determinants which contribute to a particular response.

III. SPECIFICITY REPERTOIRE OF THE bm11 ANTI-H-2K^b RESPONSE

In view of the large number of different antigenic determinants which are recognized in a T cell response against a single allogeneic H-2 molecule, it may be concluded that the high frequency of alloreactive CTL reflects the summation of precursors specific for numerous distinct determinants. It has been demonstrated in several laboratories that the frequency of CTL precursors responsive to antigenic differences in H-2 molecules caused by mutations affecting one or two

TABLE III

Reactivity by Some B10.BR Anti-H-2K^b CTL Clones on H-2K^d

	Percent ^{125}I-labeled UdR release from indicated target cells								
Clone[a]	Kb	bm8	bm1	bm3	bm4	bm9	bm10	bm11	D2.GD
1a	*42*	0	0	0	5	*50*	4	0	0
b	*70*	0	3	10	17	*58*	11	15	*43*
2a	*57*	0	6	0	*56*	*46*	*59*	0	8
b	*73*	0	13	5	*91*	*68*	*82*	16	*80*
3a	*65*	*44*	8	*68*	*59*	*40*	*54*	*74*	0
b	*74*	*70*	10	*77*	*66*	*86*	*60*	*88*	*66*
4a	*99*	9	*85*	7	*100*	*82*	*95*	21	6
b	*65*	13	*74*	7	*83*	*75*	*73*	0	*54*

[a] Methods are as described in Table I.

amino acids may be as high as the frequency of CTL precursors observed in conventional allogeneic responses (Pimsler and Forman, 1978, 1980; Widmer and MacDonald, 1980). It was, therefore, of interest to consider the diversity of CTL precursors which are specific for alloantigenic differences resulting from a single amino acid substitution. The example which was chosen for analysis was the repertoire of the bm11 anti-H-2K^b response (Sherman, 1981).

The results obtained in the analysis of 65 clones are presented in Table IV. Twenty different receptor specificities were identified using the K^b mutants and the third-party allogeneic strain D2.GD. Therefore, a minimum of 20 different determinants are created by a single amino acid change. The frequency of clones expressing third-party reactivity as determined on the basis of recognition of D2.GD is 4.5%, which is comparable to the frequency observed for the B10.BR anti-K^b repertoire. Only one clone was found which recognized the bm3 target. This is most likely due to the fact that bm3 contains two amino acid alterations,

TABLE IV

Reactivity Patterns (RP) Obtained for bm11 Anti-K^b CTL Clones[a]

	Target cells									Clones observed with
RP	Kh	bm8	bm1	bm3	bm4	bm9	bm10	bm11	D2.GD	indicated RP
1	+	·	·	·	·	·	·	·	·	16
2	+	·	·	·	·	+	·	·	·	9
3	+	·	·	·	·	·	+	·	·	5
4	+	·	·	·	+	·	·	·	·	2
5	+	·	·	·	+	+	+	·	·	5
6	+	·	·	·	+	·	+	·	·	2
7	+	·	·	·	+	+	·	·	·	4
8	+	·	·	·	·	+	+	·	·	3
9	+	·	+	·	·	+	·	·	·	4
10	+	·	+	·	·	·	·	·	·	1
11	+	·	+	·	+	+	·	·	·	1
12	+	+	+	·	·	·	·	·	·	1
13	+	+	·	·	·	·	·	·	·	3
14	+	+	·	·	·	+	·	·	·	2
15	+	+	·	·	·	·	+	·	·	1
16	+	+	·	·	·	+	+	·	·	2
17	+	·	·	+	+	·	+	·	·	1
18	+	+	·	·	·	·	+	·	+	1
19	+	·	·	·	+	·	+	·	+	1
20	+	+	+	·	+	+	+	·	+	1
										65

[a] RP are described for 65 CTL clones obtained from 14 individual bm11 responders (Sherman, 1981).

one of which occurs at the same position as the bm11 mutation (Nairn *et al.*, 1980). It is also of interest that a large proportion (25%) of CTL clones recognize only the wild type K^b molecule used for stimulation (Table IV, RP 1). Such clones describe determinant(s) on the K^b molecule which are not conserved in any of the mutants. Considering that most of the sequence changes in these mutants are scattered throughout the amino terminal half of the molecule, this suggests that a focus of the bm11 response is recognition of "fragile" determinants which are altered as a consequence of mutation in any one of a number of different positions on the molecule. This is, perhaps, most readily interpreted as the consequence of conformational alterations in the mutant molecules. In addition, bm11 anti-H-2K^b CTL clones recognize fewer mutants than do clones participating in the fully allogeneic B10.D2 and B10.BR anti-H-2K^b response. Thus, mutant recognition of wild type alloantigens is restricted to areas of the molecule which are relatively variant among the mutants (Sherman, 1981).

IV. THE C57BL/6 ANTI-bm11 CTL RESPONSE: A MODEL FOR DETERMINANT RECOGNITION

The specificity analyses described above are based on the assumption that each mutant retains at least some wild type K^b determinants. The reciprocal stimulation, K^b anti-bm11, should activate CTL precursors which bear receptors reacting with determinants shared by bm11. In view of the distal amino acid positions of most of the other mutations, it might be expected that only bm3 target cells which share an amino acid difference with bm11 would be recognized by such CTL clones. Any reactivity on other mutants would presumably reflect only shared conformationally induced determinants. Therefore, the C57BL/6 anti-bm11 response was investigated in order to determine the relative significance of recognition of such determinants created by changes in molecular conformation. As predicted, the majority of the clones (85%) included recognition of bm3 targets, and only 4% recognized either the bm4 or the bm10 mutants. This level of cross-reactivity is comparable to that observed on an allogeneic target, D2.GD (6%). However, 56% of the clones also reacted with either bm1, bm8, or bm9 targets. This level of recognition is 3- to 4-fold greater than expected for an unrelated third party alloantigen. These results suggest that as much as half of the B/6 anti-bm11 response could represent recognition of conformationally induced determinants, and that mutations in quite distant amino acid positions on the molecule may result in the creation of a determinant which can be recognized by the same receptor.

One possible explanation for such recognition would be that different mutants may share an identical determinant. Of course, this could only be true if the amino acids involved in the mutation are not part of the recognized determinant.

For example, an amino acid substitution may cause distal conformational changes which render previously tolerated or inaccessible determinants immunogenic. Thus, a specific determinant could emerge as a consequence of any of several different distal mutations. This interpretation, if correct, has far-reaching implications concerning T cell recognition in general. If a single amino acid change in H-2 molecules can result in a vigorous CTL response, due in part to "expression" of such self-determinants, it is possible that other types of perturbations of H-2 molecules may also cause immunogenic presentation of self. For example, there is evidence for interaction of H-2 molecules with viral proteins on the surface of infected cells (Schrader *et al.*, 1975; Bubbers *et al.*, 1978; Honneycut and Gooding, 1980). This type of noncovalent association may result in local conformational disturbance in H-2 molecules and thereby induce the expression of several new H-2 determinants. If such were the case, receptor recognition would appear to be virus specific even in the absence of direct involvement of viral antigens. Indeed, this is consistent with the relative difficulty in demonstrating antigen recognition, as compared with MHC recognition, by either T helper cell or CTL using antibody blocking techniques (Ellner and Rosenthal, 1975; Askonas and Webster, 1980).

V. THE INFLUENCE OF MHC ON RECEPTOR REPERTOIRE

The influence of the MHC on T cell repertoire is exemplified by MHC-linked immune response genes, by MHC restriction of T cell function, and by tolerance to self MHC antigens. Recent evidence obtained in a variety of different experimental systems suggest some of these phenomenon may reflect control on receptor repertoire selection (Zinkernagel and Doherty, 1979; Hunig and Bevan, 1980). It was, therefore, of interest to compare the anti-H-2K^b CTL specificity repertoires obtained for two congenic strains which differ at the MHC, B10.D2 and B10.BR. In view of the vast diversity of the B10.D2 response, it was anticipated that it would not be possible to compare repertoires on the basis of the presence or absence of randomly distributed specificities. Therefore, the feasibility of performing comparative studies would be dependent entirely on the availability of a nonrandom distinguishing characteristic which could then be used as a phenotypic marker for a particular repertoire. A candidate for such a marker is the predominant B10.D2 specificity which represents 20% of K^b-specific CTL precursors in this strain. The presence of this potential phenotypic marker for repertoire encouraged comparative analysis of the B10.BR repertoire.

As was found for the B10.D2 repertoire, the B10.BR receptor repertoire was highly diverse; 78 clones obtained from 17 mice defined 34 different specificities (Sherman, 1982). Among these were three highly recurrent specificities which are the most significant features of the B10.BR repertoire in comparison with the

B10.D2 repertoire (Table V). Specifically, RP A represents the adult B10.D2 predominant specificity previously discussed, while RP, B, C, and D are recurrent B10.BR specificities. Considering that these two mouse strains which differ only at the MHC express different recurrent specificities, it may be concluded that (1) the CTL specificity repertoire is a heritable trait, and (2) the MHC influences repertoire at the level of the frequency of at least some receptor specificities within the CTL precursor pool. Preliminary experiments comparing the repertoire of neonatal and adult CTL from these strains indicate that additional factors may be involved in the expression of some predominant specificities. For example, although RP A and B are represented to a comparable extent in both the adult and neonatal repertoire, RP D is highly recurrent in the repertoire of both B10.D2 and B10.BR neonates, whereas RP C appears at a low frequency in neonates of both strains.

In order to further explore the basis for MHC regulation, the anti-K^b specificity repertoire of (B10.BR × B10.D2)F_1 mice was next examined (Sherman, 1982) (Table V). Only the B10.D2 predominant specificity is maintained at a high level in F_1 individuals, although evidence has been obtained for intermediate levels of expression of RP B and D in the F_1 neonatal repertoire. The persistence of such specificities in the F_1 repertoire would imply that simple H-2-specific tolerance could not account entirely for repertoire difference or predominant expression. The complex control of repertoire is further exemplified by RP patterns E, F, and G which represent specificities which are recurrent in the F_1 repertoire but not in either parental repertoire. The existence of such specificities presumably is due to both positive and negative regulatory effects

TABLE V

Frequency of Representation of Recurrent Specificities in the Repertoires of B10.D2, B10.BR, and (B10.BR × B10.D2)F_1 Mice

Reactivity pattern	B10.D2	B10.BR	(B10.BR × B10.D2)F_1
A	++++[a]	+	+++
B	−	+++	+
C	+	++++	−
D	−	+++	+
E	−	−	+++
F	−	−	+++
G	−	−	+++

[a] Symbols represent the following range of frequencies: −, 0–2% of all clones; +, 2–5%; ++, 5–7%; +++, 7–12%; ++++, >12%. The probability of random occurrence of a particular specificity as 7% or more within any one of these three repertoires is <0.01 as determined using the Poisson distribution. Therefore, RP represented by greater than 7% of clones are considered recurrent specificities (Sherman, 1982).

attributable to MHC. Although speculation is premature, it is interesting to consider the possibility of some relationship between F_1 predominant specificities and unique F_1 antigens created by combinatorial association of *I* region gene products. In this regard, it would certainly be of interest to determine which locus within the MHC is responsible for the expression of different recurrent specificities in the parental strains.

The results presented above suggest numerous levels of complexity in regulation of the frequency of a particular specificity within the CTL precursor pool. Future experiments will be directed at identifying the mechanisms responsible for such regulation as well as continued identification of other genetic loci involved in repertoire determination. It is anticipated that this type of approach will continue to contribute significant new information concerning the T cell repertoire as well as the basis of determinant recognition.

ACKNOWLEDGMENTS

This research was supported by United State Public Health Service Grants AI-15710 and CA-25803.

REFERENCES

Askonas, B. A., and Webster, R. G. (1980). Monoclonal antibodies to hemagglutinin and to H-2 inhibit the cross reactive cytotoxic T cell population induced by influenza. *Eur. J. Immunol.* **10,** 151.

Bubbers, E. J., Chen, S., and Lilly, F. (1978). Nonrandom inclusion of H-2K and H-2D antigens in Friend virus particles from mice of various strains. *J. Exp. Med.* **147,** 340.

Ellner, J. J., and Rosenthal, A. S. (1975). Quantitative and immunologic aspects of the handling of 2,4-dinitrophenyl guinea pig albumin by macrophages. *J. Immunol.* **114,** 1563.

Goronozy, J., Schaefer, U., Eichmann, K., and Simon, M. M. (1981). Quantitative studies on T cell diversity. II. Determination of the frequencies and Lyt phenotypes of two types of precursor cells for alloreactive cytotoxic T cells in polyclonally and specifically activated splenic T cells. *J. Exp. Med.* **153,** 857.

Honneycutt, P. J., and Gooding, L. R. (1980). Solubilization of complexes between tumor associated and H-2 antigens from a cell plasma membrane. *Eur. J. Immunol.* **10,** 363.

Hunig, T., and Bevan, M. J. (1980). Self H-2 antigens influence the specificity of alloreactive cells. *J. Exp. Med.* **151,** 1288.

Johnson, N., Douglas, R., and Hood, L. (1981). Nucleic acid rearrangements in the differentiation of mouse B cells. *In* "B Lymphocytes in the Immune Response: Functional, Developmental and Interactive Properties" (N. R. Klinman, D. Mosier, I. Scher, and E. Vitetta, eds.), p. 3. Elsevier/North-Holland Publ., New York.

Klein, J. (1978). H-2 mutations: Their genetics and effect on immune function. *Adv. Immunol.* **26,** 55.

MacDonald, H. R., Cerottini, J.-C., Ryser, J.-C., Maryanski, J., Taswell, C., Widmer, M. B., and Brunner, K. T. (1980). Quantitation and cloning of cytolytic T lymphocytes and their precursors. *Immunol. Rev.* **51,** 93.

Miller, R. G., Teh, H.-S., Harley, E., and Philips R. A. (1977). Quantitative studies on the activation of cytotoxic lymphocyte precursor cells. *Immunol. Rev.* **35,** 38.

Nairn, R., Yamaga, K., and Nathenson, S. G. (1980). Biochemistry of the gene products from murine MHC mutants. *Annu Rev. Genet.* **14,** 241.

Pimsler, M., and Forman, J. (1978). Estimates of the precursor frequency of cytotoxic T lymphocytes against antigens controlled by defined regions of the *H-2* gene complex: Comparison of the effect of H-2 differences due to intra H 2 recombination vs. mutation. *J. Immunol.* **121,** 1302.

Pimsler, M., and Forman, J. (1980). Use of H-2 mutations to quantitate alloreactivity: Alloreactivity is strongest against H-2 antigens which are closest to self. *Immunogenetics* **11,** 111.

Schrader, J. W., Cunningham, B. A., and Edelman, G. M. (1975). Functional interactions of viral and histocompatibility antigens at tumor cell surfaces. *Proc. Natl. Acad. Sci. U.S.A.* **72,** 5066.

Sherman, L. A. (1980). Dissection of the B10.D2 anti-H-2K^b cytolytic T lymphocyte receptor repertoire. *J. Exp. Med.* **151,** 1386.

Sherman, L. A. (1981). Mutationally derived H-2 antigenic differences as defined by cytolytic T lymphocyte clones. *J. Immunol.* **127,** 1259.

Sherman, L. A. (1982). The influence of the major histocompatibility complex on the repertoire of allospecific cytolytic T lymphocytes. *J. Exp. Med.* **155,** 380.

Widmer, M. B., and MacDonald, H. R. (1980). Cytolytic T lymphocyte precursors reactive against mutant K^b alloantigens are as frequent as those reactive against a whole foreign haplotype. *J. Immunol.* **124,** 48.

Zinkernagel, R. M., and Doherty, P. C. (1979). MHC restricted cytotoxic T cells. *Adv. Immunol.* **27,** 51.

26

Alloreactive T Cell Clones Which Recognize Hybrid Determinants

Barbara N. Beck/C. G. Fathman

Text 325
References 328

Clones of T cells specifically reactive to alloantigens were isolated and maintained as has been described in greater detail elsewhere (Fathman and Hengartner, 1978; Hengartner and Fathman, 1980). The clonal lines were derived from long-term mixed lymphocyte cultures in which A/J lymph node cells were stimulated by irradiated (C57BL/6 × A/J)F_1 [(B6A)F_1] spleen cells. Originally, clones were obtained by picking colonies from cultures plated in soft agar, but this technique has since been supplanted by limiting dilution cloning. From the long-term A/J anti-(B6A)F_1 cultures one obtains several different types of clonal lines (Hengartner and Fathman, 1980). Some of the lines respond to B6 as well as they do to (B6A)F_1 stimulator cells, indicating that these lines are specific for H-2^b allodeterminants. Other lines respond specifically to (B6A)F_1 cells and not to B6 cells. These lines are clearly responding to hybrid determinants present only on the F_1 cells.

One would expect *a priori* that each clonal alloreactive cell line would react specifically with one MLR determinant, in analogy with the clonal specificity of immunoglobulin-producing cells. If this is true, one could potentially count the number of MLR determinants which differ between genetically different mice. We have used two ways of comparing the reactivities of our cloned alloreactive cell lines: (1) mapping the hybrid determinants by using various recombinant and F_1 mice as sources of stimulator cells and (2) using various monoclonal anti-Ia antibodies specific for the haplotype(s) of the stimulator cells to block stimulation of the clonal lines.

To date, all of the F_1-specific cloned lines which we have examined respond to determinants which map to the *I* region of *H-2* (Fathman and Hengartner, 1979).

ISOLATION, CHARACTERIZATION, AND
UTILIZATION OF T LYMPHOCYTE CLONES

ISBN 0-12-249920-4

On the basis of the mapping data, a representative example of which is displayed in Table I, these clones can be divided into two groups. One group reacts with a determinant which maps to the *I-A* region, and the expression of this determinant requires heterozygosity at this region. This is demonstrated by the ability of (B6 × B10.A(4R))F_1 cells to stimulate clone 10.39 as well as (B6A)F_1 cells do, while cells from (A/J × B10.A(4R))F_1 and (B10.MBR × A.AL)F_1 mice fail to stimulate this clone. The second group reacts with a determinant which is expressed on B10.A(3R) cells as well as on (B6A)F_1 cells. This indicates that expression of the hybrid antigen to which these clones respond depends not upon heterozygosity at any one locus, but rather upon the interaction of products from two loci. The locus contributed by the *b* haplotype maps to the left of *I-E* and the locus from the *a* haplotype maps to the right of *I-J,* based on the reactivity with B10.A(3R) cells. The failure of cells from (B10.A(4R) × A/J)F_1 and (B10.MBR × A.AL)F_1 mice to stimulate these clones indicates that the *b* haplotype contribution to the hybrid antigen expression maps to *I-A*. Precise mapping of the *a* haplotype contribution cannot be done since the proper recombinant strains do not yet exist. However, the *D* region can be ruled out on the basis of the failure of cells from B10.A(18R) mice to stimulate these clones. Since the *S* region codes for serum proteins, not cell-surface antigens, it is most likely that the locus required for the hybrid antigen expression is in either the *E* or the *C* region. For the sake of simplicity, this hybrid antigen will be designated the A-E antigen.

TABLE I

Mapping the Hybrid MLR Determinants[a]

	Haplotype								Clone	Clone 4.1.4	
Stimulator Cells	*K*	*A*	*B*	*J*	*E*	*C*	*S*	*D*	10.39	Expt. 1	Expt. 2
A	*k*	*k*	*k*	*k*	*k*	*d*	*d*	*d*	209	614	102
B6	*b*	*b*	*b*	*b*	*b*	*b*	*b*	*b*	196	381	587
(B6 × A/J)F_1	*b/k*	*b/k*	*b/k*	*b/k*	*b/k*	*b/d*	*b/d*	*b/d*	4749	7044	9777
B10.A(3R)	*b*	*b*	*b*	*b*	*k*	*d*	*d*	*d*	344	6023	10,391
(B6 × B10.A(4R))F_1	*b/k*	*b/k*	*b/b*	*b/b*	*b/b*	*b/b*	*b/b*	*b/b*	4301	2710	236
(B10.A(4R) × A/J)F_1	*k/k*	*k/k*	*b/k*	*b/k*	*b/k*	*b/d*	*b/d*	*b/d*	271	NT[b]	1577
(B10.MBR × A.AL)F_1	*b/k*	*k/k*	*k/k*	*k/k*	*k/k*	*k/k*	*k/k*	*q/d*	180	NT	278
B10.A(18R)	*b*	*b*	*b*	*b*	*b*	*b*	*b*	*d*	NT	586	NT

[a] The response, in cpm of ^{3}H-TdR incorporated, on day 2 of 1 × 10^4 cells from clones 10.39 and 4.1.4 to 1 × 10^6 stimulator spleen cells of a variety of haplotypes.

[b] NT, not tested.

These mapping data correlate very nicely with what is known serologically and biochemically about the expression of Ia antigens. Anti-Ia antisera can be generated only in donor–recipient combinations which differ either in the *A* or in the *E/C* region (Shreffler *et al.*, 1977), and, biochemically, two classes of Ia antigens can be isolated from cells, the molecules in each class being composed of two chains (Silver *et al.*, 1976, 1977). The two-chain nature of Ia molecules explains how hybrid Ia antigens can be created, namely, by the random association of α and β chains in heterozygous or the appropriate recombinant mice. Thus, it appears very likely on the basis of these data that the hybrid MLR determinants recognized by our alloreactive clones are in fact hybrid Ia antigens. We have used monoclonal anti-Ia antibodies to provide further support for this hypothesis.

It has been observed previously that stimulation in the MLR proliferative assay could be blocked by the addition to the cultures of alloantisera directed against Ia antigens on the stimulator cells (Meo *et al.*, 1975). We set out to use various monoclonal anti-Ia antibodies in a similar way to examine the relationship between the specificities recognized by these antibodies and the determinants recognized by our alloreactive T cell clones. The monoclonal antibodies used were generously provided by Dr. Günter Hämmerling, Heidelberg, Germany, and their specificities have been described (Hämmerling *et al.*, 1979). We tested the ability of a particular antibody to block stimulation of a responder T cell clone by adding a small amount into the culture. As controls we used the same quantity of antibody in cultures of responder clones which should not be blocked by that particular antibody. Thus, clones which respond to the A-E type hybrid antigen(s) should not be blocked by antibodies directed against strictly *A* region antigens and vice versa. In these studies we used several clones of each type. We found that the responder clones which recognize the I-A^k/I-A^b hybrid antigen(s) could be divided into two groups on the basis of the ability of various monoclonal anti-I-A^k antibodies to block their stimulation. As is illustrated in Table II, antibodies H116.32 (anti-Ia.19) and H118.49 (anti-Ia.2) could block the stimulation of clone 10.39, whereas H150.13 and 10–2.16, both anti-Ia.17 antibodies, could not. However, these two antibodies could block the stimulation of clone 11.19, while H116.32 and H118.49 had no effect on this clone. This dichotomy of reactivities has been true for all of the clones we have tested which are specific for the hybrid I-A^k/I-A^b antigen(s). Since the Ia antigens are composed of two chains, we would expect there to be two different hybrid antigens mapping to the *A* region, namely $A^b_\alpha A^k_\beta$ and $A^k_\alpha A^b_\beta$. It has been established that antibody 10–2.16 reacts with a specificity on the A^k_β chain (Silver *et al.*, 1980). Therefore, these data suggest that the H150.13 specificity also resides on the A^k_β chain and that clone 11.19 recognizes the hybrid antigen composed of the A^b_α chain and the A^k_β chain. This suggests that antibodies H116.32 and H118.49 recognize specificities on the A^k_α chain, and that clone 10.39 recognizes the $A^k_\alpha A^b_\beta$ hybrid antigen. We have preliminary evidence, using SDS-polyacrylamide gel elec-

TABLE II

Inhibition with Monoclonal Anti-Ia Antibodies[a]

Antibody		Expt. 1		Expt. 2	
		10.39	11.19	10.39	4.1.4
H116.32	(anti-Ia.19)	517	4424	903	7336
H118.49	(anti-Ia.2)	946	6270	—	—
H150.13	(anti-Ia.17)	5403	63	12,302	8513
10-2.16	(anti-Ia.17)	4141	75	11,682	7027
Y-17	(anti-Ia-m.44)	—	—	12,575	328
13/18	(anti-Ia.7)	—	—	10,088	164
No antibody		6727	5393	12,773	10,290

[a] The response, in counts per minute of incorporated ^{3}H-TdR, on day 2 of 1×10^4 cells from clones 10.39, 11.19, and 4.1.4 to 1×10^6 (B6A)F_1 stimulator cells in the presence of various monoclonal antibodies. The apparent specificity of each monoclonal antibody has been included next to the designation of the antibody. These antibodies have all been described previously.

trophoresis, that antibodies H116.32 and 10–2.16 do indeed precipitate different molecules from (B6A)F_1 spleen cells (Beck *et al.*, 1982).

We have also examined the ability of monoclonal antibodies to block the stimulation of clones which recognize the A-E hybrid antigen(s). We have found that both antibody 13/18 (anti-Ia.7) (Hämmerling *et al.*, 1979) and antibody Y-17 (anti-Ia-m.44) (Lerner *et al.*, 1980) are able to block the stimulation of clone 4.1.4 and all other clones in the same group which have been tested to date. Studies are underway using additional antibodies to examine whether all of these clones recognize the same determinant, or whether they too will be divisible into two or more groups.

Thus, the antibody-blocking experiments have provided strong evidence that the determinants recognized by our alloreactive T cell clones are Ia antigens. Furthermore, they have allowed us to subdivide the I-A^k/I-A^b reactive group, and to establish that, to date, we have three different types of F_1-specific alloreactive clones. We can, therefore, conclude that there are at least three unique hybrid determinants (Ia antigens) on (B6A)F_1 cells which can be recognized by A/J lymph node T cells.

REFERENCES

Beck, B. N., Frelinger, J. G., Shigeta, M., Infante, A. J., Cummings, D., Hämmerling, G., and Fathman, C. G. (1982). T cell clones specific for hybrid I-A molecules: Discrimination with monoclonal anti I-A^k antibodies. Submitted.

Fathman, C. G., and Hengartner, H. (1978). Clones of alloreactive T cells. *Nature* (London) **272,** 617.

Fathman, C. G., and Hengartner, H. (1979). Hybrid I region antigens and I region restriction of recognition in MLR. *In* "T and B Lymphocytes: Recognition and Function" (F. H. Bach, B. Bonavida, E. Vitetta, and C. F. Fox, eds.), p. 577 Academic Press, New York.

Hämmerling, G. J., Hämmerling, U., and Lemke, H. (1979). Isolation of 12 monoclonal antibodies against Ia and H-2 antigens. Serological characterization and reactivity with B and T lymphocytes. *Immunogenetics* **8,** 433.

Hengartner, H., and Fathman, C. G. (1980). Clones of alloreactive T cells. I. A unique homozygous MLR stimulating determinant present on B6 stimulators. *Immunogenetics* **10,** 175.

Lerner, E. A., Matis, L. A., Janeway, C. A., Jones, P. P., Schwartz, R. H., and Murphy, D. B. (1980). Monoclonal antibody against an *Ir* gene product? *J. Exp. Med.* **152,** 1085.

Meo, T., David, C. S., Rijnbeck, A. M., Nabholz, M., Miggiano, V., and Shreffler, D. C. (1975). Inhibition of mouse MLR by anti-Ia sera. *Transplant. Proc.* **7,** Suppl. 1, 127.

Shreffler, D. C., David, C. S., Cullen, S. E., Frelinger, J. A., and Niederhuber, J. E. (1977). Serological and functional evidence for further subdivision of the *I* region of the *H-2* gene complex. *Cold Spring Harbor Symp. Quant. Biol.* **41,** 477.

Silver, J., Cecka, J. M., McMillan, M., and Hood, L. (1976). Chemical characterization of products of the *H-2* complex. *Cold Spring Harbor Symp. Quant. Biol.* **41,** 369.

Silver, J., Russell, W. A., Reis, B. L., and Frelinger, J. A. (1977). Chemical characterization of murine Ia alloantigens determined by the I-E/I-C subregions of the *H-2* complex. *Proc. Natl. Acad. Sci. U.S.A.* **74,** 5131.

Silver, J., Swain, S. L., and Hubert, J. J. (1980). Small subunit of *I-A* subregion antigens determines the allospecificity recognized by a monoclonal antibody. *Nature (London)* **286,** 272.

27

Anti-H-2 Reactivity of Mls-Specific T Cell Clones

Susan R. Webb/Jennifer Bruce/Katherine Molnar-Kimber/ Darcy B. Wilson/Jonathan Sprent

I.	H-2 Specificity of Uncloned Mls-Reactive T Cell Lines	332
II.	Anti-H-2 and Anti-Mls Reactivity T Cell Clones	334
III.	Characteristics of Cloned Mls-Reactive T Cell Lines	336
	A. Surface Markers of Clones	336
	B. Functional Analysis of Mls-Reactive T Cell Clones	336
IV.	Conclusions	336
	References	338

The unusually high frequency of alloreactive T cells poses as yet unresolved problems concerning the relationship between T cells recognizing major histocompatibility complex (MHC)-encoded determinants and those recognizing conventional antigens. A variety of evidence, much of it indirect, has led to the notion that T cells may express dual specificity for (a) conventional antigens (antigen X) seen in association with self MHC gene products, and (b) certain MHC alloantigens (Wilson *et al.*, 1977; Heber-Katz and Wilson, 1976; Janeway *et al.*, 1980). The most direct approach to this problem is to examine the specificity of cloned lines of T cells. In this respect, recent studies of *H-2*-restricted antigen-reactive T cell clones indicate that certain of these clones also exhibit alloreactivity (von Boehmer *et al.*, 1979; Sredni and Schwartz, 1981; Braciale *et al.*, 1981). A key question here is whether the alloreactivity displayed by clones with a particular *H-2*-restricted specificity for antigen X is random or, conversely, is skewed toward recognition of only certain foreign H-2 determinants. Skewed alloreactivity would favor the notion that association of self H-2 plus antigen X mimics a particular alloantigen. To study this question, we have examined the pattern of alloreactivity displayed by lines and clones of T cells reactive to gene products of the *Mls* locus (Molnar-Kimber *et al.*, 1980; Webb *et al.*, 1981).

ISOLATION, CHARACTERIZATION, AND
UTILIZATION OF T LYMPHOCYTE CLONES

ISBN 0-12-249920-4

Mls determinants are unusual. They are coded by a locus on chromosome 1, unlinked to the *H-2* complex (Festenstein, 1973). Like H-2 determinants, they evoke strong primary mixed lymphocyte reactions (MLR), but unlike MHC antigens, they do not evoke lethal graft-versus-host reactions or cytotoxic T cell responses, and they do not appear to act as transplantation antigens (Nisbet and Edwards, 1973; Korngold and Sprent, 1978; Rollinghoff *et al.*, 1975; Sachs *et al.*, 1973; Huber *et al.*, 1973). To date it has not been possible to raise antibodies to these determinants (Tonkonogy and Winn, 1977; Dickler *et al.*, 1980). Unlike conventional antigens, in our experience (Molnar-Kimber and Sprent, 1980) Mls determinants are not recognized by T cells in an MHC-restricted fashion. Four alleles of the *Mls* locus were originally described, Mls^a, Mls^b, Mls^c, and Mls^d, although only Mls^a and Mls^d give strong primary MLR (Festenstein, 1973). From a variety of evidence, we and others have concluded that the $\mathrm{Mls}^{\mathrm{a}}$ and $\mathrm{Mls}^{\mathrm{d}}$ determinants are probably identical or are at least highly cross-reactive (Molnar-Kimber and Sprent, 1980, 1981; Ryan *et al.*, 1979; Molnar-Kimber *et al.*, 1980). Thus, there appears to be little demonstrable polymorphism in the expression of these "strong" Mls determinants.

This chapter summarizes the results of recent studies which suggest that many Mls-reactive T cells have dual specificity for allogeneic H-2 determinants, and that the recognition of these determinants shows no obvious skewing towards a particular *H-2* haplotype.

I. H-2 SPECIFICITY OF UNCLONED Mls-REACTIVE T CELL LINES

Initial experiments with uncloned T cell lines positively selected *in vitro* by repeated stimulation with $\mathrm{Mls}^{\mathrm{a}}$ determinants indicated that these lines also gave high proliferative responses to a variety of $\mathrm{Mls}^{\mathrm{a}}$-negative H-2-different stimulating cells (Molnar-Kimber *et al.*, 1980). Long-term T cell lines were obtained by repeated stimulation of BALB/c ($H\text{-}2^d$, Mls^b; hereinafter referred to as, *d,b*) lymph node cells at bimonthly intervals with irradiated H-2-identical, Mls-different DBA/2 (*d,a*) spleen cells. As expected, in analytical microcultures these T cell lines showed proliferative responses to all strains bearing the selecting strong Mls ($\mathrm{Mls}^{\mathrm{a}}$ and $\mathrm{Mls}^{\mathrm{d}}$) determinants, but in addition they reacted strongly to $\mathrm{Mls}^{\mathrm{a,d}}$-negative strains expressing a variety of *H-2* haplotypes.

These $\mathrm{Mls}^{\mathrm{a,d}}$-reactive (*d,b* anti-*d,a*) T cell lines were found to grow as effectively when stimulated with H-2-different, Mls-identical cells as with cells bearing the priming $\mathrm{Mls}^{\mathrm{a}}$ determinants. Repeated stimulation over a period of 2 months with cells from CBA/CaHn (*k,b*) or H-2-congenic BALB.K (*k,b*) donors resulted in a line which lost its reactivity to all *H-2* haplotypes other than $H\text{-}2^k$.

Significantly, this *d,b* anti-*d,a* line diverted by stimulation with *k,b* cells maintained strong reactivity to $Mls^{a,d}$ determinants, antigens to which these cells had not been exposed for 60 days. Similarly, $Mls^{a,d}$-selected, H-2-panreactive (*d,b* anti-*d,a*) lines diverted on $H\text{-}2^b$ continued to show reactivity for $Mls^{a,d}$ determinants but lost reactivity to other *H-2* haplotypes. The simplest explanation for these findings is that at least some portion of T cells are capable of recognizing both *Mls* and *H-2* gene products.

TABLE I

Specificity Patterns of T Cell Clones[a] Selected for Reactivity to H-2[b]

Stimulating[b] cells	*H-2*	*Mls*	^{3}H-TdR uptake[c] C1.3	C2.2
B10.D2	*d*	*b*	52[d]	117
DBA/2	*d*	*a*	160	31,436
D1.C	*d*	*a*	151	23,681
D1.LP	*b*	*a*	6509	30,066
CBA/J	*k*	*d*	305	27,348
AKR/Cum	*k*	*a*	149	37,729
B10	*b*	*b*	5552	10,071
B10.BR	*k*	*b*	119	107
B10.RIII	*r*	*b*	162	118
B10.M	*f*	*b*	90	149
B10.S	*s*	*b*	88	87

[a] B10.D2 (*d,b*) LN cells were stimulated five times at 10–14 day intervals with irradiated B10 (*b,b*) spleen cells. Twenty-four to 48 hr following the last stimulation, cells were cloned by limiting dilution in flat-bottom microtiter plates containing 1×10^6 irradiated (3000 R) stimulating cells, 2×10^5 irradiated (3000 R) syngeneic spleen cells, and 25% conditioned medium from 24 hr concanavalin A-stimulated Lewis rat spleen cells. Eight to 10 days later, wells positive for growth were expanded in 2-ml wells containing fresh stimulating cells, medium, and growth factor. Clones derived in this way were maintained by harvesting the cells every 10–14 days and restimulating at low cell density. Although we routinely added T cell growth factor (TCGF) for maximal proliferation in bulk cultures, these clones did not apparently have an obligatory requirement for exogenous growth factors, as all the microculture analysis was done in the absence of any added TCGF. All of the clones described in subsequent tables were derived and maintained in a similar fashion.

[b] Cells from each of these stimulating cells effectively stimulated normal B10.D2 lymph node cells in the same experiment.

[c] Response of $1\text{–}2 \times 10^4$ cloned T cells measured on day 3.

[d] Mean counts per minute of three cultures; SD were usually within 10–20% of the mean.

II. ANTI-H-2 AND ANTI-Mls REACTIVITY OF T CELL CLONES

To examine more directly this question of dual reactivity, limiting dilution techniques were employed to prepare cloned lines of T cells (Webb *et al.*, 1981) (Table I). Clones were derived from bulk cultures repeatedly stimulated with either H-2- or Mls-different cells. The proliferative specificity of two representative anti-MHC clones is shown in Table I. Of seven anti-H-2^b (*d,b* anti-*b,b*) clones tested, four reacted exclusively to *H-2^b* gene products (C1.3), whereas three reacted well to both H-2^b and $Mls^{a,d}$ determinants (C2.2); the use of appropriate H-2 recombinant mice showed that the H-2 alloreactivity of the clones mapped to the *I-A* subregion. It should be noted that the three dual-reactive clones had not been exposed previously to $Mls^{a,d}$ determinants.

The second series of clones were selected for reactivity to Mls determinants. Table II shows that of thirteen B10.D2 (*d,b*) anti-DBA/2 (*d,a*) clones tested, seven of these, for example, E7, responded to cells from all strains expressing strong $Mls^{a,d}$ determinants but showed no reactivity to five strains expressing only H-2 differences. Five other clones (E4, E8, E19, E24, and E26) showed

TABLE II

H-2 Reactivity of Mls-Reactive (B10.D2 anti-DBA/2) T Cell Clones[a]

Stimulating cells	*H-2,Mls*	^{3}H-TdR uptake of clones						
		E7	E4	E8	E19	E26	E21	E24
B10.D2	*d,b*	162	178	216	287	3620	2618	466
B10	*b,b*	246	162	169	170	218	184	477
B10.BR	*k,b*	204	162	278	289	135	173	695
B10.RIII	*r,b*	265	682	19,514	1631	536	292	401
B10.M	*f,b*	153	152	531	161	137	100	370
B10.S	*s,b*	163	124	2863	173	159	163	2768
B10.P	*p,b*	170	5508	280	223	146	117	6753
D1.LP	*b,a*	7932	6676	11,210	44,788	7105	311	7305
DBA/2	*d,a*	6729	4475	15,442	24,057	8455	2873	5907
CBA/J	*k,d*	6799	3628	13,426	35,517	16,869	179	6093
AKR/J	*k,a*	4700	2813	3870	24,165	7013	227	2270
D1.C	*d,a*	8858	3565	24,172	22,723	10,654	4748	6961
C3H/HeJ	*k,c*	242	127	157	684	157	189	225
Reactivity	*Mls*	*a,d*	*a,d*	*a,d*	*a,d*	*a,d*	—	*a,d*
Pattern	*H-2*	—	*p,r*	*r,s*	*r*	*d*	*d*	*p,s*

[a] The proliferative specificity of these various clones was examined in three independent experiments with similar results; in the experiment reported here (B10.A (4R) × B10.P)F_1 stimulating cells were substituted for B10.P. Mean counts per minute of three cultures; SD were usually within 10–20% of mean. Data adapted from Webb *et al.*, 1981.

reactivity for $Mls^{a,d}$ and one or more of the stimulating *H-2* haplotypes tested. Significantly, each of these five clones had a different pattern of anti-H-2 reactivity. The remaining clone, E21, proliferated only when tested on strains bearing $H\text{-}2^d$ (self) determinants. Specificity analyses conducted after repeated stimulation of the clones confirmed that their reactivity patterns were stable.

Many of the dual-reactive T cell clones examined have shown an appreciably weaker response on a second *H-2* haplotype (see Table II, e.g., E8). These small but detectable cross-reactivities were maintained in repeated assays of these clones. A trivial explanation for this finding is that these clones are in fact mixtures of more than one clone. As a test of our cloning procedures, one such clone, D5.16, was recloned by limiting dilution to derive four independent subclones. These were then tested against the same panel of stimulating cells as the parent clone. The results are shown in Table III. The parent clone showed equivalent reactivity against $H\text{-}2^b$ and strong Mls determinants with some degree of cross-reactivity on $H\text{-}2^f$ as well. All four subclones showed the same pattern of reactivity for $Mls^{a,d}$ and $H\text{-}2^{b,f}$, indicating that these reactivities are indeed a property of a single clone.

TABLE III

Subclones of Dual-Reactive T Cell Clones Showing Same Specificity for Mls and H-2 as Parent Clone

Stimulating cells[b]	^{3}H-TdR uptake[a]				
		Subclones			
	Parent clone D5.16[c]	D5.16/1	D5.16/2	D5.16/3	D5.16/4
B10.D2 (*d,b*)	299[d]	413	90	104	82
DBA/2 (*d,a*)	11,547	4585	3436	4948	4549
D1.LP (*b,a*)	25,041	5946	4604	10,024	13,557
CBA/J (*k,d*)	14,718	4773	2331	4897	7579
AKR/J (*k,a*)	6677	1950	1934	1415	3301
B10 (*b,b*)	10,552	4952	6620	5528	11,800
B10.BR (*k,b*)	203	253	70	99	86
B10.RIII (*r,b*)	317	339	145	186	112
B10.M (*f,b*)	4837	1317	669	470	831
B10.S (*s,b*)	447	513	189	209	138
C3H/HeJ (*k,c*)	396	389	173	346	144

[a] Response of 1–2 × 10^4 responding cells as measured on day 3. Data from Webb *et al.*, 1981.

[b] In the same experiment, cells from these strains effectively stimulated normal B10.D2 LN.

[c] D5.16 was derived from a B10.D2 (*d,b*) anti-D1.LP (*b,a*) line restimulated at 10–14 day intervals for 5 weeks prior to cloning by limiting dilution.

[d] See Table I.

III. CHARACTERISTICS OF CLONED Mls-REACTIVE T CELL LINES

A. Surface Markers of Clones

Ten of the B10.D2 (*d,b*) anti-DBA/2 (*d,a*) clones were examined for surface expression of Thy-1.2, Lyt-1.2 and Lyt-2.2 antigens using both immunofluorescence and complement-mediated cytotoxicity. With the notable exception of clone E21 (which has specificity for self H-2^d determinants), all clones were strongly Thy-1.2^+ by immunofluorescence. Plateau lysis of 80–100% was observed with anti-Thy-1.2 antibody plus complement; antibody titers tended to be somewhat lower (>10×) with the clones than with normal splenic T cells. All of the clones (including E21) were weakly Lyt-1.2^+ by immunofluorescence; only marginal lysis was observed in the presence of complement. None of these clones were positive for Lyt-2.2 by either method. The phenotypes of these clones are thus consistent with the expected profile of noncytotoxic proliferating T cells.

B. Functional Analysis of Mls-Reactive T Cell Clones

Although we have little definitive information regarding the functional capabilities of Mls-reactive T cells, two preliminary points can be made. First, none of these clones has shown cytotoxic potential as tested in a 4-hr ^{51}Cr release assay using lipopolysaccharide-stimulated blast cells as targets. The second point is that the supernatant taken from cultures of Mls-reactive T cell clones contains a factor(s) which appears to polyclonally activate normal syngeneic B cells in a 7-day culture.

IV. CONCLUSIONS

The key question emerging from these studies is the significance of the dual specificity of the clones for $Mls^{a,d}$ and H-2 determinants. To date we have observed a total of eight distinct anti-H-2 reactivity patterns by clones with anti-$Mls^{a,d}$ specificity (Table IV). The point to be emphasized is that the anti-H-2 reactivity of clones raised from bulk cultures stimulated initially against Mls determinants appears to be random, i.e., there is no obvious skewing toward particular H-2 determinants.

At face value, the most likely explanation for the dual specificity of the clones would seem to be that Mls and H-2 determinants show marked cross-reactivity. This explanation is orthodox in the sense that it argues that both ligands are recognized via the same set of receptors. Antigenic cross-reactivity readily accounts for the other examples of clones showing dual specificity; thus in the case

TABLE IV

Summary of H-2 Reactivity Patterns of $Mls^{a,d}$-Specific T Cell Clones[a]

	H-2 haplotype recognized							
Clone	*b*	*k*	*f*	*r*	*s*	*p*	*d*(self)	$Mls^{a,d}$
D5.14		++						++++
D5.16	+++		++					++++
C2.2	++							++++
E4				+		++++		++++
E8				++++	+			++++
E19				+				++++
E26							++	++++
C5.2	++	+						++++

[a] The + indicates the relative response on H-2 of each clone; the Mls response was given an arbitrary ++++. From Webb *et al.*, 1981.

of D^b-restricted H-Y-specific T killer cells which have joint specificity for D^d alloantigens (von Boehmer *et al.*, 1979), one can envisage that D^d mimics D^b + H-Y. The main problem with applying this argument to the present studies is that it fails to account for the seemingly random anti-H-2 reactivity of Mls-specific clones. To sustain this view one would be forced to argue that a multiplicity of different H-2 epitopes are represented on the $Mls^{a,d}$ molecule(s). *A priori,* this seems rather unlikely.

The alternative possibility, which we favor, is that Mls and H-2 determinants are recognized by two independent sets of receptors. If further analysis indicates that the association of anti-H-2 and anti-Mls reactivity is indeed totally random (the number of clones tested to date is limited), this would seem to be the only logical explanation for the data. Definitive evidence for this argument, however, may be difficult to obtain.

The notion that Mls and H-2 determinants are recognized by two independent sets of receptors raises the following several issues.

1. Do all anti-Mls clones have anti-H-2 reactivity? It was mentioned that 5 of 13 Mls-reactive clones showed anti-H-2 reactivity (Table II). Bearing in mind that only 5 *H-2* haplotypes were tested, i.e., only a fraction of those known to exist, it is quite conceivable that all Mls-specific clones might have anti-H-2 reactivity. Parenthetically, it should be emphasized that the converse is not true, i.e., all H-2-reactive T cells are clearly not $Mls^{a,d}$ reactive (Table I) (Molnar-Kimber and Sprent, 1980).

2. What are Mls "determinants"? It was mentioned earlier that $Mls^{a,d}$ gene products are not serologically detectable, display little if any polymorphism, and,

at least in our hands, are not recognized in an MHC-restricted fashion. Mls determinants thus differ significantly from MHC glycoproteins and most non-MHC antigens. For this reason, it does not strain credulity to imagine that the recognition of Mls determinants is fundamentally different from that of either H-2 alloantigens or conventional antigens. Elsewhere we have suggested that Mls determinants might be viewed, not as antigens, but as mitogens (Molnar-Kimber and Sprent, 1980; Molnar-Kimber *et al.*, 1980). As for phytohemagglutinin and concanavalin A, Mls determinants might thus be recognized via a separate set of "mitogen receptors."

3. Relevance to one versus two-receptor controversy. Although most workers now feel that T cells do not recognize conventional antigens via two independent sets of receptors, the controversy of a single recognition unit for neoantigenic determinants versus two linked recognition units (one for antigen X and the other for self MHC) on one "receptor" is far from resolved. At face value one might argue that the present data support the dual recogition hypothesis. The validity of this argument rests on whether Mls determinants fall into the antigen X category. For various reasons (see above), particularly the apparent lack of H-2 restriction for anti-Mls responses, it is difficult to imagine that Mls determinants do fall into this category. Hence, although we argue that anti-Mls and anti-H-2 responses are mediated via different sets of receptors, we are hesitant to step to the further conclusion that a similar process of dual recognition applies to anti-(self + X) responses.

As a final point one might mention that if recognition of Mls determinants is indeed independent of that of H-2 determinants or conventional antigen, certain T cell clones would be expected to have triple specificity, i.e., for self + X, a particular H-2 alloantigen, and for Mls determinants. Screening self + X-reactive clones for anti-Mls reactivity might reveal such specificity.

ACKNOWLEDGMENTS

This work was supported by United States Public Health Service Grants CA-15822, CA-09140, AI-10961, and AI-15393. The excellent technical assistance of Ms. Carol Reinsel is gratefully acknowledged.

REFERENCES

Braciale, T. J., Andrew, M. E., and Braciale, V. L. (1981). Simultaneous expression of H-2-restricted and alloreactive recognition by a cloned line of influenza virus-specific cytotoxic T lymphocytes. *J. Exp. Med.* **153,** 1371.

Dickler, H. B., Rosenstreich, D. L., Ahmed, A., and Sachs, D. H. (1980). Genetic linkage between *Ly M-1*, *Sas-1*, and *Mls* loci. *Immunogenetics* **10,** 93.

Festenstein, H. (1973). Immunogenetic and biological aspects of *in vitro* lymphocyte allotransformation (MLR) in the mouse. *Transplant. Rev.* **15,** 62.

Heber-Katz, E., and Wilson, D. B. (1976). SRBC specific helper activity in rat TDL populations positively selected for reactivity to specific strong histocompatibility antigens. *J. Exp. Med.* **143,** 701.

Huber, B., Demant, P., and Festenstein, H. (1973). Influence of *M* locus and *K* end and *D* end (*H-2* region) incompatibilities on heart muscle allograft survival time. *Transplant. Proc.* **5,** 1377.

Janeway, C., Jones, B., Binz, H., Frischknecht, H., and Wigzell, H. (1980). T-cell receptor idiotypes. *Scand. J. Immunol.* **12,** 83.

Korngold, R., and Sprent, J. (1978). Lethal graft-versus-host disease after bone marrow transplantation across minor histocompatibility barriers in mice. Prevention by removal of mature T cells from marrow. *J. Exp. Med.* **148,** 1687.

Molnar-Kimber, K. L., and Sprent, J. (1980). Absence of H-2 restriction in primary and secondary mixed lymphocyte reactions to strong Mls determinants. *J. Exp. Med.* **151,** 407.

Molnar-Kimber, K. L., and Sprent, J. (1981). Evidence that strong Mls determinants are non-polymorphic. *Transplantation* **31,** 376.

Molnar-Kimber, K. L., Webb, S. R., Sprent, J., and Wilson, D. B. (1980). T-cell lines with dual specificity for strong Mls and H-2 determinants. *J. Immunol.* **125,** 2643.

Nisbet, N. W., and Edwards, J. (1973). The *H-2 D* and *H-2 K* regions of the major histocompatibility system and the *M* locus of the mouse investigated by parabiosis. *Transplant. Proc.* **5,** 1411.

Rollinghoff, M., Pfizenmeier, K., Trostman, H., and Wagner, H. (1975). T cell proliferation in the mixed lymphocyte culture does not necessarily result in the generation of cytotoxic T effector cells. *Eur. J. Immunol.* **5,** 560.

Ryan, J. J., Ahmed, A., Kind, P., and Sell, K. W. (1979). Crossreactivity exists between Mls^a and Mls^d lymphocyte-activating determinants as demonstrated by the negative clonal selection of responder cells in a mixed lymphocyte reaction. *Transplant. Proc.* **11,** 1377.

Sachs, J. A., Huber, B., Pena-Martinez, J., and Festenstein, H. (1973). Genetic studies and effect on skin allograft survival of *DBA/2, DAG, Ly,* and *M* locus antigens. *Transplant. Proc.* **5,** 1385.

Sredni, B., and Schwartz, R. (1981). Antigen-specific, proliferating T lymphocyte clones. Methodology, specificity, MHC restriction and allreactivity. *Immunol. Rev.* **54,** 187.

Tonkonogy, S. L., and Winn, H. J. (1977). Further genetic and serological analysis of the Ly M-1 alloantigenic system. *Immunogenetics* **5,** 57.

von Boehmer, H., Hengartner, H., Nabholz, M., Lernhardt, W., Schreier, M. H., and Haas, W. (1979). Fine specificity of a continuously growing killer cell clone specific for H-Y antigen. *Eur. J. Immunol.* **9,** 592.

Webb, S. R., Molnar-Kimber, K. L., Bruce, J., Sprent, J., and Wilson, D. B. (1981). T cell clones with dual specificity for Mls and various MHC determinants. *J. Exp. Med.* **154,** 1970.

Wilson, D. B., Heber-Katz, E., Sprent, J., and Howard, J. C. (1977). On the possibility of multiple T-cell receptors. *Cold Spring Harbor Symp. Quant. Biol.* **41,** 559.

28

Lymphokine Production by Cytolytic and Noncytolytic Alloreactive T Cell Clones

*Andrew L. Glasebrook/Anne Kelso/Rudolf H. Zubler/
John M. Ely/Michael B. Prystowsky/Frank W. Fitch*

I. Analysis of Lymphokine Production by a Noncytolytic T Cell Clone and Its Variant upon Alloantigenic Stimulation 342
II. Analysis of Lymphokine Production by Noncytolytic and Cytolytic Alloreactive T Cell Clones after Stimulation with Mitogen 345
III. Biological Separation of Lymphokine Activities Using Different T Cell Clones 348
IV. Heterogeneity of Cell Clones Producing Lymphokines 350
V. Conclusions 352
References 353

Antigenic or mitogenic stimulation of T lymphocytes *in vitro* is often accompanied by the appearance of soluble factors (lymphokines) in the culture supernatant fluids (SF). Activities reported to be present within such culture SF include the family of interleukin (IL) molecules (IL-1, IL-2, IL-3), immune interferon (IFN-γ), macrophage activating factor (MAF), colony stimulating factors (CSF), B cell stimulating factor (BCSF), B cell helper factor (BCHF), factors affecting macrophage Ia expression (MIRF), migration inhibitory factor (MIF), and factors affecting complement synthesis. Several of these lymphokines can exert a regulatory influence on immune respones, replacing in some instances the need for direct interactions between cells. While lymphokines produced in some systems may be antigen specific, the majority appear to be nonspecific in function. Although some of these lymphokines have been separated by physicochemical techniques, it has not been clear whether discrete subpopulations of T cells

ISBN 0-12-249920-4

produce different lymphokines or whether a single cell type can produce multiple lymphokines. In addition, the role of different antigens for the induction of particular lymphokines have not been defined. Also, it has been difficult to determine whether T cells actually secrete the lymphokines or induce their production by other non-T cells which are required for antigenic or mitogenic stimulation.

Analysis of clonal T cell products offers one approach to the study of soluble mediators. Cloned antigen-responsive cells provide unique model systems for determining the range of lymphokine activities produced by a single T cell type and for characterizing the interactions involved in immune responses. We have observed that alloreactive noncytolytic and cytolytic T cell clones stimulated with allogeneic cells are quite heterogeneous in the array of lymphokines which they produce. Although most cloned cytolytic T cells (CTL) do not produce IL-2, CTL can produce other lymphokines. Some of these lymphokines can be separated biologically by differences in the kinetics of their production. Alternatively, the dissociation of various lymphokines can be achieved using different T cell clones. It has been determined that the lymphokines originate from the cloned T cells, since stimulation with concanavalin A (Con-A) after extended culture of cloned cells in IL-2 alone causes similar patterns of lymphokine release.

I. ANALYSIS OF LYMPHOKINE PRODUCTION BY A NONCYTOLYTIC T CELL CLONE AND ITS VARIANT UPON ALLOANTIGENIC STIMULATION

The derivation of noncytolytic, Thy-1$^+$, Lyt-2$^-$, T cell clones from secondary C57BL/6 anti-DBA/2 mixed leukocyte culture (MLC) has been described previously (Glasebrook and Fitch, 1979, 1980; Glasebrook *et al.*, 1981a). These T cell clones proliferated in the absence of exogenously added IL-2 when cultured with the original stimulating DBA/2 alloantigen ($H\text{-}2^d$, Mls^a). Analysis of antigenic specificity indicated that the clones were reactive toward non-MHC antigens, most likely the strongly stimulating *Mls* locus determinants ($Mls^{a,d}$). The clones were defined operationally as amplifier or helper cells, since they could cooperate with cytolytic T lymphocytes (CTL) in generating specific cytolytic activity. In addition, SF collected from cultures of alloantigen-stimulated T cell clones contained IL-2 activity equivalent to or greater than that present in secondary MLC SF (Ryser *et al.*, 1978).

One clone, designated L2, has been studied in greater detail. L2 cells were restimulated with T cell-depleted stimulating cells. Supernatant fluids were then collected over a 6–192 hr culture period and analyzed for the presence of IL-2, CSF, and BCSF (Ely *et al.*, 1981). IL-2 was quantified by measuring the proliferation of a cloned IL-2-dependent cytolytic T cell line (Gillis *et al.*, 1978). The results are expressed as units of IL-2 per milliliter as determined by comparison with a standardized preparation of IL-2 provided by S. Gillis. Colony stimulating factor was quantified by measuring the number of colonies formed by bone marrow cells incubated with a 1/20,000 dilution of SF in semisolid medium (Stanley *et al.*, 1972). The stimulation of plaque-forming cells (PFC) by a 1/15 dilution of SF in the absence of antigen was used to quantify BCSF (Glasebrook *et al.*, 1981c). For the latter two assays, these particular dilutions of SF were chosen on the basis of previous dose–response studies.

The results from a representative experiment are shown in Fig. 1. The activity of IL-2 was detected as early as 6 hr after stimulation and reached a maximum value of 15 IL-2 units/ml at 24 hr. IL-2 activity declined thereafter and was no longer detectable after 96 hr. However, CSF and BCSF reached peak levels of activity after 12–24 hr of culture and remained at near maximal values throughout the entire 192 hr culture period. Supernatant fluids collected from cultures containing only stimulating cells or L2 cells were negative for all three activities (data not shown).

The transient expression of IL-2 activity during the first 96 hr of culture was similar to that reported by Gillis *et al.* (1978). Possible explanations for the disappearance of IL-2 activity include the release of an inhibitory factor, and the absorbtion and/or degradation of IL-2 by L2 cells or stimulating cells. Only slight

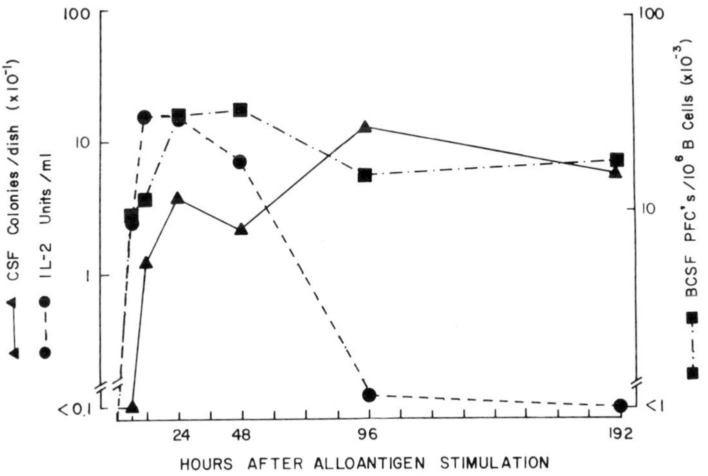

Fig. 1. Time course of lymphokine release by the cloned amplifier T cell, L2. At $t = 0$, 1×10^5 L2 cells were stimulated with 6×10^6 T-depleted CBA spleen cells in 1.1 ml of culture medium. Wells harvested at 6, 12, 24, 48, 96, and 192 hr were tested for Il-2 (●--●), CSF (▲——▲, final dilution 1/20,000), and BCSF (■—·—■, final dilution 1/15) activities. Background levels were 0.1 units/ml, 6 ± 4 colonies/dish, and 2900 PFC/10^6 B cells, respectively.

inhibition of cell proliferation induced by IL-2 was observed upon addition of 96 hr or 192 hr L2 SF (Ely *et al.* 1981). The extent of inhibition was not great enough to account for the absence of detectable IL-2 after 96 hr. These findings are consistent with those of Gillis *et al.* (1978) and suggest that the release of inhibitory substances does not account completely for the transient expression of IL-2 activity. Other results suggest that proliferation of L2 cells is due to the utilization of IL-2 released following stimulation with antigen. L2 cells will proliferate when cultured with 24-hr L2 SF but not with 96-hr L2 SF which contains high levels of other lymphokines but not IL-2. Antigen-stimulated L2 but not L2V cells can be grown without added IL-2. Thus, it is most probable that the time-dependent reduction in IL-2 titer is due to utilization by L2 cells. Although enzymatic degradation of IL-2 can not be excluded, nonspecific degradation seems unlikely, since CSF and BCSF were not similarly degraded.

Cloned L2 cells have been maintained by weekly stimulation with irradiated allogeneic spleen cells and secondary MLC SF containing IL-2; these conditions are optimal for culture of T cells *in vitro,* favoring the maintenance of a stable phenotype. These conditions, however, may not be optimal for maintaining functional properties. After an extended period of culture *in vitro,* it was observed that the levels of IL-2 activity in L2 SF gradually declined. It had been shown that variants were often generated and/or selected by culture in IL-2-containing conditioned medium (Nabholz *et al.,* 1980; von Boehmer and Haas, 1981). Therefore, it seemed possible that the presence of IL-2 in maintenance cultures of

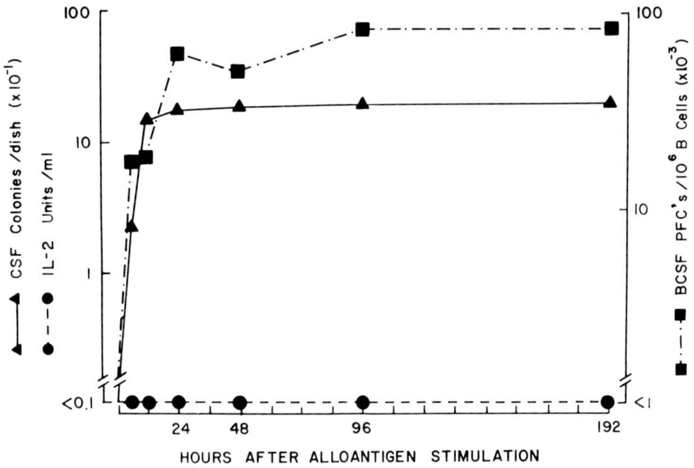

Fig. 2. Time course of lymphokine release by the variant cloned T cell, L2V. See the legend of Fig. 1 for culture conditions. Wells harvested at 6, 12, 24, 48, 96, and 192 hr were tested for IL-2 (●--●), CSF (▲——▲, final dilution 1/2000), and BCSF (■-·—·-■, final dilution 1/15) activities. Background levels were 0.1 units/ml, 3 ± 2 colonies/dish, and 3600 PFC/10^6 B cells, respectively.

TABLE I

Lymphokine Activities Secreted by T Cell Clones

	Lymphokine activity[a]								
Clone	IL-2	CSF	BCSF	IFN-γ	MIRF	MIF	FcR induction	C2/C4	IL-3
L2	+	+	+	+	+	+	+	+	+
L2V	−	+	+	+	−	−	+	−	+

[a] IL-2, interleukin 2; CSF, granulocyte/macrophage colony stimulating factor (Dr. Eugene Goldwasser); BCSF, B cell stimulating factor (Dr. José Quintans); IFN-γ, antiviral activity (interferon) (Dr. Stefanie Vogel); MIRF, macrophage Ia recruiting factor (Dr. David Beller); MIF, migration inhibitory factor (Dr. Heinz Remold); FcR induction, increase in macrophage Fc receptors (Dr. Stefanie Vogel); C2/C4, prolonged synthesis of the second and fourth components of complement by macrophages (Drs. John and Margaret Goldman); IL-3, induction of 20 α-steroid dehydrogenase in lymphocytes (Dr. James Ihle). The name within parenthesis after each factor indicates the investigator who was responsible for that assay.

L2 cells may have generated and/or selected for variants which were IL-2-dependent and did not produce IL-2. Therefore, the population of L2 cells was recloned, and a variant subclone of L2 (designated L2V) was isolated which did not produce IL-2 (Ely *et al.*, 1981). Supernatant fluids collected from cultures of the L2V variant clone stimulated with allogeneic cells were then analyzed for the presence of IL-2, CSF, and BCSF. As shown in Fig. 2, the time course of CSF and BCSF production by variant L2V cells was identical to that observed with the parent L2 clone (Fig. 1). IL-2 activity, however, was not detected in any of the samples. Therefore, the kinetics of lymphokine release together with the array of biological activities found in SF from a variant clone indicate that the molecule responsible for IL-2 activity differs from the molecules accounting for CSF and BCSF activity.

Both L2 and L2V produce additional lymphokines (Table I). L2 secretes a wide range of lymphokines affecting T cells, B cells, macrophages, hematopoietic stem cells, and fibroblasts after either antigen or mitogen stimulation. While these data show that a single T cell clone is capable of producing numerous lymphokine activities, it is not clear whether L2 represents a common or rare type of T helper cell.

II. ANALYSIS OF LYMPHOKINE PRODUCTION BY NONCYTOLYTIC AND CYTOLYTIC ALLOREACTIVE T CELL CLONES AFTER STIMULATION WITH MITOGEN

Interpretations regarding the cellular origin of the lymphokines are complicated by the need to use allogeneic spleen cells as the antigenic stimulus for lymphokine production. It cannot be excluded, for example, that some of the multiple activities may be contributed by stimulating cells. Recent reports have shown that T cell lymphomas and hybridomas can be stimulated by mitogen to secrete appreciable quantities of IL-2 (Farrar *et al.*, 1980; Gillis *et al.*, 1980; Harwell *et al.*, 1980; Shimizu *et al.*, 1980; Schrader and Clark-Lewis, 1981). These observations suggested that mitogenic stimulation of alloreactive cloned T cells might trigger a similar release of lymphokines. L2 cells were removed from culture, separated from dead cells and debris, and stimulated with various concentrations of concanavalin A (Con-A). After 24 hr, SF were collected and assayed for IL-2 activity. As shown in Fig. 3, release of IL-2 was induced by Con-A in a dose-dependent manner; 2 μg/ml stimulated a release of IL-2 similar to that observed with allogeneic spleen cells. Levels of CSF and BCSF activity induced with Con-A were also comparable to those obtained by stimulation with allogeneic cells (data not shown). Stimulation of the variant L2 clone with Con-A caused the release of CSF and BCSF comparable in activity to that obtained with alloantigenic stimulation, but did not cause the release of IL-2 (data not shown). These results strongly suggest that the lymphokine activities detected in SF from alloantigen-stimulated cloned T cells were derived from the T cells.

However, the L2 cells had been maintained with allogeneic spleen cells prior to stimulation with Con-A, and it is possible that residual stimulating cells may have contributed to lymphokine release upon Con-A stimulation. To avoid this possibility, four independently derived C57BL/6 anti-DBA/2 T cell clones were maintained for 1 month in IL-2-containing conditioned medium alone. Although

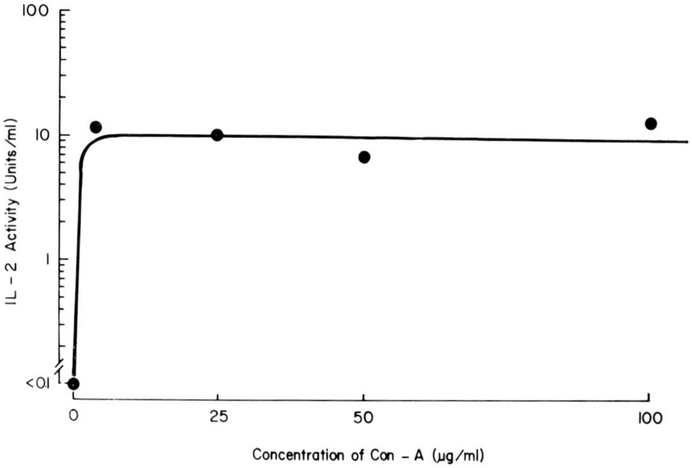

Fig. 3. Stimulation of IL-2 release from L2 cells by Con-A. 1×10^5 L2 cells were cultured with various concentrations of Con-A in 1.1 ml culture medium for 24 hr. Supernates were harvested and tested for IL-2 activity.

in our hands, T cell clones grow optimally in the presence of antigen/feeder cells as well as a source of IL-2, cloned T cells can be grown in IL-2-containing conditioned medium alone, although cell recoveries are at least 5- to 10-fold lower. After 1 month culture in IL-2, these T cell clones were stimulated with either T cell-depleted DBA/2 spleen cells or Con-A for 24 hr, and the SF were collected and analyzed for IL-2, MAF, IFN-γ and B cell helper factor (BCHF) (Glasebrook *et al.*, 1982a). Macrophage activating factor was quantified by measuring the activation of macrophage-mediated cytotoxicity against tumor target cells. Immune interferon levels were determined by measuring the ability of SF to protect L cells from the cytopathic effect of encephalomyocarditis virus and the data were converted to units of IFN-γ by comparison with the NIH standard. The assay for BCHF activity measured the ability of SF to induce IgG SRBC-specific plaque-forming cells (PFC) in cultures containing B cells, macrophages, SRBC, and lipopolysaccharide (Zubler and Glasebrook, 1982).

As shown in Table II, lymphokine release was not constitutive but could be induced by stimulation with either allogeneic cells or Con-A. More importantly, the patterns of lymphokine release upon antigenic or mitogenic stimulation were identical. Preferential release of a particular lymphokine could not be stimulated with allogeneic cells or Con-A. Three clones (AD5, M5, and D3) are noncytolytic and proliferate when stimulated with appropriate allogeneic cells in the absence of IL-2. Stimulation of these three clones (AD5, D3, M5) with allogeneic cells resulted in approximately 3- to 10-fold higher titers in lymphokine activity relative to the levels observed after stimulation with Con-A. In contrast, stimulation of a highly cytolytic, IL-2-dependent clone (L3C5) with allogeneic cells resulted in 4-fold lower titers of MAF and IFN-γ when compared to stimulation with Con-A. It is not readily apparent why such differences were observed. The majority of cloned T cell SF also contained higher levels of lymphokine compared to secondary MLC SF. This is especially significant since the number of cloned T cells used for SF production was tenfold lower than the number of responding cells in secondary MLC. Whether this reflects simply an enrichment of lymphokine-producing cells or the absence of regulatory cells normally present in MLC populations, mitogenic stimulation of cloned helper T cells provides a simple model system for study of the kinetics and heterogeneity of lymphokine release while avoiding possible contribution of stimulating cells to lymphokine production.

Since other investigators had observed that Con-A did not stimulate long-term cultured T cell lines or T cell clones to proliferate (Fathman and Hengartner, 1978; Watson, 1979), it is somewhat surprising that lymphokine production by antigen-reactive T cells can be stimulated with Con-A. However, similar results have been reported recently by Marcucci *et al.* (1981; Chapter 21 in this treatise) who found that hapten-reactive T cell clones maintained in IL-2 also could be stimulated with Con-A to release several biologically different lymphokines. It is

TABLE II

Lymphokine Production by Alloreactive T Cell Clones after Culture for 1 Month in IL-2 Alone[a]

T cell clone	Stimulation	Units of activity/ml			
		IL-2	MAF	IFN-γ	BCHF
AD5	Con-A	3.3	1208	1300	9
	Allogeneic cells	20.0	3325	5200	92
	Medium	<0.1	<2	<10	<0.2
M5	Con-A	4.0	191	640	38
	Allogeneic cells	27.0	388	1300	150
	Medium	<0.1	<2	<10	<0.2
D3	Con-A	0.7	1524	2600	8
	Allogeneic cells	5.3	3478	5200	25
	Medium	<0.1	<2	<10	<0.2
L3C5	Con-A	<0.1	376	640	<0.2
	Allogeneic cells	<0.1	109	160	<0.2
	Medium	<0.1	<2	<10	<0.2
—	Con-A	<0.1	<2	<10	<0.2
	Allogeneic cells	<0.1	<2	<10	<0.2
Secondary MLC SF	—	16.0	100	1300	100

[a]< T cell clones were maintained in secondary MLC SF (IL-2) in the absence of antigen/feeder cells for 1 month prior to stimulation. Approximately 10^5 cloned cells were stimulated with 2 μg Con-A or 5 × 10^6 irradiated T cell-depleted allogeneic spleen cells in a total volume of 1.0 ml culture medium (Glasebrook and Fitch, 1980). SF were harvested after 24 hr of culture and tested for the various lymphokine activities. Adapted from Glasebrook *et al.* (1982a).

interesting to note that although Con-A triggers the release of large amounts of lymphokines including IL-2, cells proliferate poorly if at all after stimulation with Con-A (A. L. Glasebrook, unpublished observation). The mechanism by which Con-A triggers lymphokine release is not known. The lectin may bind to the receptor for antigen and mimic antigen binding.

III. BIOLOGICAL SEPARATION OF LYMPHOKINE ACTIVITIES USING DIFFERENT T CELL CLONES

The previous section demonstrated that a noncytolytic T cell clone (L2) and its variant could be used to dissociate the molecular species responsible for different lymphokine activities. Such an analysis requires the isolation of variants which arise either spontaneously or after mutagenesis treatment. This procedure is time consuming and may not always be possible. An alternative approach would be to screen a large number of independently derived T cell clones for those which release some but not all lymphokines. We have carried out such an analysis using alloreactive T cell clones which were derived by limiting dilution or micromanipulation (Glasebrook *et al.*, 1981a). After subcloning, the lines were maintained continuously *in vitro* by stimulation with alloantigen and secondary MLC SF.

Analysis of SF collected from cultures of independently derived cloned T cell lines stimulated with T cell-depleted allogeneic cells indicated considerable heterogeneity in lymphokine release. None, few, or many lymphokine activities could be detected in SF from cloned T cells. Results obtained from six representative clones are summarized in Table III and demonstrate the biological separation of lymphokine activities which can be achieved. Identical patterns of lymphokine release were also observed when several of these clones were maintained only in IL-2-containing medium and then stimulated with mitogen (Table II and data not shown). Several dissociations are readily apparent. SF from clone M5 contained all five lymphokine activities (I1-2, IFN-γ, MAF, BCHF, and CSF), while SF from clone V4 contained only IL-2, BCHF, and CSF activity. This clear separation of IFN-γ and MAF activities from IL-2, BCHF, and CSF activity was also observed with clone L3C5 SF which contained IFN-γ, MAF activity but not IL-2, BCHF, or CSF activity. Evidence that the molecules responsible for IL-2 and BCHF activity are not identical was provided by analysis of SF from clones AB1 and AF3; SF from AB1 contained IL-2 activity but no detectable BCHF activity, while SF from clone AF3 contained BCHF but not IL-2.

We have only recently begun to examine CSF activity and have not yet analyzed all SF from all T cell clones for this lymphokine activity. So far CSF activity has been dissociated only from IFN-γ, MAF activity, although results

TABLE III

Multiple Patterns of Lymphokine Production by Alloreactive T Cell Clones[a]

T cell clone	Cytolytic activity	Lymphokine activities detected in SF				
		IL-2	IFN-γ	MAF	BCHF	CSF
M5	−	+	+	+	+	+
V4	−	+	−	−	+	+
AB1	−	+	+	+	−	n.t.
AF3	+	−	+	+	+	n.t.
L3C5	+	−	+	+	−	−
CH80	+	−	−	−	n.t.	n.t.

[a] Approximately 10^5 cloned T cells were cultured with 5×10^6 T cell-depleted allogeneic spleen cells in a total volume of 1.5 ml culture medium. SF were harvested after 24 hr of culture and tested for the presence of the various lymphokines. n.t., not tested.

obtained with the L2 cell clone and its variant demonstrated that CSF and IL-2 activity were separable. IFN-γ and MAF activity have not been separated in any of the cloned T cell SF tested. This may be associated with a selection of T cells which grow well *in vitro*. However, Krammer *et al.* (Chapter 21 in this treatise) have reported dissociation of IFN-γ and MAF activity in SF from subclones of a picryl chloride-reactive T cell clone. It should be noted that cytolytic as well as noncytolytic T cell clones could release an array of lymphokines. Cytolytic T cell clones have been examined by others for their ability to release IL-2 and were found to be negative. We observed however that cytolytic cells could release a variety of lymphokines other than IL-2. This was observed with several different cytolytic clones (Glasebrook *et al.*, 1982a). Collectively, our results would indicate then that at least three different molecules are responsible for IL-2, BCHF/CSF, and IFN-γ/MAF activities.

IV. HETEROGENEITY OF CELL CLONES PRODUCING LYMPHOKINES

Considerable heterogeneity was observed among the lymphokine-producing T cell clones when analyzed for the expression of cytolytic activity and the ability to proliferate to specific antigenic stimulation in the absence of added IL-2 (Glasebrook *et al.*, 1981b). Table IV summarizes the results obtained with 26 different alloreactive T cell clones which differ according to the strain of origin, antigenic specificity, and Lyt expression. All T cell clones could be functionally placed into at least 11 different subgroups. In most instances each subgroup contained two or more clones. SF collected from some Lyt-2^+ T cell clones were devoid of lymphokine activity. However, all Lyt-2^- T cell clones could be stimulated with allogeneic cells to release one or more lymphokines. In terms of cytolytic function, three distinct groups of clones were observed; those which were directly cytolytic (Lyt-2^+), those which required lectin for the expression of nonspecific cytolytic activity (Lyt-2^- or Lyt-2^+), and those which were totally noncytolytic, either in the presence or absence of lectin (Lyt-2^-). Clones from all three groups could be stimulated to release IFN-γ and MAF although the majority of IL-2-secreting T cell clones were noncytolytic and Lyt-2^-. We have derived lectin-dependent (Lyt-2^-) or directly cytolytic (Lyt-2^+) T cell clones which secrete IL-2, although the frequency of such cells in primed MLC cell populations is much lower compared to noncytolytic IL-2-producing cells (Glasebrook *et al.*, 1982b). Further subdivisions became apparent based on the antigen-specific proliferation of T cel! clones. All IL-2-secreting T cell clones could proliferate when stimulated with antigen in the absence of added conditioned medium, although not all T cell clones which proliferated when stimulated with alloantigen secreted detectable IL-2.

TABLE IV

Heterogeneity of Lymphokine Production by Phenotypically Different T Cell Clones

Cytolytic activity	IL-2-independent antigen-specific proliferation	Antigenic specificity	Lyt expression	Lymphokines detected in SF[a]		
				IL-2	IFN-γ	MAF
Cytolytic	+	H-2^d (I?)	1^+2^+	+	+	+
	+	H-$2D^d$		±	+	+
	+	H-$2K^k$	1^-2^+, 1^+2^+	−	+	+
	−	H-$2D^d$		−	+	+
	−	H-$2K^k$	1^-2^+, 1^+2^+	−	−	−
Lectin-dependent cytolytic	+	Mls^a		+	+	+
	+	H-2^d				
	+	H-$2I^k$	1^-2^-, 1^+2^-	−	+	+
	−	H-$2K^k$	1^+2^+	−	−	−
Noncytolytic	+	Mls^a		+	+	+
			1^+2^-			
	+	H-$2I^k$		+	−	−
	±	H-2^d	1^+2^-	−	+	+

[a] Cloned T cell SF were produced as described in Table III. Adapted from Glasebrook *et al.* (1981b).

All antigens toward which the clones were reactive appeared equally effective at inducing the release of IFN-γ and MAF activity. However, only strong *Mls* locus of *I* region determinants could stimulate the release of appreciable IL-2 activity. H-2K,D antigens stimulated the release of little or no detectable IL-2 activity. Other investigators have reported that production of IL-2 in response to H-2K,D stimulation in primary MLC required the presence of Lyt-2^+ T cells (Okada and Henney, 1980; Andrus *et al.*, 1981). We have been unable to reproduce these results in several different strain combinations over a wide dose–response range (A. L. Glasebrook, unpublished results). While it has been possible to isolate cytolytic (Lyt-2^+) T cell clones specific for H-2K,D antigens which proliferate to antigenic stimulation in the absence of added IL-2, these clones release little or no detectable IL-2 activity. Conversely, a cytolytic T cell clone with similar growth properties but which was not specific for H-2K,D secreted amounts of IL-2 comparable to that observed for noncytolytic T cell clones. Cells responsive to H-2K,D stimuli may proliferate autonomously or produce IL-2 at a rate which is only slightly greater than their rate of utilization. Cells responsive to *Mls* locus or *I* region antigens, however, secrete an excess of IL-2 which is detectable in SF. Thus, particular antigens appear to stimulate preferentially IL-2 production. The role which IL-2 or other growth-promoting lymphokines may play in those genetic combinations where IL-2 production is low or not detectable remains to be determined. It is of interest, however, that repeated attempts to derive IL-2-secreting T cell clones in the syngeneic male H-Y system have so far been unsuccessful (O. Kanagawa, personal communication).

The T cell clones used in this study often have been derived for other purposes (cytolytic activity, IL-2 production, etc.) and have been maintained continuously *in vitro*. This surely has selected clones with particular properties which may have influenced the patterns of lymphokine release observed. The considerable heterogeneity observed even in this selected panel of clones, however, suggests that the true heterogeneity of T cells which secrete lymphokines will be much greater and more complex. Another approach to analysis of T cells is by limiting dilution (Chapter 21 in this treatise), although with this approach, there may be a problem in determining whether the cells actually originated from a single precursor. To avoid this problem, we have begun to analyze lymphokine production using cells isolated from MLC by micromanipulation. Cloning efficiencies are often greater than 40% with this method, and one is sure of clonality. It is possible to determine frequencies of lymphokine-producing cells and to define dissociations of the production of multiple lymphokines. Preliminary results are encouraging and appear to offer an alternative to limiting dilution.

V. CONCLUSIONS

Antigenic or mitogenic stimulation of T cell clones provides a simple model system for study of the kinetics and heterogeneity of lymphokine release by T cells. Both cytolytic and noncytolytic T cell clones can be induced to release a variety of lymphokines. Analysis of clonal specificity and function has provided information regarding the ability of certain antigens to stimulate release of specific lymphokine activities and the phenotype of the producing T cells. Culture systems allowing for the derivation and maintenance of a large number of short-term T cell clones and development of microassays will facilitate analysis of lymphokine production by T cells and enable more definitive characterization of the cellular phenotype of the secreting T cells and the antigens to which they respond.

The availability of lymphokine-secreting T cell clones also offers the possibility of obtaining homogeneous lymphokine free from contaminating activities. Many of the lymphokine activites which are proving difficult to separate and purify to homogeneity using physicochemical methods appear to be secreted differentially by some T cell clones. Lymphokine levels found in SF from cloned

T cells are often greater than that found in bulk cell cultures, and this may reflect the lack of regulatory controls which operate at the populational cell level.

T cell clones which release known lymphokines upon stimulation also should facilitate study of the role of lymphokines *in vivo* and the interactions between cells and molecules involved in generation of an immune response. Other than proliferation, the only discernible function of the noncytolytic clones described above is the secretion of biologically active lymphokines, and these cells appear to be regulatory T cells. It is surprising, however, that cytolytic T cell clones which function as effector cells in immune response could also function to secrete lymphokines, sometimes including even IL-2. It has been difficult to show directly that cytolytic T cells are the actual effector cells in allograft injection and tumor immunity. However, it is not hard to imagine how specific antigenic stimulation of cytolytic cells to release nonspecific lymphokines inhibiting virally infected cells or activating macrophages which have been observed selectively to infiltrate allografts would then facilitate an immune response *in vivo*. Expression of cytolytic activity may then be secondary to recruitment of other cells and release of antiviral activity. What regulatory mechanisms exist *in vivo* to control such responses is not known. Having defined reagents is a step toward answering such questions, and clones should prove very valuable in this regard.

REFERENCES

Andrus, L., Prowse, S. J., and Lafferty, K. J. (1981). Interleukin-2 production by both $Ly2^+$ and $Ly2^-$ T-cell subsets. *Scand. J. Immunol.* **13,** 297.

Ely, J. M., Prystowsky, M. B., Eisenberg, L., Quintans, J., Goldwasser, E., Glasebrook, A. L., and Fitch, F. W. (1981). Alloreactive cloned T cell lines. V. Differential kinetics of IL-2, CSF, and BCSF release by a cloned T amplifier cell and its variant. *J. Immunol.* **127,** 2345.

Farrar, J. J., Fuller-Farrar, J., Simon, P. L., Hilfiker, M. L., Stadler, B. M., and Farrar, W. L. (1980). Thymoma production of T cell growth factor (Interleukin 2). *J. Immunol.* **125,** 2555.

Fathman, C. G., and Hengartner, H. (1978). Clones of alloreactive T cells. *Nature (London)* **272,** 617.

Gillis, S., Ferm, M. M., Ou, W., and Smith, K. A. (1978). T cell growth factor: Parameters of production, and a quantitative microassay for activity. *J. Immunol.* **121,** 2168.

Gillis, S., Scheid, M., and Watson, J. (1980). Biochemical and biologic characterization of lymphocyte regulatory molecules. III. The isolation and phenotypic characterization of interleukin-2 producing T cell lymphomas. *J. Immunol.* **125,** 2570.

Glasebrook, A. L., and Fitch, F. W. (1979). T-cell lines which cooperate in generation of specific cytolytic activity. *Nature (London)* **278,** 171.

Glasebrook, A. L., and Fitch, F. W. (1980). Alloreactive cloned T cell lines. I. Interactions between cloned amplifier and cytolytic T cell lines. *J. Exp. Med.* **151,** 876.

Glasebrook, A. L., Sarmiento, M., Loken, M. R., Dialynas, D. P., Quintans, J., Eisenberg, L., Lutz, C. T., Wilde, D., and Fitch, F. W. (1981a). Murine T lymphocyte clones with distinct immunological functions. *Immunol. Rev.* **54,** 225.

Glasebrook, A. L., Kelso, A., MacDonald, H. R., and Engers, H. D. (1981b). Heterogeneity of T cell clones. *Transpl. Clin. Immunol.* **13,** 63.

Glasebrook, A. L., Quintans, J., Eisenberg, L., and Fitch, F. W. (1981c). Alloreactive cloned T cell lines. II. Polyclonal stimulation of B cells by a cloned helper T cell line. *J. Immunol.* **126,** 240.

Glasebrook, A. L., Kelso, A., Zubler, R. H., MacDonald, H. R., Engers, H. D., and Brunner, K. T. (1982a). Heterogeneity of soluble factor production by cytolytic and non-cytolytic alloreactive T cell clones. (Submitted for publication.)

Glasebrook, A. L., MacDonald, H. R., Kelso, A., and Brunner, K. T. (1982b). IL-2-independent proliferating cytolytic T cell clones. I. Frequency, specificity, and phenotype. (Submitted for publication.)

Harwell, L., Skidmore, B., Marrack, P., and Kappler, J. (1980). A concanavalin A inducible, interleukin 2 producing T cell hybridoma. *J. Exp. Med.* **152,** 893.

Marcucci, F., Walter, M., Kirchner, H., and Krammer, P. (1981). Production of immune interferon by murine T-cell clones from long-term cultures. *Nature* (*London*) **291,** 79.

Nabholz, M., Conzelmann, A., Acuto, O., North, M., Haas, W., Pohlit, H., von Boehmer, H., Hengartner, H., Mach, J.-P., Engers, H., and Johnson, J. P. (1980). Established murine cytolytic T-cell lines as tools for a somatic cell genetic analysis of T-cell functions. *Immunol. Rev.* **51,** 125.

Okada, M., and Henney, C. S. (1980). The differentiation of cytotoxic T cells *in vitro*. II. Amplifying factor(s) produced in primary mixed lymphocyte cultures against K/D stimuli require the presence of Lyt 2^+ cells but not Lyt 1^+ cells. *J. Immunol.* **125,** 300.

Ryser, J.-E., Cerottini, J.-C., and Brunner, K. T. (1978). Generation of cytolytic T lymphocytes *in vitro*. IX. Induction of secondary CTL responses in primary long-term MLC by supernatants from secondary MLC. *J. Immunol.* **120,** 370.

Schrader, J. W., and Clark-Lewis, I. (1981). T cell hybridoma-derived regulatory factors. I. Production of T cell growth factor following stimulation by concanavalin A. *J. Immunol.* **126,** 1101.

Shimizu, S., Kanaka, Y., and Smith, R. (1980). Mitogen-initiated synthesis and secretion of T cell growth factors by a T lymphoma cell line. *J. Exp. Med.* **152,** 1436.

Stanley, E. R., Metcalf, D., Marite, J. S., and Yeo, G. F. (1972). Standardized bioassay for bone marrow colony stimulating factor in human urine: Levels in normal man. *J. Lab. Clin. Med.* **79,** 657.

von Boehmer, H., and Haas, W. (1981). H-2 restricted cytolytic and noncytolytic T cell clones: Isolation, specificity and functional analysis. *Immunol. Rev.* **54,** 27.

Watson, J. (1979). Continuous proliferation of murine antigen-specific helper T lymphocytes in culture. *J. Exp. Med.* **150,** 1510.

Zubler, R. H., and Glasebrook, A. L. (1982). Requirement for three signals in "T-independent" (lipopolysaccharide-induced) as well as in T-dependent B cell responses. *J. Exp. Med.* **155,** 666.

VI

Murine T Cell Clones Reactive with Soluble Antigens

29

An Overview

C. Garrison Fathman

Text 357
References 364

It was not until recent years that cloning of T lymphocytes became possible. Why was it not done earlier? In large part, cellular biologists were deluded by the ease with which clones of cells from the B lymphocyte lineage could be derived following myelomatous change. Such transformation resulted in cells retaining many relevant immunologically functional elements from their normal counterparts. From such cells, it was quite easy to isolate their antigen binding receptors (immunoglobulins). Remarkable strides have been made in the understanding of immunoglobulin structure, function, and molecular genetics due to the availability of myelomas providing large numbers of replicate copies of individual cells. One of the obvious advantages of isolating clones of T lymphocytes is the propagation of replicate copies of a single cell with a given immunological function.

In great part, the inability of cellular immunologists to clone or study T cells was due to the following two points: First, despite the existence of a large number of transformed cells of T lymphocyte lineage, it is not entirely clear that many of these cells shed or secrete immunologically relevant products. This is in distinct contrast to myeloma cells which almost invariably secrete the immunologically relevant product they are programmed to make. The inability of cell biologists to isolate "T cell receptors" from transformed T cell lines was due not only to the fact that such cells did not seem to secrete such products, but also to a complete lack of understanding of what such receptor products are. The second point was that T lymphocytes, which had not undergone transformation, required growth supporting factors produced by other immunologically competent cells. It was only with the discovery that such "T cell growth factors" were required for T cell growth and division that cellular immunologists were

ISBN 0-12-249920-4

finally able to solve the elusive problem of perpetuating T cell growth *in vitro*. Now that we have begun to isolate and study clones of individual T lymphocytes, what questions have been addressed?

Some parts of this book have been devoted to discussion of the isolation and characterization of the factors which allow the growth and ultimate isolation and propagation of such T lymphocyte clones. Other parts have dealt with somatic cell hybridization as a means of generating transformed populations of T lymphocytes with immunologically relevant products or functions. This part will deal with murine T cell clones which recognize and respond to soluble antigens. Using available technology, various laboratories have begun to address basic questions concerning immunocompetent cellular interactions. These include certain questions which will be outlined briefly in this introductory chapter, and many which have not yet been adequately answered.

One question which has perplexed cellular immunologists for a decade is the relationship between T cell recognition of alloantigen and other foreign antigens such as soluble proteins (Simonsen, 1967). Due to the high frequency of alloreactive T lymphocytes, many investigators have felt that the two T cell populations must be overlapping (Heber-Katz and Wilson, 1976; Lemonnier *et al.*, 1977; Bevan, 1977; Burakoff *et al.*, 1978). It was quite clear that this question could be addressed at the single cell level by asking whether alloreactive T cell clones recognize nominal antigens and whether clones of T cells recognizing nominal antigens can be stimulated by alloantigens. The first demonstration that such overlap might be possible was made by von Boehmer *et al.* (1979). In these studies, it was shown that clones selected for cytotoxicity against the H-Y antigen in association with D^b alloantigens also would lyse specifically male or female target cells carrying the D^d alloantigens. Additional studies which suggested that the populations of alloreactive and antigen-specific T cell clones were overlapping were provided by Sredni and Schwartz (1980) and will be discussed in Chapter 31 by Schwartz and Sredni. Basically, these studies showed that clones, selected for reactivity to nominal antigens and restricted by *I* region determinants, exhibited independent alloractivity against haplotype dissimilar stimulating cells. For example, clones selected for recognition of DNP-OVA, whose recognition was restricted by the *I-A* subregion of syngeneic B10.A antigen-presenting cells, could equally well be stimulated by alloreactive stimulator cells bearing $I\text{-}A^s$ alloantigens. The fact that alloreactivity of an *I-A* subregion restricted antigen-specific clone is directed at an *I-A* subregion product and that alloreactivity of a *D*-region restricted cytotoxic clone is directed at a *D*-region product suggests that the two specificities are not randomly associated. Thus, T cell clones have allowed an unequivocal answer to one of the perplexing problems of cellular immunology concerning the overlap of alloreactive and soluble antigen reactive T cell sets. The interesting and perplexing problem raised by Webb *et al.* (Chapter 27 in this treatise) concerning Mls recognition in the context of allorecognition adds a new wrinkle to the previous question. Their discussion of possible receptor interactions is of considerable interest.

A second question which could be addressed directly following the isolation of antigen specific murine T cell clones was whether helper T cells activated *in vivo* by one species of erythrocytes could help an antibody response directed against an unrelated antigen, provided that both antigens were present at the same time (Hartmann, 1970). Initial studies which addressed this question were by Max Schreier (Schreier *et al.*, 1980, for review) and his collaborators using murine T cell clones reactive with sheep erythrocytes. It was a consistent finding that clones or lines of specific helper T cells promoted antibody response to homologous and unrelated antigens to the same extent provided both antigens were present in culture. These findings argued strongly against an obligatory antigen-mediated T cell–B cell contact and hapten carrier linkage. They also presumably argued against antigen-specific T cell factors as well. This question will be addressed at the level of responses of antigen-specific murine T cell clones *in vitro* by Hodes *et al.* in Chapter 32 and Theze *et al.* in Chapter 33 of this treatise. It is quite clear in the studies presented by Hodes and his collaborators that there is no hapten-specific nor obligatory antigen-mediated T cell–B cell interaction for B cell IgM anti-hapten responses (see Chapter 32 in this treatise). These results support the earlier findings of Hartmann (1970). The basic observation was that (T,G)-A--L specific T cell clones would allow primary responses to KHL-TNP providing that (T,G)-A--L was also added to the culture. Their assay was the primary IgM response to the hapten DNP. On the face of it, these results would support the concept that hapten–carrier interaction is not obligatory for the elaboration of help for primary DNP-specific responses. On the other hand, the data reported by Theze and his collaborators in Chapter 33 of this treatise seem contradictory. In their system, the clones are GAT-specific, but they have been derived in a manner identical to that for the (T,G)-A--L specific clones used by Hodes. Again, their assay is a DNP-specific response, but, unlike Hodes, theirs is a secondary response and requires priming of the hapten-responsive B cell population. In their studies, it is quite clear that hapten–carrier linkage is required for appropriate hapten-specific responses. That is, GAT-specific T cell clones do not allow secondary (IgG) anti-TNP responses in the presence of GAT and KLH-TNP. The same clones gave antigen-specific and MHC restricted help when there was hapten-carrier linkage, i.e., challenge with GAT-TNP (see Chapter 32 in this treatise). The simplest explanation for these apparent discrepancies is that help for primary responses proceeds through a pathway which requires neither obligate hapten–carrier linkage nor (according to data by Hodes and collaborators) T cell–B cell MHC-restricted interactions. However, for secondary IgG responses, the data presented by Theze and his collaborators would suggest that once B cells have become primed, there is a second pathway which requires hapten–carrier linkage and *H-2* restricted recognition between the helper T cells and the antigen-primed B cells.

These findings are reminiscent of data recently reported by Asano *et al.* (1981) which characterized the requirements for MHC restricted T cell recognition of B cells and antigen presenting cells (APC) which cooperate *in vitro* for T cell-dependent antibody responses to the antigen TNP-KLH. There were two populations of responses recognized. In one population, helper T cells uniformly recognized *H-2* products on antigen-presenting cells, but were not required to recognize H-2 determinants expressed on B cells. These IgM responses were apparently mediated through Lyb-5-positive B cells, whereas the IgG responses were characterized by obligate T cell–B cell MHC restriction and hapten–carrier linkage. This IgG response was mediated by the Lyb-5-negative B cell population. Results presented by Hodes *et al.* (Chapter 32 in this treatise) support this interpretation. The same KHL-specific clone which allowed Lyb-5^+ IgM responses, which were not MHC-restricted at the level of T cells and B cells and did not require hapten–carrier linkage, allowed IgG responses which required hapten–carrier linkage and MHC identity among APC, T cells, and Lyb-5^- B cells.

The third question that has been addressed using murine T cell clones is the question of *I* region restriction of recognition. This phenomenon is an extrapolation of the elegant studies by Zinkernagal and Doherty (1974), Shearer (1974), and Bevan (1975), which suggested that cytotoxic T lymphocytes much recognize target cells bearing class I molecules identical with those of immunizing cells in addition to bearing the appropriate antigen "X." Recent studies have suggested that helper cells exhibit a similar type of restricted antigen recognition, restricted by class II molecules rather than by class I molecules. Such *I* region restricted recognition will be discussed by several of the chapters that follow. Some of the important observations which have been made on *I* region restriction of antigen recognition required the use of antigen-reactive T cell clones. One of the initial observations made with murine alloreactive T cell clones is the recognition of hybrid *I* region antigens as alloantigens and has been discussed by Beck (Chapter 33 in this treatise). Basically, these observations were centered around the isolation of alloreactive murine T cell clones which recognize "hybrid Ia antigens." Such hybrid Ia antigens were formed by free combinatorial association of the α and β chains controlled by the *I-A* or the *I-A* and *I-E* subregions. Alloreactive clones reactive against hybrid Ia determinants recognized stimulating alloantigens controlled by subregions of the *I* region which were expressed only on cells from heterozygous or recombinant mice and were not present on cells from the allogeneic parent. The description and characterization of the number of products of the *I* subregions have been facilitated by studies using cloned T cells in addition to the elegant biochemical studies of Jones *et al.*

(1978), Silver *et al.* (1980), and Uhr *et al.* (1979). Studies discussed by Infante in Chapter 30 in this treatise will show that such hybrid *I* region products can also be used to restrict the recognition of soluble antigens. Simplistically, certain antigen reactive murine T cell clones derived from (A × B)F_1 mice recognize antigen only if presented by antigen-presenting cells having heterozygous *I* regions. Such clones will not recognize antigen presented either by antigen-presenting cells of parent A or parent B. These and similar data suggested that the same hybrid *I* region products which were recognized as alloantigens served to restrict the recognition of murine T cell clones reactive with soluble antigens (Fathman *et al.*, 1981). These observations allowed the subsequent development of two separate sorts of experiments. The first of these dealt with the question of whether or not a single *I* region molecule could present more than one antigenic epitope, and could a single antigeneic epitope be presented by more than one *I* region molecule. If both or either of these suppositions proved correct, the strictest interpretation of determinant selection theories would be untenable (Rosenthal, 1978). Data presented by Infante suggests that such is the case, i.e., data obtained from murine T cell clones derived from (B6A) F_1 mice have shown that one cyanogen bromide cleavage fragment of myoglobin can be recognized in association with more than one *I* region molecule, and that a single *I* region molecule can restrict the recognition of more than one epitope of a synthetic polypeptide (e.g., GAT or (T,G)-A--L). Using T cell clones, it has been possible to document the following points: (1) that there exist multiple subsets of T cell clones reactive with a given antigen, each of which is restricted by a single *I* region molecule; (2) that on cells from hybrid mice there exist more molecules than can be accounted for by the simple summation of parental *I* region products, (data conclusively show that these new products are functional and are formed by free combinatorial association of α and β chains); (3) that single *I* region restriction sites can present more than one antigenic epitope; and (4) provisionally these data suggest that one epitope (as defined by a cyanogen bromide cleavage fraagment of sperm whale myoglobin) can be presented by more than one *I* region molecule.

Another question which has been addressed through the use of T cell clones has been the question of functional activity of proliferating T cells. For years, cellular immunologists have uscd antigen-induced T cell proliferation as a means of assessing immune response. As shown in Chapter 32 by Hodes *et al.* and Chapter 33 by Theze *et al.*, such antigen-specific proliferating T cells provide help for the differentiation of B cells into antibody-secreting plasma cells. Such help is antigen specific and MHC-restricted at the level of antigen presentation, but, depending upon the assay involved, can or cannot show obligate hapten–carrier linkage and requisite *I* region restriction between T and B cells. One point that emerges from the data of Theze *et al.* is that these particular T helper cells do not help only one isotype, i.e., the response generated to GAT-TNP can be measured in all three conventional IgG isotypes. The work presented by Hodes and his collaborators furthermore suggests that supernatants derived from antigen-specific MHC-restricted reactions serve as polyclonal activators when recultured with a source of virgin B cells. Thus, although there is an antigen-specific and *I* region restricted step involved in the generation of T cell help, it is quite clear from these studies that there are several pathways such help might follow. To date, we have not isolated T cell clones which modulate or drive such responses into selected isotypy or idiotypy. Work from other investigators would certainly suggest that there are allotype-specific and/or idiotype-specific T helper and T suppressor cells. The search for such elusive T helper cells or modifiers of the core T helper circuit is in progress.

Despite the inability of these two investigators to find antigen-specific or MHC-restricted factors, data by Cantor (Chapter 34 in this treatise) and his co-workers have pointed out the elegance of isolating T cell clones of the effector lineage, i.e., T suppressor cells specific for selected antigen. These cells, specific for sheep red blood cell glycophorin, secrete or shed an antigen-specific factor that is extremely interesting and has potential implications for future studies on immunotherapy. Their data suggest that a suppressor factor is composed of two parts: one is a 25,000 dalton peptide which has antigen-binding specificity, but does not possess suppressing capabilities. The second is a 45,000 dalton peptide which is a nonspecific suppressor of antigen-induced help, yet has no antigen specificity. Put together, these two products form a molecule which is both antigen-specific and suppressive. These studies suggest that there might exist suppressor molecules, very much analogous to immunoglobulin molecules in that they have an antigen-binding "Fab" portion and an effector portion "Fc." Thus, unlike "helper factors" from T cell clones, it is quite clear that the suppressor T cell clones elaborate an antigen specific factor.

Studies with murine T cell clones reactive with soluble antigens have allowed Theze and his collaborators (Chapter 33 in this treatise) to address the question of whether or not such helper T cell clones bear idiotype on their surface. There has been a long-standing debate concerning the expression of immunoglobulin idiotype on T cell surfaces. It seems quite clear that T cells do not express conventional immunoglobulin molecules. However, it is also clear in many systems that there is an apparent immunoglobulin idiotype present on T cells, be they of helper or suppressor T lineage (Harvey *et al.*, 1979). Studies by Theze and his workers are the first to demonstrate conclusively that, at the clonal level, T cell inducer clones specific for GAT bear on their surface a product which can be recognized by anti-idiotype "anti-C-GAT" antibodies. These data would quite firmly support the concept that there is sharing of idiotope, if not idiotype, between antibodies to GAT and T cell inducer clones which recognize GAT in association with *I* region products. As will be apparent to readers of this treatise to date there has been no biochemical characterization of T cell receptors; however, functional characterizations have been carried out.

One of the most perplexing problems faced by cellular immunologists to date is the characterization of T cell receptors for antigen. The initial impetus for cloning T cells was in large part directed at a solution to the problem of characterizing T cell receptors.

One basic tenet of the clonal selection theory is that each antigen-specific T cell bears surface receptors with predetermined antigen specificity having a given affinity for antigen. In the context of receptors for T cells, it is somewhat difficult to talk about receptor affinity; however, it might be possible to deal with avidity of antigen binding to the T cell which presumably reflects composite multi-point attachment of antigen to cell bound receptors, each presumably possessing identical affinity. If the receptors expressed on antigen-specific T cell clones have binding properties similar to those of antibodies, then minor modifications in the antigen or epitope presented to such T cells may reveal effects on antigen-specific T cell reactions that are reminiscent of cross-reactions of antibodies to slightly modified determinants. In an attempt to document such T cell receptor "affinity," experiments were performed in my laboratory which examined the ability of isolated T cell clones from mice immunized with one synthetic polypeptide to cross-react with various other synthetic polypeptides. Data obtained might support the concept that antigen-reactive T cell clones do express a different avidity for cross-reactive antigens which can be measured as a "weaker" proliferative response of the T cell to the cross-reactive antigen. These data are presented in Fig. 1 which compares the proliferative response of a clone derived from a mouse immunized with (T,G)-A--L which has cross-reactive recognition for the synthetic polymer GAT to a second clone derived from a mouse immunized with GAT which has cross-reactive recognition of the synthetic polymer GA. As can be seen from these results, the response of the clone to (T,G)-A--L is approximately twice as great as the response of the clone to the cross-reactive antigen GAT. The simplest explanation is that this is not a true clone, yet multiple cloning and subcloning experiments have demonstrated that

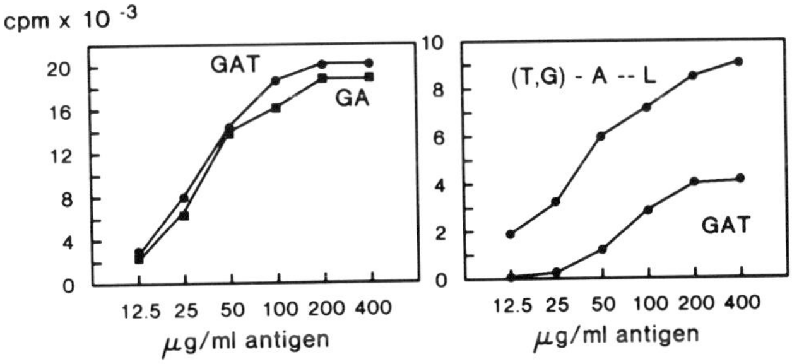

Fig. 1. Response measured as counts per minute (cpm) of incorporation of 2 μCi of tritiated thymidine following an overnight pulse of 1×10^4 antigen reactive T cell clones, one of which is from an animal primed with GAT which cross-reacts on the synthetic polymer GA, the second which is from an animal primed to (T,G)-A--L which cross-reacts on the synthetic polymer GAT.

all progeny of this cell behave in an identical manner (data not presented). Thus, these data support the observation that the response of this particular clone to (T,G)-A--L is simply better than the response of this clone to GAT. It has been proposed that cooperativity between receptors and ligands in a fluid membrane constitutes the basis for effective T cell interaction with antigen-presenting cells. If such interaction results in T cell triggering, this might require multiple receptor–ligand interactions at contact areas and a time-dependent threshold for triggering. Thus, it is entirely possible that the avidity of the T cell for GAT or the affinity of the individual receptors for GAT is lower than it is for (T,G)-A--L, and a triggering threshold is achieved less frequently with the weak avidity interaction. Alternatively it is possible that there are simply differences in epitope density between (T,G)-A--L and GAT. The weaker response of the clone to GAT may reflect the presence of fewer (T,G)-A--L-like epitopes on GAT than on (T,G)-A--L.

This chapter has given a brief review of some of the important questions which have been addressed using murine T cell clones reactive with soluble antigen. The following chapters will present these points in more detail. It is hoped that this treatise will serve as an impetus for other workers in the field to explore unanswered questions concerning immunocompetent cellular interactions. In particular, questions such as the mechanism of "antigen processing," the biochemical nature of the T cell receptor for antigen and/or the receptor for *I* region or *K* region restricting determinants, the biochemical events underlying blastogenesis, and the multitude of products generated by antigen reactive cloned cells need to be examined.

REFERENCES

Asano, Y., Singer, A., and Hodes, R. J. (1981). Role of the major histocompatibility complex (MHC) in T-cell activation of B cell subpopulations. MHC restricted and unrestricted B cell responses are mediated by distinct B cell subpopulations. *J. Exp. Med.* **154,** 1100.

Bevan, M. J. (1975). The major histocompatibility complex determines susceptibility to cytotoxic T-cells directed against minor histocompatibility antigens. *J. Exp. Med.* **142,** 1349.

Bevan, M. J. (1977). Killer cells reactive to altered self antigens can also be alloreactive. *Proc. Natl. Acad. Sci. U.S.A.* **74,** 2094.

Burakoff, S. J., Finberg, R., Glimcher, L., Lemonnier, F., and Cantor, H. (1978). The biologic significance of alloreactivity. The ontogeny of T cell sets specific for alloantigens or modified self antigens. *J. Exp. Med.* **148,** 1414.

Fathman, C. G., Kimoto, M., Melvold, R., and David, C. S. (1981). Reconstitution of *Ir* genes I-A antigen and mixed lymphocyte reaction determinants by gene complementation. *Proc. Natl. Acad. Sci. U.S.A.* **78,** 1853.

Hartmann, K. U. (1970). Induction of a hemolysin response *in vitro*. Interaction of cells of bone marrow origin and thymic origin. *J. Exp. Med.* **132,** 1267.

Harvey, M. A., Adorini, L., Miller, A., and Sercarz, E. (1979). Lysozyme induced T suppressor cells and antibodies have a predominant idiotype. *Nature (London)* **281,** 594.

Heber-Katz, E., and Wilson, D. B. (1975). Collaboration of allogeneic T and B lymphocytes in the primary antibody response to sheep erythrocytes in vitro. *J. Exp. Med.* **142,** 928.

Jones, P. P., Murphy, D. B., and McDevitt, H. O. (1978). Two-gene control of the expression of a murine Ia antigen. *J. Exp. Med.* **148,** 925.

Lemonnier, F., Burakoff, S. J., Germaine, R. N., and Benacerraf, B. (1977). Satellitic thymus derived lymphocytes specific for allogenic stimulator cells cross-react with chemically modified syngeneic cells. *Proc. Natl. Acad. Sci. U.S.A.* **74,** 1229.

Rosenthal, A. S. (1978). Determinant selection and macrophage function in genetic control of the immune response. *Immunol. Rev.* **40,** 136.

Schreier, M. H., Iscove, N. N., Tees, R., Aarden, L., and von Boehmer, H. (1980). Clones of killer and helper T cells: Growth requirements, specificity, and retention of function in long-term culture. *Immunol. Rev.* **51,** 215.

Shearer, G. M. (1974). Cell mediated cytotoxicity to trinitrophenyl modified syngeneic lymphocytes. *Eur. J. Immunol.* **4,** 527.

Silver, J., Swain, S. L., and Hubert, J. J. (1980). Small subunit of *I-A* subregion antigens determines the allospecificity recognized by a monoclonal antibody. *Nature* (*London*) **286,** 272.

Simonsen, M. (1967). The clonal selection hypothesis evaluated by grafted cells reacting against their hosts. *Cold Spring Harbor Symp. Quant. Biol.* **32,** 517.

Sredni, B., and Schwartz, R. H. (1980). Alloreactivity of an antigen specific T cell clone. *Nature* (*London*) **287,** 855.

Uhr, J. W., Capra, J. D., Vitetta, E. S., and Cook, R. G. (1979). Organization of the immune response genes. *Science* **206,** 292.

von Boehmer, H., Hengartner, H., Nabholz, M., Lernhardt, W., Schreier, M. H., and Hass, W. (1979). Fine specificity of a continuously growing killer cell clone specific for H-Y antigen. *Eur. J. Immunol.* **9,** 592.

Zinkernagal, R. M., and Doherty, T. C. (1974). Restriction of an *in vitro* T-cell mediated cytotoxicity in lymphocytic choriomeningitis within a syngeneic or semi-allogeneic system. *Nature* (*London*) **248,** 701.

30

An Analysis of T Cell Antigen Recognition Utilizing T Cell Clones

A. J. Infante/M. Kimoto/C. G. Fathman

I.	Experimental Design	368
II.	T Cell Antigen Specificity	368
III.	Conformational Requirements of T Cell Antigen Recognition	369
IV.	Antigen-Presenting Cell Function	370
V.	*Ia* Restriction and *Ir* Gene Function	371
VI.	Conclusions	373
	References	373

Despite the considerable effort of a number of investigators, perhaps no other area of immunological investigation remains as speculative and inferential as studies aimed at understanding the chemical structure and mechanism of action of the "T cell receptor." Indeed, evidence suggests that the T helper, T suppressor, and T cytotoxic cell receptors may differ considerably from one another and be best considered as three distinct structures. In large part, the frustration felt by those engaged in T cell receptor studies is exacerbated by the relative ease with which receptor binding of B cells (i.e., immunoglobulins) can be studied. Nevertheless, a number of creative approaches have been utilized to gain insight into the structure and mechanism of action of T cell receptors. In this chapter we will review selected aspects of T cell antigen recognition, emphasizing recent data obtained in our laboratory through the analysis of T cell clones reactive to soluble antigens. These data demonstrate how functional aspects of T cell receptor action can be studied utilizing monoclonal techniques. The analytical power of these techniques derives from the ability to isolate monoclonal T cells and thus receptors of monoclonal specificity; the receptors themselves need not be isolated chemically.

ISOLATION, CHARACTERIZATION, AND
UTILIZATION OF T LYMPHOCYTE CLONES

ISBN 0-12-249920-4

I. EXPERIMENTAL DESIGN

We have isolated clones of murine antigen-reactive T cells by a general method (Kimoto and Fathman, 1980) which appears to generate T helper–inducer cells (Hodes *et al.*, 1981). Basically, draining lymph node cells are harvested after priming *in vivo* with antigen in adjuvant and propagated *in vitro* in long-term culture. The cells are serially restimulated with antigen in the presence of fresh media and nonimmune, syngeneic whole spleen cells (3300 R irradiated). Clones are derived by soft-agar colony formation or limiting dilution techniques. Clonality is measured by Poisson distribution analysis, subcloning, and functional assessment. Assay of T cell reactivity is done by measuring [^{3}H]thymidine uptake of T cells in the presence of antigen and irradiated spleen cells (see Appendix for methods).

Using the above techniques we have derived stable long-term cultures and clones of murine T cells reactive to GAT (Kimoto and Fathman, 1980), (T,G)-A--L (Kimoto and Fathman, 1981), sperm whale myoglobin (Mb) (Infante *et al.*, 1981), and keyhole limpet hemocyanin (KLH) (Shigeta and Fathman, 1981). Most commonly, the clones were derived from mice of strain (C57BL/6 × A/J)F_1 [(B6A)F_1] in order to map *Ia* restriction specificity (*vide infra*). Other strains used have included A/J, C57BL/6, DBA/2, and (C57BL/6 × C3H)F_1. In addition to utilizing normal, whole spleen cells as antigen-presenting cells (APC), we have also used to advantage a number of lymphoid cell tumors to study accessory cell function (McKean *et al.*, 1981a).

II. T CELL ANTIGEN SPECIFICITY

T cells from long-term culture show very clear specificity for the immunizing antigen. In addition, multiple epitopes which are recognized by monoclonal T cells can be defined for synthetic and naturally occurring protein antigens, e.g., Mb-reactive clones can be shown to specifically respond to one of three cyanogen bromide (CNBr) fragments. Clones have been isolated which react with either the CNBr fragment comprising residues 1–55 or that consisting of 56–131 (Infante *et al.*, 1981).

Similarly, GAT-reactive clones can be divided into two groups: one group recognizes GAT and the related polymer GA; the second recognizes GAT, but not GA (Kimoto *et al.*, 1981b). Thus, monoclonal T cells have specificity for individual epitopes on a single antigen. We are presently attempting to define the size and chemical nature of T cell epitopes by utilizing Mb-reactive clones and synthetic peptides representing regions of myoglobin.

Since antibody molecules demonstrate cross-reactivity to closely related antigens (as measured by different affinities of a single combining site for antigens of

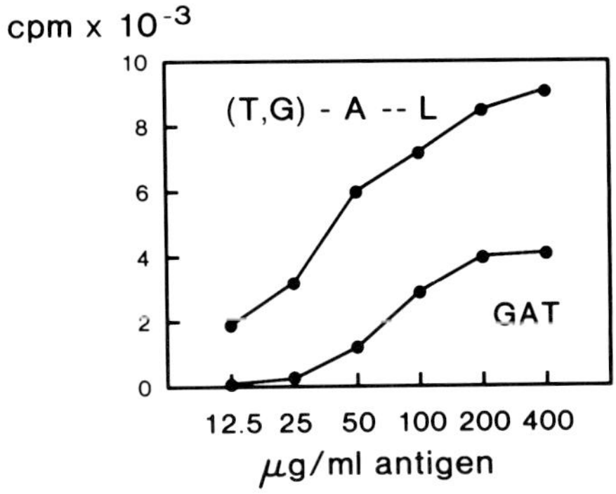

Fig. 1. Response of the (T,G)-A--L reactive clone 2eSA.12 to the immunizing antigen (T,G)-A--L and the cross reactive antigen GAT.

similar structure), we asked whether T cell receptors demonstrated a similar phenomenon. Myoglobin-reactive clones (i.e., reactive to sperm whale Mb) showed no cross-stimulation with dog and horse myoglobin (A. J. Infante, unpublished observations). Certain T cell clones reactive to (T,G)-A--L (TGAL), however, could recognize GAT (Fig. 1), although less efficiently (Fathman *et al.*, 1981a). These clones were subcloned to be sure that they did not consist of two populations of cells, one of which recognized TGAL alone and one which recognized TGAL and GAT equally well. Since the subclones continued to recognize TGAL strongly and GAT weakly, we hypothesized that there was true cross-reactivity of a cloned T cell receptor for two similar antigens.

III. CONFORMATIONAL REQUIREMENTS OF T CELL ANTIGEN RECOGNITION

Several lines of evidence have indicated that antibodies recognize antigens in a manner which is strictly conformation dependent. It has been asserted that T helper (T_H) cells, on the other hand, recognize native and denatured forms of the same antigen equally well (Endres and Grey, 1980). One measure of this difference is seen in the response to Mb. Serum antibodies raised against (native) Mb can be quantitatively removed from antisera by precipitation with Mb or its CNBr fragments (Atassi and Saplin, 1968). However, a four- to tenfold molar excess of CNBr fragments (relative to native Mb) was required for complete precipitation. It was concluded that the difference in binding was due to the fact that antibodies bound native conformational determinants, and a greater amount of the relatively denatured CNBr fragments was required to reach saturation of Mb-binding sites in the antisera.

In contrast, Mb-reactive T cells could respond equally well to native Mb and

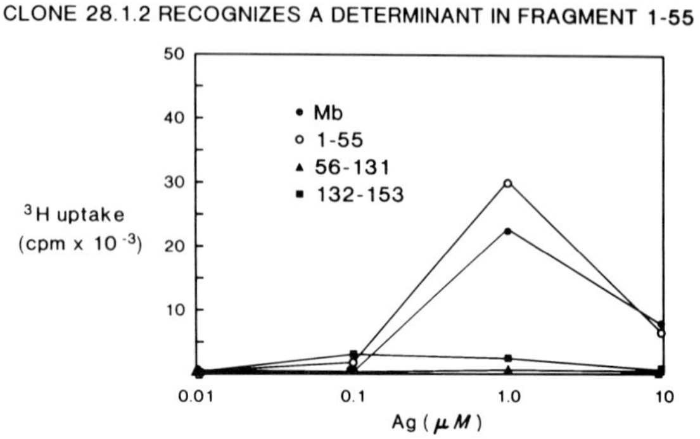

Fig. 2. Response of the Mb-reactive clone 28.1.2 to Mb and its three CNBr fragments.

the appropriate CNBr fragment (Fig. 2), as measured by dose–response curves (Infante *et al.*, 1981). Although interpretation of these results is complicated by the effects of antigen presentation by accessory cells (see below), it is clear that the T cells do not differentiate between Mb and CNBr fragments in the way that antibodies do. Thus, T cells may recognize antigen in a "non-native" conformation. Further evidence for this is provided by the failure of high-titered antisera to myoglobin (both syngeneic and xenogeneic) to inhibit T cell proliferation in response to myoglobin presented on APC which have been pulsed with Mb and then washed extensively (A. J. Infante and D. J. McKean, unpublished observations). The same antisera markedly diminish the T cell response when T cells, APC, Mb, and antisera are mixed simultaneously.

IV. ANTIGEN-PRESENTING CELL FUNCTION

T helper cells recognize antigen only in the context of antigen presentation by accessory cells. T cell recognition of antigen is "restricted" and requires in addition recognition of Ia antigen epitopes on APC. Various mechanisms, none entirely satisfactory, have been invoked to explain the obligate role of Ia in antigen presentation (e.g., proteolysis of antigen by Ia, specific association of antigen and Ia). We have utilized long-term T cell lines and clones to study antigen presentation by a series of lymphoblastoid cell lines (McKean *et al.*, 1981a). These lines function effectively as APC's, although somewhat less efficiently than splenic adherent cells. Since the APC lines we have studied lack detectable phagocytic and enzymatic functions attributable to macrophages (the "classic" APC), these functions may not be involved in antigen presentation.

One postulated mechanism of antigen presentation is that Ia molecules on the APC bind to certain regions of an antigen, thus orienting it in three-dimensional space and allowing T cell recognition of particular epitopes. Since Mb-reactive T cell clones respond equally well to Mb and an appropriate CNBr fragment of Mb, presentation of an antigen epitope on one CNBr fragment cannot depend on APC binding to other parts of the Mb molecule. This seems to restrict the possible ways in which an APC might directly interact with an antigen.

The role of Ia in APC function may in some respects be quantitative as well as qualitative. For example, when certain (B6A)F_1 Mb-reactive T cell clones were stimulated with Mb on a panel of splenic APC, homozygous (B6) APC were approximately 2–3 times more effective (^{3}H-TdR incorporation) than (B6A)F_1 heterozygous APC (Table I). When stimulated with 3-fold more antigen, the response with (B6A)F_1 APC reached the previous level seen with B6 APC. Thus, the level of expression of Ia on the APC surface may be an important controlling factor in determining the magnitude of an immune response, assuming a gene dosage effect resulting in less I-A^b on F_1 compared to homozygous cells. We can also suggest that this effect is susceptible to modulation, since lipopolysaccharide (LPS) stimulation of APC lymphoblastoid lines increases their efficiency of APC function roughly in proportion to the increase in the quantity of Ia expressed on the cell surface (McKean *et al.*, 1981). Results such as these have also been found in a similar experimental system (P. P. Jones, personal communication).

V. *Ia* RESTRICTION AND *Ir* GENE FUNCTION

Analysis of immune responses by techniques involving T cell clones has had possibly its greatest impact on the understanding of *Ir* gene control mechanisms. We have shown that hybrid Ia molecules of (B6A)F_1 mice (i.e., $A_\alpha{}^b A_\beta{}^k$ and $A_\alpha^k A_\beta{}^b$) exist on APC and function to "restrict" the responses of certain T cell clones (Kimoto and Fathman, 1980). Thus, *I-A* heterozygous animals are able to generate increased possibilities for immune recognition relative to homozygous animals. Furthermore, a mutation within an Ia molecule can eliminate certain immune responses while preserving others (Fathman *et al.*, 1981b). This was shown by the ability or inability of (B6A)F_1-restricted T cell clones to react to antigen presented by APC of (B6A)F_1 versus (bm12 × B10.A)F_1 (bm12 = B6.C-H-2^{bm12}) mice. The *I* regions of these two hybrids are identical except for a mutation in the A_β^{bm12} chain (McKean *et al.*, 1981b). All T cell clones reactive to GAT could recognize GAT equally well on (B6A)F_1 and (bm12 × B10.A)F_1 APC. T cell clones reactive to (T,G)-A--L, however, fell into two groups: one group recognized antigen presented by both types of hybrid APC; the second group reacted to (T,G)-A--L only when presented by (B6A)F_1 APC. We concluded that a mutation in one chain of an Ia molecule could lead to genetically determined nonresponsiveness at the T cell level. This is perhaps the strongest

TABLE I

Clone 28.1.2.: (B6A)F_1, Mb-Reactive T Cells[a]

[Mb]	APC strain	MHC regions *K*	*A*	*E*	*D*	cpm
3 μM	B6	*b*	*b*	*b*	*b*	47,709
3 μM	(B6A)F_1	*b/k*	*b/k*	*b/k*	*b/k*	8120
10 μM	(B6A)F_1	*b/k*	*b/k*	*b/k*	*b/k*	39,586
3 μM	B10.MBR	*b*	*k*	*k*	*q*	257

[a] Conditions: 10^4 T cells and 10^6 whole, irradiated spleen cells (APC) in 0.2 ml medium. Soluble antigen added at time 0 and ^{3}H-TdR incorporation measured at day 3.

evidence to date that the serologically detected Ia antigens are the *Ir* gene products and solely responsible for *Ir* gene function (Table II).

It has been shown in our laboratory, as well as others, that *I-E* subregion products also restrict the response of certain T cell clones. Based on *Ir* gene studies, responsiveness to certain antigens may map to *I-A* (e.g., GAT), *I-E* (GLϕ), both *I-A* and *I-E* (Mb), or neither (i.e., no MHC controlled response variations, e.g., KLH). Using T cell clone restriction mapping, we sought to explain these results on the basis of T cell ''associative'' recognition of antigen and Ia. In the case of GAT, no clones have been found which are restricted to the *I-E* subregion. Myoglobin-reactive clones are restricted to either *I-A* or *I-E*. We found that T cell clones responding to the NH_2 terminal CNBr fragment of Mb were of two types: one type is restricted by *I-A*, another by *I-E* (Infante *et al.*, 1981). A similar result was found for clones reactive to the central CNBr peptide. It is presently unclear how many T cell epitopes are present on a given Mb fragment, so definitive conclusions cannot be drawn. Hopefully, future results may allow us to choose between two alternative models: in one, a specific Ia antigen on the APC is recognized in a unique combination with each epitope of a

TABLE II

Clones 2e.LD.2 and 2e.SA.13: (B6A)F_1, TGAL-Reactive T Cells[a]

APC strain	MHC regions *K*	*A*	*E*	*D*	cpm 2e.LD.2	2e.SA 13
(B6A) F_1	*b/k*	*b/k*	*b/k*	*b/k*	14,779	22,702
[B10.A(4R) × B6]F_1	*k/b*	*k/b*	*b/b*	*b/b*	15,202	22,293
(bm12 × B10.A)F_1	*b/k*	*b*/k*	*b/k*	*b/d*	893	16,241

[a] Conditions: same as Table I.

multideterminant antigen; alternatively, all combinations of Ia and soluble antigen epitopes are possible and selection for responsiveness occurs at the T cell receptor level.

We have obtained some evidence to indicate that in two separate cases genetically determined low responsiveness *in vivo* is not due to failure of APC function. We have found certain $(B6A)F_1$ T cell clones which respond to (T,G)-A--L when presented by splenic APC of low responder strain A (Kimoto *et al.*, 1981a). Similarly, certain $(B6A)F_1$ clones reactive to Mb are restricted by APC of low responder strain B6 (Infante *et al.*, 1981). In both cases, low responsiveness *in vivo* should not be due to failure of APC to effectively present antigen. Either the low responder strain lacks T cells (T cell receptors?) which can recognize the appropriate Ia + antigen association or such T cells are suppressed *in vivo*.

Finally, we could show genetic restriction of the response of individual T cell clones to KLH, despite a lack of genetically mapped low versus high responsiveness *in vivo* (Shigeta and Fathman, 1981). For KLH (as for Mb) responsiveness to the whole antigen may be assured by recognition of multiple epitopes. Response to each individual epitope may well exhibit *Ir* gene control.

Another level of complexity occurs at the T cell level, i.e., antigen-specific suppressor cells. What is their receptor repertoire? As clearly shown for the anti-lysozyme response (Adorini *et al.*, 1979) and as recently postulated in the anti-myoglobin response (Atassi *et al.*, 1981), specific suppressor inducing epitopes may exist on complex antigens. By applying techniques for generating T suppressor (T_S) clones, we hope to isolate ''suppressor epitope'' specific cells. We might then hope to analyze specific T cell circuits *in vitro*.

VI. CONCLUSIONS

The use of soluble antigen-reactive T cell clones as immunological tools has created a burst of new information bearing on a wide variety of issues, as sampled above. Although in some cases definitive answers have not been found, some basic experimental systems have been defined which will allow us to approach some fundamentally important questions. The most important of these appears to be, ''what is the mechanism of genetically controlled responsiveness and unresponsiveness?'' The answer may have far-reaching implications not only for basic research but clinical medicine as well.

REFERENCES

Adorini, L., Harvey, M. A., Miller, A., and Sercarz, E. E. (1979). Fine specificity of regulatory T cells. II. Suppressor and helper T cells are induced by different regions of hen egg-white lysozyme in a genetically non-responder mouse strain. *J. Exp. Med.* **150,** 293.

Atassi, M. Z., and Saplin, B. J. (1968). Immunochemistry of sperm whale myoglobin. I. The specific interaction of some tryptic peptides and peptides containing all the reactive regions of the antigen. *Biochemistry* **7,** 688.

Atassi, M. Z., Yokuta, S., Twining, S. S., Lehmann, H., and David, C. S. (1981). Genetic control of the immune response to myoglobin. VI. Inter-site influences in T-lymphocyte proliferative response from analysis of cross-reactions of ten myoglobins in terms of substitutions in the antigenic sites and in environmental residues of the sites. *Mol. Immunol.* (in press).

Endres, R. O., and Grey, H. M. (1980). Antigen recognition by T cells. I. Suppressor T cells fail to recognize cross-reactivity between native and denatured ovalbumin. *J. Immunol.* **125,** 1515.

Fathman, C. G., Howard, J., Shigeta, M., and Kimoto, M. (1981a). Antigen reactive T cell clones. V. An affinity dependent step in the activation of antigen specific T cell clones. (In preparation.)

Fathman, C. G., Kimoto, M., Melvold, R., and David, C. S. (1981b). Reconstitution of *Ir* genes. Ia antigens and MLR determinants by gene complementation. *Proc. Natl. Acad. Sci. U.S.A.* **78,** 1853.

Hodes, R. J., Kimoto, M., Hathcock, K. S., Fathman, C. G., and Singer, A. (1981). Functional helper activity of monoclonal T cell populations. Antigen specific and H-2 restricted cloned T cells provide help for *in vitro* antibody responses to trinitrophenyl-poly-L-(Try,Glu)-poly-D,L-Ala--poly-L-Lys. *Proc. Natl. Acad. Sci. U.S.A.* **78,** 6431.

Infante, A. J., Atassi, M. Z., and Fathman, C. G. (1981). T cell clones reactive with sperm whale myoglobin. Isolation of clones with specificity for individual determinants on myoglobin. *J. Exp. Med.* **154,** 1342.

Kimoto, M., and Fathman, C. G. (1980). Antigen reactive T cell clones. I. Transcomplementing hybrid *I-A* region gene products function effectively in antigen presentation. *J. Exp. Med.* **152,** 759.

Kimoto, M., and Fathman, C. G. (1981). Antigen reactive T cell clones. II. Unique homozygous and (high responder × low responder)F_1 hybrid antigen-presenting determinants detected using poly(Tyr,Glu)-poly-D,L-Ala—poly-Lys-reactive T cell clones. *J. Exp. Med.* **153,** 375.

Kimoto, M., Krenz, T., and Fathman, C. G. (1981a). Antigen reactive T cell clones. III. Low responder antigen presenting cells function effectively to present antigen to selected T cell clones derived from (high responder × low responder)F_1 mice. *J. Exp. Med.* **154,** 883.

Kimoto, M., Krenz, T., Cummings, D., and Fathman, C. G. (1981b). Antigen reactive T cell clones. IV. Evidence that one *I* region restriction determinant can associate with multiple antigenic epitopes. (Submitted for publication.)

McKean, D. J., Infante, A. J., Nilson, A., Kimoto, M., Fathman, C. G., Walker, E., and Warner, N. (1981a). MHC restricted antigen presentation to antigen reactive T cells by B lymphocyte tumor lines. *J. Exp. Med.* **154,** 1419.

McKean, D. J., Melvold, R. W., and David, C. S. (1981b). Tryptic peptide comparison of 1a antigen α and β polypeptides from the 1-A mutant B6.C-H-$2^{bm/2}$ and its congenic parental strain B6. *Immunogenetics* **14,** 41.

Shigeta, M., and Fathman, C. G. (1981). *I*-region restrictions imposed upon the recognition of KLH by murine T cell clones. *Immunogenetics* **11,** 493.

31

Alloreactivity of Antigen-Specific T Cell Clones

Ronald H. Schwartz/Benjamin Sredni

Text 375
References 382

The frequency of T cells which recognize and respond to antigens of the major histocompatibility complex (MHC) of other members of the species is quite high (Simonsen, 1967; Bach *et al.*, 1969; Wilson, 1974; Ford *et al.*, 1975; Binz and Wigzell, 1975; Skinner and Marbrook, 1976; Fischer-Lindahl and Wilson, 1977; Ryser and MacDonald, 1979). On the order of 1–5% of the whole T cell population reacts in a mixed lymphocyte reaction against any given allogeneic haplotype. This observation is in contrast to the frequency of T cells which respond to other foreign antigens (Tse *et al.*, 1980). In the latter case, frequency estimates of 0.05–0.1% have been obtained for antigen-primed populations. If one postulates that priming has achieved a 10-fold expansion of the cells, then an estimate of the difference in frequencies in the unprimed animal of T cells specific for alloantigens and those specific for other foreign antigens is 100- to 500-fold.

The relationship between the two subpopulations of T lymphocytes is not clear. Many early investigators (Simonsen, 1967; Wilson, 1974) felt that because the frequency of alloreactive cells was so high and because the number of allogeneic haplotypes was so large (potentially 50 to 100, Götze *et al.*, 1980), all the T cells must have at least one allospecificity. If so, then the alloreactive population would be overlapping with the foreign antigen-specific population. In contrast, Jerne (1971) postulated that the high frequency of alloreactive cells was a consequence of the germ line genes encoding for the lymphocyte receptors. In this model, each lymphocyte initially expresses an anti-MHC antigen receptor directed against a particular alloantigen of the species. In the thymus, those T cells with receptors specific for self-MHC antigens are stimulated to divide. During this process they undergo somatic mutation and are negatively selected

ISBN 0-12-249920-4

against self specificity. Those variants which have mutated sufficiently to escape the negative selection emerge from the thymus as the foreign antigen-specific subpopulation. Those lymphocytes which express receptors specific for other alloantigens of the species are unaffected by the thymic selection and emerge as the alloreactive subpopulation. Thus, the two subpopulations are nonoverlapping in this model.

Experiments to distinguish between these two points of view have been carried out on whole populations of T lymphocytes. Cytotoxic T cell populations specific for TNP-modified self (Shearer *et al.*, 1976; Burakoff *et al.*, 1976), viral (Finberg *et al.*, 1978), or minor histocompatibility (Bevan, 1977) antigens in association with self MHC molecules have shown cross-reactive lysis on certain allogeneic targets differing only at the MHC. This allogeneic cross-reactive lysis could be competed for in cold target inhibition studies by unlabeled cells bearing only the foreign antigen and self MHC molecules. Reciprocal experiments have also been reported in which alloreactive T cells were shown to produce cross-reactive lysis of target cells bearing TNP-modified self antigens (Lemonnier *et al.*, 1977). All these results suggest that the same T cell can possess specificity for both an alloantigen and another foreign antigen.

Additional evidence to support this conclusion has come from radiation-induced bone marrow chimeras of the type $(A \times B)F_1$ marrow transferred into irradiated parental recipients ($F_1 \rightarrow P_A$) (Hünig and Bevan, 1980). T cells from such chimeras recognize foreign antigens in association with MHC gene products of parent A and not with MHC gene products of parent B. The cells also show no alloreactivity against either parent A or B cells. In the experiments on cross-reactive lysis, alloreactivity was generated against third party (anti-C) MHC gene products and the cells tested for cytotoxicity against TNP-modified parent A or B cells. Alloreactive T cells from such chimeras showed preferential cross-reactive killing against TNP-modified parent A cells. The result demonstrated that allospecificity was influenced by radiation-resistant cells of the host (presumably in the thymus, based on other experiments) (Zinkernagel *et al.*, 1978; Fink and Bevan, 1978) in the same manner as the repertoire of T cells specific for other foreign antigens. This observation is inconsistent with the Jerne hypothesis and suggests that all T cells are similarly influenced by the thymus.

The most direct experimental approach to this problem has been with T cell cloning. This technology has provided the means for demonstrating unequivocally that a single T cell has specificity for both an alloantigen and another foreign antigen in association with a self MHC gene product. The first demonstration of this was in a cytotoxic system by von Boehmer and colleagues (1979). They isolated a cytotoxic T cell clone specific for the male antigen, H-Y, in association with the self MHC product, D^b, using the approach of generating a long-term T cell line followed by limiting dilution cloning. This antigen specific clone also killed equally well allogeneic targets bearing D^d, even from female donors, i.e., in the absence of the H-Y antigen. Cold target inhibition studies demonstrated that unlabeled allogeneic D^d-bearing cells could compete as well as unlabeled male, D^b-bearing cells to inhibit the killing of labeled male, D^b-bearing cells. This confirmed the fact that the same cell had both specificities and suggested that the same receptor might be used to mediate both types of killing. However, the possibility that the unlabeled allogeneic target bound to one receptor and sterically prevented the labeled target from binding to a second, independent receptor, could not be excluded.

Although the experimental data on this cytotoxic clone were very convincing, the authors were hesitant to conclude that this was a typical cell for two reasons. First, attempts to enrich for alloreactive, D^d-specific cells from bulk cultures primed and stimulated *in vitro* with male H-2^b-bearing cells were unsuccessful. This raised the possibility that the clone was an abnormal somatic variant which arose in culture. Second, the cytotoxic clone could only be assayed for its specificity in killing and not for its specificity of induction, because cytotoxic clones are factor addicted, i.e., withdrawal of the growth factor (IL-2) leads to death of the cells in 24–48 hr. This left open the possibility that the cross-reactivity was a degeneracy of receptor specificity seen only in binding to the target cell for killing and that it did not represent a true allogeneic cross-reaction, which would be degeneracy at the level of cellular activation.

Both of these reservations were overcome when an antigen-specific proliferative T cell clone was also shown to possess alloreactivity (Sredni and Schwartz, 1981). This clone was derived using the soft agar cloning technique (Sredni *et al.*, 1980) 3 days after secondary stimulation of primed B10.A lymph node T cells *in vitro* with dinitrophenylated ovalbumin (DNP-OVA). This method of T cell cloning avoids the prolonged stimulation of long-term T cell lines *in vitro*

TABLE I

Alloreactivity of an Antigen-Specific T Cell Clone

Irradiated spleen cells	DNP-OVA 100 μg/ml	Proliferative response of subclone 5.6 (cpm ± SEM)
B10.A	–	180 ± 52
B10.A	+	39,200 ± 1950
B10	–	233 ± 116
B10.D2	–	410 ± 35
B10.M	–	46 ± 8
B10.P	–	230 ± 41
B10.Q	–	60 ± 20
B10.RIII	–	53 ± 12
B10.S	–	36,300 ± 1900
B10.PL	–	80 ± 39

TABLE II

Allostimulation in the Absence of Exogenous IL-2

IL-2 (%, v/v)	Proliferative response (cpm ± SEM) of clone 5 (B10.A anti-DNP-OVA) to	
	10^4 B10.S spleen	10^5 B10.S spleen
0	6,600 ± 500	15,100 ± 800
5	14,300 ± 400	21,800 ± 1400
10	18,900 ± 2600	40,200 ± 1200

and thus reduces the chances of selecting out unusual somatic variants or minor subpopulations. The original colonies were recloned in soft agar several times at high plating efficiency to assure that the dual specificity was the property of a single cell. The proliferative response of a subclone from this study, 5.6, is shown in Table I.

This clone responded equally well to DNP-OVA in association with B10.A irradiated spleen cells (the source of nonimmune antigen-presenting cells) and B10.S irradiated spleen cells without DNP-OVA (alloreactivity). No other allogeneic spleen cell population tested stimulated at all. As demonstrated in Table II, the proliferative T cell clone could be stimulated with allogeneic B10.S spleen cells in the absence of any added T cell growth factor, although addition of small amounts of IL-2 to the culture increased the magnitude of the proliferative response. Furthermore, the clone could be propagated in culture using B10.S spleen cells instead of DNP-OVA and B10.A spleen cells. Thus, in contrast to the cytotoxic clone, the proliferative T cell clone could be activated to divide by both the foreign protein antigen and the alloantigen.

The allostimulation was shown to be due to a direct presentation of alloantigen by the irradiated spleen cells and not to a back reaction, i.e., recognition of the clone by alloreactive T cells in the spleen cell population with subsequent recruitment of the clone to give the proliferative response. This was demonstrated

TABLE III

Allostimulation by a Macrophage Line

Macrophage colony	T cell clone	DNP-OVA 100 μg/ml pulse	Proliferation (cpm ± SEM)
B10.S	−	−	40 ± 10
B10.S	+	−	12,100 ± 500
B10.S	+	+	12,400 ± 900

in two ways. In the first experiment, the T cells were removed from the splenic population by treatment with a monoclonal anti-Thy-1 and complement (Sredni *et al.*, 1981b); no effect was observed on the subsequent allostimulation of the clone by this depleted population. In the second experiment, macrophage lines devoid of T cells were derived from bone marrow colonies and used as allostimulators (Sredni and Schwartz, 1981). As shown in Table III, a B10.S macrophage colony could stimulate a proliferative response from the B10.A anti-DNP-OVA clone 5 in the presence of 5% IL-2. Pulsing the macrophages with DNP-OVA did not increase or decrease the magnitude of this response. These results strongly suggested that a T cell-dependent back reaction could not account for the allostimulation.

The MHC gene products involved in both the allogeneic $H\text{-}2^s$ and the DNP-OVA plus syngeneic $H\text{-}2^a$ stimulations were mapped using MHC (*H-2*) recombinant strains (Sredni *et al.*, 1981a; Sredni and Schwartz, 1981). As shown in Table IV, experiment 1, DNP-OVA-induced T cell proliferation required antigen-presenting cells syngeneic with the B10.A T cell clone at the $I\text{-}A^k$ subregion. Thus, spleen cells from the B10.A(4R) and A.TL recombinant mice supported a proliferative response but spleen cells from the B10.A(5R) did not. A similar analysis for allostimulation (Table IV, experiment 2) implicated the $I\text{-}A^s$

TABLE IV

***I-A* Subregion Gene Products Are Required for Both Allogeneic and Antigen-Specific Stimulation of T Cell Clone 5**

Expt. No.	Antigen-presenting cells: Source	Antigen-presenting cells: MHC alleles[a]	DNP-OVA 100 μg/ml	Proliferation (cpm ± SEM)
1	B10.A	*k k k k k d d d*	−	20 ± 3
	B10.A	*k k k k k d d d*	+	7000 ± 500
	B10	*b b b b b b b b*	+	20 ± 5
	B10.A(4R)	*k k b b b b b b*	−	20 ± 3
	B10.A(4R)	*k k b b b b b b*	+	7200 ± 700
	B10.A(5R)	*b b b k k d d d*	+	20 ± 1
	A.TL	*s k k k k k k d*	−	15 ± 3
	A.TL	*s k k k k k k d*	+	7100 ± 1100
2	B10.A	*k k k k k d d d*	−	150 ± 100
	B10.A	*k k k k k d d d*	+	14,700 ± 2300
	B10.S	*s s s s s s s s*	−	15,900 ± 2000
	B10.S(9R)	*s s ? k k d d d*	−	15,700 ± 800
	A.TL	*s k k k k k k d*	−	90 ± 20
	A.TH	*s s s s s s s d*	−	15,700 ± 2300

[a] Letters refer to the haplotype source of origin of the *K*, *I-A*, *I-B*, *I-J*, *I-E*, *I-C*, *S*, and *D* regions and subregions of the murine major histocompatibility complex (MHC).

or $I\text{-}B^s$ subregion as spleen cells from the B10.S(9R) and A.TH recombinant mice stimulated a proliferative response in the absence of DNP-OVA, but spleen cells from the A.TL mice did not. Because the major allogeneic lymphocyte activating determinant locus has been mapped to the *I-A* subregion in other mouse strains (Shreffler and David, 1975) and because the existence of an *I-B* subregion has been recently questioned (Baxevanis *et al.*, 1981), it seems reasonable to conclude that the relevant genetic subregion required for allostimulation of the T cell clone is $I\text{-}A^s$. Furthermore, since the same Ia antigens are known to be involved in both allostimulation and MHC restriction of antigen recognition (Schwartz, 1981), it seems reasonable to conclude from these data that a single T cell can respond equally to DNP-OVA in association with a gene product of $I\text{-}A^k$ and an (allelic ?) gene product of $I\text{-}A^s$ in the absence of antigen.

Since these early studies, a number of investigators have confirmed the existence of T cell clones with dual specificity for an alloantigen and another foreign antigen in association with self MHC gene products (Cerottini, 1981; Braciale *et al.*, 1981; Janeway and Conrad, 1981). The next important task then became to determine how frequent such clones were in the whole T cell population. We approached this question by immunizing three different MHC-congenic strains, B10.A, B10, and B10.S, with DNP-OVA and isolating 20 to 40 antigen-specific colonies from each strain using the soft agar cloning technique (B. Sredni and R. H. Schwartz, unpublished results). The expanded colonies were then screened for alloreactivity against spleen cells bearing one of eight independent MHC haplotypes. The results of this experiment are shown in Table V. The first

TABLE V

Frequency of Antigen-Specific T Cell Colonies with Alloreactivity

Allogenic spleen cells	Number of alloreactive colonies from		
	B10.A	B10	B10.S
B10.A	—	1	0
B10	0	—	0
B10.D2	2	1	0
B10.M	1	1	6[a]
B10.P	0	1	3
B10.Q	0	0	2[a]
B10.RIII	1	0	1
B10.S	4	0	—
B10.PL	0	0	2
Total	8/38	4/21	14/32
Frequency (%)	21	19	44

[a] One colony had reactivity against both B10.M and B10.Q spleen cells.

striking aspect of the data is the high frequency of T cell colonies that displayed both antigen specificity and alloreactivity: 8 out of 38 B10.A colonies (21%), 4 out of 21 B10 colonies (19%), and 14 out of 32 B10.S colonies (44%). Similar data have been generated by Janeway and Conrad (1981), who found that 6 out of 29 OVA specific T cell colonies (20%) from BALB/c mice (*H-2*^{d}) also had alloreactivity. If one expresses the data as a function of the number of independent haplotypes tested (number of alloreactive colonies/number of antigen-specific colonies/number of allogeneic haplotypes tested) the frequencies range from 2.5 to 5%. This correlates with the frequency of alloreactive proliferative cells to any given haplotype in whole T cell populations and suggests that the clones are a representative sample of this population. Furthermore, when one considers that only 8 MHC haplotypes were used to screen for alloreactivity, whereas up to 50 independent haplotypes are estimated to exist in the species (Götze *et al.*, 1980), it seems reasonable to conclude that even the T cell colonies which did not show alloreactivity would have shown it if all haplotypes had been tested.

The second striking aspect of the data was the nonrandom distribution of the allogeneic specificites in two of the three strains tested. DNP-OVA specific colonies from B10.A mice showed a tendency (3 or more colonies) for alloreactivity to B10.S, whereas DNP-OVA specific colonies from B10.S mice showed a tendency for alloreactivity to B10.M and B10.P. These results suggest a relationship between the antigen specificity of the T cell and its alloreactivity. Furthermore, it appears that this relationship is not just an intrinsic property of a given antigen, since the dominant alloreactivity changes with the MHC haplotype of the strain from which the colonies were derived.

Even though these data represent only the beginning of our exploration of the relationship between the alloreactive and foreign antigen-specific T cell repertoires, they already have important implications for theories of T cell receptor specificity. The high frequency of T cell colonies with dual specificity, coupled with the demonstrations of overlap at the whole population level, proves that a large percentage (at least 20%) of the T cells perform both functions. These results are directly contradictory to the prediction of nonoverlap made by the Jerne model (1971) and strongly suggest that this aspect of the model is wrong.

If a single T cell possesses both specificities, what is the relationship between the receptors which mediate each component of recognition? There are two potential solutions: two independent receptors or one receptor unit with cross-reactivity. The observation that two of the four series of OVA-specific colonies examined so far show a nonrandom distribution of alloreactivity suggests that the antigen and allospecificities are related. However, this does not necessarily mean that there is only one receptor unit. It is possible that the association between a particular set of alloreceptors and a particular set of antigen receptors results from linkage at the DNA level, e.g. minigene families of receptors whose expression is regulated by MHC genes. Furthermore, the nonrandom nature of the preliminary data may turn out to be simply a sampling artifact. Clearly, further studies are needed to firmly establish the observation of nonrandomness as an experimental fact.

It should be obvious from this summary of one small area of cellular immunology how powerful the T cell cloning technology can be. It has firmly established the dual specificity of single T cells for both alloantigen and other foreign antigens in association with self MHC products. In a similar manner, in other studies, it has firmly established MHC restriction as a property of the T cell receptor for antigen (Sredni *et al.,* 1981a) and anti-Ia antisera inhibition as a disruption of macrophage–T cell interaction rather than a secondary consequence of suppressor T cells (Sredni *et al.,* 1981b). In the future, T cell clones will most certainly provide the biochemical materials (proteins and DNA) from which the structural nature and composition of the T cell receptor(s) will be defined. Because of this the clones will undoubtedly be considered the major technological advance responsible for achieving an understanding of the specificity and function of the T cell receptor.

REFERENCES

Bach, F. H., Bock, H., Graupner, K., Day, E., and Klosterman, H. (1969). Cell kinetic studies in mixed leukocyte cultures: An *in vitro* model of homograft reactivity. *Proc. Natl. Acad. Sci. U.S.A.* **62,** 377.

Baxevanis, C. N., Nagy, Z. A., and Klein, J. (1981). A novel type of T–T cell interaction removes the requirement for *I-B* region in the *H-2* complex. *Proc. Natl. Acad. Sci. U.S.A.* **78,** 3809.

Bevan, M. J. (1977). Killer cells reactive to altered-self antigens can also be alloreactive. *Proc. Natl. Acad. Sci. U.S.A.* **74,** 2094.

Binz, H., and Wigzell, H. (1975). Shared idiotypic determinants on B and T lymphocytes reactive against the same antigenic determinants. II. Determination of frequency and characteristics of idiotypic T and B lymphocytes in normal rats using direct visualization. *J. Exp. Med.* **142,** 1218.

Braciale, T. J., Andrew, M. E., and Braciale, V. L. (1981). Simultaneous expression of *H-2*-restricted and alloreactive recognition by a cloned line of influenza virus-specific cytotoxic T lymphocytes. *J. Exp. Med.* **153,** 1371.

Burakoff, S. J., Germain, R. N., and Benaceraf, B. (1976). Cross-reactive lysis of trinitrophenyl (TNP)-derivatized H-2 incompatible target cells by cytolytic T lymphocytes generated against syngeneic TNP spleen cells. *J. Exp. Med.* **144,** 1609.

Cerottini, J.-C. (1981). Clonal analysis of cytolytic T lymphocytes and their precursors. *Prog. Immunol.* **4,** 622.

Finberg, R., Burakoff, S. J., Cantor, H., and Benacerraf, B. (1978). Biological significance of alloreactivity: T cells stimulated by Sendai virus-coated syngeneic cells specifically lyse allogeneic target cells. *Proc. Natl. Acad. Sci. U.S.A.* **75,** 5145.

Fink, P. J., and Bevan, M. J. (1978). H-2 antigens of the thymus determine lymphocyte specificity. *J. Exp. Med.* **148,** 766.

Fischer-Lindahl, K., and Wilson, D. B. (1977). Histocompatibility antigen-activated cytotoxic T lymphocytes. II. Estimates of the frequency and specificity of precursors. *J. Exp. Med.* **145,** 508.

Ford, W. L., Simmonds, S. J., and Atkins, R. C. (1975). Early cellular events in a systemic graft-vs-host reaction. II. Autoradiographic estimates of the frequency of donor lymphocytes which respond to each Ag-B-determined antigenic complex. *J. Exp. Med.* **141,** 681.

Götze, D., Nadeau, J., Wakeland, E. K., Berry, R. J., Bonhomme, F., Egorov, I. K., Hjorth, J. P., Hoogstraal, H., Vives, J., Winking, H., and Klein, J. (1980). Histocompatibility-2 system in wild mice. X. Frequencies of H-2 and Ia antigens in wild mice from Europe and Africa. *J. Immunol.* **124,** 2675.

Hünig, T., and Bevan, M. J. (1980). Self H-2 antigens influence the specificity of alloreactive cells. *J. Exp. Med.* **151,** 1288.

Janeway, C. A., Jr., and Conrad, P. J. (1981). Degeneracy in the response of individual T cells to non-self major histocompatibility complex antigens. *Behring Inst. Res. Comm.* (in press).

Jerne, N. K. (1971). The somatic generation of immune recognition. *Eur. J. Immunol.* **1,** 1.

Lemonnier, F., Burakoff, S. J., Germain, R. N., and Benacerraf, B. (1977). Cytolytic thymus-derived lymphocytes specific for allogeneic stimulator cells crossreact with chemically modified syngeneic cells. *Proc. Natl. Acad. Sci. U.S.A.* **74,** 1229.

Ryser, J. E., and MacDonald, H. R. (1979). Limiting dilution analysis of alloantigen-reactive T lymphocytes. I. Comparison of precursor frequencies for proliferative and cytolytic responses. *J. Immunol.* **122,** 1691.

Schwartz, R. H. (1981). Functional properties of *I* region gene products and theories of immune response (Ir) gene function. *In* "Ia Antigens and their Analogues in Man and Other Animals." (S. Ferrone and C. S. David, eds.). CRC Press, Boca Raton, Florida (in press).

Shearer, G. N., Rehn, T. G., and Schmitt-Verhulst, A. (1976). Role of murine major histocompatibility complex in the specificity of *in vitro* T cell-mediated lympholysis against syngeneic trinitrophenyl-modified targets. *Transplant. Rev.* **29,** 222.

Shreffler, D. C., and David, C. S. (1975). The H-2 major histocompatibility complex and the *I* immune response region: Genetic variation, function, and organization. *Adv. Immunol.* **20,** 125.

Simonsen, M. (1967). The clonal selection hypothesis evaluated by grafted cells reactive against their host. *Cold Spring Harbor Symp. Quant. Biol.* **32,** 317.

Skinner, M. A., and Marbrook, J. (1976). An estimation of the frequency of precursor cells which generate cytotoxic lymphocytes. *J. Exp. Med.* **143,** 1562.

Sredni, B., and Schwartz, R. H. (1981). Antigen-specific, proliferating T lymphocyte clones. Methodology, specificity, MHC restriction and alloreactivity. *Immunol. Rev.* **54,** 187.

Sredni, B., Tse, H. Y., and Schwartz, R. H. (1980). Direct cloning and extended culture of antigen-specific, MHC-restricted, proliferating T lymphocytes. *Nature (London)* **283,** 581.

Sredni, B., Tse, H. Y., Chen, C., and Schwartz, R. H. (1981a). Antigen-specific clones of proliferating T lymphocytes. I. Methodology, specificity and MHC-restriction. *J. Immunol.* **126,** 341.

Sredni, B., Matis, L. A., Lerner, E. A., Paul, W. E., and Schwartz, R. H. (1981b). Antigen-specific T cell clones restricted to unique F_1 major histocompatibility complex determinants. Inhibition of proliferation with a monoclonal anti-Ia antibody. *J. Exp. Med.* **153,** 677.

Tse, H. Y., Schwartz, R. H., and Paul, W. E. (1980). Cell–cell interactions in the T cell proliferative response. I. Analysis of the cell types involved and evidence for nonspecific T cell recruitment. *J. Immunol.* **125,** 491.

von Boehmer, H., Hengartner, H., Nabholz, M., Lernhardt, W., Schreier, M. H., and Haas, W. (1979). Fine specificity of a continuously growing killer cell clone specific for H-Y antigen. *Eur. J. Immunol.* **9,** 592.

Wilson, D. B. (1974). Immunologic reactivity to major histocompatibility alloantigens: HARC, effector cells and the problem of memory. *Prog. Immunol.* **2,** 145.

Zinkernagel, R. M., Callahan, G. N., Althage, A., Cooper, S., Klein, P. A., and Klein, J. (1978). On the thymus in the differentiation of "H-2 self recognition" by T cells: Evidence for dual recognition? *J. Exp. Med.* **147,** 882.

32

Mechanism of B Cell Activation by Monoclonal T Helper Cell Populations

Richard J. Hodes/Yoshihiro Asano/Minoru Shigeta/
Karen S. Hathcock/Masao Kimoto/C. Garrison Fathman/
Alfred Singer

I. KLH-Specific Cloned T Cells Provide *H-2* Restricted Help for Antibody Responses to TNP-KLH 386
II. Cloned T_h Cells Can Be *H-2* Restricted in Their Recognition of Accessory Cells But Not B Cells 388
III. After Specific Activation T Cell Clones Can Provide Antigen-Nonspecific Helper Activity 389
IV. Cloned T_h Cell Supernatant Mediates Antigen Nonspecific Help . . 389
V. Cloned T_h Cells Can Function through a Pathway Requiring Lyb-5^+ B Cells . . . .
VI. The Same Cloned T_h Cells Function through Pathways Which Are 390
Either Restricted or Unrestricted for T_h Cell Recognition of B Cell MHC Determinants 391
VII. The Same Cloned T_h Cells Function through Pathways Which Activate Different B Cell Subpopulations 393
VIII. Conclusions 394
References 395

It has been demonstrated recently that alternate pathways exist for B cell activation in T-dependent antibody responses (Asano *et al.*, 1981; Singer *et al.*, 1981). Conventional heterogeneous T cell populations activate Lyb-5^- B cells via a pathway which requires *H-2* restricted T cell recognition of B cells as well as accessory cells and which requires covalent carrier–hapten linkage. In contrast, these same T cell populations activate Lyb-5^+ B cells through a different activation pathway which requires *H-2* restricted T cell recognition only of

ISBN 0-12-249920-4

accessory cells, but not B cells. It has not been determined whether the same individual T cells can function to activate both B cell subpopulations or whether distinct T cell subpopulations specifically interact with each.

The use of cloned T lymphocyte populations has provided a recent addition to the available approaches for study of a number of T cell functions. Monoclonal T cell lines have been established which are antigen specific and major histocompatibility complex (MHC) restricted in their proliferative responses (Kimoto and Fathman, 1980; Kimoto and Fathman, 1981; Sredni *et al.*, 1980) or in the generation of cytotoxic T lymphocytes (von Boehmer *et al.*, 1980). More recently, T cell clones have been characterized which are competent as antigen-specific T helper (T_h) cells for antibody responses to erythrocytes (Watson, 1979) or to soluble antigens (Cammisuli and Schreier, 1981; Hodes *et al.*, 1981; Jones and Janeway, 1981). From studies of these cloned T_h populations, it has been concluded that single T_h cells are competent to provide antigen-specific help for antibody responses to both particulate and soluble antigens, although the mechanism of such help remains incompletely characterized.

In the present study, cloned T_h cells specific for the antigen keyhole limpet hemocyanin (KLH) were employed to study the mechanism or mechanisms by which individual T cell populations function in triggering B cell responses. It was demonstrated that a single monoclonal T_h cell population was capable of activating B cells through two functionally distinct activation pathways which differed in their genetic requirements and which resulted in the activation of distinct B cell subpopulations.

I. KLH-SPECIFIC CLONED T CELLS PROVIDE *H-2* RESTRICTED HELP FOR ANTIBODY RESPONSES TO TNP-KLH

The KLH reactivity and *H-2* restriction of several T cell clones derived from (B6 × C3H)F_1 ($H\text{-}2^b$ × $H\text{-}2^k$) mice were first demonstrated by assays of proliferation. All clones tested proliferated specifically in response to KLH and syngeneic (B6 × C3H)F_1 antigen-presenting cells (Table I). In addition, clone 16 responded to KLH in the presence of B6 ($H\text{-}2^b$) but not C3H ($H\text{-}2^k$) presenting cells, while clone 1 responded in the presence of C3H but not B6 presenting cells. Clone 11 demonstrated a third restriction pattern in that it responded to TNP-KLH in the presence of F_1 antigen-presenting cells, but not in the presence of presenting cells from either parent. Thus, KLH-reactive clones were either $H\text{-}2^b$ restricted, $H\text{-}2^k$ restricted, or ($H\text{-}2^b$ × $H\text{-}2^k$)F_1 restricted in their proliferative responses to that antigen. Antigen specificity was demonstrated by the inability of these cells to respond to ovalbumin or PPD (data not shown).

The functional T_h activity of these KLH-specific T cell clones was first as-

TABLE I

T Cell Clones Are Genetically Restricted in Their Proliferative Responses to KLH

		Thymidine incorporation (cpm)		
		Antigen-presenting cells		
	Antigen	B6	C3H	(B6 × C3H)F_1
Clone 1	—	323	508	659
	KLH	426	3756	6090
Clone 16	—	209	502	577
	KLH	5071	485	8969
Clone 11	—	261	484	332
	KLH	172	510	21,189

sessed by assaying their ability to activate unprimed TNP-specific B cells in responses to TNP-KLH. Activation of unprimed TNP-specific B cells in microcultures generally requires relatively high doses (5–20 μg/ml) of antigen. Each of the six clones tested provided efficient helper activity for IgM plaque forming cell (PFC) responses to TNP-KLH under these experimental conditions. The

TABLE II

Cloned Cells Function as *H-2* Restricted Helper Cells

		Anti-TNP PFC/culture[a]		
		(B + accessory) cells[b]		
Cloned T cells/culture		B10 (*H-2b*)	B10.BR (*H-2k*)	(B10 × B10.BR F_1
Clone 1	3×10^2	0	12	3
	10^3	0	145	68
	3×10^3	0	344	218
Clone 16	3×10^2	73	0	8
	10^3	269	5	169
	3×10^3	255	0	186
Clone 7	3×10^2	2	8	115
	10^3	2	3	313
	3×10^3	0	6	276

[a] Geometric mean response of triplicate cultures in the present of 15 μg/ml TNP-KLH. Responses in the absence of antigen or in the absence of added T cells were <5 PFC/culture.

[b] 4×10^5 anti-Thy-1.2+C treated unprimed spleen cells per culture.

patterns of *H-2* restriction observed for this helper activity are demonstrated in Table II. Clone 1 was capable of cooperating with $H\text{-}2^k$ (or F_1) but not $H\text{-}2^b$ (B + accessory) cells; clone 16 cooperated with $H\text{-}2^b$ (or F_1) but not $H\text{-}2^k$ cells; and clone 7 cooperated only with $(H\text{-}2^b \times H\text{-}2^k)F_1$ (B + accessory cells. These findings demonstrate that KLH-specific and *H-2* restricted F_1 T cell clones are competent to provide help for responses to soluble TNP-KLH, a finding which is consistent with results previously reported for homozygous T_h cell clones specific for either SRBC (Watson, 1979) or soluble antigens (Cammisuli and Schreier, 1981; Hodes *et al.*, 1981; Jones and Janeway, 1981). The present results also demonstrate that monoclonal F_1 T_h cells may be restricted in their recognition of unique F_1 specific as well as parental restricting elements expressed on the B cells and/or accessory cells with which they cooperate.

II. CLONED T_h CELLS CAN BE *H-2* RESTRICTED IN THEIR RECOGNITION OF ACCESSORY CELLS BUT NOT B CELLS

Further experiments were carried out in order to determine whether the *H-2* restriction demonstrated above reflects a requirement for T_h cell recognition of B cells, accessory cells, or both. $H\text{-}2^k$ restricted clone 14 T cells cooperate with unprimed (B + accessory) cells from B10.BR but not B10 (Table III). However, when B10.BR SAC were present in culture as accessory cells, clone 14 T cells were efficient helpers of responses by B10 B cells. Thus, in the presence of accessory cells expressing the appropriate *H-2*, cloned T_h cells appeared unrestricted in their ability to activate unprimed B cells. These results demonstrate

TABLE III

Cloned T Helper Cells Can Be *H-2* Restricted in Their Cooperation with Accessory Cells But Not B Cells

Clone 14 T cells/culture	SAC	Anti-TNP PFC/culture[a] (B + accessory) cells[b] B10	B10.BR
3×10^3	None	0	479
3×10^3	4×10^4 B10	0	—
3×10^3	4×10^4 B10.BR	283	—

[a] See Table II.
[b] See Table II.

that cloned T_h cells can function through a pathway of B cell activation which requires *H-2* restricted recognition of accessory cells, but not B cells.

III. AFTER SPECIFIC ACTIVATION T CELL CLONES CAN PROVIDE ANTIGEN-NONSPECIFIC HELPER ACTIVITY

In order to further evaluate the mechanism by which KLH-specific T cell clones provide help, it was determined whether a requirement exists for covalent linkage between the carrier KLH and the hapten TNP in responses mediated by cloned T_h cells. T cells from clone 14 were efficient in helping TNP-specific responses to TNP-KLH, but did not support significant PFC responses in the presence of free carrier KLH alone or in the presence of TNP-(T,G)-A--L (TGAL) [an active immunogen for TGAL specific cloned T_h cells (Hodes *et al.*, 1981)] (Table IV). However, when both KLH and TNP-TGAL were simultaneously present in culture, clone 14 T cells supported highly significant TNP-specific responses. These results suggest that while T_h cell activation is KLH specific for the clones studied, help once activated is in fact antigen nonspecific, allowing responses to unrelated antigens such as TNP-TGAL. One mechanism by which such helper activity could be mediated is through the generation of antigen-nonspecific soluble helper factors which would be released following *H-2* restricted interaction of T_h cells with accessory cells and specific antigen.

TABLE IV

Activation of B Cells by Cloned Helper Cells Does Not Require Carrier–Hapten Linkage

		Anti-TNP PFC/culture[a]			
Clone 14 T cells/culture	(B + accessory) cells[b]	TNP-KLH	TNP-(T,G)-A--L	KLH	KLH + TNP-(T,G)-A--L
10^3	(B10 × B10.BR)F_1	253	0	15	82
3×10^3	(B10 × B10.BR)F_1	289	0	15	196

[a] See Table II. TNP-KLH or KLH was present at 15 μg/ml, and TNP-(T,G)-A--L at 0.8 μg/ml.
[b] See Table II.

IV. CLONED T_h CELL SUPERNATANT MEDIATES ANTIGEN NONSPECIFIC HELP

The possibility that helper activity can be mediated by soluble products of cloned T_h cells was directly tested by assaying the activity of supernatants from

TABLE V

Supernatant of Antigen-Stimulated Cloned T_h Cells Mediates Antigen-Nonspecific Help

Dilution[1] clone 1a36 supernatant[c]	Anti-TNP PFC/culture[a] B10 (B + accessory) cells[b] TNP-KLH	No Ag
—	0	0
2	106	3
4	163	0
8	101	0
16	25	0
32	3	0

[a] See Table II.
[b] See Table II.
[c] Supernatant of clone 1a36 T cells stimulated for 4 days with 100 μg/ml TGAL.

cultured T_h cells. B6 derived TGAL-specific clone 1a36 T cells, which have been shown to provide help for responses to TNP-TGAL but not TNP-KLH (Hodes *et al.*, 1981), were cultured for 4 days in the presence of irradiated syngeneic filler cells and 100 μg/ml TGAL. The resulting supernatant was assayed for its ability to help responses to TNP-KLH by T-depleted syngeneic spleen populations. The addition of clone 1a36 supernatant reconstituted in a dose-dependent manner the responsiveness of anti-Thy-1.2 + C-treated B10 spleen cells to TNP-KLH, an antigen unrelated to the specificity of this clone; the supernatant did not stimulate a TNP-specific PFC response in the absence of added antigen (Table V). These findings demonstrate that these cloned T_h cells, once activated by specific antigen, generate a soluble product which is capable of helping (B + accessory) cells in antigen-nonspecific fashion.

V. CLONED T_h CELLS CAN FUNCTION THROUGH A PATHWAY REQUIRING Lyb-5$^+$ B CELLS

Previous studies have demonstrated that the activation pathway which is involved in T cell-dependent antibody responses is determined by the B cell subpopulation(s) which is activated under given experimental conditions. It has been shown that the activation of Lyb-5$^-$ B cells requires MHC restricted T–B cell interactions (Asano *et al.*, 1981; Singer *et al.*, 1981), whereas the activation of

TABLE VI

Cloned T_h Cells Functioning Through a Pathway Requiring Lyb-5$^+$ B Cells

	Anti-TNP PFC/culture[a]	
	(B + accessory) cells[b]	
Clone 1 T cells/culture	CBA/N (Lyb-5$^-$)	CBA/CaHN (Lyb-5$^+$ and Lyb-5$^-$)
0	0	9
3×10^2	0	113
10^3	0	281
3×10^3	18	312

[a] See Table II.
[b] See Table II.

Lyb-5$^+$ B cells does not require restricted T–B interaction (Asano *et al.*, 1981; Singer *et al.*, 1981). It was therefore of interest to determine whether the MHC unrestricted activation of B cells by the T_h cell clones presented here under high antigen dose conditions also activated only the Lyb-5$^+$ B cell subpopulation. Clone 1 T cells, which were *H-2*^{k} restricted KLH-specific helpers, were assayed for their ability to help (B + accessory) cells derived from CBA/N (a mutant defective *H-2*^{k} strain expressing only Lyb-5$^-$ B cells) or CBA/CaHN (a normal *H-2*^{k} strain expressing both Lyb 5$^+$ and Lybt-5$^-$ B cells). Under these experimental conditions, clone 1 T cells were sufficient to induce T-dependent responses in CBA/CaHN but not CBA/N B cells (Table VI). In contrast, both (B + accessory) populations were activated by the T-independent type 1 antigen TNP-*Brucella abortus* (data not shown). Thus, under these experimental conditions, T_h cell clones only activated B cell populations which contained the Lyb-5$^+$ subset.

VI. THE SAME CLONED T_h CELLS FUNCTION THROUGH PATHWAYS WHICH ARE EITHER RESTRICTED OR UNRESTRICTED FOR T_h CELL RECOGNITION OF B CELL MHC DETERMINANTS

In order to test the possibility that the same cloned T_h cells can function in multiple B cell activation pathways, these cloned T_h cells were also studied under other experimental conditions known to activate Lyb-5$^-$ B cells (Asano *et al.*, 1981). Specifically, T_h cell clones were assayed for the ability to cooperate with

TABLE VII

Cloned T Helper Cells Function Through Pathways which are Either Restricted or Unrestricted for T Cell Recognition of B Cells

Concentration of TNP-KLH	T cells/culture	Accessory cells	Anti-TNP PFC/culture (B + accessory) cells[a]	
			B10	CBA/CaHN
20 μg/ml[b]	1×10^4 clone 14	None	60	1553
	1×10^4 clone 14	(B10 × B10.BR)F_1	895	1620
	1×10^4 clone 16	None	823	252
	1×10^4 clone 16	(B10 × B10.BR)F_1	756	1356
0.001 μg/ml[c]	1×10^4 clone 14	None	9	3048
	1×10^4 clone 14	(B10 × B10.BR)F_1	4	2991
	1×10^4 clone 16	None	3196	0
	1×10^4 clone 16	(B10 × B10.BR)F_1	1435	120

[a] 3×10^6 RAMB+C treated TNP-primed spleen cells/culture.
[b] Responses are presented as mean direct (IgM) PFC/culture.
[c] Responses are presented as mean indirect (IgG) PFC/culture.

TNP-primed (rather than unprimed) (B + accessory) cell populations for responses to TNP-KLH at low concentrations of antigen (0.001 μg/ml) as well as high concentrations (20 μg/ml). Cloned T_h cells were competent to help under either antigen condition, with predominantly IgM responses generated at the higher antigen concentration and predominantly IgG responses at the lower concentration (Table VII). Under both conditions, T_h function was MHC restricted, with clone 14 T cells cooperating with CBA/CaHN but not B10 (B + accessory) cells and clone 16 T cells showing the reciprocal restriction pattern.

TABLE VIII

Activation of B Cells by Cloned Helper Cells Requires Carrier–Hapten Linkage at Low Concentrations of Antigen

Clone 16 T cells/culture	(B + accessory) cells[b]	Anti-TNP PFC/culture[a]			
		TNP-KLH	TNP-FGG	KLH	KLH + TNP-FGG
1×10^4	B10	3196	14	0	81

[a] TNP-KLH, TNP-FGG, or KLH was present in culture at 0.001 μg/ml. Responses are presented as mean indirect (IgG) PFC/culture.
[b] See Table VII.

It was next determined whether the MHC restrictions demonstrated under these conditions reflected requirements for T_h cell recognition of B cells, accessory cells, or both. In the presence of (B10 × B10.BR)F_1 ($H\text{-}2^{b/k}$) accessory cells, clone 14 or clone 16 T cells cooperated efficiently with either B10 or CBA/CaHN B cells for responses to 20 μg/ml TNP-KLH (Table VII), confirming that under these conditions, cloned T_h cells were restricted only in their recognition of accessory cells and not B cells. In contrast, for the response to 0.001 μg/ml TNP-KLH, the restriction of cloned T_h cell activity was not reversed by F_1 accessory cells, suggesting that the function of the same T_h cells under these conditions required recognition of MHC products expressed by B cells (Table VII).

Further characterization of the helper function mediated at low concentrations of TNP-KLH was carried out by testing the requirements for covalent carrier–hapten linkage in these responses. Clone 16 T cells supported responses to 0.001 μg/ml TNP-KLH, but no significant responses were stimulated by 0.001 μg/ml KLH or by 0.001 μg TNP-fowl γ-globulin (FGG), itself immunogenic in the presence of FGG-specific T_h cells (data not shown) (Table VIII). In contrast to the findings for responses to high concentrations of KLH (Table V), there was no significant response by cloned T_h cells to 0.001 μg/ml TNP-FGG + 0.001 μg/ml KLH (Table VIII). Thus, the activation of TNP-primed B cells under low antigen dose conditions required both MHC restricted T_h–B cell interaction and carrier hapten linkage.

VII. THE SAME CLONED T_h CELLS FUNCTION THROUGH PATHWAYS WHICH ACTIVATE DIFFERENT B CELL SUBPOPULATIONS

The findings reported above indicate that, under different conditions of antigen stimulation, the same cloned T_h cells can activate TNP-primed B cells via two distinct activation pathways, one which is not MHC restricted and one which is genetically restricted. The identity of the B cell subpopulations activated by T_h cells under these conditions was next determined. TNP-primed CBA/CaHN (Lyb-5^+ and Lyb-5^- B cells) and CBA/N (Lyb-5^- B cells only) (B + accessory) cells were cultured with clone 14 T cells and assayed for responses to either 20 or 0.001 μg/ml TNP-KLH. At high antigen concentration, CBA/CaHN but not CBA/N B cells were responsive, consistent with a requirement for Lyb-5^+ B cells in these responses (Table IX). In marked contrast, for responses to 0.001 μg/ml TNP-KLH, CBA/CaHN and CBA/N B cells were both efficient responders, demonstrating that Lyb-5^- B cells were activated in these cultures. These results demonstrate that the same cloned T_h cells can function through at least

TABLE IX

Cloned T Helper Cells Function through Pathways Which Activate Different B Cell Subpopulations

Concentration of TNP-KLH[a]	Clone 14 T cells/culture	Anti-TNP PFC/culture (B + accessory) cells[a] CBA/N ($Lyb\text{-}5^-$)	CBA/CaHN ($Lyb\text{-}5^+$ and $Lyb\text{-}5^-$)
20 μg/ml	3×10^3	72	1766
	1×10^4	36	1689
0.001 μg/ml	3×10^3	1574	2870
	1×10^4	1646	3148

[a] See Table VII.

two distinct pathways of B cell activation which result in the activation of different B cell subpopulations.

VIII. CONCLUSIONS

Recent findings have demonstrated the existence of two distinct pathways for B cell activation in T dependent antibody responses. These pathways were shown to differ from one another in terms of the carrier specificity of effective T cell help, in terms of requirements for MHC restricted versus unrestricted T cell–B cell interactions and in the identity of the B cell subpopulations activated. The studies presented here have employed monoclonal T_h cell populations to further characterize these mechanisms of B cell activation.

It was demonstrated that at low concentrations of TNP-KLH, T_h cell clones cooperated with hapten-primed (B + accessory) populations to generate predominantly IgG responses. For these responses, help was carrier-specific, and T_h cells were MHC restricted in their interaction with B cells. The $Lyb\text{-}5^-$ B cell subpopulation was activated by this pathway. These findings suggest that cloned T_h cells can function through direct interaction with responding ($Lyb\text{-}5^-$) B cells, and that this interaction is mediated by T_h cell recognition of B cell MHC determinants as well as by carrier–hapten bridging between T and B cells. At high concentrations of TNP-KLH, the same T cell clones cooperated with primed or unprimed B cells to generate predominantly IgM responses. Although T_h cell activation was antigen specific in these responses, helper activity once triggered was nonspecific and could be mediated by the supernatant product of cloned T_h cells stimulated with a high dose of antigen. T_h cell–B cell interactions were not

MHC restricted under these conditions, and this pathway of responses required the participation of Lyb-5^+ B cells.

The results presented here thus demonstrate that a single T cell population is able, under appropriate experimental conditions, to provide help which is either carrier specific or nonspecific, for which T cell–B cell interaction is either MHC restricted or unrestricted, and which results in the activation of either Lyb-5^- or Lyb-5^+ B cell subsets. These findings imply that the different genetic requirements for activating Lyb-5^- and Lyb-5^+ B cells need not result from differences in the identity of the T_h cells which interact with each B cell subset, but rather result from differences in the ability of each B cell subpopulation to respond to activation signals provided by a single T_h cell.

REFERENCES

Asano, Y., Singer, A., and Hodes, R. J. (1981). Role of the major histocompatibility complex (MHC) in T cell activation of B cell subpopulations. MHC restricted and unrestricted B cell responses are mediated by distinct B cell subpopulations. *J. Exp. Med.* **154,** 1100.

Cammisuli, S., and Schreier, M. H. (1981). Individual clones of carrier-specific T cells help idiotypically and isotypically heterogeneous anti-hapten B-cell responses. *Immunology* **43,** 581.

Hodes, R. J., and Singer, A. (1977). Cellular and genetic control of antibody response *in vitro*. I. Cellular requirements for the generation of primary IgM responses to soluble antigens. *Eur. J. Immunol.* **7,** 892.

Hodes, R. J., Kimoto, M., Hathcock, K. S., Fathman, C. G., and Singer, A. (1981). Functional helper activity of monoclonal T cell populations. Antigen-specific and *H-2* restricted cloned T cells provide help for in vitro antibody respones to trinitrophenyl-poly-L-(Tyr, Glu)-D,L-Ala--poly-L-Lys. *Proc. Natl. Acad. Sci. U.S.A.* **78,** 6431.

Jones, B., and Janeway, C. A. (1981). Cooperative interaction of B lymphocytes with antigen-specific helper T lymphocytes in MHC restricted. *Nature (London)* **292,** 547.

Kimoto, M., and Fathman, C. G. (1980). Antigen-reactive T cell clones. I. Transcomplementing hybrid *I-A*-region gene products function effectively in antigen presentation. *J. Exp. Med.* **152,** 759.

Kimoto, M., and Fathman, C. G. (1981). Antigen-reactive T cell clones. II. Unique homozygous and (high responder × low responder)F_1 hybrid antigen-presenting determinants detected using poly(Tyr,Glu)-poly-D,L-Ala-poly-Lys-reactive T cell clones. *J. Exp. Med.* **153,** 375.

Shigeta, M., and Fathman, C. G. (1981). *I* region genetic restrictions imposed upon the recognition of KLH by murine T cell clones. *Immunogenetics* **14,** 415.

Singer, A., Morrissey, P. J., Hathcock, K. S., Ahmed, A., Scher, I., and Hodes, R. J. (1981). Role of the major histocompatibility complex (MHC) in T cell activation of B cell subpopulations. Lyb-5^+ and Lyb-5^- B cell recognition. *J. Exp. Med.* **154,** 501.

Sredni, B., Tse, H. Y., and Schwartz, R. H. (1980). Direct cloning and extended culture of antigen-specific MHC-restricted, proliferating T lymphocytes. *Nature (London)* **283,** 581.

von Boehmer, H., Haas, W., Pohlit, H., Hengarner, H., and Nabholz, M. (1980). T cell clones: Their use for the study of specificity, induction and effector function of T cells. *Springer Semin. Immunopathol.* **3,** 23.

Watson, J. (1979). Continuous proliferation of murine antigen-specific helper T lymphocytes in culture. *J. Exp. Med.* **150,** 1510.

33

T Cell Lines and T Cell Clones Bearing Cross-Reactive Idiotype

Jacques Thèze/Masao Kimoto/Marie-Lise Gougeon/
Jean-Louis Moreau/Gerard Somme/
Lise Leclercq/C. Garrison Fathman

I.	Functional Characterization of the Helper Activity of Cell Line L.14	398
II.	L.14 Cells Express Idiotype-Like Determinants	400
III.	Effect of Anti-Idiotypic Serum B658 on the Activity of Clone C.14.14	401
IV.	Conclusions	402
	References	403

A considerable amount of work has been devoted toward understanding the mechanisms by which helper T cells (T_h) regulate the activation of B cells in T-dependent antibody responses. T_h cells recognize both specific antigen and "self" major histocompatibility complex products on antigen presenting cells and/or B cells (Sprent, 1978). Very little is known about the precise molecular nature of the T cell receptor(s) which controls these recognition events. Evidence supporting the existence of shared idiotypic determinants on T_h and B cells of the same specificity has been reported (Rajewsky and Eichmann, 1977). In addition the T_h cell population appears to be heterogeneous. Experiments showing the role of T_h specific for idiotypic (Woodland and Cantor, 1978), allotypic (Herzenberg *et al.*, 1976) and isotypic determinants (Kishimoto and Ishizaka, 1973) have been reported.

The availability of large numbers of idiotype-positive T_h cells should facilitate the purification and characterization of the molecules involved in T cell recognition. Taking advantage of recent progress in T cell culture technology which allows long term *in vitro* propagation of antigen specific T helper cells we have established lines and clones of poly(Glu^{60}-Ala^{30}-Tyr^{10}) (GAT) specific T helper cells. It was demonstrated that these cells were highly efficient in providing help for IgG response to DNP-GAT *in vitro* (Gougeon *et al.*, 1982). Furthermore all

ISBN 0-12-249920-4

our lines are able to induce IgG_1, IgG_{2a}, and IgG_{2b} anti-DNP plaque-forming cell (PFC) responses in presence of DPN-GAT indicating that T_h cells selected on the basis of antigen specificity do not select immunoglobulin isotypes. This has been confirmed by the isolation of T_h clones; these clones are able to induce IgM, IgG_3, IgG_1, IgG_{2a}, and IgG_{2b} anti-DNP PFC responses *in vitro* (Seman and Thèze, 1981). Supernatants of our cultured T cell lines in our experimental conditions do not contain detectable specific helper factor(s) able to replace the T_h cells.

In parallel we have obtained a series of anti-idiotypic reagents made against anti-GAT antibodies. All reagents confirm the existence of a major idiotype (C.GAT) in the anti-GAT response of the mouse (Thèze and Moreau, 1978; Ju *et al.*, 1978). This idiotype has been dissected into a variety of specificities (Somme *et al.*, 1981). We have demonstrated that a syngeneic anti-idiotypic antiserum made in BALB/c against BALB/c anti-GAT antibodies can specifically block the helper function of GAT-specific helper T cells (Gougeon *et al.*, 1982).

To illustrate our findings and to describe our experimental approach, we will describe in this chapter the results obtained with a GAT-specific cell line (L.14) and a GAT-specific cell clone (C.14.14) derived from C57BL/6 mice (B6) (Kimoto and Fathman, 1980).

I. FUNCTIONAL CHARACTERIZATION OF THE HELPER ACTIVITY OF CELL LINE L.14

Assessment of the helper activity of such long-term lines or cloned cells was made *in vitro* (Gougeon *et al.*, 1982). Cultures contained 5×10^5 DPN-primed B cells and varying numbers of T cells to be tested. B cells were from animals primed with DNP-ovalbumin (DNP-OVA) in Maalox (Laboratoires Rorer, France) and *B. pertussis* vaccine (Institut Pasteur Production Paris, France). Animals were boosted 8 days before the culture. The B cells were prepared by treating spleen cells with monoclonal anti-Thy-1.2 antibodies (Olac-Bicester, Oxom, England) and guinea pig complement.

Table I shows the titration of the helper activity of line 14. The maximum activity is obtained with 5×10^3 cells/well; 5×10^2 cells/well still exhibit a very significant helper activity. This activity is specific since no response is obtained in presence of DNP conjugated to human γ-globulin (DNP-HGG) in conditions where 5×10^5 HGG primed LNC gave a very significant response. In addition these cells are not able to activate anti-DNP PFC response in culture in presence of GAT plus DNP-HGG; these cells require a hapten–carrier bridge to provide help to B cells.

TABLE I

Characteristics of the Helper Activity of Cell Line L.14

Number of cells added per well	DNP-specific PFC response/10^6 viable cells in presence of[a]					
	DNP-GAT[b]				DNP-HGG	DNP-HGG + GAT
	Total response	IgG_1	IgG_{2a}	IgG_{2b}	Total response	Total response
L.14						
10^4	910	530	310	124	0	0
5×10^3	2180	968	710	792	30	75
2.5×10^3	1750	926	640	642	0	0
5×10^2	270	—[c]	—	—	0	0
10^2	30	—	—	—	0	0
HGG-specific T cell						
5×10^5	83	—	—	—	3882	3563

[a] 5×10^5 DNP-OVA primed, T depleted spleen cells were cultured in triplicate together with various numbers of L.14 cells or HGG primed lymph node cells in presence of optimal concentrations of DNP-GAT (5 μg/ml), DNP-HGG (4 μg/ml), or DNP-HGG plus GAT. After 5 days in culture the numbers of anti-DNP PFC were evaluated. The numbers reported represent the arithmetic means of the responses from triplicate cultures. The background response obtained in the absence of antigen has been determined and was subtracted from the results reported. No IgM response was detected under our experimental conditions.

[b] The total anti-DNP response was measured in the presence of a multivalent rabbit anti-mouse immunoglobulin antisera. IgG_1, IgG_{2a}, and IgG_{2b} were measured with isotype specific rabbit antisera.

[c] Not done.

L.14 cells can induce IgG_1, IgG_{2a}, and IgG_{2b} anti-DNP PFC response *in vitro* (Table I). Whatever the concentration of T cells used the proportion of the three isotypes tested remains roughly constant. This seems to indicate that there is no heterogeneity of cell line L.14 concerning the capacity of the cells to induce a response of IgG_1, IgG_{2a}, and IgG_{2b} type. This is in agreement with our previous results obtained with other T cell lines (Gougeon *et al.*, 1982) and with MHC restricted, GAT-specific T helper cell clones of BALB/c origin (Seman and Thèze, 1981). Similar data have been obtained with clones specific for fowl γ-globulin (Cammisuli and Schreier, 1981) and (Tyr-Glu)-Ala-Lys (TGAL) (Hodes *et al.*, 1981).

L.14 cells cannot provide help to histoincompatible B cells. Whatever the concentration of T cells tested, no significant anti-DNP PFC response is generated *in vitro* in the presence of 5×10^5 primed splenic B cells from BALB/c origin. As a positive control, T cells from a BALB/c GAT-specific cell line provide very efficient help to BALB/c B cells (data not shown).

TABLE II

Effect of Syngeneic Anti-C.GAT Serum on L.14 Helper Activity

Sera added to the cultures[a]	DNP-specific PFC response/10^6 viable cells[b]		
	IgG_1	IgG_{2a}	IgG_{2b}
Experiment 1: (2500 cells/well)			
0	1015	255	250
anti-C.GAT	*208*	174	214
ads. anti-C.GAT[c]	1060	322	380
anti-X24[d]	1024	270	204
Experiment 2: (3000 cells/well)			
0	1144	1052	890
anti-C.GAT	*293*	666	855
anti-X24	1384	920	715
NMS	1265	515	706
Experiment 3: (5000 cells/well)			
0	1070	810	915
anti-C.GAT	*252*	499	432
ads. anti-C.GAT	1452	877	795
NMS	1452	730	642

[a] The various sera were added at a final dilution of 1:240 on day 0 of the culture. All sera have been extensively adsorbed with mouse lymphocytes before use.

[b] The cells were cultured and the responses were measured as indicated in Table I. The results reported represent the arithmetic means of the responses from triplicate cultures.

[c] Anti-C.GAT syngeneic serum was adsorbed on hybridoma protein with anti-GAT activity coupled to cyanogen bromide activated Sepharose 4B. The efficiency and specificity of the adsorption were verified as indicated in the text.

[d] Syngeneic anti-idiotypic serum prepared against myeloma protein X24 (anti-galactan).

II. L.14 CELLS EXPRESS IDIOTYPE-LIKE DETERMINANTS

A syngeneic anti-idiotypic serum (B658) was made by immunizing BALB/c mice with affinity purified BALB/c anti-GAT antibodies coupled to keyhole limpet hemocyanin (KLH). B658 specifically precipitates Fab fragments from BALB/c anti-GAT antibodies or Fab fragments from a hybridoma protein with anti-GAT activity. This binding was specifically inhibited by anti-GAT sera and not by sera with unrelated activity. An assay measuring inhibition of idiotype binding assay was used to study the genetic distribution of the idiotype recognized by this serum. As previously described with xenogeneic sera made in rabbit (Thèze and Moreau, 1978) or in guinea pig (Ju *et al.*, 1978), the idiotypic structure identified by this reagent is present in all strains of mice irrespectively of their allotypic markers. The serum also recognizes all the hybridoma proteins which have an anti-GAT activity (L. Leclercq *et al.*, unpublished results).

In some experiments an unrelated syngeneic anti-idiotypic serum was used as control. This serum was prepared by Dr. P. A. Cazenave in BALB/c mice against the myeloma protein X24. This protein has an anti-galactan activity.

The effects of B658 on the helper activity of L.14 cells were studied. Three experiments are reported in Table II. In each experiment, a different number of T_h cells was used and the isotypic pattern of the anti-DNP response obtained on day 5 of the culture was determined. It can be seen that in all experiments the IgG_1 response is dramatically affected by addition of serum B658 into the cultures. The percentage of inhibition of the IgG_1 response is between 75 to 80%. The IgG_{2a} and IgG_{2b} responses are less inhibited.

Additional controls are included in these experiments. In experiments 1 and 2 the effect of an unrelated anti-idiotypic antiserum has been assayed. No effect of the syngeneic serum directed against myeloma protein with anti-galactan activity is observed on the activity of the L.14 cells. In experiments 1 and 3, the effect of anti-idiotypic antiserum B658 after adsorption on hybridoma protein with anti-GAT activity has been studied. From the results it is clear that adsorption removes the inhibitory capacity of serum B658, thus showing that the anti-idiotypic activity is responsible for the inhibition of the GAT-specific helper activity.

III. EFFECT OF ANTI-IDIOTYPIC SERUM B658 ON THE ACTIVITY OF CLONE C.14.14

A clone of GAT-specific cells was derived from line 14 as previously described (Kimoto and Fathman, 1980). Its helper activity was assessed as well as

TABLE III

Effect of Syngeneic Anti-C.GAT Serum on the Helper Activity of Clone C.14.14

Sera added to the cultures[a]	DNP-specific response/10^6 viable cells[b]		
	IgG_1	IgG_{2a}	IgG_{2b}
0	1713	339	338
Anti-C.GAT	*331*	424	480
Anti-X24	1316	436	499

[a] The sera were added on day 0 of the helper assay as indicated in Table II.

[b] The cells were cultured and the responses were measured as indicated in Table I; 10^4 T helper cell from clone C.14.14 were added per well. The results reported represent the arithmetic means of the responses from triplicate cultures.

the isotypic pattern of the secondary response induced in presence of DNP primed B cells and DNP-GAT (Table III). The cloned cells induce IgG_1, IgG_{2a}, and IgG_{2b} anti-DNP PFC responses *in vitro*. When the effect of serum B658 was assayed on the helper activity of C.14.14 cells, the IgG_1 response is inhibited of 80%, while the IgG_{2a} and IgG_{2b} responses are not significantly affected. As control the effect of the anti-idiotypic serum directed against myeloma protein X24 is shown; it does not alter the total immune response to DNP-GAT nor the isotypic pattern of the response (Table III).

IV. CONCLUSIONS

Long-term cultured T cell lines and clones have been studied. Their ability to function as T helper cells for antibody responses to DNP-GAT*in vitro* has been demonstrated. The helper activity is carrier specific and requires a hapten–carrier bridge in order to deliver the helper specific signals to DNP-primed B cells (Gougeon *et al.*, 1982). In the supernatants of the GAT cell line we were not able to detect specific helper factor(s) able to replace the T_h cells in our assays. L.14 cells have been shown to act only on histocompatible B cells.

All the GAT-specific T cell lines and clones isolated are able to induce *in vitro* IgG_1, IgG_{2a}, and IgG_{2b} anti-DNP PFC in the secondary response to DNP-GAT. When the helper activity of the T cell line is titered, the proportion of the three isotypes remains constant, suggesting that each helper cell selected on the basis of its antigen specificity does not select immunoglobulin isotype (Gougeon *et al.*, 1982). These results have been confirmed by GAT-specific T cell clones from BALB/c mice (Seman and Thèze, 1981) and by clone C.14.14 derived from B6 mice. The experiment has been performed with B cell populations depleted of T cells with anti-Thy-1.2 treatment. Therefore, only one type of T_h cell is sufficient to provide help to DNP-primed B cells. Furthermore these results indicate that a monoclonal T cell population can induce all types of B memory cells independently of the isotype of their receptors. These data are strong arguments against a stringent requirement for idiotypic-, allotypic-, or isotypic-specific T_h cells for the induction of a response to T-dependent antigens. This tends to indicate that Ig determinant-specific T cells, when they exist, are involved in modulating the immune response initiated by antigen-specific and MHC restricted T cells.

L.14 T cell lines as the other GAT-specific cell lines derived from BALB/c and B6D2 mice (Gougeon *et al.*, 1982) express idiotype-like determinants, and their helper function can be specifically blocked by anti-idiotypic antiserum directed against the C.GAT idiotype. A syngeneic serum prepared in BALB/c mice against BALB/c anti-GAT antibodies was used in these experiments. Blockade of helper functions was found with B6 helper cells, although these mice bear different allotypic markers than BALB/c animals. Therefore at the T cell level, as at the B cell level, the C.GAT idiotypic determinants are broadly distributed.

The blockade observed is never total; only 50% of the total response induced by L.14 is affected. However, when the blockade is examined at the isotypic level we found that 100% of the IgG_1 specific response of BALB/c mice (data not shown) and about 80% of the IgG_1 response induced by L.14 cells are blocked. The IgG_{2a} and IgG_{2b} responses are always less inhibited. This raises the question of the mechanism of the inhibition of the helper activity by the anti-idiotypic serum.

Since the same preferential inhibition of the IgG_1 response has been found with clone C.14.14, this effect cannot be simply attributed to a heterogeneity of the helper cell population. Furthermore we have shown that all helper T cells from our lines have the same potential to induce IgG_1, IgG_{2a}, and IgG_{2b} responses. One could consider that interactions between GAT-specific T_h cells and IgG_{2a} and IgG_{2b} DNP-primed B cells may be more difficult to inhibit than the interactions with IgG_1 DNP-primed B cells. This can be explained if the amount of antigen bound to the IgG_{2a} and IgG_{2b} B cells is higher either because their receptors have greater affinity for DNP or because the number of their receptors is higher. Therefore, the dilution of serum used in these experiments may have been optimal for inhibiting the interactions between T_h cells and IgG_1 anti-DNP B cells but may have been suboptimal for preventing the interactions of the helper cells with IgG_{2a} and IgG_{2b} specific B cells. Alternatively the isotype of the anti-idiotypic serum itself may play some indirect role in the selective inhibition of the IgG_1 response; this possibility will be investigated with isotypically defined monoclonal anti-idiotypic antibodies.

REFERENCES

Cammisuli, S., and Schreier, M. H. (1981). Individual clones of carrier specific T cells help idiotypically and isotypically heterogeneous anti-hapten B cell responses. *Immunology* **43,** 581.

Gougeon, M. L., Leclercq, L., Lowy, I., Bismut, G., Somme, G., and Thèze, J. (1982). In vitro inhibition of the helper activity of GAT specific T cell lines by a syngeneic anti-idiotypic serum: Preferential effect on the IgG_1 response. *Cell. Immunol.* (in press).

Herzenberg, L. A., Okumura, K., Cantor, H., Sato, V. L., Shen, F. W., Boyse, E. A., and Herzenberg, L. A. (1976). T cell regulation of antibody response: Demonstration of allotype-specific helper T cells and their specific removal by suppressor T cells. *J. Exp. Med.* **144,** 330.

Hodes, R. J., Kimoto, M., Hathcock, K. S., Fathman, C. G., and Singer, A. (1981). Functional helper activity of monoclonal T cell populations. Cloned T cells provide antigen-specific and H-2 restricted help for *in vivo* antibody responses to TNP-TGAL. *Proc. Natl. Acad. Sci. U.S.A.* **78,** 6431.

Ju, S.-T., Kipps, T., Thèze, J., Benacerraf, B., and Dorf, M. E. (1978). Idiotypic analysis of anti-GAT antibodies. I. Presence of common idiotypic specificities in both responder and nonresponder mice. *J. Immunol.* **121,** 1034.

Kimoto, M., and Fathman, G. (1980). Antigen reactive T cell clones. I. Transcomplementing hybrid *I-A* region gene products function effectively in antigen presentation. *J. Exp. Med.* **152,** 759.

Kishimoto, T., and Ishizaka, K. (1973). Regulation of antibody response *in vitro*. VI. Carrier specific helper T cells for IgG and IgE antibody response. *J. Immunol.* **111,** 720.

Rajewsky, K., and Eichmann, K. (1977). Antigen receptors of T helper cells. *Contemp. Top. Immunol.* **7,** 69.

Seman, M., and Thèze, J. (1981). *H-2* restricted carrier specific T cell clones do not select immunoglobulin isotypes. *ICN/UCLA Symp. Mol. Cell. Biol.* **20,** 523.

Somme, G., Leclercq, L., Petit, C., and Thèze, J. (1981). Genetic control of the immune response to the GAT terpolymer. V. Three types of idiotypic specificities on BALB/c anti-GAT antibodies. *Eur. J. Immunol.* **11,** 493.

Sprent, J. (1978). Restricted helper function of F_1 hybrid T cells positively selected to heterologous erythrocytes in irradiated parental strain mice. II. Evidence for restrictions affecting helper cell induction and T-B collaboration, both mapping to the *K*-end of the *H-2* complex. *J. Exp. Med.* **147,** 1159.

Thèze, J., and Moreau, J. L. (1978). Genetic control of the immune response to the GAT terpolymer. I. Interstrains and interspecies cross-reactive idiotype. *Ann Immunol.* (*Paris*) **129C,** 721.

Woodland, R., and Cantor, H. (1978). Idiotype specific T helper cells are required to induce idiotype-positive B memory cells to secrete antibody. *Eur. J. Immunol.* **8,** 600.

34

Specific Regulation of Immune Responses by Products of T Cell Clones

Harvey Cantor

Text 405
References 408

The intensity and type of an immune reaction do not simply reflect the numbers of antigen-specific cells. The response is regulated by two major types of T cells: inducer cells and suppressor cells. Although these T cells are morphologically indistinguishable, inducer and suppressor T cells express characteristic patterns of glycoproteins at their cell membrane (Cantor and Gershon, 1979). Examination of inducer and suppressor T cells after separation according to these molecular labels had indicated that both express receptors for antigen and that cell supernatants or cell extracts can mimic the antigen-specific functions of intact cells (Germain and Benacerraf, 1980). However, analyses of these materials have not defined the genes and molecules responsible for antigen-specific T cell function.

These questions have been difficult to answer largely because of technical reasons. A biochemical explanation of the function and specificity of antibodies has come from analyses of neoplastic B cell clones (myeloma cells) that secrete different types of immunoglobulins. Unfortunately, neoplastic T cell lines have not proved so useful. Many do not grow well in continuous culture, and very few express immunologic function. A more successful approach has come from fusion of normal T cells to T cell lymphomas, with polyethylene glycol. Several groups have reported that such fusions can produce hybrid cells that suppress or induce antibody response (Taniguchi *et al.*, 1979; Sproviero *et al.*, 1980). However, hybrids resulting from fusion of T cells with T cell lymphomas usually express the phenotype of the tumor cell partner and tend to lose chromosomes in

ISBN 0-12-249920-4

cell cultures. Biochemical analysis of stable hybrids that express antigen-specific T cell functions has also been hindered to date by the extremely small amounts of antigen-specific material synthesized by T hybrid cells.

Using a method that allows production of large numbers of continuously propagatable cloned cells, we have defined both helper and suppressor T cell clones (Nabel *et al.*, 1981). C1.Lyt-23/4 is an SRBC-specific T suppressor clone that expressed surface receptors for the glycophorin expressed by sheep erythrocytes (Fresno *et al.*, 1981b). Analysis of this T cell clone has suggested that these cells share several major characteristics with antibody-forming B cells. Suppressor T cells and B cells display similar numbers of surface receptors that bind to antigen in the absence of MHC products. Both respond to signals from inducer T cells by secretion of antigen-binding proteins. C1.Lyt-23/4 in Lyt-2^+ secretes 70 kilodalton proteins that bind to antigen and mediate suppression. Picogram amounts of purified antigen-binding proteins specifically inhibit productions of antibody in response to the antigen (Fresno *et al.*, 1981c). In addition to the 70 kilodalton protein, 45 and 24 kilodalton proteins have been routinely observed under conditions where proteolysis was not carefully controlled (Fresno *et al.*, 1981b). Fractionation of biosynthetically labeled supernatant proteins by size in Sephacryl S-200 frequently demonstrated small amounts of 24 kilodalton peptides that bound specifically to SRBC but did not suppress as well as 45 kilodalton peptides without binding activity but capable of suppressing PFC responses to all erythrocytes tested (albeit less efficiently than the 70 kilodalton fraction) (Fresno *et al.*, 1981c). Interaction of the 70 kilodalton protein with antigen markedly increases its susceptibility to degradation, resulting in breakdown into two major peptides, 45 and 24 kilodalton, according to mobility in sodium dodecyl sulfate-polyacrylamide gel electrophoresis (SDS-PAGE).

Degradation of immunoglobulins with proteolytic enzymes has provided important insights into the structural basis of this molecule's biological activity and specificity for antigen (Edelman, 1971; Natvig and Kunkel, 1973). We used this approach to study the functional organization of the 70 kilodalton suppressor protein (Fresno *et al.*, 1981a). We found that although the 70 kilodalton protein is sensitive to digestion by several different proteases, including pepsin and trypsin, papain yielded the most reproducible cleavage: this enzyme splits the 70 kilodalton antigen-binding molecule into two peptide subunits of 45 and 24 kilodaltons. These subunits were relatively resistant to further degradation and represented 70–85% of the digested product after 5–120 min of digestion. Since this restricted cleavage of the 70 kilodalton protein was a reproducible characteristic of the protein, we defined the biologic activity of the two cleavage products. The 45 kilodalton subunit retained suppressive activity, although activity was 5- to 50-fold less potent than the intact 70 kilodalton peptide; the 24 kilodalton peptide bound specifically to SRBC but did not suppress. Thus, the two breakdown products obtained after papain digestion displayed the same size and biologic activities as the 45 and 24 kilodalton peptides obtained after incubation of 70 kilodalton material with antigen. The two peptides were also distinguished serologically. An antiserum made against myeloma proteins MOPC 315 that probably recognizes framework regions in V_H sequences reacted with the 70 kilodalton parent molecules and the 24 kilodalton peptide. A rabbit serum prepared against TNP-specific T cell suppressor factor, which reacts with determinants on several T cell suppressor factors specific for different antigens (Gershon *et al.*, 1981), reacted with the 70 kilodalton molecule and the 45 kilodalton subunit, but not the 24 kilodalton subunit.

The combined activities of the separate 45 and 24 kilodalton peptides after papain digestion of the 70 kilodalton protein accounted for the biologic activity of the parent molecule, and the peptides probably represent two distinct domains of the T suppressor (T_S) protein (Table I). However, it is formally possible that the 24 kilodalton peptide is a breakdown product of the 45 kilodalton peptide. This is unlikely, since the ratio between the 45 and 23 kilodalton peptides remains approximately equal and constant throughout the entire period of papain digestion (5–60 min). Moreover, if the peptides resulted from sequential cleavage, the "first" enzymatic cut of the 70 kilodalton protein must result in a 45 kilodalton product that has lost both antigen binding sites and V_H determinants, while a "second" cleavage of the 45 kilodalton protein yields a 23 kilodalton peptide which reexpresses both sites. Nonetheless, definitive evidence that the 45 and 23 kilodalton peptides represent independent regions of the 70 kilodalton parent molecule requires amino acid sequencing or peptide mapping of the three molecules.

Papain digestion of Ig chains produces two fragments, Fc and Fab. The Fab monomer (H chain) has a size of 22 kilodaltons, carries the antigen-binding site, and contains sequences encloded by V_H genes. The Fc fragment has a size of 50 kilodaltons, carries the biologic activity of different classes of immunoglobulins, and is encoded by C genes. Each C gene product displays characteristic "isotypic" determinants and can be serologically defined by antibodies. T sup-

TABLE I

Properties of Two Different Domains of T Suppressor (T_S) Molecules

				Suppression		Serologic reaction	
	MW	PI	Antigen binding	Antigen specific	Nonspecific	αTSF	αFv
Purified T_S	70,000	5.0	++	++	−	+	+
Peptide A	45,000	5.6	−	−	+	+	−
Peptide B	24,000	?	+	−	−	−	+

pressor (T_S) molecules purified from cloned T cells also appear to consist of two functionally distinct domains formed after cleavage by papain: A V region (23 kilodaltons) that binds specifically to antigen but lacks suppressive activity and a second C region (45 kilodaltons) that does not bind antigen but suppresses antibody responses to a variety of antigens. The 45 kilodalton portion of this molecule appears to share serologic determinants with partially purified T_s proteins that are likely to be specific for other antigens (Fresno *et al.*, 1981a). Since these determinants are not detected on proteins synthesized by cloned inducer T cells, they may represent isotypic determinants on T cell molecules that suppress immune responses.

Picogram amounts of a purified monoclonal 70 kilodalton protein suppresses the entire antibody response to a complex cellular antigen (Fresno *et al.*, 1981b,c). The structural properties of this molecule suggest the following mechanism to account for "global" suppression by single T cell molecule: binding of the 70 kilodalton protein to T helper cells that display the correct antigenic determinant is followed by increased sensitivity of the T_s molecule to surface protease on target T helper cells and release of the 45 kilodalton subunit. This subunit suppresses both antigen-specific target T helper cells as well as other Lyt-1 T helper cells which have bound to closely associated determinants displayed by the foreign erythrocyte. The net effect of this reaction is suppression of an immune response to a complex foreign protein by T_s molecules specific for one or several sites on the foreign protein. An important feature of this mechanism is that it ensures efficient regulation of immunity to a large array of foreign molecules by a relatively small number of T_s clones.

REFERENCES

Cantor, H., and Gershon, R. K. (1979). Immunological cell circuits: Cellular composition. *Fed. Proc., Fed. Am. Soc. Exp. Biol.* **38,** 2058.

Edelman, G. M. (1971). Antibody structure and molecular immunology. *Ann. N.Y. Acad. Sci.* **190,** 5.

Fresno, M., McVay-Boudreau, L., and Cantor, H. (1981a). Antigen specific T-lymphocyte clones. III. Papain splits purified T suppressor molecules into two functional domains. (Submitted for publication.)

Fresno, M., Nabel, G., McVay-Boudreau, L., Furthmayer, H., and Cantor, H. (1981b). Antigen specific T lymphocyte clones. I. Characterization of a T lymphocyte clone expressing antigen-specific suppressive activity. *J. Exp. Med.* **153,** 1246.

Fresno, M., McVay-Boudreau, L., Nabel, G., and Cantor, H. (1981c). Antigen specific T lymphocytes clones. II. Purification and biological characterization of an antigen-specific suppressive protein synthesized by cloned T cells. *J. Exp. Med.* **153,** 1260.

Germain, R. N., and Benacerraf, B. (1980). Helper and suppressor T cell factors. *Springer Simin. Immunopathol.* **3,** 93.

Gershon, R. K., Iverson, G. M., Janeway, C. A., Rosenstein, R. W., Cone, R. E., Cantor, H., Fresno, M., Muttingly, J. A., Wigzell, H., Binz, H., Frischnecht, H., and Ptak, W. (1981). *Proc. Natl. Acad. Sci. U.S.A.* (in press).

Nabel, G., Fresno, M., Chessman, A., and Cantor, H. (1981). Use of cloned populations of mouse lymphocytes to analyze cellular differentiation. *Cell* **23,** 19.

Natvig, J. B., and Kunkel, H. G. (1973). Human immunoglobulin: Classes, subclasses, genetic variants, and idiotypes. *Adv. Immunol.* **16,** 1.

Sproviero, J. A., Imperiale, M. J., and Dauderer, M. (1980). Clonal analysis of F_1 hybrid helper T cells restricted to parental or F_1 hybrid major histocompatibility determinants. *J. Exp. Med.* **152,** 920.

Tanaguchi, M., Saito, T., and Tada, T. (1979). Antigen specific suppressor factor produced by a transplantable I-J-bearing T cell hybridoma. *Nature* (*London*) **278,** 555.

VII

Human T Cell Clones

35

Cloning of T Lymphocytes in Man

*Fritz H. Bach/Hartwig Bunzendahl/Siew-Lin Wee/
Jun Iwaki/Miriam Segall*

I. PLT-Reactive Clones 414
II. Cytotoxic (CTL) Clones 417
A. Cytotoxic (Tc) Cloning in Agarose versus Cloning by Limiting Dilution 417
B. Plating Efficiency in Limiting Dilution 418
C. Growth Profile of Cytotoxic Clones 419
D. Functional Specificities of Cloned Cytotoxic Cells 419
E. Cell Surface Phenotype of Cloned Cytotoxic Cells 421
III. Conclusions 422
References 423

The impetus for cloning of human T lymphocytes of different functional subcategories derives not only from the enormous potential offered for increased understanding of T cell reactivities and interactions (true for any species), but also, in the case of man, from the possibility of utilizing cloned, and thus maximally antigen specific, cells for immunotherapy, i.e., to manipulate the immune system of man *in vivo*. Although factors that promote the growth of T lymphocytes *in vitro* have been described for many years, it was the specific description in man and mouse of a T cell growth factor (TCGF)-containing lymphocyte culture supernatant, which would allow ''normal'' peripheral blood lymphocytes (Ruscetti *et al.*, 1977) as well as specifically sensitized cells (Gillis and Smith, 1977; Charmot *et al.*, 1980) to multiply for prolonged periods of time, which led to the recent flurry of activity including the cloning of T lymphocytes in mouse (Gillis and Smith, 1977; Fathman and Hengartner, 1978; Nabholz *et al.*, 1978;) and man (Bach *et al.*, 1979; Goulmy *et al.*, 1980; Kornbluth and Dupont, 1980; Lotze *et al.*, 1980; Malissen *et al.*, 1980; Segall *et al.*, 1980; Inouye *et al.*, 1981).

Our emphasis, in man, has been on obtaining clones that show primed lymphocyte typing (PLT) reactivity (Bach *et al.*, 1979), i.e., following growth in TCGF-containing medium, the cells can be ''washed free'' of TCGF and then

ISOLATION, CHARACTERIZATION, AND
UTILIZATION OF T LYMPHOCYTE CLONES

ISBN 0-12-249920-4

show a proliferative response to the allosensitizing antigens (Bach *et al.*, 1979, 1981; Inouye *et al.*, 1980). In addition, we have attempted to develop methodologies for the generation and maintenance of cytotoxic T lymphocyte (CTL) clones (Bach *et al.*, 1979, 1981; Inouye *et al.*, 1980; Wee *et al.*, 1981). Pertinent to this second category of effort has been both our concern with the definition of HLA encoded determinants recognized by CTL, i.e., the cytotoxicity defined (CD) determinants as potentially being different from those recognized by antisera, as well as the desire to generate cytotoxic cells maximally specific for autologous abnormal cells, such as Epstein-Barr virus transformed lymphoblastoid cell lines (LCLs) (Bunzendahl *et al.*, 1982) or leukemia cells.

It is the purpose of this chapter to discuss some of the immunogenetic and functional aspects of this work. Although PLT-reactive clones have been used primarily for immunogenetic analysis of determinants associated with HLA-D genes, we believe that at least some of the PLT-reactive clones may be helper T lymphocytes (Th) (S. L. Wee and F. H. Bach, in preparation).

In many experiments, we have attempted to grow human T lymphocytes under conditions such that the probability of having progeny of two or more cells included in a given population is >0.05. We shall utilize the word "colony" when we discuss cell populations obtained in such cases or following picking colonies from agarose, where quantitative statements about the probability of having a clone are difficult. The word "clone" is reserved for populations where Poisson statistics predict a likelihood of clonality of >95%.

I. PLT-REACTIVE CLONES

Primed lymphocyte typing-reactive clones proliferate when stimulated with the sensitizing alloantigen in the absence of exogenous TCGF. For the most part it would appear that such clones recognize determinants controlled by HLA-D region (Inouye *et al.*, 1981), analogous to the proliferative response elicited by these determinants in primary MLC and bulk PLT reagents (Sheehy *et al.*, 1975). PLT-reactive clones (or colonies) can be expanded to yield very large numbers of cells indeed; utilizing as feeder cells LCL from the donor of the clonal population or the initial sensitizing cells, it would be possible to obtain in excess of 1×10^{10} cells per clone or colony had all the cells been left in culture for continued growth for 7 to 8 weeks (Hank *et al.*, 1980). More recently, T lymphocytes expanded in TCGF and irradiated prior to use have also been used as feeder cells. Clones give highly reproducible patterns of reactivity when tested against a given panel for the first 7 weeks; we have performed relatively few experiments beyond that time period.

Technically, it is possible, with only 1250 or 2500 responding cells of a PLT-reactive colony or clone, to obtain highly significant proliferative responses

TABLE I

Responses of PLT-Reactive Colonies[a]

			Restimulating cells							
Colonies	R[b]	S[c]	2	3	4	5	6	7	8	9
1. 2-23(5)	160	29,158	133	144	462	596	206	160	512	166
2. 2-11(5)	342	5,872	1,520	296	470	259	3,342	562	288	246
3. 1-26(50)	212	4,890	3,384	922	446	637	632	468	162	100
4. 1-29(50)	312	178,552	7,148	606	14,450	649	1,450	1,206	442	9,022
5. 3-75(5)	902	117,514	144,798	326	252	705	14,820	764	22,158	484
6. 2-4(0.5)	284	66,898	73,196	1,792	2,926	5,463	5,358	428	230	204
7. 1-37(50)	564	147,996	154,444	2,016	698	644	104,136	906	290	414
8. 4-7(5)	100	133	552	154	238	35,294	226	902	100	150

[a] Counts per minute.
[b] R, original responding cell.
[c] S, original sensitizing cell.

as assayed by labeling with radioactive thymidine from 40 to 48 hr after restimulation. Examples of this type of data are presented in Table I.

It should be noted that in many cases control responses, i.e., restimulation with autologous X-irradiated cells, are in the range of 300–500 cpm, where specific restimulation with the allosensitizing cells can be in excess of 150,000 cpm. To interpret these data, it is essential to recognize that these are all colonies; the number within parentheses following designation of each colony indicates the number of cells plated per well initially. Even with an average of 0.5 cells/well, we probably are dealing with a colony rather than a clone. Differential responses to different restimulating cells can thus be attributed to the presence of more than a single clone in the PLT responding population. Colonies 1 and 2, seeded at 5 cells/well initially, gave relatively specific responses; colony number 1 responded only to the initial sensitizing cell and colony number 2 responded significantly to two other stimulating cells. Colony number 3, initially seeded at 50 cells/well, shows a similar pattern except that the magnitude of the response to several of the restimulating cells is significantly lower than 3000–5000 cpm, which is clearly positive, but significantly greater (range 623–922) than the response to autologous stimulating cells (212 cpm); these values are difficult to interpret. In a quantitative sense, responses of colonies 4 and 5, seeded at 50 and 5 cells/well, respectively, give a different pattern of response in terms of those cells of the panel which led to restimulation. However, the initial sensitizing cell produced strong stimulation, and highly significant but clearly intermediate responses were observed with other stimulating cells. Similar results were observed with colonies 6 and 7 which demonstrate highly significant responses against restimulating cells 1 and 2 in one case, and 1, 2, and 6 in the other case; colony 6, in addition, shows some intermediate values of restimulation. Colony number 8 shows a phenomenon seen in a few instances; there is a reproducibly high response to a stimulating cell from the panel but no significant response to the initial sensitizing cell.

It should be noted that what we have referred to as intermediate responses in colonies such as 4, 5, 6, and possibly 7 (responses to the initial sensitizing cell varying from 66,898 to 178,522 cpm) might not be recognized as being above background with colonies such as numbers 2 and 3 if the level of response to the various stimulating cells remains proportional to the maximum restimulation. It is not known to what extent these different levels of response are due to the presence of several clones in the responding cell population, or to (i) different

TABLE II

Patterns of PLT Reactivity in Colonies

	DR	D	SB	1	2	3	4	5	6	7[a]
1	8?	9	4	+	–	–	–	–	–	+
2	1,4	1,10	ND	+	–	–	–	–	–	ND
3	1,4	1,4	ND	+	–	–	–	–	–	+
4	4	4,—	4	+	–	–	–	–	–	+
5	6,4	6	2,3	+	+	+	+	ND	ND	+
6	1,6	1,6	2,3	+	+	+	+	–	–	+
7	3,—	3,—	2	+	+	+	+	+	+	+
8	4	4,40	2	–	+	+	+	+	–	+
9	4,7	4,7	2	–	+	+	+	–	–	+
10	1,4	1,—	ND	–	+	+	+	ND	ND	ND
11	1,7	1,7	2,3	–	+	+	+	+	+	+
12	4,—	4,—	2,4	–	+	+	+	ND	ND	+
13	1,2	1,2	2,4	–	+	+	+	–	–	+
14	2,4	2,—	ND	–	+	+	+	+	–	ND
15	6	6,—	2,4	–	+	+	+	+	–	+
16	4,7	4,7	2,4	–	+	+	+	+	+	±
17	1,7	1,7	2,4	–	+	+	+	+	+	+
18	1,4	1,4	2,4	–	+	+	+	ND	ND	+
19	1,4	1,40	2,4	–	+	+	+	±	–	+
20	2,7	2,7	2,4	–	+	+	+	+	+	+
21	2	2	ND	ND	ND	ND	ND	ND	ND	ND
22	2,3	2,3	2,4	ND	ND	ND	ND	ND	ND	+
23	7,4	7,40	4±	–	–	–	–	–	–	+
24	3,8	3,8	4	–	–	–	–	+	+	–
25	2,5	2,5	ND	–	–	–	–	+	+	±
26	3,6	3,—	4±	–	–	–	–	+	+	ND
27	1,2	1,2	4	–	–	–	–	–	–	–

[a] Bulk PLT reagent.

densities of the same antigenic determinant on different allogeneic cells or (ii) recognition of cross-reactive antigenic determinants with which the receptor of the PLT-reactive cell combines with different affinities.

The cloning of PLT cells has allowed the beginning of a fine structure analysis of the HLA-D region with the "splitting" of the antigenic clusters defined with homozygous typing cells (HTC) as well as the definition of new determinants not definable with presently available antisera or groups of HTC. The extent of dissection of HLA-D region encoded determinants that can be detected currently with cloned PLT-reactive cells is illustrated in Table II. In this experiment, the priming bulk MLC was prepared using cells from two family members who shared one haplotype and were identical (serologically and with HTC) for their HLA-DR and HLA-D antigens of the second haplotype as responding and sensitizing cells, respectively. The reactivity of a series of different clones is presented in Table II. It was known, based on previous typing with bulk PLT reagents, that the stimulating cells carried the SB-2 antigen (Shaw *et al.*, 1980) and the responding cells did not. Several clones were obtained that responded to SB-2-positive cells and not to cells lacking SB-2. In addition, however, other clones were obtained whose reactivity was not associated with the presence of SB-2 on the restimulating cells. Findings such as these illustrate that cloning of PLT reactive cells makes it possible to define determinants other than those can be distinguished with serology (DR), homozygous typing cells (Dw), and bulk PLT reagents (e.g., SB).

II. CYTOTOXIC (CTL) CLONES

A. Cytotoxic (Tc) Cloning in Agarose versus Cloning by Limiting Dilution

After initial sensitization in MLC to allogeneic cells, we have derived CTL clones reactive both to alloantigens (Bach *et al.*, 1979; Wee *et al.*, 1981) and to autologous Epstein-Barr virus-transformed, lymphoblastoid cell lines (LCL) (Bunzendahl *et al.*, 1982). Clones with both types of reactivity can be derived either by initially plating either bulk sensitized or isolated blasts in agarose or initially plating day 4 or day 5 blasts in limiting dilution (LD).

Although we have not performed extensive experiments attempting to compare the two methods of cloning, the results we have obtained indicate that the cloning efficiency for CTL is higher in agarose than in LD. Shown in Table III is an experiment where cells to be cloned were sensitized to a pool of stimulating cells from 20 allogeneic donors used as stimulators; blasts were separated on day 4 of the priming MLC and plated either in agarose or into wells of a microtiter plate. The cultures were picked on day 7 after plating, grown for an additional week

TABLE III

Frequency of CTL Colonies after Allostimulation

Cloning in agarose			Cloning in limiting dilution		
	No. of clones	Percent		No. of clones	Percent
0.5– 5%	21	21.8	0.5– 5%	102	30.4
5.1–10%	42	43.8	5.1–10%	68	20.2
>10%	26	27.1	>10%	30	8.9
Neg.	7	7.3	Neg.	136	40.5
Total	96		Total	336	

in microwells, and tested for their cytolytic capacity against the autologous LCL. Of those colonies derived from agarose, 43.7% produced lysis between 5.1 and 10%, and 21.1% at greater than 10%. In contrast, of the colonies derived by limiting dilution, 20.2% gave between 5.1% and 10% lysis, and only 8.9% gave greater than 10% lysis. Further, only 7.3% of colonies from agarose did not give significant lysis, whereas 40.5% of those colonies derived from plating in limiting dilution were negative in cytotoxicity.

From these and similar results, we tentatively suggest that both the agarose and the limiting dilution methods are capable of yielding cytotoxic populations that can lyse both allogeneic targets and autologous abnormal cells, such as an LCL. Further, plating in agarose may yield a higher percentage of cytotoxic colonies (based on the total number of growing colonies) with a higher lytic efficiency, as compared with colonies obtained from limiting dilution.

B. Plating Efficiency in Limiting Dilution

We have performed more than 15 different experiments in which day 4 blasts have been isolated from an MLC and plated at 0.2 cells/well with 5×10^3 X-irradiated "pooled allogeneic feeders" per well and TCGF obtained from spleen. Under these conditions, cloning efficiency has been 15–25%. We have performed only three experiments in which "unseparated" day 4 MLC cells were seeded directly into the wells of microtiter plates at an average density of 1 cell per well. Under these conditions, 3–7% of the wells yielded proliferating cells.

In contrast, a wide range of plating efficiencies has been noted when blasts that have been grown for various periods of time as bulk cultures in TCGF-containing medium are plated under limiting dilution conditions. Between 10 and 50% of wells yielded proliferating cells when plating was carried out at an average density of 1 cell/well. It is not clear whether this variation is related to the age of the bulk culture being propagated in the TCGF-containing medium or to other factors.

C. Growth Profile of Cytotoxic Clones

Using the cloning technique described above for the generation of T cell clones from *in vitro* sensitized primary or secondary bulk cultures, we have observed a marked difference in growth potential between the antigen-reactive (PLT) clones and the cytotoxic clones in most experiments. Fast-growing clones are almost always antigen reactive and noncytotoxic. These clones double every 24 hr or less and can be expanded to large numbers in flask cultures. In contrast, the majority of cytotoxic clones show very slow growth. At about 15 days after primary sensitization, they double every 48 hr or more, and slowly decline in growth rate until, by the end of a month, many clones only double every 3–4 days. At about this time, a great number of them are lost, while the surviving few appear to grow better only with more frequent changes of medium and addition of fresh feeder cells. Whereas, PLT clones need be fed no more than once every 6–7 days, the cytotoxic clones are maintained by periodic medium change every other day and with addition of fresh feeder cells every third day.

Some CTL clones and colonies derived from allosensitized, day 4 blast populations show growth characteristics more similar to those of PLT-reactive clones and can be propagated for more than 60 days. One colony, plated at a density of 0.2 cells/well, was studied quantitatively starting on day 12, at which time an estimated 1×10^4 cells were present in the colony. Based on this initial cell number estimate, on day 15 there were 5×10^4 cells, which were replated at 2.5×10^4 cells/well in cluster wells. Twelve days later, on day 27, there were slightly more than 6×10^5 cells in the cluster wells; these cells were replated at 2×10^5 cells/well, and their growth assayed on later days. Cells were frozen at various times to compare growth characteristics of frozen and thawed cells with cells continuously propagated. The frozen cells, plated after thawing, grew at a rate not significantly different from cells maintained continuously in culture.

We interpret these data to indicate that the rate of cell growth during at least the first 45–50 days of culture is approximately the same. Subsequently, growth slows, although cytotoxic activity is maintained, until approximately 65–67 days following initiation of culture, at which time the cells of this colony could no longer be propagated under the conditions used. Surviving and rapidly dividing colonies appear usually to retain their cytolytic potential, although the extent of lysis may vary considerably.

D. Functional Specificities of Cloned Cytotoxic Cells

We have previously generated CTL colonies in agarose and tested them against a panel of target cells which shared none, one, or more of the sensitizing

TABLE IV

Cytolytic Specificity of Alloactivated Colonies[a]

			Percent lysis against ^{51}Cr-labeled targets							
			Autol. RG	Specific NO	DD	GP	DS	KB	KJ	SO
Colony number	Test[b]	E/T ratio	— —	A3,B7 DR1,2	A3,B7 DR1[c]	A3,B7 —	B7 DR1	A3 DR1,2	— DR1,2	— —
S73	1	ND[j]	3 S.D.[d]	49	40	35	29	(−1)	(0)	(−3)
	2	10:1	NT[e]	NT	36	NT	24	(5)	(5)	NT
		1:1	(0)[f]	NT	10	20	9	(7)	(4)	(0)
		0.1:1	(2)	NT	(4)	11	(3)	(−2)	(2)	(−4)
S94	1	ND	3 S.D.	17	12	7	(1)	6	(5)	(−3)
	2	10:1	(1)	NT	18	12	(−1)	11	(3)	(2)
		1:1	(0)	NT	6	10	(0)	(7)	(4)	(−3)
		0.1:1	(2)	NT	(0)	(2)	(1)	(7)	(0)	(1)
S93	1	ND	3 S.D.	52	34	32	(−2)	25	30	(−1)
	2	ND	(−3)	NT	40	27	(0)	29	34	(4)
S19	1	ND	3 S.D.	53	18	17	(2)	9	(4)	11
	2	ND	(4)	NT	8	16	(2)	10	(2)	NT
S80	1	ND	3 S.D.	40	23	26	19	(1)	49	(1)
	2	ND	(0)	NT	21	36	18	(5)	10	(2)
S45	1	ND	3 S.D.	45	23	16	(4)	(−2)	(−1)	(−1)
S27	1	ND	3 S.D.	28	(−3)	(4)	(5)	(−1)	(−4)	(−1)
S78	1	ND	3 S.D.	40	25	31	30	18	(0)	(−2)
Test 1		SR[g] (cpm)	212	120	185	131	174	129	113	107
			±30	±11	±29	±18	±19	±14	±13	±14
		MR[h] (cpm)	NT	750	1531	1258	1109	1148	748	584
			NT	±66	±196	±154	±90	±153	±111	±18
		MPR[i] (%)	NT	5	7	5	6	4	6	9
Test 2		SR (cpm)	140	NT	203	134	252	160	133	103
			±20	NT	±24	±12	±37	±25	±17	±11
		MR (cpm)	1112	NT	1423	694	1822	1116	1130	700
			±154	NT	±365	±82	±217	±140	±172	±174
		MPR (%)	6	NT	6	7	7	8	5	6

[a] HLA types of donors: RG(A1,A2,B14,B21,C(blank),DR7); NO(A3,B7,C(blank),DR1,DR2); DD(A1,A3, B7,B8,C(blank),DR1,DR4); GP(A28,A3,B7,C(blank),DR7); DS(A28,A32,B7,B27,C1,DR1,DR7); KB(A3, A25,B18,B35,C4,DR1,DR2); KJ(A10,A11,B18,B12,C(blank),DR2); SO(A2,A24,B51,B15,C3,DR4,DR5). Adapted from Wee *et al.* (1981). Copyright Elsevier North-Holland.

[b] Test 1, assayed on day 14 following initiation of MLC; test 2, assayed on day 18 following initiation of MLC.

[c] HLA antigens given are those shared with sensitizing cell NO.

[d] ^{51}Cr release 3 S.D. above mean SR.

[e] NT, not tested.

[f] Percent lysis is MPR on the given target.

[g] SR, spontaneous release.

[h] MR, maximum release.

[i] MPR, minimum positive response, calculated as: [3 S.D. above mean SR − (MR − SR)] × 100.

[j] ND, not determined.

TABLE V

Lysis of the Autologous LCL and Allogeneic Cells after Allosensitization

	Lysis on targets (%)			
Clone	Autologous LCL	Autologous normal PBL	Allogeneic LCL	Allogeneic LCL
1	78.1	4.6	9.4	93.9
2	8.3	4.9	75.4	25.2

antigens. An example of the reactivity patterns is shown in Table IV. These results show that cloned CTL populations exhibit more specific lytic patterns than observed normally with bulk cultures. These patterns correlate with specific HLA-A or HLA-B class I antigens. The results also suggest that, in some instances, the determinants recognized by the CTL populations may differ from those recognized by alloantisera.

Following allosensitization *in vitro,* we also have isolated clones that are lytic not only to certain allogeneic cells but also to the autologous lymphoblastoid cell line (LCL) used as a target (Bunzendahl *et al.,* 1982). One example of such a clone (clone 1) is given in Table V. This clone is highly lytic to the autologous LCL (78.1% lysis at an effector–target ratio of 25 : 1), does not lyse autologous normal peripheral blood lymphocytes, and lyses one of two allogeneic LCL targets showing little or no lysis on the other allogeneic LCL target. Data from a second clone are included to illustrate that certain clones show very little if any lysis on either the autologous LCL or the autologous normal peripheral blood lymphocytes used as targets but do lyse allogeneic targets. The data presented in Table V demonstrate that these clones have specificity associated with CTL function.

E. Cell Surface Phenotype of Cloned Cytotoxic Cells

Monoclonal antibodies produced in mice and directed at human lymphocyte cell surface antigens have proved useful in differentiating functional subcategories of these cells. The general correlation seen, using the OKT antibodies (Zarling *et al.,* 1981), has been that helper (amplifier) T cells are $OKT4^+$, $OKT8^-$ and cytotoxic/suppressor T cells are $OKT4^-$, $OKT8^+$. Our own results studying the OKT phenotype of cells present on day 6 or 7 of a primary MLC have been consistent with these rules; essentially all cytotoxic activity directed at either the allosensitizing target or an autologous LCL target can be ablated by treatment with OKT8 antiserum plus complement.

The CTL clones that were derived after sensitization to alloantigens and subsequently found to be lytic not only to the allosensitizing target but also to the autologous LCL were OKT3$^+$, OKT4$^+$, OKT8$^-$, and OKT9$^\pm$. Of a total of 12 clones tested, eight have failed to show any evidence of the presence of OKT8 antigen by FACS analysis; the remaining four have shown a very low level presence of the OKT8 antigen as compared with the high level expressed by a given percentage of the cells obtained on day 6 of a primary MLC and grown in TCGF for an additional 4 days.

The results we have obtained to date do not allow us to differentiate among three possible explanations for this finding: First, it is possible that there is loss of OKT antigen expression; cells from which the CTL clones are derived may have been OKT4$^+$, OKT8$^+$ initially and during the cloning procedure have lost OKT8 expression. Second, may be that the cloned OKT4$^+$, OKT8$^-$ cells were derived from a very small subpopulation of precursor CTL which carry that phenotype. Third, it is possible that there is a change in the OKT phenotype of the cytotoxic cells; cells could "start out" on day 4 (when the MLC blasts are separated and plated in limiting dilution) as OKT4$^-$, OKT8$^+$ and, subsequently, during the cloning procedure changed to an OKT4$^+$, OKT8$^-$ phenotype.

In mouse, CTL directed at CD determinants on class II antigens, specifically of the *I-A* subregion, are Lyt-1$^+$, 2$^-$ (Swain, 1981) in contrast to class I directed CTL that are Lyt-1$^+$, 2$^+$ or Lyt-1$^-$, 2$^+$. To the extent that we can extrapolate from the Lyt phenotype in mouse to the OKT phenotype in man, it may be that OKT4$^+$, OKT8$^-$ CTL are ones directed at CD specificities on class II molecules. Further studies will be needed to resolve these various issues.

III. CONCLUSIONS

It is clear from our results that it is possible to clone at least two major functional subcategories of T lymphocytes: PLT-reactive cells (that are, at least in some cases, helper T lymphocytes) and cytotoxic T lymphocytes. Whether, in man, we have achieved cloning of what are functionally different subpopulations of CTL, as has been observed in mouse (see Parts V and VI in this treatise; Widmer and Bach, 1981) has yet to be evaluated.

The PLT-reactive clones and colonies have allowed a dissection of the HLA-D complex that has been impossible to obtain with the currently available reagents including sera, homozygous typing cells, or bulk PLT reagents. Such a dissection has potential applicability and relevance to transplantation and to studies concerned with association of histocompatibility antigens with particular disease states. Specifically, it allows the definition of series of antigenic determinants that are homologous with the various loci that have been defined genetically and functionally in mouse.

The availability of cloned CTL will allow the types of dissection that we have attempted previously (Wee *et al.*, 1981) to evaluate whether there is a separate determinant polymorphism for those epitopes recognized by CTL as opposed to those recognized serologically. Once again, such findings are important not only to transplantation and disease association studies but to other areas on which MHC immunogeneic impacts.

These studies in man have one other application which may be of the greatest importance, i.e., the adoptive transfer of cells reactive with specific antigens. In this context, it is essential to keep in mind that not only is immunotherapy of tumors involved but also the possible manipulation of the immune system in other diseases. It is especially important to recognize that helper T lymphocytes, or perhaps other T lymphocytes yet to be cloned and adequately characterized functionally, may be able to provide greater insights into antigen-specific delayed-type hypersensitivity reactions that play major roles in a variety of disease states.

ACKNOWLEDGMENTS

This work was supported by NIH Grants AI/GM 17687, AI 18326, CA 27826, and AI 15486 and March of Dimes Grant 6-255. Hartwig Bunzendahl was supported by the Deutsche Forschungsgemeinschaft. This is manuscript 276 from the Immunobiology Research Center, University of Minnesota, Minneapolis.

REFERENCES

Bach, F. H., Inouye, H., Hank, J. A., and Alter, B. J. (1979). Human T lymphocyte clones reactive in primed lymphocyte typing and cytotoxicity. *Nature (London)* **281,** 307.

Bach, F. H., Alter, B. J., Widmer, M. B., Segall, M. S., and Dunlap, B. (1981). Cloned cytotoxic and non-cytotoxic lymphocytes in mouse and man: Their reactivities and a large cell surface membrane protein (LMP) differentiation marker system. *Immunol. Rev.* **54,** 5.

Bunzendahl, H., and Bach, F. H., (1982). Submitted for publication.

Charmot, D., Malissen, B., Ghiotto, M., and Mawas, C. (1980). Expansion of human lymphocyte populations expressing specific immune reactivities. II. A comparison of immune reactivities in human T lymphocyte lines derived from allogeneically primed cultures and maintained with lectins or conditioned medium. *Tissue Antigens* **15,** 297.

Fathman, C. G., and Hengartner, H. (1978). Clones of allo-reactive T cells. *Nature (London)* **272,** 617.

Gillis, S., and Smith, K. A. (1977). Long-term culture of tumour-specific cytotoxic T cells. *Nature (London)* **268,** 154.

Goulmy, E., Blockland, E., van Rood, J. J., Charmot, D., Malissen, B., and Mawas, C. (1980). Production, expansion and clonal analysis of T cells with specific HLA restricted male lysis. *J. Exp. Med.* **152,** 182s.

Hank, J. A., Inouye, H., Guy, L. A., Alter, B. H., and Bach, F. H. (1980). Long term maintenance of "cloned" human PLT cells in TCGF with LCL cells as a feeder layer. *J. Supramol. Struct.* **13,** 525.

Inouye, H., Hank, J. A., Chardonnens, X., Segall, M., Alter, B. J., and Bach, F. H. (1980). Cloned PLT reagents in the dissection of HLA-D. *J. Exp. Med.* **152,** 143s.

Inouye, H., Hank, J., Chardonnens, X., Alter, B. J., Reinsmoen, N. L., Segall, M., and Bach, F. H. (1981). Cloned human T lymphocytes in PLT analysis of the HLA-D complex. *Transplant. Proc.* **9,** 1030.

Kornbluth, J., and Dupont, B. (1980). Cloning and functional characterization of primary alloreactive human T lymphocytes. *J. Exp. Med.* **152,** 164s.

Lotze, M. T., Strausser, J. L., and Rosenberg, S. A. (1980). *In vitro* growth of cytotoxic human lymphocytes. II. Use of T cell growth factor (TCGF) to clone human T cells. *J. Immunol.* **124,** 2972.

Malissen, B., Charmot, D., Goulmy, E., Blockland, E., Liabeuf, A., Goridis, T. C., Mawas, C., and Kourilsky, F. M. (1980). Alloreactive monofunctional human T cell clones expressing cytotoxic or primed lymphocyte typing reactivity as well as restricted immunogenetic specificity. *In* "New Trends in Human Immunology and Cancer Immunity" (B. Serrou and C. Rosenfeld, eds.), p. 138. Doin, Paris.

Nabholz, M., Engers, H. D., Collavo, D., and North, M. (1978). Cloned T-cell lines with specific cytolytic activity. *Curr. Top. Microbiol. Immunol.* **81,** 176.

Ruscetti, F. W., Morgan, D. A., and Gallo, R. C. (1977). Functional and morphologic characterization of human T cells continuously grown *in vitro*. *J. Immunol.* **119,** 131.

Segall, M., Reinsmoen, N. L., Noreen, H. J., and Bach, F. H. (1980). Complexity of the HLA-D region studied by primed lymphocyte test. *J. Exp. Med.* **152,** 156s.

Shaw, S., Johnson, A. H., and Shearer, G. M. (1980). Evidence for a new segregant series of B cell antigens that are encoded in the HLA-D region and that stimulate secondary allogeneic proliferative and cytotoxic responses. *J. Exp. Med.* **152,** 565.

Sheehy, M. J., Sondel, P. M., Bach, M. L., Wank, R., and Bach, F. H. (1975). HL-A LD (lymphocyte defined) typing: a rapid assay with primed lymphocytes. *Science* **188,** 1308.

Swain, S. L. (1981). Significance of class I and class II major histocompatibility complex antigens: Help to allogeneic K and D antigen does not involve I recognition. *J. Immunol.* **126,** 2307.

Wee, S. L., Wu, S., Alter, B. J., and Bach, F. H. (1981). Early detection and specificity analysis of human cytolytic T lymphocyte (CTL) colonies generated in soft agarose culture: A potential assay for definition of CTL defined (CD) determinants. *Hum. Immunol.* **3,** 45.

Widmer, M. B., and Bach, F. H. (1981). Antigen-driven helper cell-independent cloned cytolytic T lymphocytes. *Nature (London)* **294,** 750.

Zarling, J. M., Bach, F. H., and Kung, P. C. (1981). Sensitization of lymphocytes against pooled allogeneic cells. II. Characterization of effector cells cytotoxic for autologous lymphoblastoid cell lines. *J. Immunol.* **126,** 375.

36

Human T Cell Clones: Function, Specificity, and Cell Surface Markers

Bernard Malissen/Claude Mawas

I. T Cell Clones Obtained Following Sensitization *in Vitro* 426
A. MLC-Derived T Cell Clones 426
B. Soluble Antigen-Specific T Cell Clones 429
II. T Cell Clones following *in Vivo* Immunization 430
A. MHC Restricted Anti-H-Y Cytotoxic Clones 430
B. MHC Specificity of Alloreactive Cytotoxic T Cell Clones Derived from Recipients Immunized *in Vivo* 431
III. Surface Markers of Human T Cell Clones: Monoclonal Antibodies (mAB) Interacting with the Cytolytic Function 433
IV. Conclusions 435
References 435

The discovery by P. C. Nowell (1960) that lymphoid cells stimulated by phytohemagglutin (PHA) would undergo division and blastic transformation was the first demonstration that human lymphoid cells could be grown in culture. The subsequent development of tissue culture conditions appropriate for the growth of lymphoid tissue *in vitro* has been a key to the study and understanding of the role of subsets of human T cells. By 1964, mixed leukocyte culture (MLC) had been discovered (Bain *et al.*, 1964; Bach and Hirschhorn, 1964) leading to a revolution among cell biologists interested in studying the functions of cultured lymphoid cells. MLC and cell-mediated lympholysis (CML) became tools which provided insight into complex immune reactions. Specific proliferation to soluble antigens (Bergholtz and Thorsby, 1977), one way MLC (Bach and Voynow, 1966), CML assays (Häyry and Defendi, 1970; Solliday and Bach, 1970), secondary MLC (Sheehy *et al.*, 1975), and cytotoxic T lymphocyte (CTL) responses (Charmot *et al.*, 1975) became standard assays to study the relationships between MHC products and *in vitro* phenomenology.

As described in the preceding chapters, Morgan *et al.* (1976) and Ruscetti *et al.* (1977) reported that factors present in "conditioned medium" (CM) could

ISOLATION, CHARACTERIZATION, AND
UTILIZATION OF T LYMPHOCYTE CLONES

ISBN 0-12-249920-4

support the growth of T cells and maintain two main functions expressed *in vitro*, i.e., specific proliferation (Pappas *et al.*, 1979; Charmot *et al.*, 1980) or cytotoxicity (Bonnard *et al.*, 1978; Gillis *et al.*, 1978; Strausser and Rosenberg, 1978). This technology allowed the isolation of functional T cell clones either through soft agar cloning or through limiting dilution (LD) using conditioned medium as promoter of T cell growth.

I. T CELL CLONES OBTAINED FOLLOWING SENSITIZATION *IN VITRO*

A. MLC-Derived T Cell Clones

Following a one way MLC, *in vitro* assays can measure the level of lysis by specific cytotoxic T cells against their relevant target antigens as well as the proliferation of T cells specific for the D/DR antigens of the priming cells. Helper/inducer activities or suppressor activities also can be qualified through *in vitro* assays, but they are far less reproducible than the assays mentioned above. The direct relationship between a complex population of T cells and any given function has primarily been studied through T cell surface markers (for review, see Chess and Schlossman, 1977; Reinherz and Schlossman, 1980). Similarly the technology of cloning has allowed characterization of T cell subsets involved in cooperation or effector functions.

Following a primary MLC, with or without a secondary specific stimulation, limiting dilutions of MLC cells are plated in microtiter wells containing 5×10^4 γ-irradiated (4000 R) PBL, autologous to the responder population of lymphocytes. Growth promotion is obtained through a T cell lectin stimulation (leukoagglutinin, 1 μg/ml), thought to act upon the irradiated feeder (PBL) which then locally produces the right proportion of the required interleukins (Malissen *et al.*, 1981a). Ten to fifteen days later, colony growth was visually inspected in all microwells, and sizable colonies are then transferred to cluster plate wells. Further expansion is obtained using either conditioned supernatant or lectin and irradiated PBL as feeders. As soon as sufficient cell numbers have been obtained, each growing colony is screened for its cytotoxic or proliferative function. In most instances, if cloning occurs a few days following the secondary boost (10 to 14 days primary culture), many more proliferating (PLT) than cytotoxic (CTL) clones are found.

1. *Cytotoxic Clones*

Such clones are derived from primary growing colonies shown to specifically lyse targets autologous to the priming cells but not to the responder cells. Further expansion allows testing of a panel of target cells, including unrelated individuals and family members to study MHC segregation as well as the fine target specificity. As far as the CTL clones themselves are concerned, their specificity is usually clearly related to known serologically defined class I HLA specificities, but often the clones show cross-reactions between serologically well-defined HLA alleles (Malissen *et al.*, 1981a). CTL clones in general are highly lytic, and in most instances at an effector to target (E/T) ratio of 1 to 1, specific ^{51}Cr release is still well above 30%.

Growth and expansion of CTL clones depends upon the quality of the batch of CM used. We found that the most reproducible secure long-term growth schedule was obtained by using serial two 4-day cycles of CM alone followed by a 3–4 day passage on irradiated PBL in the presence of lectin. Such clones are absolutely dependent for their growth upon extrinsic or intrinsic CM (as provided by lectin stimulated irradiated PBL): they do not proliferate in the presence of their specific target cells. The specificity of the killing remains stable, but most CTL clones derived *in vitro* tend to lose their killing activity.

2. *HLA-D Region Specific Proliferative Clones or PLT Clones*

Due to the technical ease of the primed lymphocyte assay (PLT), many clones can simultaneously be analyzed and compared to the proliferative pattern of the original primed population; the reactivity pattern of each clone can then be related to the known HLA-D/DRw alleles of the stimulator cells. In Table I, we have analyzed some clones obtained from an unrelated MLC: individual Fue. is the responder (HLA-D/DRw: 6 and 8) and the stimultor is Chap. (HLA-D/DRw 1 and 7). To analyze the specificity as well as the haplotype segregation, only family members were chosen for the assay. Although PLT clones were expected to correlate either with DR1 or DR7, most of the clones tested were essentially correlated with DR7; this has been a consistent finding. At the population level, this combination was restimulated strongly by DR7 cells and weakly by DR1 cells. Therefore, the outcome of the cloning could be a genuine reflection of the clonal size involved in the primary response in this combination. The correlation with DR7 was variable: some clones reacted strongly against the stimulator but only reacted with some of the DR7 (C22.1); others were strongly correlated with DR7 as C22.2 and C22.9; yet others showed cross-reactivity with DR5 or 4 (C1.26). Such patterns of reactivity are consistent with the recently proposed model of the HLA-D region, consisting of at least two regions and coding for at least four allospecificities per haplotype (Charmot *et al.*, 1981).

An example of a so-called "wild" clone C1.30 is apparent in Table I: although clone C1.30 was initially found to be negative on the specific stimulator cell (Chap.), this clone was found to segregate with a given HLA haplotype when tested against family members: d, in family Schr. (DR2); d, in family Fr. although weakly (also DR2), and a in family Del. (also DR2). The most likely interpretation at this point is transtimulation during the primary MLC and isolation of an anti-DR2 clone during the cloning procedure.

The recent demonstration of a new segregant series of DR-like antigens separable through recombination (Shaw *et al.*, 1981) or DR-loss variants (Kavathas *et al.*, 1981) should allow the use of PLT clones to isolate reagents specific for products of different loci within the classical D region. Preliminary data from

TABLE I

Proliferative Responses of Five PLT Clones Derived from Secondary MLC (Fue.Chap$_2$) to Members of Several HLA-DR Typed Families

			Thymidine incorporation (cpm × 10^{-3}) PLT clones[a]				
Stimulators[b]		HLA-DR	C22.1	C22.2	C22.9	C1.26	C1.30
Fue.		6/8	0.3	0.1	0.4		0.09
Chap.		1/7	*30.4*	*30.4*	*31.2*	*16.6*	0.3
Family Fr.	a/b	–/7	*9.7*	*17.6*	*32.4*	*12.6*	0.07
	c/d	1/2	1.1	0.3	0.1	0.5	*1.8*
	a/c	–/1	1.5	0.1	0.3	1.0	0.03
	a/d	–/2	0.6	0.4	4.6	0.1	1.2
	b/c	7/1	*2.2*	*11.4*	*15.5*	*10.7*	0.6
Family Var.	a/b	7/2	2.7	*6.3*	*9.9*	NT	NT
	c/d	–/1	0.3	0.2	0.6	NT	NT
	a/c	7/–	1.3	*19.4*	*28.2*	NT	NT
	a/d	7/1	2.6	*11.9*	*24.0*	NT	NT
	b/d	2/1	2.4	0.7	0.6	NT	NT
Family Schr.	a/b	6/1	3.1	1.5	0.6	1.0	0.8
	c/d	1/2	1.9	0.2	1.3	1.2	*4.4*
	a/c	6/1	NT[c]	NT	NT	0.2	0.05
	a/d	6/2	NT	NT	NT	0.4	*4.0*
	b/d	1/2	NT	NT	NT	0.5	*3.9*
	b/c	1/1	NT	NT	NT	1.0	0.1
Family Fich.	a/b	5/4	NT	NT	NT	*12.8*	1.1
	c/d	5/7	NT	NT	NT	*8.3*	0.3
Family May.	a/b	1/6	NT	NT	NT	1.1	0.9
	c/d	4/6	NT	NT	NT	1.2	0.3
Family Del.	a/b	2/7	NT	NT	NT	*13.8*	*1.8*
	c/d	1/5	NT	NT	NT	*10.5*	0.3

[a] 1 × 10^4 responding cells from clones C22.1, C22.2, C22.9, C1.26, and C1.30 were restimulated by 1 × 10^5 irradiated cells from members of different families. Data for ^{3}H-TdR incorporation are mean cpm × 10^{-3} after 48-hr cultures. Italic values represent significant stimulation.

[b] See text for explanation of stimulators.

[c] NT, not tested.

N. L. Reinsmoen (personal communication), P. Wernet (personal communication), and D. Charmot (unpublished data) are very promising, indicating the isolation of clones specific for SB1 and SB4. Cloning PLT combinations should also allow definition of hybrid specificities (See Chapter 26 by Beck and Fathman), either through trans complementation or even cis complementation using the few recombinant families between D/DR and SB loci (Mawas *et al.*, 1980).

B. Soluble Antigen-Specific T Cell Clones

Most human T cell populations are reactive *in vitro* to a wide variety of soluble antigens, either because humans have been immunized against naturally occurring antigens (streptolysin, streptodornase, etc.) or through vaccination [tetanus toxoid, tuberlin purified protein derivative (PPD) etc.]. This reaction is clearly monocyte dependent as well as HLA-D/DR restricted (Sønderstrup Hansen *et al.*, 1978). The study of the HLA restriction at the population level has been hampered by two fundamental technical problems (Bergholtz and Thorsby, 1977): (1) incomplete monocyte depletion (i.e., nonresponse of T cells could be achieved only for suboptimal doses of antigens), and (2) complementation studies using allogeneic monocytes caused an allogeneic MLC, necessitating the substraction of this background proliferation from the counts observed in the presence of both the allogeneic monocytes and the antigen. Following the work of Kurnick *et al.* (1979, 1980), it has become clear that long-term maintenance of T cells specific for soluble antigen utilizing the optimal dose of antigen with the elimination of background proliferation induced by allogeneic monocytes can be achieved. Therefore immunogenetic studies became very clean. In Table II, an example of a soluble antigen-reactive T cell clone is given. A PPD-specific T cell clone was derived from the same donor used above to generate PLT or CTL clones. The analysis of the reactivity of clone C6.1, restimulated by either autologous or allogeneic PBL, confirms the sharpness of the observed discrimination: no background proliferation is observed in the absence of antigen either in the presence or absence of autologous PBL; furthermore, no MLC is observed. In the presence of antigen, only one allogeneic cell reconstitutes the response at the level of the autologous PBL, and this cell shares DR7 with the responder T cell. Most other cells only partially complement the response: complementing cells tend to belong to DR groups 5 and 1. However, not all cells DR7, 5, or 1 do complement. Further information will require larger panel studies or better family studies.

In conclusion, this technique allows fine genetic studies in a very clean system, without any background noise. It is yet limited to antigens toward which the individuals have been immunized *in vivo*. An exception is the proliferative response to DNP- or TNP-derivatized autologous lymphocytes: here there is apparently a primary response, whatever its origin is.

TABLE II

HLA-D Restricted Proliferation of a PPD-Specific T Cell Clone (C6.1)[a]

Presenting cells	HLA-DR	Antigen added	
		None	PPD
None	—	1.6	1.1
Chap.(self)	1/7	0.8	22.0
Fue.	6/8	0.5	7.3
014	7/–	1.5	22.4
213	5/5	1.7	10.6
223	3/5	2.0	2.9
040	6/3	1.1	4.5
086	2/5	1.5	7.6
072	2/5	1.3	10.8
022	3/7	0.7	5.9
222	1/5	1.0	9.0
Schr.Da	1/2	0.9	4.2
Schr.De	1/6	0.7	9.0
Fr.A.	1/2	0.2	11.8

[a] Peripheral blood lymphocytes from individual Chap. were stimulated with PPD (2 μg/ml) for 7 days, cloned by limiting dilution (0.1 cell/well) and expanded as previously described. Twenty-eight days after the onset of cloning, 10^4 cells from clone C6.1 were restimulated with or without antigen (2 μg/ml) by 10^5 irradiated (2000 R) PBL from panel members. Data for ^{3}H-TdR incorporation are mean cpm $\times 10^{-3}$ after 48-hr cultures.

A limitation in the cloning of T cells to soluble antigen already observed with the PLT clones is their relative instability with time, in contrast to cytotoxic clones. Furthermore the insight into the functional role of D/DR products for soluble antigens presentation should be greatly facilitated by the combined use of specific proliferative T cell clones and monoclonal antibodies to HLA-D/DR products.

II. T CELL CLONES FOLLOWING *IN VIVO* IMMUNIZATION

A. MHC Restricted Anti-H-Y Cytotoxic Clones

In an earlier work, Goulmy *et al.* (1977, 1979) have shown that from aplastic anemia patients who expressed the H-Y HLA restricted phenomenon toward more than one specificity, cytotoxic T cells could be separated, both on the basis of specific monolayer absorptions, as well as cold target inhibition studies,

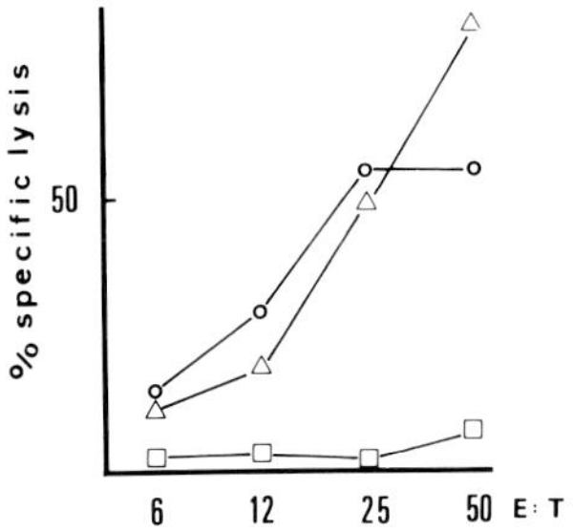

Fig. 1. CTL clone with anti-HY-HLA-2 restricted specificity. △ and ○, HLA-A2 positive male individuals; □, HLA-A2 positive female individual. The results are expressed as percent specific ^{51}Cr release at four different effector to target (E:T) ratios.

suggesting a clonal expression of the cytotoxic effectors. Furthermore, in one patient, at the population level, strong H-Y HLA-A2 specific cytotoxicity was expressed in association with a weaker cytotoxicity toward two HLA-A2 positive females (Goulmy *et al.*, 1977). Attempts to clone specific H-Y HLA-A2 restricted cytotoxic effectors yield a collection of stable CTL clones, none of which were found cytotoxic toward cells from these two females (Goulmy *et al.*, 1980).

In Fig. 1, an example of the specificity of such clones if given. The HLA-A2 female target represents one of the extra reactions observed at the population level. These clones have been stable for 2 years now, and the activity is well preserved after freezing and thawing according to standard procedures. None were found to be specifically proliferative in the presence of their specific target cells.

B. MHC Specificity of Alloreactive Cytotoxic T Cell Clones Derived from Recipients Immunized *in Vivo*

From donor AR5, a volunteer hyperimmunized against one selected donor, a collection of clones were derived after a secondary *in vitro* MLC (Malissen *et al.*, 1981b). None were found to proliferate in response to the original stimulating cells. However, many were cytotoxic toward the specific target cell. Many clones had no additional detectable function, with the exception of clone C4.9 which was found to suppress polyclonal B lymphocyte proliferation following pokeweed mitogen stimulation (Kristensen *et al.*, 1981). This suppression was restricted to B cells of the donor and of his HLA identical brother and not seen with B cells of the parents nor of a large panel of unrelated individuals.

Among the CTL clones, clones specific for all the expected HLA specificities (HLA-A2, Cw3 and B40) toward which the donor should have been sensitized were found, with the exception of clones specific for HLA-DRw6. All have been

TABLE III

Reactivity of C4.22.1 Compared to Relevant Serological HLA-A, B, C Assignments[a]

	Vs.	++	+−	−+	−−	χ^2	r	p^b
C4.22.1	A2	4	4	3	29	7.32	0.43	**
	B40	9	0	3	28	27.10	0.82	***
	Bw60	9	0	0	31	40.00	1.00	***
	Bw61	0	9	3	28	−0.94	−0.15	
	B7	0	8	7	25	−2.12	−0.23	
	B13	1	7	4	28	0	0	
	B27	0	8	3	29	−0.81	−0.14	
	B47	0	8	1	31	−0.26	−0.08	
	Cw3	7	0	8	24	13.65	0.59	***

[a] Clone defining a serological split of HLA-B40, HLA-Bw60.
[b] **, $0.001 < p < 0.01$; ***, $p < 0.001$.

stable for more than 16 months. The absence of anti-HLA-DRw6 specific cytotoxic clones is probably due to the screening procedure, and emphasis is now given to isolate such clones using appropriate DRw6 positive targets (Albrechtsen *et al.*, 1979; Feighery and Stastny, 1979; Johnsen, 1980). Furthermore, we have been able to qualify the anti-B40 cytotoxic clones as being specific for a HLA serologic split of B40, i.e., Bw60 (Table III). The accuracy of such reagents used as typing reagents was excellent compared to the serological typing, with r values of 1.0.

It was somewhat surprising to find that the T cell repertoire was indistinguishable from the classic B cell repertoire defining the serological HLA specificities. In contrast to cytotoxic clones derived from *in vitro* MLC, few clones were cross-reactive or gave unexpected killing. An hypothesis, which can be further verified in the near future, is that the apparent identity of both repertoires is due to the fact that the T cell clones were derived from an hyperimmune donor. At the present, we do not understand why no PLT clones could be derived from this hyperimmune recipient.

These CTL clones have been very stable with time, with no alteration in their fine specificity. They have so far remained entirely conditioned medium dependent. None of them proliferate in presence of their specific target cells. Few CTL clones still under investigation were found to be cross-reactive with peculiar patterns, i.e., all HLA-A2 positive targets but very few of the HLA-A28 positive cells (unpublished data).

III. SURFACE MARKERS OF HUMAN T CELL CLONES: MONOCLONAL ANTIBODIES (mAB) INTERACTING WITH THE CYTOLYTIC FUNCTION

As expected, all of our CTL clones studied to date are E rosette-positive; Fc and C3b, d receptors negative; surface immunoglobulin negative; and HLA-A,B,C, and β2m positive (Malissen *et al.*, 1981b). From our earlier cloning experiments, we also know that they are HLA-DR positive, whether using alloantibodies (Goulmy *et al.*, 1980) or xeno-monoclonal antibodies (Malissen *et al.*, 1982).

In an attempt to raise mAb against membrane structures unique to CTL clones, we have used the protocol outlined in Fig. 2. The supernatants obtained from the cloned hybridomas were screened for their ability to inhibit the cytolysis of the

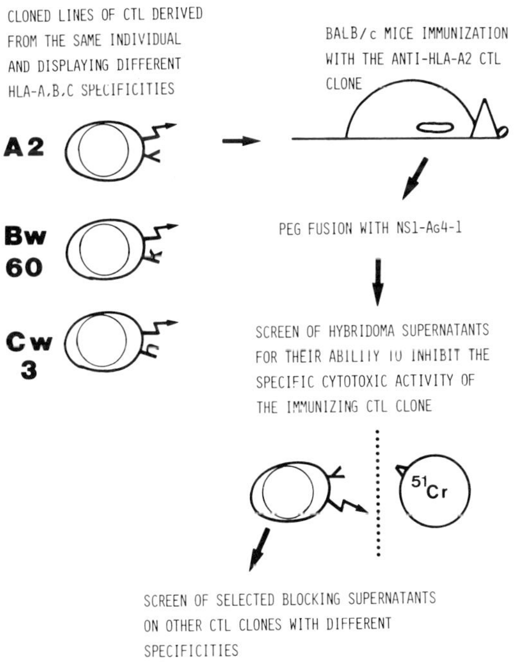

Fig. 2. Protocol used to obtain monoclonal antibodies interacting with the lytic function. From a panel of three CTL clones, each with a different target specificity, one CTL clone anti-HLA-A2 specific is used to immunize BALB/c mice. After fusion with NS1-Ag4.1 myeloma line, hybridoma supernatants are screened at the appropriate time for their ability to block the cytotoxic activity of the three different CTL clones.

TABLE IV

Inhibition of Specific T Cell-Mediated Cytolysis of a Cloned Anti-HLA-A2 CTL Line (C5.6)[a]

mAb added[b]	Specific ^{51}Cr release (%)	Inhibition (%)
None	69	0
B9.1.1	22.5	68
B9.2.4	22	68
B9.3.1	16	77
B9.4.1	5	93
B9.7.6	9	87
B9.8.3	16	77
B9.11.10	6	91
B1.1.G6 (anti-human β2m mAb)	12	82
B8.12.2 (anti-HLA-DR monomorphic mAb)	67	3

[a] A panel of mAb (B9.1.1 to B9.11.10) directed against C5.6 cell surface structures was used.
[b] Cytotoxic assay was performed as described (Malissen *et al.*, 1981a) for 4 hr at 37°C, using as ^{51}Cr-labeled target cells 4 day PHA blasts, The effector to target ratio used in this experiment was 5 : 1. Effector cells were incubated for 30 min at 37°C with the different mAb supernatants at a final dilution of 1 : 2 before adding the target cells.

immunizing clone and of two other CTL clones of different allospecificity. In theory, such a protocol could generate mAb against structures involved either in the lytic machinery of the CTL clones or in the recognition process. Additional screening using binding assays and appropriate targets allows to select for T cell-specific mAb of different types. In Table IV seven mAb (B9.1.1 to B9.11.10) selected on the basis of their strong inhibition of the lytic process of the immunizing CTL clone are shown and compared to the activity of mAb anti-β2m (Liabeuf *et al.*, 1981) and anti-HLA-DR. These monoclonal antibodies bind to about 20% of PBL T cells, 20–25% of T cells from day 6 MLC, and 100% of CTL clones; all are negative on PLT clones. These antibodies do not bind to any lymphoblastoid B cell line tested so far. Furthermore they are negative on B cell blasts induced by pokeweed mitogen. Those tested immunoprecipitate, after reduction, a membrane protein of 30,000 MW, indicating that they could be human equivalent of Lyt-2,3 antigens (Malissen *et al.*, 1982).

In conclusion, using CTL clones as immunogens and screening mAb for functional blocking of lysis, it has been possible to derive a number of Mab directed to lymphocyte function associated antigens, some of which are clear candidates for the human equivalent of the murine Lyt-2,3 structure. Further work is required to compare these mAb and elucidate the mechanism of the lytic block that they mediate.

IV. CONCLUSIONS

We have noticed that the functional types and proportions of T clones obtained were very much dependent upon the timing of cloning and whether we start from *in vitro* sensitization or *in vivo* immunization. More systematic studies are required in order to analyze the meaning of such observations and to draw conclusions about the use of cloning to monitor ongoing immune responses.

We have failed so far to find helper T clones complementing CTL clones for growth in presence of the specific sensitizing cell, in the absence of external source of conditioned medium.

Except for one clone interfering with polyclonal B cell proliferation, we have not isolated any clone with a genuine helper or suppressor activity, a reflection perhaps of the lack of reproducible assays for testing such functions.

T cell hybridization attempts using CTL clones both in our laboratory or in J. Zeuten's laboratory at the Basel Institute for Immunology have so far been unsuccessful. New attempts should allow derivation of functional T lymphocyte hybridomas both to overcome the problem of growing T cell clones in the presence of conditioned medium and to allow easy access to the study of cytolytic mechanism, isolation of T cell receptors, or various lymphokines.

In our attempts, using specific CTL clones as a starting population to raise xeno-mAb against them, many monoclonals were found against a structure of 30,000 MW resembling the murine Lyt-2,3 structure. In the future, such monoclonals will be used to derive mutants negative for the 30,000 MW structure and analyze the functional role of such membrane structure in the lytic process.

Finally it is possible that mAb which interfere with T cell effector functions might be used to prevent graft rejection or graft versus host in patients, replacing therefore ALS or chemotherapeutical immunosuppression.

ACKNOWLEDGMENTS

Supported in part by INSERM (CRL 79.5.118.1) and DGRST (80.7.0218).

REFERENCES

Albrechtsen, D., Arnesen, E., and Thorsby, E. (1979). Cell-mediated lymphocytotoxicity directed against HLA-D gene products. *Transplantation* **27,** 338.

Bach, F. H., and Hirschhorn, K. (1964). Lymphocyte interaction: A potential histocompatibility test *in vitro*. *Science* **143,** 813.

Bach, F. H., and Voynow, N. K. (1966). One-way stimulation in mixed leukocyte cultures. *Science (Washington, D.C.)* **153,** 545.

Bain, B., Vaz, M. R., and Lowenstein, L. (1964). The development of large immature mononuclear cells in mixed lymphocyte cultures. *Blood* **23,** 108.

Bergholtz, B. O., and Thorsby, E. (1977). Macrophage-dependent response of immune human T lymphocytes to PPD *in vitro*. Influence of HLA-D histocompatibility. *Scand. J. Immunol.* **6,** 779.

Bonnard, G. D., Schendel, D. J., West, W. H., Alvarez, J. M., Maca, R. D., Yasaka, K., Fine, R. L., Herberman, R. B., de Landazuri, M. O., and Morgan, D. A. (1978). Continued growth of normal human T lymphocytes in culture with retention of important functions. *In* "Human Lymphocyte Differentiation. Its Application to Cancer" (B. Serrou and C. Rosenfeld, eds.), pp. 319. Elsevier/North Holland, Amsterdam.

Charmot, D., Mawas, C. E., and Sasportes, M. (1975). Secondary response of *in vitro* primed human lymphocytes to allogeneic cells. II. Role of HLA, mixed lymphocyte reaction stimulation determinants and non-specific mitogens in the generation of secondary cytotoxic effectors. *Immunogenetics* **2,** 465.

Charmot, D., Malissen, B. Ghiotto, M., and Mawas, C. (1980). Expansion of human lymphocyte populations expressing specific immune reactivities. II. A comparison of immune reactivities in human T lymphocyte lines derived from allogeneically primed cultures and maintained with lectins or conditioned medium. *Tissue Antigens* **15,** 297.

Charmot, D., Mawas, C., Kristensen, T., and Mercier, P. (1981). The HLA-D system: At least two loci and four distinct phyotypic traits per haplotype. Introduction to component typing in families and population by primed lymphocyte typing. *Immunogenetics* **13,** 57.

Chess, L., and Schlossman, S. F. (1977). Human lymphocyte subpopulations. *Adv. Immunol.* **25,** 213–241.

Feighery, C. R., and Stastny, P. (1979). Specific inhibition of T-cell-mediated cytolysis by alloantiserum against HLA-D related (DR) antigens. *Transplant. Proc.* **11,** 708.

Gillis, S., Baker, P. E., Ruscetti, F. W., and Smith, K. A. (1978). Long-term culture of human antigen-specific cytotoxic T cell lines. *J. Exp. Med.* **148,** 1093.

Goulmy, E., Termijtelen, A., Bradley, B. A., and van Rood, J. J. (1977). Y-antigen killing by T cells of women is restricted by HLA. *Nature (London)* **266,** 544.

Goulmy, E., Hamilton, J. D., and Bradley, B. A. (1979). Anti-self HLA may be clonally expressed. *J. Exp. Med.* **149,** 545.

Goulmy, E., Blockland, E., van Rood, J. J., Charmot, D., Malissen, B., and Mawas, C. (1980). Production, expansion and clonal analysis of T cells with specific HLA restricted male lysis. *J. Exp. Med.* **152,** 182s.

Häyry, P., and Defendi, V. (1970). Mixed lymphocyte culture produces effector cells: Model *in vitro* for allograft rejection. *Science* **168,** 133.

Johnsen, H. E. (1980). Human B blast specific target determinants in CML. A panel study. *Tissue Antigens* **15,** 199.

Kavathas, P., Demars, R., Bach, F. H., and Shaw, S. (1981). HLA-SB: A new human histocompatibility gene defined using HLA-mutant cell lines. *Nature (London)* **293,** 747.

Kristensen, T., Malissen, B., Madsen, M., and Mawas, C. (1981). A cloned human T lymphocyte suppressing polyclonal B lymphocyte proliferation with exquisite genetic restriction. *In* "Mechanism of Lymphocyte Activation" (Resch and Kirchner, eds.), pp. 518–520. Elsevier/North-Holland Publ., New York.

Kurnick, J. T., Gronvik, K. J., Kimura, A. K., Lindblom, J. B., Skoog, V. T., Sjoberg, O., and Wigzell, H. (1979). Long term growth *in vitro* of human blasts with maintenance of specificity and function. *J. Immunol.* **122,** 1255.

Kurnick, J. T., Altevogt, P., Lindblom, J. Sjöberg, O., Danneus, A., and Wigzell, H. (1980). Long-term maintenance of HLA-D restricted T cells specific for soluble antigens. *Scand. J. Immunol.* **11,** 131.

Liabeuf, A., LeBorgne, C., Kourilsky, F. M., Malissen, B., Manuel, Y., and Sanderson, A. R. (1981). An antigenic determinant of human 2-microglobulin masked by the association with HLA-heavy chains at the cell surface: Analysis using monoclonal antibodies. *J. Immunol.* **127,** 1542.

Malissen, B., Charmot, D., and Mawas, C. (1981a). Expansion of human lymphocyte populations expressing specific immune reactivities. III. Specific colonies, either cytotoxic or proliferative obtained from a population of responder cells primed *in vitro*. Preliminary immunogenetic analysis. *Hum. Immunol.* **2,** 1.

Malissen, B., Kristensen, T., Goridis, C., Madsen, M., and Mawas, C. (1981b). Clones of human cytotoxic T lymphocytes derived from an allosensitized individual. HLA specificity and cell surface markers. *Scand. J. Immunol.* **14,** 213.

Malissen, B., Rebai, N., Liabeuf, A., and Mawas, C. (1982). Human cytotoxic T cell structures associated with expression of cytolysis. I. Analysis at the clonal cell level of the cytolysis inhibiting effect of seven monoclonal antibodies. *Eur. J. Immunol.* (in press).

Mawas, C., Charmot, D., and Mercier, P. (1980). Split of HLA-D into two regions α and β by a recombination between HLA-D and GLO. I. Study in a family and primed lymphocyte typing for determinants coded by the region. *Tissue Antigens* **15,** 458.

Morgan, D. A., Ruscetti, F., and Gallo, R. (1976). Selective *in vitro* growth of T lymphocytes from normal human bone marrow. *Science* **193,** 1007.

Nowell, P. C. (1960). Phytohaemagglutinin: An initiator of mitosis in cultures of normal human leukocytes. *Cancer Res.* **20,** 462.

Pappas, F., Bonnard, G. D., Hartzman, R. J., and Strong, D. M. (1979). Human PL cells grown as continued T cell cultures. *Transplant. Proc.* **11,** 1986.

Reinherz, E. L., and Schlossman, S. F. (1980). The differentiation and function of human T lymphocytes. *Cell* **19,** 821.

Ruscetti, F. W., Morgan, D. A., and Gallo, R. C. (1977). Functional and morphologic characterization of human T cells continuously grown *in vitro*. *J. Immunol.* **119,** 131.

Shaw, S., Kavathas, P., Pollack, M. S., Charmot, D., and Mawas, C. (1981). Family studies define a new histocompatibility locus, SB between HLA-DR and GLO. *Nature* (*London*) **293,** 745.

Sheehy, M. J., Sondel, P. M., Bach, M. L., Wank, R., and Bach, F. H. (1975). HLA-D (LD) typing: A rapid assay with primed lymphocytes. *Science* **188,** 1308.

Solliday, S., and Bach, F. H. (1970). Cytotoxicity: Specificity after *in vitro* sensitization. *Science* **170,** 1406.

Sønderstrup Hansen, G., Rubin, B., Sørensen, S. F., and Svejgaard, A. (1978). Importance of HLA-D antigens for the cooperation of HLA-D antigens for the cooperation between human monocytes and T lymphocytes. *Eur. J. Immunol.* **8,** 520.

Strausser, J. L., and Rosenberg, S. A. (1978). *In vitro* growth of cytotoxic human lymphocytes. I. Growth of cells sensitized *in vitro* to alloantigens. *J. Immunol.* **121,** 1491.

37

Human T Cell Clones Reactive with Soluble Antigens: Methodology, Specificity, and MHC Restriction

Benjamin Sredni/David Volkman/
Ronald H. Schwartz/Anthony S. Fauci

I. Antigen Specificity of Soft Agar Colonies of Human T Cells 440
II. Genetic Requirements for Antigen Stimulation 442
References 445

One of the major goals of immunologists for the past 5 years has been to obtain cloned populations of antigen-specific T lymphocytes. During the past year this goal has been realized by several laboratories (von Boehmer *et al.*, 1979; Watson, 1979; Glasebrook and Fitch, 1979; Schreier and Tees, 1980; Sredni *et al.*, 1980, 1981c; Kimoto and Fathman, 1980) including our own. However, it is important to point out that many other laboratories have contributed significant technological advances in this area which were essential in achieving the final outcome. In particular, the early work of MacDonald *et al.* (1974) on alloreactive T cells and Ben-Sasson *et al.* (1975) on antigen-specific T cells demonstrated that T lymphocytes could be propagated and enriched for specificity by repeated exposure to antigen *in vitro*. At about this time, innovations in soft agar technology (Rozenszajn *et al.*, 1975; Sredni *et al.*, 1975, 1976) allowed for the cloning of mitogen responsive T cells. Finally, the discovery and characterization of T cell growth factor (TCGF, also called interleukin-2) (IL-2) (Ruscetti *et al.*, 1977; Gillis and Smith, 1977; Farrar *et al.*, 1980) made it possible to maintain *in vitro* cultures of antigen-specific (Schrier *et al.*, 1979; Watson, 1979; Augustin *et al.*, 1979; Apte *et al.*, 1981) and alloreactive (Watanabe *et al.*, 1977) T cells for long periods of time. Improvement in technology allowed for the progression from T cell lines to T cell clones, and it soon became possible

ISBN 0-12-249920-4

to obtain antigen-reactive clones, first for alloantigens, (von Boehmer *et al.*, 1979; Fathman and Hengartner, 1978; Hengartner and Fathman, 1980), then for particulate antigens such as sheep red blood cells (Schreier and Tees, 1980), and finally for soluble protein antigens (Sredni *et al.*, 1980, 1981b; Kimoto and Fathman, 1980, 1981).

Attempts to create monoclonal T cell populations generally employ the techniques of repeated antigen stimulation *in vitro* in the presence of IL-2 followed by cloning in soft agar or by limiting dilution in the presence of IL-2. Potential problems with this approach are the possibility of bias in *in vitro* selection of a subset of T cells possessing the ability to grow well in culture, selective stimulation of T cells responsive to IL-2 that are not antigen specific, and selection of a subset of T cells with a skewed set of specificities for the antigen. All of these problems could result in the selecting out and ultimate loss of certain T cell subpopulations before the cloning step is carried out. In order to reduce this possibility to a minimum, we devised a method in which the cells were cloned in soft agar after only 5 days of antigen stimulation *in vitro*. This method uses soluble antigen as the selecting agent in the agar and does not introduce IL-2 until the colonies are picked for expansion. The procedure, which is outlined in the Appendix, is basically a modification of the soft agar cloning technique developed for cloning mitogen and antigen reactive T cells in the mouse (Sredni *et al.*, 1976, 1980; Sredni and Schwartz, 1981). By taking this approach, we have been able to monitor the antigen specificity of the cells from the beginning of their expansion *in vitro* and have demonstrated that they maintain this specificity throughout expansion and recloning.

I. ANTIGEN SPECIFICITY OF SOFT AGAR COLONIES OF HUMAN T CELLS

When the colonies reached the 50- to 100-cell stage in soft agar (see Appendix), they were picked and transferred to microtiter wells for subsequent expansion. Growth in liquid culture was carried out with antigens, antigen presenting cells (APC) in the form of irradiated peripheral blood mononuclear cells (PBMNC), and 20% IL-2. It is important to point out that omission of any one of these components resulted in death of the cells within days. Cultures were then fed every 3 days for several weeks with 50% IL-2. In addition, they were intermittently restimulated with antigen and PBMNC until the T cells had increased in number of 1 to 2 $\times$ 10^5. At this point, the cells were examined for antigen specificity.

The colonies which had originally been selected for keyhole limpet hemagglutinin (KLH) reactivity could be stimulated to incorporate [^{3}H]thymidine only by KLH and not by tetanus toxoid, and only when the appropriate antigen (KLH) was presented with fresh irradiated autologous

TABLE I

Maintenance of Antigen Specificity on Recloning[a]

	Proliferative response (cpm) (±SEM)						
	Original colony	Clones			Subclones		
Stimulant[b]	L.S.1	1.3	1.4	1.7	1.3.3	1.3.6	1.3.9
Medium	140(±23)	60(±16)	93(±13)	80(±10)	85(±17)	93(±19)	80(±36)
Autologous APC alone	173(±56)	63(±19)	83(±32)	63(±7)	65(±15)	53(±22)	70(±6)
KLH alone	147(±29)	40(±6)	60(±10)	140(±35)	53(±30)	60(±15)	80(±21)
Autologous APC + KLH	20,000(±2488)	12,523(±638)	10,187(±445)	7,663(±170)	11,170(±1365)	8,977(±1699)	9,770(±243)
TT alone	130(±38)	70(±15)	77(±12)	80(±32)	70(±15)	130(±35)	110(±32)
Autologous APC + TT	132(±28)	90(±25)	63(±12)	67(±9)	52(±7)	55(±12)	97(±27)

[a] Data represent [^{3}H]thymidine uptake expressed as mean (±SEM) cpm for three separate determinations per experiment.

[b] 1×10^5 APC were added in culture to 5×10^3 cloned or subcloned T cells. TT, tetanus toxoid.

PBMNC (Table I). Of note is the fact that L.S. was immune to tetanus toxoid as determined by tetanus-induced *in vitro* blastogenic responses of her fresh PBMNC.

II. GENETIC REQUIREMENTS FOR ANTIGEN STIMULATION

The concept of major histocompatibility complex (MHC) restriction in the recognition of foreign antigens by thymus-derived (T) lymphocytes (Paul and Benacerraf, 1977; Zinkernagel and Doherty, 1979) has been an area of intensive interest and study in immunobiology over the past decade. According to this concept, T lymphocytes, in order to be stimulated by antigen, must simultaneously encounter both the foreign antigen and certain gene products of the MHC.

Using heterogeneous populations of cells, the critical evidence in support of the concept of MHC restriction is the finding that in F_1 mice there are distinct subsets of T cells which recognize the same antigen, but only in association with one or the other of the parental MHC gene products (Paul *et al.,* 1977; Zinkernagel and Doherty, 1975; Sprent, 1978; Kappler and Marrack, 1976).

More recently, the concept of MHC restriction in mouse has been unequivocally proved through the use of T cell cloning technology (Sredni *et al.,* 1980, 1981b; Kimoto and Fathman, 1980). Antigen-specific T cell clones have been developed in several laboratories, and it has been shown that the progeny of a single cell bears receptors specific for the antigen only in association with self-MHC-gene products (von Boehmer *et al.,* 1979; Schreier and Tees, 1980; Sredni *et al.,* 1980; Kimoto and Fathman, 1980). In addition, studies employing clones from F_1 animals have demonstrated that separate and distinct T cells recognize the antigen in association with each of the parental MHC gene products (Kimoto and Fathman, 1980, 1981; Sredni *et al.,* 1981a; Fathman and Kimoto, 1981).

Acceptance of the concept of genetic restriction of human T cell responses has met with skepticism and resistance. Studies on pokeweed mitogen-induced immunoglobulin synthesis indicated that allogeneic as well as autologous T lymphocytes could provide help to B lymphocytes (Keightley *et al.,* 1976; Saxon *et al.,* 1977; Hirano *et al.,* 1977). Furthermore, the same lack of genetic restriction was shown for the monocytes which were required for this response (Blaese *et al.,* 1977; Fauci *et al.,* 1981). However, more recent studies of antigen-induced proliferative responses of human T cells have suggested that MHC restriction is operable in monocyte–T lymphocyte interactions. Several groups have demonstrated a requirement for HLA-D compatibility between T cells and monocytes in the generation of a proliferative response to PPD, tetanus toxoid, and other soluble protein antigens (Bergholtz and Thorsby, 1978; Dattner and Levis, 1978; Sønderstrup-Hansen *et al.,* 1978). In addition, it has been demonstrated that histocompatibility at the HLA-D locus is required to stimulate a factor-independent proliferative response from long-term T cell lines maintained in culture with T cell growth factor (TCGF) (Kurnick *et al.*, 1980).

With regard to the human T cell clone under current study, the requirement for antigen-presenting cells in the form of irradiated PBMNC is shown in Table I. In the absence of these cells, no antigen-induced proliferative response was observed from the T cell colony, clones, or subclones. We investigated what the histocompatibility requirements were for stimulating the KLH-specific human T cell clone. The obvious logistic constraints of the human system with the lack of genetically defined inbred strains (which are available in the mouse model) render it impossible to unequivocally delineate the gene products required in the genetic restriction of antigen-specific human T cell responses. However, one can at least implicate particular loci by correlation analyses on samplings from the general population. Thus, we obtained PBMNC from eight unrelated donors, typed the cells to identify their histocompatibility antigens, and then used these cells to present KLH to the antigen-specific T cell subclones (Table II).

As can be seen, sharing of alleles at the HLA-A, B, or C locus was not sufficient for presentation of KLH by the presenting cells to the clones. For example, PBMNC donor 3 shared only HLA-A3 in common with the donor of the T cell clone, and PBMNC donor 2 shared only HLA-B8, yet neither PBMNC population supported a proliferative response. In contrast, histocompatibility at the DRw locus was sufficient for antigen presentation. PBMNC donor 4 shared only HLA-DRw2 in common with the donor of the T cell clone, yet it supported a proliferative response as well as autologous PBMNC. A total of three of the eight PBMNC donors were DRw2-positive, and all three were capable of presenting KLH to the clone. Thus, it appears that histocompatibility for the DRw2 allele (or closely linked genes) is required to stimulate the KLH-specific clone, as suggested by this absolute correlation.

It is important to point out that the donor of the T cell clone was heterozygous at the DRw locus, possessing both the DRw6Y and DRw2 alleles. In this regard, PBMNC from neither of the two donors sharing DRw6Y and not DRw2 with the donor of the clone (Nos. 7 and 8), was capable of supporting a KLH-induced proliferative response. Thus, it would appear that only one of two alleles at the DRw locus is required to stimulate the KLH-specific clone. This was clearly demonstrated in studies utilizing PBMNC from the parents of the donor of the T cell clone for antigen-presenting activity. PBMNC from one parent LR ($DRw2^{+}6Y^{-}$), presented KLH to the T cell clone as well as PBMNC from random $DRw2^{+}$ donors (Table III). In contrast, PBMNC from the other parent, FS ($DRw2^{-}6Y^{+}$), did not present KLH to the clone. These results demonstrate that the T cell clone is restricted to recognizing KLH only in association with the gene product of the DRw2 allele (or closely linked gene). This observation strongly suggests a direct analogy with the situation in the F_1 mouse, and it is highly likely that as additional antigen-specific human T cell clones are de-

TABLE II

Relationship of Antigen-Specific Clonal Proliferation to the MHC Antigens of Presenting Cells

Presenting cells[a]	HLA antigens A	B	C	DRw	Antigen in culture[b]	Clone LS 1.3[c]	Subclone LS 1.3–4
Experiment 1							
L.S.	3,26	7.8	-	2,6Y	−	80 ± 30	60(± 20)
					+	12,600 ± 100	13,100 ± 2600
1	28,31	7,35	4	1,2	−	100 ± 10	70 ± 20
					+	9,100 ± 500	8,800 ± 1300
2	1,2	8,27	1	1,3	−	50 ± 3	50 ± 10
					+	100 ± 30	50 ± 5
3	3,-	15,13	-	4,5	−	50 ± 20	90 ± 30
					+	80 ± 40	120 ± 60
Experiment 2							
1	28,31	7,35	4	1,2	−	180 ± 60	100 ± 20
					+	10,300 ± 500	8,700 ± 700
4	2,-	50,-	6	2,7	−	80 ± 60	80 ± 40
					+	9,900 ± 800	9,100 ± 600
5	30,33	5,14	-	2,-	−	100 ± 10	100 ± 30
					+	9,800 ± 600	9,100 ± 600
6	26,-	38,44	-	4,-	−	50 ± 15	170 ± 40
					+	170 ± 20	80 ± 40
Experiment 3							
4	2,-	50,0	6	2,7	−	140 ± 35	170 ± 20
					+	10,200 ± 500	50,800 ± 5000
7	2,-	7,56	-	4,6Y	−	170 ± 20	90 ± 3
					+	140 ± 10	90 ± 10
Experiment 4							
1	28,31	7,35	4	1,2	−	170 ± 10	120 ± 50
					+	10,400 ± 700	10,200 ± 1100
8	3,31	35,40	3,4	4,6Y	−	190 ± 2	150 ± 20
					+	120 ± 60	120 ± 20

[a] Irradiated PBMNC (1×10^5 APC) were cultured with 5×10^5 cloned cells. Each number in this column refers to a different individual. Certain individuals were studied in separate experiments as indicated. Donor L.S. was immunized with KLH as noted. However, as a control within APC, donors 1 and 6 were also immunized with KLH.

[b] KLH was added to cultures at a concentration of 100 μg/ml when indicated by +. No KLH was added to cultures designated −.

[c] Data represent mean ± SEM of cpm per 10^4 cloned cells in culture for three separate determinations per experiment.

TABLE III

Testing PBML from the Parents of the Donor of the T Cell Clone LS 1.3-4 for Antigen Presenting Activity[a]

PBML donor	A	B	C	DRw	Antigen in culture	Lymphocyte clone LS 1.3-4
4	3,2–	50,–	6	2,7	–	100 ± 10
					+	42,800 ± 5500
LR (mother)	3,–	7,62	-	2,–	–	400 ± 40
					+	49,300 ± 3200
FS (father)	3,34	8,35	4	1,6Y	–	500 ± 400
					+	50 ± 6
LS[a]	3,26	7,8	-	2,6Y	–	60 ± 20
					+	13,100 ± 2600

[a] These results are from experiment 1, Table II.

veloped, it will become evident that any given human T cell clone in a heterozygous individual can only recognize antigen in association with one of the sets of HLA-D gene products. Although we have only demonstrated that the proliferating human T cell is HLA-D restricted in its antigen recognition, it seems reasonable to generalize from the mouse that cytotoxic, helper, and delayed-type hypersensitivity-mediating T cells will also be restricted. Experiments now in progress are attempting to isolate from a single DRw heterozygous individual a large number of T cell clones specific for the same antigen in the hopes of identifying T cell clones possessing each of the three different types of restriction specificities (P_A P_B and F_1) that have been found in the mouse. Future studies employing this system of antigen specific human T cell clones will hopefully allow investigators to pursue the delineation of the mechanisms of activation and immunoregulation of human lymphocyte subsets with heretofore unavailable precision.

REFERENCES

Apte, R. N., Lowy, I., Baeteilier, P. D., and Mozes, E. (1981). Establishment and characterization of continuous helper T cell lines specific to poly(L-Tyr,L-Glu)-poly(D,L-Ala)—poly(L-Lys). *J. Immunol.* **127,** 25.

Augustin, A. A., Julius, M. H., and Cosenza, H. (1979). Antigen-specific stimulation and transstimulation of T cells in long-term culture. *Eur. J. Immunol.* **9,** 665.

Ben-Sasson, S. Z., Paul, W. E., Shevach, E. M., and Green, T. (1975). *In vitro* selection and extended culture of antigen-specific T lymphocytes. II. Mechanisms of selection. *J. Immunol.* **115,** 1723.

Bergholtz, B. O., and Thorsby, E. (1978). HLA-D restriction of the macrophage-dependent response of immune human T lymphocytes to PPD *in vitro:* Inhibition by anti-HLA-DR antisera. *Scand. J. Immunol.* **8,** 63.

Blaese, R. M., Lawrence, E. C., and Poplack, D. G. (1977). A critique of techniques of macrophage-monocyte depletion in studies of human peripheral blood mononuclear leukocyte (MNL) function. *In* "Regulatory Mechanisms in Lymphocyte Activation" (D. O. Lucas, ed.), p. 579. Academic Press, New York.

Dattner, A. M., and Levis, W. R. (1978). Clonal priming of human lymphocytes with soluble microbial antigens. High dose paralysis, restoration and autologous leukocyte preference. *Scand. J. Immunol.* **8,** 403.

Farrar, J., Farrar, J. F., Simon, P. L. Hilfiker, M. L., Stadler, B. M., and Farrar, W. L. (1980). Thymoma production of T cell growth factor, Interleukin-2. *J. Immunol.* **125,** 2555.

Fathman, C. G., and Hengartner, H. (1978). Clones of alloreactive T cells. *Nature* (*London*) **277,** 617.

Fathman, C. G., and Kimoto, M. (1981). Studies utilizing murine T cell clones; *Ir* genes, Ia antigens and MLR stimulating determinants. *Immunol. Rev.* **54,** 57.

Fauci, A. S., Stevenson, H. C., Whalen, G., and Andrysiak, P. (1981). Immunoregulation of human B cell function. Monocyte–T cell interactions in the modulation of B cell reactivity. *In* "New Trends in Human Immunology and Cancer Immunotherapy" (B. Serrou and C. Rosenfeld, eds.), p. 580. Doin, Paris.

Gillis, S., and Smith, K. A. (1977). Long-term culture of tumour-specific cytotoxic T cells. *Nature* (*London*) **268,** 154.

Glasebrook, A. L., and Fitch, F. W. (1979). T-cell lines which cooperate in generation of specific cytolytic activity. *Nature* (*London*) **280,** 171.

Hengartner, H., and Fathman, C. G. (1980). Clones of alloreactive T cells. I. A unique homozygous MLR-stimulating determinant present on B6 stimulators. *Immunogenetics* **10,** 175.

Hirano, T., Kuritani, T., Kishimoto, T., and Yamamura, Y. (1977). *In vitro* immune response of human peripheral lymphocytes. I. The mechanism(s) involved in T cell helper functions in the pokeweed mitogen-induced differentiation and proliferation of B cells. *J. Immunol.* **119,** 1235.

Kappler, J. W., and Marrack, P. C. (1976). Helper T cells recognise antigen and macrophage surface components simultaneously. *Nature* (*London*) **262,** 797.

Keightley, R. C., Cooper, M. D., and Lawton, A. R. (1976). The T cell dependence of B cell differentiation induced by pokeweed mitogen. *J. Immunol.* **117,** 1538.

Kimoto, M., and Fathman, C. G. (1980). I. Transcomplementing hybrid *I-A* region gene products function effectively in antigen presentation. *J. Exp. Med.* **152,** 759.

Kimoto, M., and Fathman, C. G. (1981). Unique homozygous and (high responder × low responder)F_1 hybrid antigen-presenting determinants detected using poly (Tyr, Glu)-poly D, L—Ala—poly-Lys-reactive T cell clones. *J. Exp. Med.* **153,** 375.

Kurnick, J. T., Altevogt, P., Lindblom, J., Oberg, S. O., Danneus, A., and Wigzell, H. (1980). Long-term maintenance of HLA-D restricted T cells specific for soluble antigens. *Scand J. Immunol.* **11,** 131.

MacDonald, H. R., Engers, H. D., Cerottini, J.-C., and Brunner, K. T. (1974). Generation of cytotoxic T lymphocytes *in vitro.* II. Effect of repeated exposure to alloantigens on the cytotoxic activity of long-term mixed leukocyte cultures. *J. Exp. Med.* **140,** 718.

Paul, W. E., and Benacerraf, B. (1977). Functional specificity of thymus-dependent lymphocytes. *Science* (*Washington, D.C.*) **195,** 1293.

Paul, W. E., Shevach, E. M., Pickeral, S., Thomas, D. W., and Rosenthal, A. S. (1977). Independent populations of primed F_1 guinea pig T lymphocytes respond to antigen-pulsed parental peritoneal exudate cells. *J. Exp. Med.* **145,** 618.

Rozenszajn, L. A., Shoham, D., and Kalechman, I. (1975). Clonal proliferation of PHA-stimulated human lymphocytes in soft agar culture. *Immunology* **29,** 1041.

Ruscetti, F. W., Morgan, D. A., and Gallo, R. C. (1977). Functional and morphologic characterization of human T cells continuously grown *in vitro*. *J. Immunol.* **119,** 131.

Saxon, A., Stevens, R. H., and Ashman, R. F. (1977). Regulation of immunoglobulin production in human peripheral blood leukocytes: Cellular interactions. *J. Immunol.* **118,** 1872.

Schreier, M. H., and Tees, R. (1980). Clonal induction of helper T cells: Conversion of specific signals into nonspecific signals. *Int. Arch. Allergy Appl. Immunol.* **61,** 227.

Schreier, R. D., Skidmore, B. J., Kurnick, J. T., Goldstine, S. N., and Chiller, J. M. (1979). Propagation of antigen-specific T cell helper function *in vitro*. *J. Immunol.* **123,** 2525.

Sønderstrup-Hansen, G., Rubin, B., Sørenson, S. F., and Svejgaard, A. (1978). Importance of HLA-D antigens for the cooperation between human monocytes and T lymphocytes. *Eur. J. Immunol.* **8,** 250.

Sprent, J. (1978). Role of *H-2* gene products in the function of T helper cells from normal and chimeric mice *in vitro*. *Immunol. Rev.* **42,** 108.

Sredni, B., and Schwartz, R. H. (1981). Antigen-specific, proliferating T lymphocyte clones. Methodology, specificity, MHC restriction, and alloreactivity. *Immunol. Rev.* **54,** 187.

Sredni, B., Rozenszajn, L. A., Kalechman, Y., and Michlin, H. (1975). Clonal proliferation in soft agar of mitogen-stimulated mouse T lymphocytes. *Exp. Hematol.* (*Copenhagen*) **4,** Suppl., 45.

Sredni, B., Kalechman, Y., Michlin, H., and Rosenszajn, L. A. (1976). Development of colonies *in vitro* of mitogen-stimulated mouse T lymphocytes. *Nature* (*London*) **259,** 130.

Sredni, B., Tse, H. Y., and Schwartz, R. H. (1980). Direct cloning and extended culture of antigen-specific MHC-restricted, proliferating T lymphocytes. *Nature* (London) **283,** 581.

Sredni, B., Matis, L. A., Lerner, E. A., Paul, W. E., and Schwartz, R. H. (1981a). Antigen-specific T cell clones restricted to unique F_1 MHC determinants: Inhibition of proliferation with a monoclonal anti-Ia antibody. *J. Exp. Med.* **153,** 677.

Sredni, B., Tse, H. Y., Chen, C., and Schwartz, R. H. (1981b). Antigen-specific clones of proliferating T lymphocytes. I. Methodology, specificity and MHC restriction. *J. Immunol.* **126,** 341.

Sredni, B., Volkman, D., Schwartz, R. H., and Fauci, A. S. (1981c). Antigen-specific human T-cell clones: Development of clones requiring HLA-DR-compatible presenting cells for stimulation in presence of antigen. *Proc. Natl. Acad. Sci. U.S.A.* **78,** 1858.

von Boehmer, H., Hengartner, H., Nabholz, M., Lernhardt, W., Schreier, M. H., and Haas, W. (1979). Fine specificity of a continuously growing killer cell clone specific for H-Y antigen. *Eur. J. Immunol.* **9,** 592.

Watanabe, T., Fathman, C. G., and Coutinho, A. (1977). Clonal growth of T cells *in vitro*: Preliminary attempts at a quantitative approach. *Immunol. Rev.* **35,** 3.

Watson, J. (1979). Continuous proliferation of murine antigen-specific helper T lymphocytes in culture. *J. Exp. Med.* **150,** 1510.

Zinkernagel, R. M., and Doherty, P. C. (1975). *H-2* compatibility requirement for T-cell-mediated lysis of target cells infected with lymphocyte choriomeningitis virus. Different cytotoxic T-cell specificities are associated with structures coded for in *H-2-D* or *H-2D*. *J. Exp. Med.* **141,** 1427.

Zinkernagel, R. M., and Doherty, P. C. (1979). MHC-restricted cytotoxic T cells: Studies on the biological role of polymorphic major transplantation antigens determining T-cell restriction specificity, function and responsiveness. *Adv. Immunol.* **27,** 51.

VIII

Future Perspectives in the Utilization of T Cell Clones

38

Potential Use of Expanded T Lymphoid Cells and T Cell Clones for the Immunotherapy of Cancer

Steven A. Rosenberg

I. Traffic *in Vivo* of Cells Grown in T Cell Growth Factor 453
II. Effect *in Vivo* of Adoptively Transferred Cells Expanded in T Cell Growth Factor 456
III. Isolation of T Lymphocyte Clones Specifically Reactive with Tumor 459
IV. The Lysis of Fresh Syngeneic or Autologous Tumor Cells by Lymphoid Cells Expanded in T Cell Growth Factor 463
V. Conclusions 465
References 465

In a recent review of the adoptive immunotherapy of cancer, Rosenberg and Terry (1977) summarized the evidence that the adoptive transfer of immunologically reactive lymphoid cells was capable of causing the regression of established tumors. An analysis of examples of successful adoptive immunotherapy of murine tumors revealed several factors that seemed essential for successful treatment. Three important factors were: (1) obtaining highly sensitized cells with specific anti-tumor reactivity; (2) obtaining large numbers of sensitized cells (at least 10^8 cells to treat a 1 cm diameter tumor in a mouse); and (3) use of syngeneic cells for therapy. Early attempts at adoptive immunotherapy of human tumors fell far short of meeting each of the above three criteria.

The development of techniques to expand T lymphoid cells to large numbers *in vitro* using T cell growth factor (TCGF) has, however, provided a means for overcoming many previous problems in the adoptive immunotherapy of human tumors (Table I). The potential now exists for isolating, from a cancer-bearing human, reactive lymphoid cells that can be cloned and expanded to large numbers for subsequent reinfusion into the autologous host. This approach to the adoptive immunotherapy of human tumors has great appeal, though major problems to its successful application must still be overcome.

ISOLATION, CHARACTERIZATION, AND
UTILIZATION OF T LYMPHOCYTE CLONES

ISBN 0-12-249920-4

TABLE I

Adoptive Immunotherapy of Cancer

Requirements for adoptive immunotherapy	Possible approaches in man
1. Specificity for tumor cells	Clone T lymphoid cells with appropriate specificity
2. Large cell numbers	Expand cells in T cell growth factor
3. Cells that will not be rejected by the recipient	Utilize autologous lymphoid cells from the cancer-bearing human

The generation of large numbers of lymphoid cells in TCGF presents no major difficulty because of the rapid expansion of both murine and human cells in TCGF *in vitro*. An example of the number of cells that can be generated from human cells growing in culture is shown in Table II using data from an actual experiment in our laboratory (Strausser and Rosenberg, 1978). Starting with 10^5 cells, after 2 months of growth more than 9.3×10^{13} (or 90 kg of packed cells) can be obtained if all cells in these cultures were to be saved. Though technical problems exist in developing large-scale culture techniques, these problems seem to be surmountable.

A greater problem is the development of techniques for identifying lymphoid

TABLE II

Kinetics of Human Cytotoxic Cell Growth *in vitro* in TCGF[a]

Number of days in culture	Time to cutback to 1×10^5 cells/cm^3 (days)	Cell number increase $\times 10^5$ (from 10^5 cells/cm^3) $\pm$ S.D.	Potential total cell number (if all cells were saved)
6	6	7.3 ± 0.5	7.3×10^5
10	4	8.0 ± 1.8	5.8×10^6
15	5	11.6 ± 0.9	6.8×10^7
20	5	8.7 ± 1.4	5.9×10^8
25	5	10.2 ± 1.2	6.0×10^9
30	5	5.9 ± 0.6	3.5×10^{10}
37	7	8.0 ± 0.6	2.8×10^{11}
44	7	5.8 ± 0.3	1.6×10^{12}
50	6	4.1 ± 0.6	6.8×10^{12}
57	7	3.5 ± 0.4	2.3×10^{13}
65	8	3.9 ± 0.8	9.3×10^{13}
73	8	9.1 ± 1.1	8.4×10^{14}

[a] Cells were sensitized to alloantigens in secondary MLC and grown in human TCGF. (Adapted from Strausser and Rosenberg, 1978).

cells with antitumor reactivity. The poor immunogenicity of tumor antigens in both the mouse and the human presents considerable difficulties in attempting to isolate the very rare T cell clones that may have specific reactivity to tumor antigens. In addition, questions have been raised concerning the effects *in vivo* of cells grown in TCGF. Though appropriately reactive cells have been shown to kill tumor cells *in vitro,* the effect of these cells *in vivo* has been poorly studied.

This chapter deals with our attempts to study some of these problems.

I. TRAFFIC *IN VIVO* OF CELLS GROWN IN T CELL GROWTH FACTOR

As a prelude to studying the immunologic effects *in vivo* of cells expanded in TCGF we have studied in detail the distribution of these cells when injected *in vivo* both in the mouse and in the human (Lotze *et al.*, 1980). For these studies, we have used murine splenocytes expanded in TCGF and reinjected into animals of the syngeneic strain. For the corresponding human studies, we have expanded peripheral blood lymphoid cells from tumor-bearing humans in TCGF and then reinjected them into the autologous host.

In the mouse, splenocytes were labeled with chromium-51, and the traffic of either fresh splenocytes or splenocytes cultured in TCGF made in either fetal calf serum or mouse serum were compared. At varying times after injection of cells, visceral organs were removed and counted for the presence of radioactivity. The results of a typical experiment are presented in Fig. 1. The distribution *in vivo* of cells expanded in TCGF containing either fetal calf serum or syngeneic mouse serum was substantially different from that of uncultured splenocytes. During the first 24 hr uncultured splenocytes distributed almost equally to both the liver and spleen. Presumably, cells that traffic to the liver are cleared from the circulation, though at least some cells that traffic to the spleen enter the recirculating lymphocyte pool. In contrast, splenocytes cultured and expanded in TCGF exhibited significant distribution to the lung, and from 40 to 50% of cells are found in the lung 2 hr after injection. These are slowly cleared from the lung over the next 24 hr and distribute predominately to the liver, with only approximately 5% of cells distributing to the spleen. When splenocytes are grown in TCGF containing only syngeneic mouse serum, a somewhat higher percentage (almost 10%) distributes to the spleen with less initial distribution in the lung than cells grown in medium containing fetal calf serum.

Thus, a marked increase in the relative number of cells distributing to the liver occurred following expansion of cells in TCGF. Though we have previously shown that the traffic of xenogeneic cells to the liver can be somewhat decreased by the use of reticuloendothelial system inhibitors such as carageenan, these effects were small and are not likely substantially to effect the traffic of cells grown in TCGF.

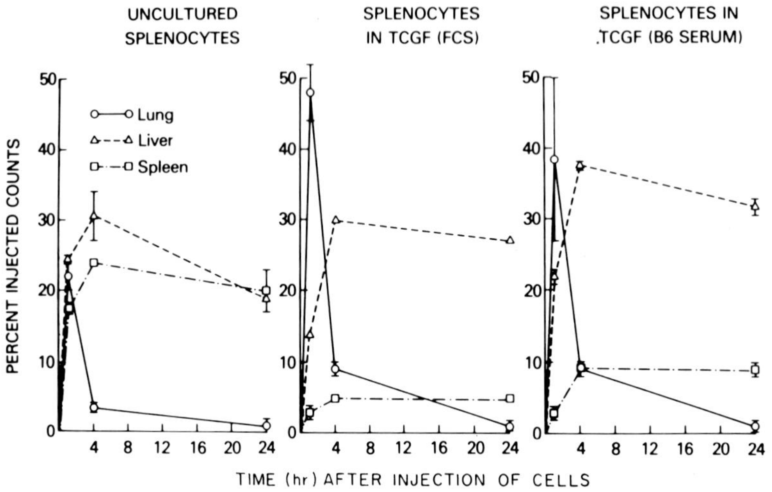

Fig. 1. Traffic of normal splenocytes (left) or splenocytes cultured in TCGF made with fetal calf serum (middle) or syngeneic mouse serum (right). Splenocytes were labeled with ^{51}Cr and then injected *in vivo*. At varying times, organs were excised and the radioactivity counts in each organ determined. Uncultured splenocytes distributed primarily to the liver and spleen. Splenocytes cultured in TCGF distributed predominantly to the lung with clearing after about 2–4 hr with distribution of lymphoid cells predominantely to the liver. More splenocytes distributed to the spleen following culture in TCGF-containing mouse serum then when lymphocytes were grown in TCGF -containing fetal calf serum (from Lotze *et al.*, 1980).

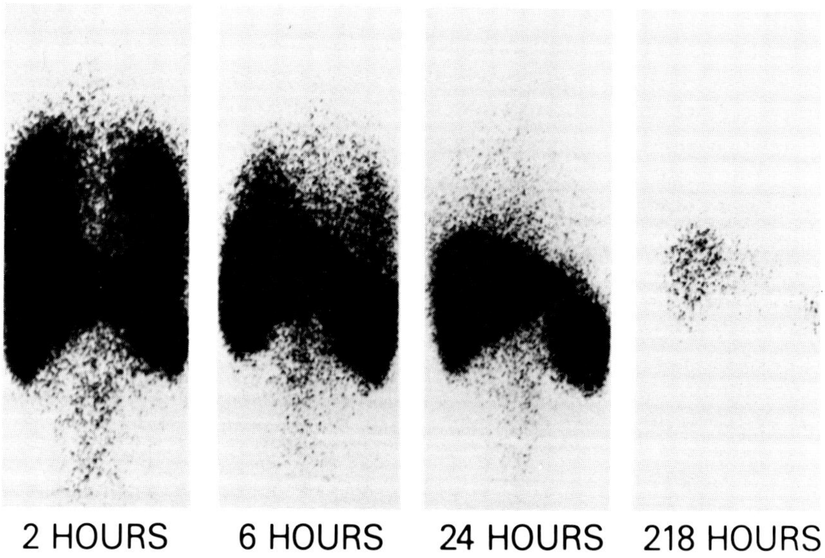

Fig. 2. Sequential rectilinear scans following injection of indium-111 labeled cells expanded in TCGF. The scan was made from neck to pelvis at similar machine settings for each sequential scan. By 2 hr cells are present in the lung, liver, and spleen. The lung clears quite rapidly, and by 24 hr counts are confined almost exclusively to liver and spleen (from Lotze *et al.*, 1980).

To determine the distribution of human cells expanded in TCGF and reinjected into the autologous host, peripheral blood lymphoid cells from tumor-bearing patients were expanded up to 20,000-fold in TCGF preparations containing human serum. These cells were then labeled with either gallium-67 or indium-111, and the organ distribution of injected cells was noninvasively measured by several techniques (Lotze *et al.*, 1980). These included measurement by rectilinear scanning using a whole body imager (Fig. 2), point counting over individual organs with a collimated whole body scanner, and use of a computer interfaced gamma camera to assess the total organ distribution of measured radioactivity. In addition, blood and urine samples were measured at varying intervals following cell injection.

The distribution *in vivo* of human cells expanded in TCGF (Fig. 3) was similar to that seen in the mouse. In the first 4 hr following injection, over 30% of cells distributed to the lung, with substantial clearance from the lung over the first 48 hr. During the first 2 days following injection, cells accumulated predominately in the liver, though approximately 25% of injected cells distributed to the spleen. Traces of radioactivity could be found in the liver and spleen up to 10 days following injection of indium-111 labeled cells. Also of interest was the rapid clearance of these cells from the peripheral blood in the human. By 20 min after injection only 5–6% of cells cultured in TCGF could be recovered from the peripheral blood. Although we did not study the distribution of labeled autologous normal lymphocytes, a recent report described that up to 50% of indium-111 labeled normal lymphocytes could be detected in the peripheral blood shortly

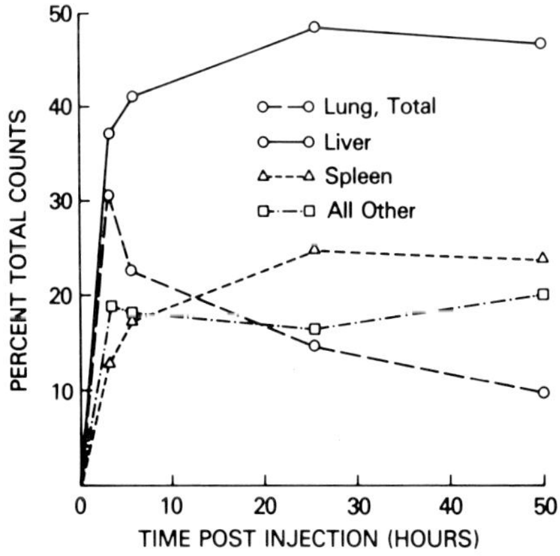

Fig. 3. Traffic of lymphoid cells expanded in TCGF following reinjection intravenously into the human. Peripheral blood lymphocytes were grown in T cell growth factor and labeled with indium-111. These lymphocytes were then injected intravenously. At varying times gamma camera views of the thorax and abdomen were obtained. The total activity in the lung, spleen, liver, and all remaining areas is expressed at a percentage of the total counts in the camera field (from Lotze *et al.*, 1980).

after iv infusion (Lavender *et al.*, 1977). The distribution of normal autologous lymphocytes exhibited a liver to spleen ratio of 1.5 to 2 seen in our studies of cells expanded in TCGF.

It is likely that the larger cultured lymphocytes growing in TCGF are removed from the circulation initially by the lung because this is the first capillary bed traversed following intravenous injection. These cells appeared to clear from the lung and redistribute to the liver and spleen during the days after intravenous injection. One to 2% of injected counts continue to exist in the peripheral circulation for up to 2 days following intravenous injections. Though cells expanded in TCGF show a substantially different pattern from that of normal cells, sufficient numbers of cells expanded in TCGF remain in the circulation and lymphoid organs to potentially mediate immunologic effects.

II. EFFECT *IN VIVO* OF ADOPTIVELY TRANSFERRED CELLS EXPANDED IN T CELL GROWTH FACTOR

The unusual pattern *in vivo* of cells expanded in TCGF raises some concerns about the function of these immune cells when reinjected into the host. There have been few studies of the effects *in vivo* of lymphoid cells expanded in TCGF. Tees and Shreier (1980) demonstrated that cloned helper cells expanded in TCGF were capable of restoring the plaque forming cell response of nude mouse when the cells expanded in TCGF were adoptively transferred *in vivo*. This reconstitution appeared to be immunologically specific. Though nude mice are incapable of producing TCGF, it was hypothesized that these cells survived for prolonged periods *in vivo,* since mice reconstituted with cloned helper cells continued to respond to antigen for up to 21 days after the adoptive transfer.

The first demonstration that immune lymphoid cells expanded in TCGF were capable of mediating tissue rejection *in vivo* were the studies of Rosenstein *et al.*, (1981). These workers utilized a skin allograft rejection model to study the effect of specifically allosensitized lymphoid cells expanded in TCGF. This model is valuable in establishing the factors that are required for the successful adoptive transfer of the ability to reject tissue using cells expanded in TCGF. These workers used (B6A) F_1 mice transplanted with skin from B10.BR mice. These two mouse strains differ at the *I-C* subregion as well as the *D* end of the *H-2* complex. Skin grafts between these two strains are rejected in approximately 14 days. The adoptive transfer of anti-B10.BR cells, sensitized either *in vivo* or *in vitro,* 1 day after application of the skin graft causes the accelerated rejection of these skin grafts from 14 to approximately 8 days (Chang and Sugarbaker, 1980). Rosenstein *et al.* (1981) sensitized cells *in vitro* and expanded them in TCGF and demonstrated that from 1.5×10^7 to 3×10^7 cells treated in this way were capable of mediating the accelerated rejection of B10.BR skin grafts on (B6A) F_1 mice.

A typical experiment is seen in Fig. 4. Untreated (B6A) F_1 mice receiving B10.BR skin grafts rejected their skin at 12.6 ± 0.2 days (mean ± 1 standard error). The adoptive transfer of 3×10^7 (B6A) F_1 anti-B10.BR cells sensitized *in vitro* and expanded in TCGF resulted in the accelerated rejection of these skin grafts at 8.0 ± 0.7 days. This reaction was immunologically specific. (B6A) F_1 anti-B10.D2 or nonsensitized (B6A) F_1 cells expanded in TCGF were incapable of accelerating graft rejection. The rejection time of the mice receiving B5AF1 anti-B10.BR cells were significantly different than that of any other group ($p < .01$) (Fig. 4).

Of further interest, Rosenstein *et al.* (1981) demonstrated that irradiation with 2000 R of cells grown in TCGF prior to adoptive transfer, completely abrogated the ability of these cells to accelerate rejection of skin grafts. It thus appears that proliferation of cells *in vivo* is necessary for their immunologic effect following injection *in vivo*. The inability of irradiated cells to cause graft rejection and the 7 day delay between the injection of the cells and the rejection of the skin grafts provide circumstantial evidence that prolonged survival of cells expanded in TCGF exists following injection *in vivo*.

	Donor	Recipient	Cells Transferred	MST + SE (N)	P Valve	Fold Expansion
——	B10.BR	B6AF₁	No Treatment	12.6+.24 (5)	p< 0.0005	NA
— —			3×10⁷ B6AF₁ Anti-B10.BR	8.0+.71 (4)	p< 0.005	6.6X
—·—			3×10⁷ B6AF₁ Anti-B10.D₂	13.0+.57 (4)	p< 0.01	5.8X
—··—			3×10⁷ Nonsensitized B6AF₁	11.4+.75 (5)		6.1X

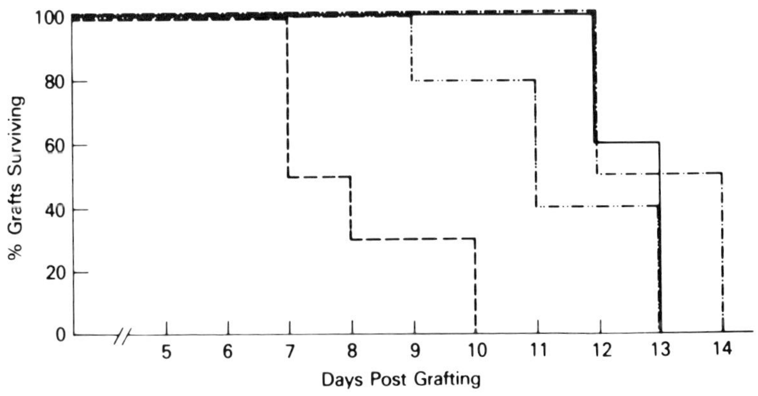

Fig. 4. Specificity of skin allograft rejection following adoptive transfer of cells expanded in TCGF. Accelerated rejection of B10.BR skin grafts on (B6A) F_1 recipient mice occurs following adoptive transfer of (B6A) F_1 anti-B10.BR lymphoid cells expanded in TCGF. The survival of skin graft of mice receiving adoptive transfer of cells expanded in TCGF that were sensitized to other alloantigens or that were nonsensitized is not different from that of mice receiving no treatment (from Rosenstein *et al.*, 1981).

The treatment of mice with disseminated lymphoma using lymphoid cells sensitized *in vitro* and expanded in TCGF has been explored by Cheever *et al.* (1981) and Eberlein *et al.* (1981). These workers have used a chemoimmunotherapy model developed by Fass and Fefer (1972), who demonstrated that the combination of cytoxan plus lymphocytes immunized *in vivo* was capable of curing mice with a disseminated lymphoma when treatment was instituted 5 days after intraperitoneal injection of lymphoma. The coculture of immunized splenocytes with FBL-3 lymphoma *in vitro* followed by expansion in TCGF resulted in the generation of cells that were also capable of curing mice when administered in conjunction with cyclophosphamide chemotherapy (Cheever *et al.*, 1981 Eberlein *et al.*, 1981).

Cheever *et al.* (1981) showed that a 7-fold expansion of immunized lymphocytes over a 19-day period in TCGF resulted in cells that were effective in treating mice with this disseminated lymphoma. Eberlein *et al.* (1981) extended these observations by demonstrating that cells cultured for over 2.5 months and expanded over 10,000-fold were also capable of curing mice with this lymphoma. A typical experiment is presented in Fig. 5. As can be seen, the injection of tumor intraperitoneally resulted in the death of all mice. Treatment with cyclophosphamide alone or cyclophosphamide plus nonsensitized cells expanded in TCGF were incapable of curing mice. However, treatment with immunized cells expanded in TCGF administered in conjunction with cyclophosphamide 5 days after intraperitoneal tumor injection was capable of curing mice with disseminated lymphoma. Eberlein *et al.* (1981) further demonstrated that irradiation

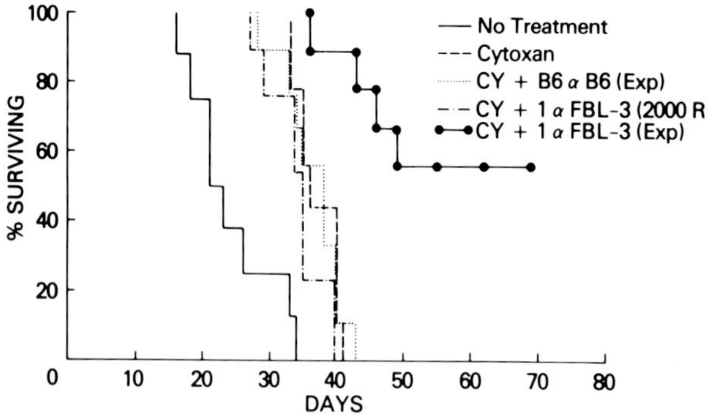

Fig. 5. Treatment of mice bearing disseminated FBL-3 lymphoma with appropriately sensitized lymphoid cells expanded for 2.5 months in TCGF. Only mice receiving cytoxan (Cy) plus appropriately sensitized cells expanded in TCGF are cured of disseminated lymphoma (Cyt+1 α FLB-3). Mice receiving cytoxan plus normal cells expanded in TCGF for this same period of time (Cy+B6 α B6) survive no differently than mice receiving cytoxan alone. Also included in this experiment are sensitized cells expanded in TCGF and then irradiated with 2000 R prior to adoptive transfer. This irradiation completely abrogates the ability of these cells to cure mice with this disseminated lymphoma (from Eberlein *et al.*, 1981).

of lymphoid cells prior to intraperitoneal injection abrogated their immunotherapeutic effect and that adoptive transfer of cloned cells isolated and expanded in TCGF was also capable of prolonging the survival of mice with FBL-3 lymphoma. These experiments demonstrate that immunized lymphoid cells expanded in TCGF are capable of reducing the growth of tumor *in vivo,* and in some instances of curing mice with disseminated tumor. Attempts to extend these observations to other solid tumors are currently in progress.

III. ISOLATION OF T LYMPHOCYTE CLONES SPECIFICALLY REACTIVE WITH TUMOR

It has been extremely difficult to identify lymphoid cells with strong reactivity against tumor cell surface antigens. The poor immunogenicity of tumor antigens as well as the probable presence of sensitization defects in the tumor-bearing host probably account for the presence of a very low incidence of lymphoid cells with specific antitumor reactivity. The use of cloning techniques in conjunction with methods for enhancing the relative incidence of antitumor reactive cells offers promise for the identification of cells that may be useful in adoptive immunotherapy. Cloning of T cells may also enable the removal, from the expansion of reactive cells from single effector T lymphoid cells, of other lymphoid cell subpopulations that might suppress or otherwise modulate antitumor reactivity.

We have developed several techniques that appear promising for the isolation of T lymphoid clones with antitumor reactivity. These techniques involve the cloning of T lymphoid cells from mixed tumor lymphocyte cultures as well as techniques for cloning T lymphoid cells that directly infiltrate solid murine and human tumors.

The reactivity of cloned cells is screened directly from limiting cultures (Eberlein *et al.*, 1981). T lymphoid cells are plated at limiting dilution in the wells of flat bottom 96-well microtiter trays in medium containing TCGF. An attempt is made to plate a sufficient number of cells to cause growth in approximately 30% of wells in the microtiter plate. Using the Poisson distribution one can calculate that approximately 80% of such wells with growth will have arisen from an individual starting cell. Using this technique interesting "clones" can be identified and recloned. After growth for 10 days a multiple tipped automatic pipettor is used to remove an aliquot from each well which is added to a replica plate containing between 10^3 and 10^4 chromium-labeled tumor target cells. Additional media is added to the original cloning plates to keep these cells alive until after the assay. The chromium release assay plate is then incubated from 4 to 18 hr, and the lysis of tumor cells in each well is measured using an automated harvester. Wells with significant tumor lysis are identified, and those "interesting" wells on the original plate are then harvested and grown for subsequent studies. These cells are then immediately recloned. This technique can be used to simultaneously test for reactivity against two or more target cells by utilizing multiple smaller aliquots from each well of the original cloning plate.

Utilizing this technique approximately 1000 clones can be assayed for antitumor reactivity on a single day. An example of the use of this technique to isolate clones with specific anti-FBL-3 lymphoma tumor reactivity from C57BL/6 mice is shown in Fig. 6, taken from the work of Eberlein *et al.* (1981). Spleens from mice immunized *in vivo* with the FBL-3 tumor were cocultured with FBL-3 tumor *in vitro* for 5 days and then cloned. After 10 days of growth each well in these limiting dilution plates was then tested for lytic activity directed against the FBL-3 tumor target. Simultaneously, normal splenocytes that had been cocultured with normal syngeneic lymphoid cells were also cloned and screened using these techniques. The results of a characteristic experiment are shown on Fig. 6. As can be seen, the control nonsensitized cultures show a distribution of lytic clones against the FBL-3 tumor (left). However, the cloned

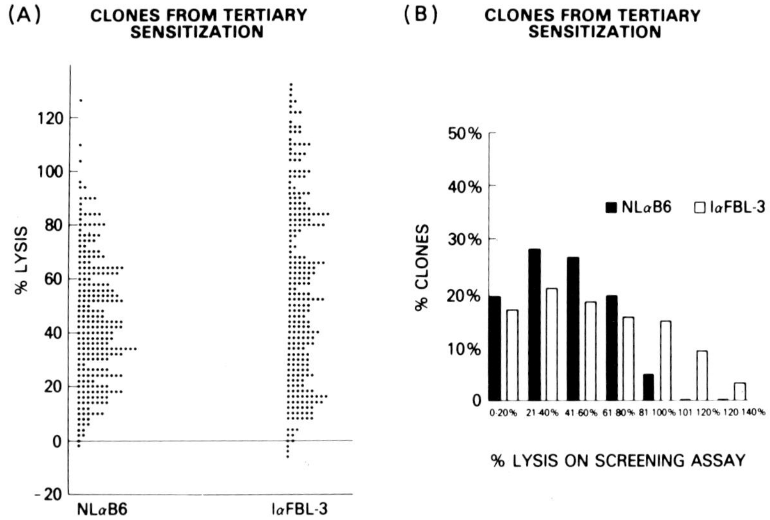

Fig. 6. Screening of multiple clones for anti-FBL-3 tumor reactivity. Splenocytes from immunized mice were sensitized three times to FBL-3 tumor *in vitro* and then cloned using limiting dilution techniques. Using the screening technique described in the text, the lytic capacity of each clone was tested. (Left): Each dot represents the percent lysis of an individual clone in an 18 hr chromium release assay. The cloning of normal cells sensitized *in vitro* to normal lymphocytes (NL α B6) and cloning of immunized cells sensitized *in vitro* to FBL-3 tumor (I α FBL-3) is also shown. (Right): The distribution of lytic clones in both control and *in vitro* sensitized cultures. As can be seen a much larger number of highly lytic clones are seen in the *in vitro* immunized cultures compared to controls (from Eberlein *et al.*, 1981).

cells sensitized *in vitro* showed a small number (approximately 5%) of cells that had substantial levels of anti-FBL-3 cytotoxic reactivity that were not seen in the control cultures. These cells were harvested and expanded and retained their anti-FBL-3 reactivity. Similar techniques may be of use in identifying human clones with for reactivity for autologous tumor. These studies are currently in progress.

A second approach to the isolation of lymphoid cells with specific antitumor reactivity is the isolation of lymphoid cells directly infiltrating solid tumors (Yron *et al.*, 1980). Most solid tumors contain about 5% of host lymphoid cells,

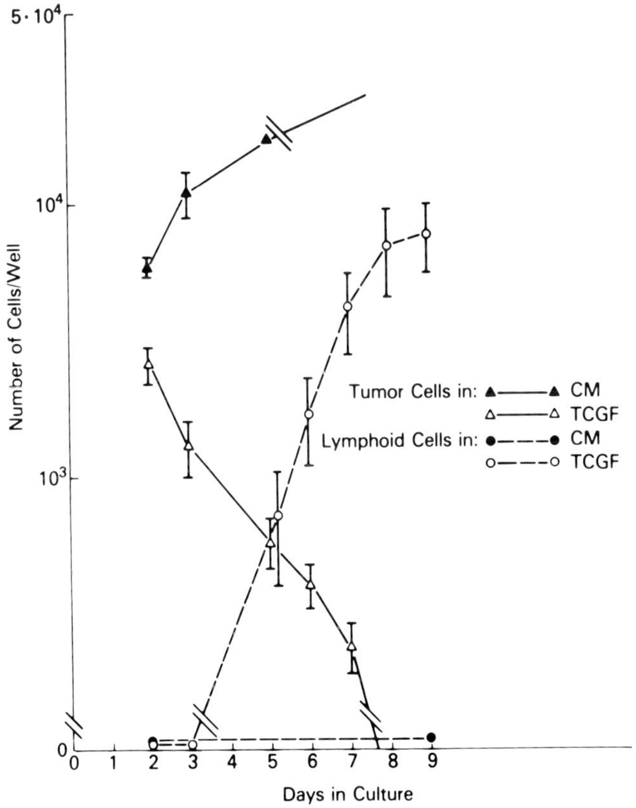

Fig. 7. Isolation of lymphoid cells infiltrating a solid human tumor. TCGF was used to isolate lymphoid cells infiltrating a solid methylcolanthrene induced tumor. The solid tumor was digested for short times in trypsin and collagenase and then placed in culture in medium containing TCGF. In the absence of TCGF tumor cells grew into confluent cultures. In the presence of TCGF the growth of lymphoid cells was seen beginning on about the third day. As lymphoid cells grew the tumor cells died and by 8 days a pure culture of tumor infiltrating lymphocytes was present in the culture (from Yron *et al.*, 1980).

and several workers have claimed that lymphoid cells have unique antitumor reactivities. Yron *et al.* (1980) have developed a rapid and simple technique for isolating and purifying lymphoid cells directly infiltrating mouse tumors that also is effective for the isolation of lymphocytes infiltrating solid human tumors. This technique is based on the unique ability of T lymphoid cells to grow in TCGF and the ability of these cells to lyse cultured tumor cells. Solid tumor fragments were exposed for short times to trypsin and collagenase, and the resulting tumor and infiltrating lymphoid cell suspensions placed in tissue culture medium containing TCGF (see Fig. 7). After approximately 8 days of culture, the lymphoid cells grew to large numbers. The tumor cells in the suspension were lysed by the expanding lymphoid cells. By 8 days after initiation of the culture a pure population of tumor-infiltrating lymphoid cells was present. Yron *et al.* (1980) have

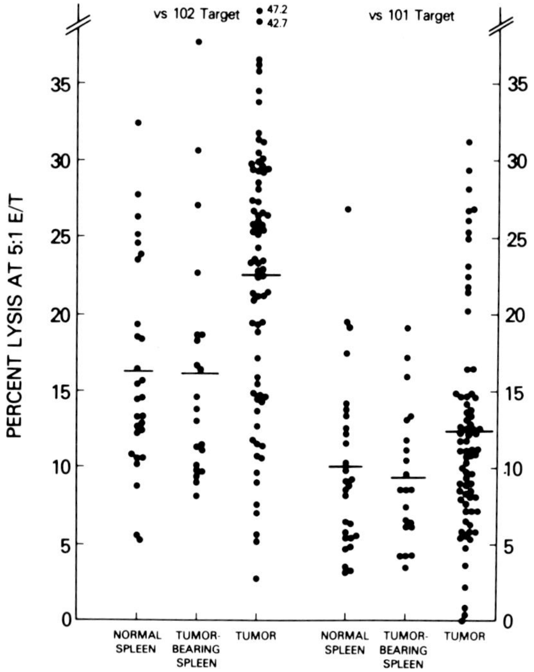

Fig. 8. The cloning of lymphoid cells directly from solid methylcholanthrene-induced tumor (MCA-102). Using limiting dilution techniques lymphoid cells were cloned directly from the solid MCA-102 tumor. Single cells suspensions were made from tumor, and limiting numbers of cells were plated in the wells of microtiter plates such that limiting numbers of lymphocytes were added to each well. In the presence of TCGF, only wells containing lymphoid cells exhibited growth. These clones were then individually tested for lysis in a 4-hr ^{51}Cr release assay against the 102 tumor target (left), as well as against the MCA-101 tumor (right), a non-cross-reactive tumor. Simultaneously cells were cloned from the spleens of both tumor-bearing and normal mice. As can be seen, a larger percentage of clones obtained from the solid tumor were highly lytic against the specific 102 target.

extensively studied the phenotypic cell surface markers and functional characteristics of the tumor-infiltrating lymphoid cells isolated in this manner.

We have recently utilized this technique to clone, in TGCF, T lymphoid cells that directly infiltrate murine tumors. This can be readily accomplished by plating tumor cell suspensions into the wells of microtiter plates at cell concentrations such that the number of infiltrating T lymphoid cells is limiting. Wells that contain T lymphoid cells exhibit growth of these lymphoid cells while the tumor cells in these wells are lysed. Visual screening of the wells identifies the T lymphoid clones which can then be individually harvested and expanded. An example of an experiment in which T lymphoid cells infiltrating a methylcholanthrene-induced sarcoma in C57BL/6 mice were cloned is shown in Fig. 8. In this experiment spleen cells from the tumor-bearing mouse and normal spleen cells were also cloned. As can be seen, the lymphocytes which have infiltrated the tumor appeared to have a larger percentage of clones with high antitumor reactivity than was seen in either the tumor-bearing or the normal spleen. M. T. Lotze *et al.* (unpublished observations) has shown that similar techniques are applicable to the study of lymphoid cells infiltrating solid human tumors.

IV. THE LYSIS OF FRESH SYNGENEIC OR AUTOLOGOUS TUMOR CELLS BY LYMPHOID CELLS EXPANDED IN T CELL GROWTH FACTOR

An interesting finding that deserves discussion in a review of the cloning of antitumor T lymphoid cells in TCGF is the observation, made first by Yron *et al.* in the mouse (1980) and Lotze *et al.* in the human (1980, 1981), that lymphoid cells from either normal or tumor-bearing individuals, when expanded in TCGF, are capable of lysing fresh syngeneic or autologous tumor cells as well as virtually all cultured normal and tumor target cells. Yron *et al.* (1980) demonstrated that C57BL/6 splenocytes from either normal or tumor-bearing mice expanded in TCGF were capable of killing a wide variety of fresh malignant cells in a 4-hr chromium release assay (see Fig. 9). Normal syngeneic splenocytes were not killed by cells grown in TCGF. This lytic capacity for fresh autologous tumor arises after a 3-day exposure to TCGF and is mediated by Lyt-$1^{-}2^{+}$ cells. Because these killer cells can lyse fresh autologous tumor in short-term assays and because they are Lyt-2^{+}, it does not appear that they are related to conventional natural killer cells.

Similar observations were made by Lotze *et al.* (1980, 1981) and E. A. Grimm *et al.* (unpublished observations) who demonstrated that peripheral blood lymphoid cells from patients bearing a variety of tumors were capable of killing fresh autologous tumor following expansion of these lymphoid cells in TCGF (See

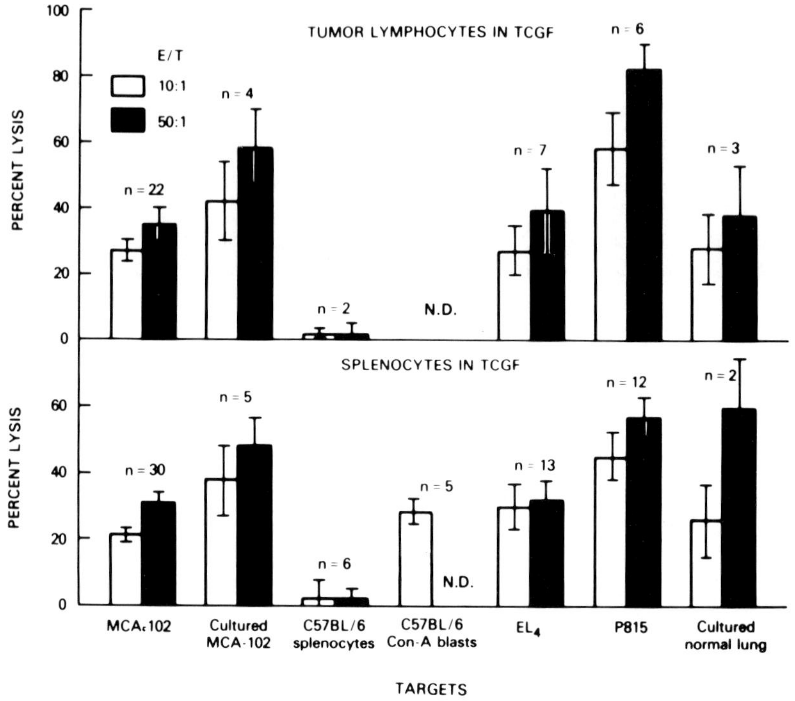

Fig. 9. Cytotoxic activity of murine lymphoid cells grown in TCGF. Lymphoid cells from the spleens of normal animals (lower), as well as lymphoid cells infiltrating a solid tumor (upper) were expanded in T cell growth factor and checked for cytotoxicity against a variety of target cells. Lymphoid cells expanded in TCGF were lytic for a variety of fresh syngeneic tumors in the C57BL/6 mouse (MCA-102 and EL-4). These cells were also lytic for an allogeneic tumor (P815) as well as for a cultured normal and tumor cell line, but not for fresh syngeneic splenocytes (from Yron *et al.*, 1980).

Fig. 10). In both the mouse and human, lysis of fresh cells appears limited to malignant cells, though virtually all cultured cell targets are lysed. In preliminary cloning experiments, Lotze (1981) has demonstrated that only selected lymphoid cells expanded in TCGF can lyse fresh autologous tumor.

The biologic significance of the lysis of fresh autologous tumor by normal lymphoid cells expanded in TCGF is not clear. In the human, this lysis appears to be a property of unsensitized cells, since this reactivity is manifested in the absence of any exposure to foreign antigen or xenogeneic serum. The antitumor reactivity of these cells may be of interest in studies of immune surveillance against tumors and perhaps for the development of cloned lymphoid cells of value in adoptive immunotherapy. The presence of this natural antitumor reactivity that appears when cells are grown in TCGF must be considered when cloned cells are used in the search for lymphocytes with unique antitumor specificities.

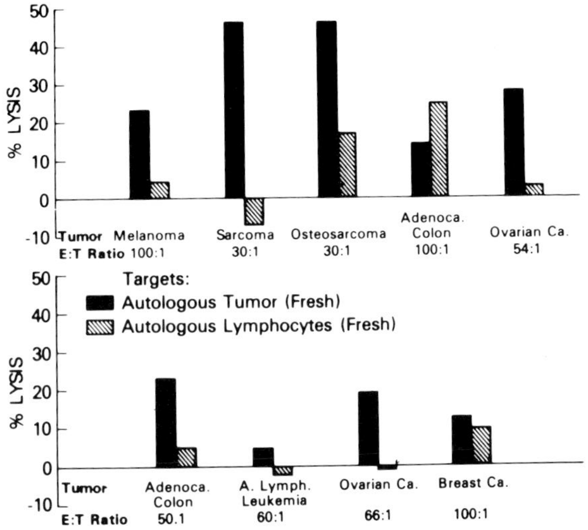

Fig. 10. Lysis of fresh human tumor and fresh lymphocytes by autologous lymphocytes cultured in TCGF. Peripheral blood lymphocytes from cancer patients were grown in TCGF and then tested for cytotoxicity using a 4-hr chromium release assay against autologous fresh tumor as well as autologous lymphocytes. Patients with a variety of tumors were tested. In most patients, substantial lysis of autologous fresh tumor cells were seen (from Lotze *et al.*, 1981).

V. CONCLUSIONS

Examples of successful adoptive immunotherapy of murine tumors have spurred efforts to develop approaches to the specific adoptive immunotherapy of cancer in man. The recent development of techniques for cloning and expanding T lymphoid cells *in vitro,* using TCGF, opens new promising approaches to the development of successful adoptive immunotherapies for human cancer. An approach to adoptive immunotherapy based on the cloning and expansion of tumor-reactive lymphoid cells from the tumor-bearing host represents an approach to adoptive immunotherapy that theoretically overcomes many of the objections to successful treatment. The demonstration in murine systems that lymphoid cells expanded in TCGF can mediate the rejection both of skin allografts as well as a syngeneic disseminated lymphoma provides encouraging evidence that the adoptive transfer of appropriately reactive cells is capable of mediating tissue rejection *in vivo*.

REFERENCES

Chang, A. E., and Sugarbaker, P. H. (1980). Assessment of T cell function with a skin allograft assay. *Transplantation* **29**, 381.

Cheever, M. A., Greenberg, P. D., and Fefer, A. (1981). Specific adoptive therapy of established leukemia with syngeneic lymphocytes sequentially immunized *in vivo* and *in vitro* and non-specifically expanded by culture with interleukin 2. *J. Immunol.* **126,** 1318.

Eberlein, T. J., Rosenstein, M., Spiess, P. J., and Rosenberg, S. A. (1981). The generation of long term T-lymphoid cell lines with specific cytotoxic reactivity for a syngeneic murine lymphoma. *J. Immunol.* (submitted for publication).

Fass, L., and Fefer, A. (1972). Studies of adoptive chemoimmunotherapy of a Friend virus-induced lymphoma. *Cancer Res.* **32,** 997.

Lavender, J. P., Goldman, J. M., Arnot, R. N., and Thakur, M. L. (1977). Kinetics of Indium-111 labeled lymphocytes in normal subjects and patients with Hodgkin's disease. *Br. Med. J.* **2,** 797.

Lotze, M. T., Strausser, J. L., Line, B. R., and Rosenberg, S. A. (1980). Tumor lysis by human T lymphocytes in long term culture and their distribution *in vivo:* Implications for immunotherapy. *Surg. Forum* **30,** 404.

Lotze, M. T., Strausser, J. L., and Rosenberg, S. A. (1981). *In vitro* growth of cytotoxic human lymphocytes. IV. Lysis of fresh and cultured autologous tumor by lymphocytes cultured in T cell growth factor (TCGF). *Cancer Res.* (in press).

Rosenberg, S. A., and Terry, W. (1977). Passive immunotherapy of cancer in animals and man. *Adv. Cancer Res.* **25,** 323.

Rosenstein, M., Eberlein, T., Kemeny, M. M., Sugarbaker, P. H., and Rosenberg, S. A. (1981). *In vitro* growth of murine T cells. VI. Accelerated skin graft rejection caused by adoptively transferred cells granted in T cell growth factor. *J. Immunol.* **127,** 566.

Strausser, J. L., and Rosenberg, S. A. (1978). *In vitro* growth of cytotoxic human lymphocytes. I. Growth of cells sensitized *in vitro* to alloantigens. *J. Immunol.* **121,** 1491.

Tees, R., and Shreier, M. H. (1980). Selective reconstitution of nude mice with long-term cultured and cloned specific helper cells. *Nature* (*London*) **283,** 780.

Yron, I., Wood, T. A., Spiess, P., and Rosenberg, S. A. (1980). *In vitro* growth of murine T cells. V. The isolation and growth of lymphoid cells infiltrating syngeneic solid tumors. *J. Immunol.* **125,** 238.

39

Cloned T Cells as a Tool for Molecular Geneticists: Approaches to Cloning Genes Which Encode T Cell Antigen Receptors

Mitchell Kronenberg/Ellen Kraig/
Suzanna J. Horvath/Leroy E. Hood

I. Immunoglobulin Expression in Cloned T Cells 468
A. J_L and C_L Gene Expression in B Lymphocytes 469
B. J_L and C_L Gene Expression in T Lymphocytes 469
C. J_H and C_H Gene Expression in B Lymphocytes 470
D. J_H and C_H Gene Expression in T Lymphocytes 470
E. V_H Gene Expression in T Lymphocytes 473
F. Summary 480
II. Cloning Nonimmunoglobulin Genes from T Cells 480
A. Selection of a cDNA Clone through Assay of Its Corresponding RNA and Protein Product 481
B. Selection of a Clone Using Partial Amino Acid Sequence and Oliogonucleotide Synthesis 483
C. Characterization of a Protein Encoded by a Cloned DNA Sequence 485
III. Conclusions 486
References 487

In the past decade, there have been profound advances in our understanding of the organization and regulation of immunoglobulin genes in B cells. This was due largely to the refinement of recombinant DNA technology and the availability of relatively stable and homogeneous B cells (myelomas and lymphomas). Previous studies on the molecular basis of T cell function were limited either to heterogeneous T cell sources, often enriched from spleen, thymus, or lymph node, or to T lymphomas, whose antigen specificities and T cell functional class were usually unknown. However, as described elsewhere in this treatise, several groups have now succeeded in cloning T cells. Most of the clones

ISBN 0-12-249920-4

maintain functions characteristic of the appropriate T cell subclass, are antigen specific, and are often MHC restricted in their action. Such T cell clones provide well-defined, homogeneous material for molecular analyses of the T cell receptor gene structure, organization, and regulation.

In this chapter, we will begin with a review of the attempts by our group and others to analyze the gene(s) encoding the T cell antigen-binding receptor. Thus far, the primary approach has been the use of immunoglobulin gene probes to detect rearrangement or transcription of immunoglobulin gene segments. However, since it is possible that the T cell antigen receptor will not utilize any immunoglobulin gene segments, we will also discuss general approaches to cloning genes from T cells. Though we will concentrate on the T cell antigen-binding receptor, the strategies described may pertain equally well to the isolation of other genes from cloned T cells, such as lymphokines and T cell differentiation antigens.

I. IMMUNOGLOBULIN EXPRESSION IN CLONED T CELLS

To characterize the T cell antigen receptor, we wished to determine whether immunoglobulin gene segments were expressed by T cells. This was a logical approach for several reasons. First, there have been reports that T cells synthesize polypeptides or RNA molecules containing immunoglobulin constant regions (Marchalonis, 1975; Storb, 1978; Lahat *et al.*, 1978). Much evidence showing the absence of constant region expression also exists (Binz and Wigzell, 1977; Loor, 1977; Rajewsky and Eichmann, 1977), and this question had not been settled. Second, serological and immunogenetic data indicated that T cells responding to carbohydrates (Eichmann and Rajewsky, 1975), MHC alloantigens (Binz and Wigzell, 1975), haptens (Cosenza *et al.*, 1977), and either natural or synthetic polypeptides (Harvey *et al.*, 1979; Germain *et al.*, 1979) expressed idiotypic determinants. Anti-idiotypic sera affected T cell functions, bound to antigen-specific secreted products of T cells, and in some cases could be used to purify antigen-binding molecules (reviewed in Eichmann, 1978; Germain and Benacerraf, 1980). While these data are not completely convincing, a number of established laboratories independently arrived at the concluson that T cells express antigenic determinants of heavy chain variable regions. Third, the presence of idiotypes on T cells appeared consistent with network and circuit theories of immunoregulation (Jerne, 1974; Herzenberg *et al.*, 1980). Fourth, a variety of cloned B cell immunoglobulin DNA probes was already available. The rearrangement of these genes and their patterns of transcription had been well characterized in B cells, and the presence of a particular variable region RNA in an antigen-specific T cell would in itself provide strong evidence that the receptor had been identified. Thus, with the appropriate cloned T cells, the initial experiments would be relatively simple technically and could be quite fruitful.

A. J_L and C_L Gene Expression in B Lymphocytes

The light chains are encoded by two unlinked gene families (λ and κ), each of which contains three different types of genetic elements, V, J, and C. The C_L gene encodes the constant region and is separated from the cluster of J_L gene segments by a kilobase (1000 nucleotides) or more of intervening DNA sequence (Fig. 1). During B cell differentiation, the two gene segments encoding the variable region (V_L and J_L) are joined to form the light chain transcription unit (Bernard *et al.*, 1978). In the λ and κ families, highly conserved sequences adjacent to V_L and J_L mediate joining of these gene segments (Max *et al.*, 1979; Sakano *et al.*, 1979). The intervening sequence which separates J_L and C_L is subsequently removed from the initial RNA transcript by splicing to produce the functional mRNA (Gilmore-Hebert and Wall, 1978; Gilmore-Hebert *et al.*, 1978). Therefore, it should be possible to look in T cells for evidence of light chain gene rearrangement as well as transcription and processing of light chain RNA.

B. J_L and C_L Gene Expression in T Lymphocytes

To look for gene rearrangement, a Southern blot is used (Southern, 1975). Briefly, the T cell DNA is digested with a restriction enzyme which cuts at specific nucleotide sequences. The resulting DNA fragments are separated by size on a gel, denatured, and subsequently transferred to nitrocellulose paper.

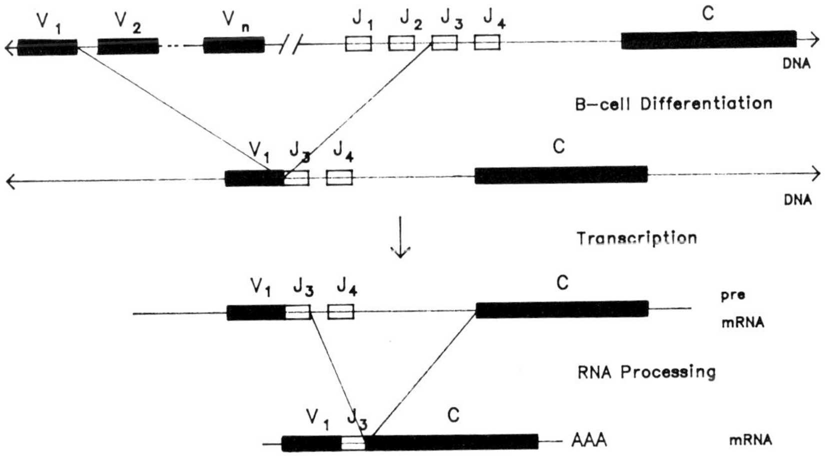

Fig. 1. The DNA rearrangement, transcription, and RNA processing steps necessary for light chain gene expression are depicted. Rectangles represent V_L, J_L, and C_L gene coding sequences, while the thin horizontal line denotes the intervening sequences. DNA and RNA sequences are not drawn to scale.

The denatured DNA can then be hybridized to a radioactive probe. To examine the transcripts in a T cell, a Northern blot is used (Alwine *et al.*, 1977). RNA is extracted and the poly(A)-containing fraction is purified by oligo(dT)-cellulose chromatography. The poly$(A)^+$ RNA is then separated by size on a denaturing gel and transferred to paper for hybridization with a radioactive probe.

Using light chain gene probes, Kronenberg *et al.* (1980) demonstrated that C_κ, J_κ, C_λ, J_λ are not rearranged in a cloned helper and a cloned killer T cell line. Similar results have been reported for a number of killer T cell lines (Forster *et al.*, 1980; Cayre *et al.*, 1981), T cell hybridomas (Zuniga *et al.*, 1982), as well as T lymphomas (Kemp *et al.*, 1980a). In addition, there was no evidence for transcription of light chain constant region sequences in any homogeneous T cell tested (Kronenberg *et al.*, 1980; Kemp *et al.*, 1980a). We conclude, therefore, that light chain J and C genes are not expressed by cloned T cells.

C. J_H and C_H Gene Expression in B Lymphocytes

The murine heavy chain gene family consists of a large number of V_H gene segments, an unknown number of D (diversity) gene segments, four functional J_H gene segments, and at least eight C_H genes. During early B cell differentiation, two DNA rearrangements, V_H–D and D–J_H joining, lead to the formation of a complete variable gene (Fig. 2). The joining of heavy chain gene segments deletes the intervening DNA and is mediated by DNA sequences homologous to those employed in V_L–J_L joining (Early *et al.*, 1980a). These data suggest that a similar joining mechanism is employed in the three antibody gene families. The heavy chain transcription unit formed by this DNA joining includes a complete variable gene (V–D–J) separated by about 8 kilobases from the C_μ gene. RNA splicing removes the large intervening sequence between the J_H and C_μ coding regions, as well as the short introns (intervening sequences) between the four exons (coding sequences) of the C_μ gene. Alternative RNA processing of μ chain mRNA also is involved in the differential expression of the membrane and secreted forms of the C_μ heavy chain (Rogers *et al.*, 1980; Early *et al.*, 1980b). In addition, the heavy chain transcription unit may be altered during B cell differentiation by a heavy chain class switch in which the C_μ gene is deleted and replaced by one of the other constant region genes (Davis *et al.*, 1980a). This DNA rearrangement is mediated by switch sequences which flank the C_H genes and which are not homologous to the sequences involved in V_L–J_L or V_H–D–J_H joining (Davis *et al.*, 1980b; Hood *et al.*, 1981).

D. J_H and C_H Gene Expression in T Lymphocytes

In two cloned T cells, a helper and a killer, the C_μ and C_α genes are not rearranged (Kronenberg *et al.*, 1980). Furthermore, the C_μ genes and 5′ flanking sequences are also in the germline configuration in a number of other cloned

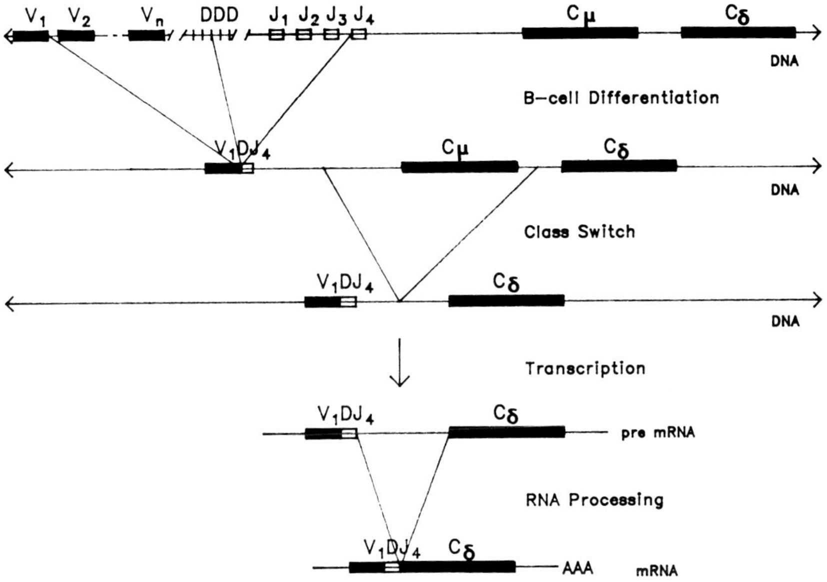

Fig. 2. Expression of heavy chain genes. Some steps in heavy chain gene expression are shown. Rectangles represent V_H, J_H and C_H exons (coding sequences), short vertical lines represent the *D* gene segments, and the thin horizontal line indicates introns (intervening DNA sequences). Introns between the exons encoding the C_H domains and the separate membrane exons have been omitted for the sake of simplicity. Sequences are not drawn to scale.

killer T cells (Forster *et al.*, 1980; Cayre *et al.*, 1981) and several T lymphomas (Cory *et al.*, 1980). However, it is possible that in cloned T cells, C_μ or other C_H genes have been deleted on one homolog as they are in B cells which have switched from expression of C_μ to expression of other C_H genes. If so, this deletion would have to occur via a mechanism different from the B cell heavy chain class switch, since the switch sequences adjacent to C_μ are not rearranged (Kronenberg *et al.*, 1980).

We have found that J_H gene segments are not rearranged in three out of the four functional monoclonal T cell lines we examined (Kronenberg *et al.*, 1980, and Fig. 3). Since all of these cells respond to antigen, J_H gene segment rearrangement cannot be a requirement for antigen receptor biosynthesis. Similarly, J_H gene segments are found to be rearranged in some, but not all, killer T cell clones (Forster *et al.*, 1980; Cayre *et al.*, 1981; Kurosawa *et al.*, 1981), T cell hybridomas (Zuniga *et al.*, 1982), and T lymphomas (Cory *et al.*, 1980).

The DNA rearrangement in two killer T cell clones has been analyzed in detail. Although the rearranged J_H gene segment was joined to a *D* gene segment, no V_H gene segment was present (Kurosawa *et al.*, 1981). In normal B cells, the immunoglobulin DNA on the unexpressed homolog is often rearranged in a nonproductive manner (Coleclough *et al.*, 1981; Nottenburg and Weissman,

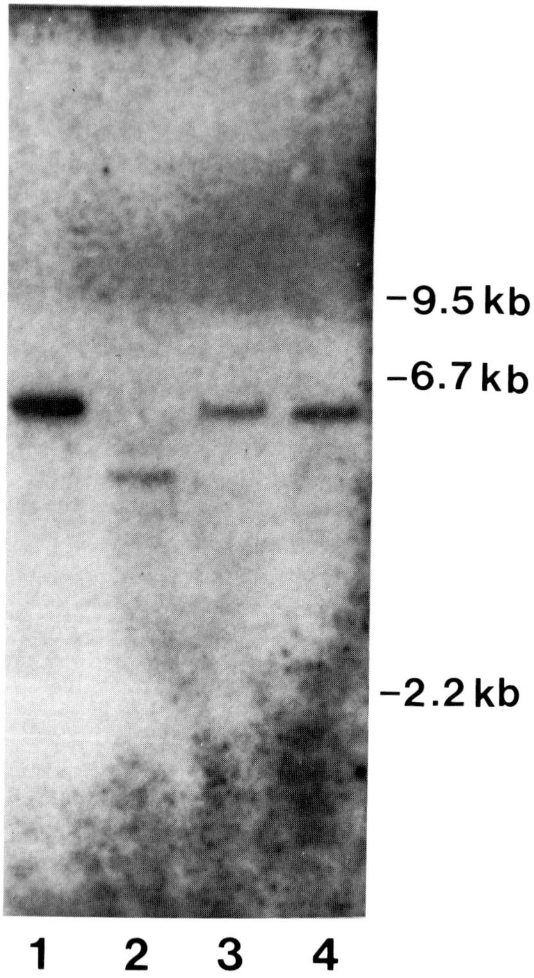

Fig. 3. J_H gene segments are rearranged in some cloned T cells. DNA was prepared from (1) AKR T lymphoma BW5147, (2) a cloned B10. A suppressor cell line, (3) B10.A liver, (4) a cloned B10.A T cell line. All cell lines were provided by Dan Hansburg and Ron Schwartz. The DNA samples were digested with *Eco*RI, blotted onto nitrocellulose filters, and hybridized with a probe containing all four J_H gene segments. The migration distance of molecular weight markers is shown. kb, kilobase.

1981), as the resulting DNA sequences are not capable of encoding a functional variable region. This probably occurs either because the gene segments are joined in the wrong translational reading frame (Altenburger *et al.*, 1980; Max *et al.*, 1980) or as a consequence of partial joining of D–J_H without V_H (Sakano *et al.*, 1981; Early and Hood, 1981). Nonproductive rearrangements are not observed in DNA from sperm or whole embryo (Coleclough *et al.*, 1981; Nottenburg and Weissman, 1981) and it has been hypothesized that these rearrangements result in B cells from attempts at V_L–J_L and V_H–D–J_H joining to form functional variable region genes. There are two points we wish to make concerning J_H rearrangement in T cells. First, because many functional T cells do not rearrange J_H gene segments and because of the partial (D–J_H) joining observed in two killer T cell clones, it appears likely that J_H rearrangements which have been observed on Southern blots but have not been further characterized by DNA sequencing also are nonproductive. Second, DNA rearrangements in T cells involve only the heavy chain and not the light chain gene families, and therefore the specific mechanism of heavy chain variable region gene formation was activated at some point in the development of these cells. This suggests, but does not prove, that productive rearrangements which form transcripts containing V_H gene segments occur in T cells.

We found no evidence for transcription of J_H, C_μ, and C_α sequences in cloned T cells (Kronenberg *et al.*, 1980). C_μ transcripts have, however, been found in thymocytes (Kemp *et al.*, 1980b), some T lymphomas (Kemp *et al.*, 1980a), and T cell hybridomas (Zuniga *et al.*, 1982). These transcripts are similar to those in immature B cells (Kemp *et al.*, 1980c). Although the RNA is spliced and polyadenylated, there is no evidence that it contains V gene segments. Furthermore, the C_μ sequence present in the T cell RNA is not translated into protein which can be immunoprecipitated by anti-μ antibody (Walker and Harris, 1980). Thus, we conclude that B cell J_H and C_H gene segments are not employed by the T cell receptor.

E. V_H Gene Expression in T Lymphocytes

We are currently using two approaches to demonstrate V_H gene expression in T cells. (1) We have isolated clones containing the variable region DNA from idiotype-positive B cells. The cloned DNA can then be used to probe RNA from T cells expressing the same idiotype. (2) We have synthesized DNA probes capable of detecting almost any V_H sequence which may be used by a T cell.

1. V Region Probes from Idiotype-Positive B Lymphocytes

To test whether T cells use the same V_H repertoire as B cells, it is necessary to obtain a V_H DNA probe from idiotype-positive B cells as well as RNA from cloned idiotype-positive T cells. On the assumption that T cells will use the V_H repertoire in a manner similar to B cells, it is advantageous to choose a system of limited heterogeneity at the B cell level. This approach would maximize the probability that the B cell probe will cross-hybridize with the T cell RNA. Therefore, we are examining the response to phosphorylcholine (PC) and the response to GAT, a linear polymer of glutamic acid, alanine, and tyrosine.

In BALB/c mice, the antibody response to phosphorylcholine predominantly has the idiotype of the PC-binding myeloma protein T15 (Lee *et al.*, 1974). In addition, the complete V_H sequences of 19 PC-binding myeloma and hybridoma heavy chains indicate that these V_H regions are very closely related to one another, regardless of whether or not they display the T15 idiotype (Gearhart *et al.*, 1981). A cDNA synthesized in this laboratory which contains the T15 V_H gene sequence is capable of hybridizing with heavy chain RNA from any of the 19 analyzed hybridomas and myelomas (Early *et al.*, 1979). Furthermore, T15 idiotype-positive, PC-responder T cells have been described (Cosenza *et al.*, 1977). Unfortunately, PC-responsive T cells from BALB/c mice do not grow well *in vitro* (J. Watson, personal communication). In collaboration with James Watson, we were able to obtain small amounts (10–50 μg) of total cellular RNA from nine uncloned PC-responding T cell lines. Although immunofluorescence indicated that the cells were almost entirely Thy-1 positive, we found significant amounts of C_κ and C_μ RNA in our preparations. The molecular weights of these molecules were characteristic of those seen in mature B cells. Control experiments indicated that irradiated feeder spleen cells were probably the source of some, if not all, of this immunoglobulin RNA.

In two T cell lines, we found RNA which hybridized with a T15 V_H probe. This result could not be reproduced with a second RNA preparation. It is not clear whether this discrepancy occurred because the uncloned PC-responding cell population had changed or because of a hybridization artifact on our earlier Northern blot. However a cloned, T15 idiotype-positive, PC-specific suppressor cell does not have any RNA which hybridizes with a T15 V_H probe (T. Honjo, personal communication).

A second suitable system for studying the molecular basis of T cell antigen recognition is the immune response to GAT. In fact, cloned GAT-responding T cells have been generated in several laboratories (Kapp *et al.*, 1980; Sredni *et al.*, 1980), and idiotypic determinants have been reported on GAT-specific suppressor factor from spleen cells (Germain *et al.*, 1979). In addition, GAT-binding immunoglobulins appear restricted in diversity as assessed by reaction with anti-idiotypic sera and N-terminal sequence analysis of the heavy chain proteins (Tonelle *et al.*, 1981). We have recently generated a cDNA clone containing the V_H region from a cell-producing GAT-binding immunoglobulin. We describe the synthesis and selection of this GAT V_H cDNA probe, since it is a model for our attempts to be able to probe T cell cDNA libraries for any variable region (see Section I,E,2). An idiotype-positive IgM-producing hybridoma, F9-238.9, was kindly provided by Ron Germain. Poly(A) RNA was prepared from these cells and approximately 3% encoded the heavy chain. As summarized in Fig. 4, a complementary DNA strand was synthesized from the RNA template by the enzyme, reverse transcriptase (Efstratiadis *et al.*, 1976). Oligo(dT) is commonly used to prime this reaction, but was not suitable for this case, since the *V* region, at the 5′ end of the heavy chain message, is 2 kilobases from the poly(A) sequence at the 3′ end, and cDNA molecules synthesized by conventional techniques are generally shorter than 2 kilobases. We used calf thymus DNA, sheared to an average length of 10–15 nucleotides, as a primer. The short stretches of sequence homology between the calf thymus DNA and the RNA template allow priming in many places along an RNA molecule (Taylor *et al.*, 1976). Therefore, we could hope to obtain clones containing the 5′ sequences of the heavy chain message. Double-stranded cDNA was synthesized with DNA

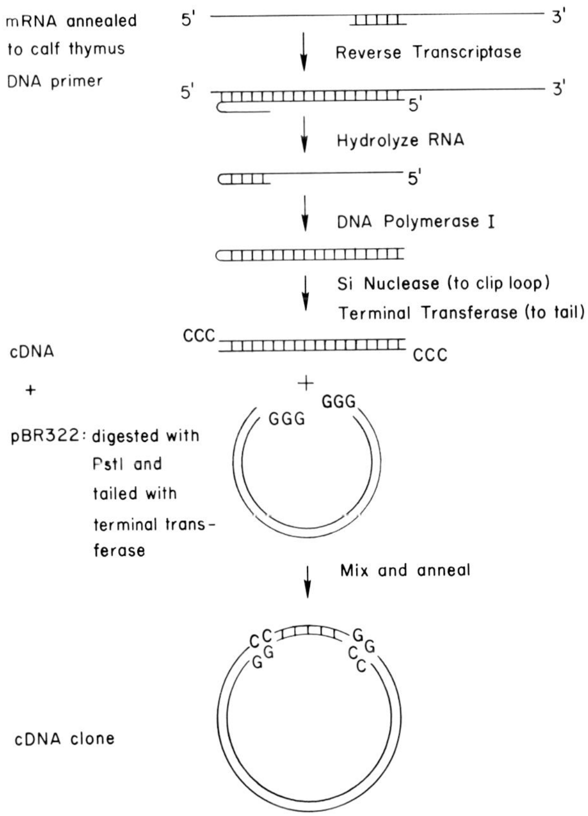

Fig. 4. A scheme for constructing cDNA clones.

polymerase I (Efstratiadis *et al.*, 1976; Villa-Komaroff *et al.*, 1978). After S1 nuclease digestion, nucleotide homopolymer tails containing cytosine were added to the cDNA with the enzyme terminal transferase. The cDNA was then annealed to plasmid DNA which had been tailed with guanine-containing nucleotides, and bacteria were transformed with the resulting recombinant molecules (Villa-Komaroff *et al.*, 1978).

Several thousand clones were obtained and screened with three different probes: (1) Cloned J_H DNA fragment: We purified a DNA fragment containing the four J_H gene segments and this fragment hybridized most strongly to one of the GAT B cell cDNA clones we screened (Fig. 5A). (2) Specifically primed spleen cDNA: A 2 kilobase restriction fragment containing the four J_H gene segments was cut with the restriction enzymes *Dde*I, *Pst*I, *Hae*III, and *Rsa*I. This digestion with all four enzymes cuts the DNA into about 35 fragments. Four of these fragments contain J_H DNA and no intervening DNA sequence (Fig. 6) and should therefore hybridize to immunoglobulin mRNA. The hybridized fragments will prime synthesis of radioactive cDNA containing a mixture of the variable regions present in the spleen RNA. To demonstrate this a single-stranded cDNA made in this way was hybridized to a Southern blot of three clones containing

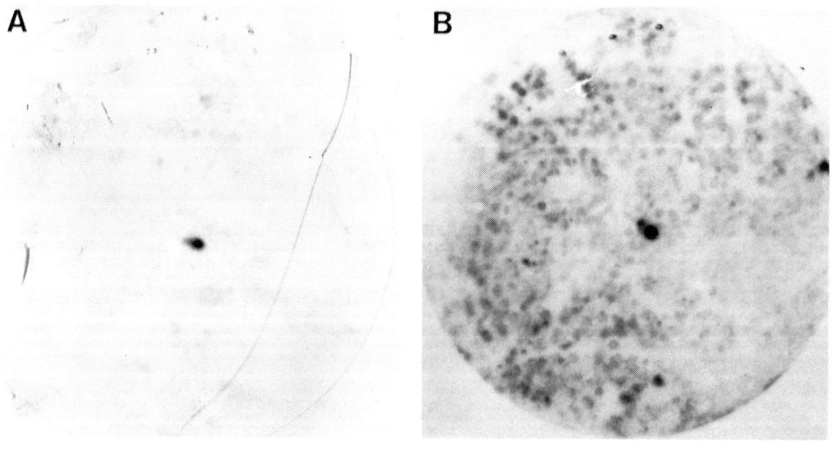

Fig. 5. Hybridization of radioactive probes to GAT B cell cDNA clones. cDNA clones were constructed as described in Fig. 4. Filter-bound DNA from several thousand clones was hybridized with the probes described (Section I, E, 2) and the filters were autoradiographed. (A) Hybridization with radioactive DNA fragment containing the J_H gene segments. The autoradiograph shows one filter which contains DNA from about 800 clones. (B) A replica of the filter in (A) was hybridized with a radioactive spleen single-stranded cDNA which had been specifically primed with J_H restriction fragments. A single cDNA clone, located near the center of the filter, hybridized strongly with both probes, and this DNA has been shown to contain a V_H gene.

J_1 5' TACTGGTACTTCGATGTCTGGGGCGCAGGGACCACGGTCACCGTTTCCTCA 3'

RsaI DdeI

J_2 5' TACTTTGACTACTGGGGCCAAGGCACCACTCTCACAGTCTCCTCA 3'

HaeIII DdeI

J_3 5' GCCTGGTTTGCTTACTGGGGCCAAGGGACTCTGGTCACTGTCTCTGCA 3'

HaeIII PstI

J_4 5' TACTATGCTATGGACTACTGGGGTCAAGGAACCTCAGTCACCGTCTCCTCA 3'

DdeI DdeI

Fig. 6. J_H primer fragments. The sequence of the primer fragments, used to generate the spleen cDNA probe, is shown (Sakano *et al.*, 1980). A 2 kilobase fragment containing the four J_H gene segments was digested with the restriction enzymes *Dde*I, *Hae*III, *Pst*I and *Rsa*I. The digestion generates four separate fragments containing the J_H coding sequences and about 30 fragments from sequences flanking or between the J_H gene segments. Only the J_H coding sequences are shown. Restriction enzyme sites are indicated with vertical lines and the primer fragments generated are enclosed in rectangles.

V_H, but not J_H, gene sequences: (a) the germline T15 V gene segment; (b) two closely linked V_H gene segments (V14A and V14B), one identical and the other similar to the V gene found in the levan-binding myeloma J606 (S. Crews, personal communication); and (c) Mu2. V1, a V_H region about 85% homologous to the dextran-binding MOPC l04E heavy chain (P. Early, personal communication). Table I shows that these V gene segments share little homology to each other. Figure 7A shows a photograph of an agarose gel in which the DNA has been stained with ethidium bromide. Figure 7B includes an autoradiograph of the resulting Southern blot which had been hybridized with the spleen single-

TABLE I

Homology Relationship between V_H Gene Segments Which Were Hybridized with the Spleen cDNA Probe[a]

	V14B	T15	Mu2.V1
V14A	89	73	59
V14B	100	74	57
T15		100	58
Mu2.V1	—	—	100

[a] Table shows percent homologous residues. The V14B gene segment did not hybridize with the probe.

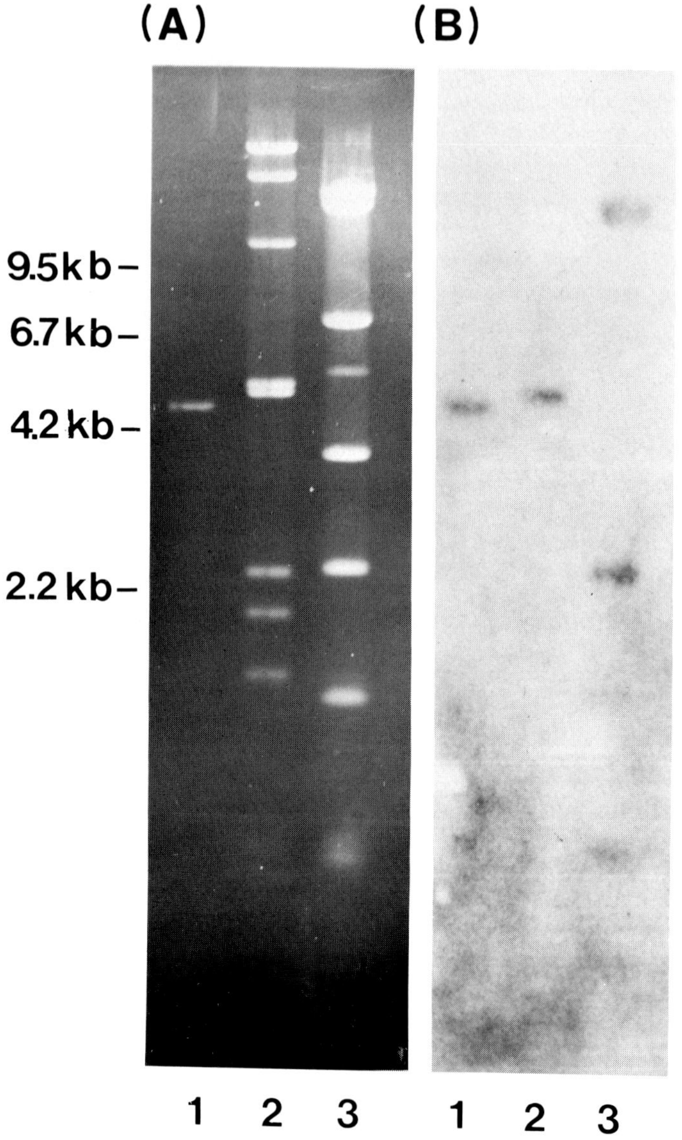

Fig. 7. Hybridization of specifically primed spleen cDNA to clones that contain V_H genes. (A) Agarose gel stained with ethidium bromide. 1, *Bam*HI digest of plasmid containing Mu2.VI sequence. 2, *Eco*RI digest of a bacteriophage λ clone containing two *V* gene segments, *V14A* and *V14B*. These *V* genes should be located on separate restriction fragments 5.0 and 2.0 kilobases long. 3, *Bam*HI digest of a bacteriophage λ clone containing the T15 V_H gene segment. The T15 V_H sequence is located on a 2.4 kilobase restriction fragment. (B) Southern blot of DNA in (A) hybridized to the specifically primed spleen cDNA. Three fragments containing *V* gene segments gave detectable hybridization. In lane 2, the 2.0 kilobase fragment containing a *V* gene segment did not hybridize. The higher molecular weight fragment in lane 3 may be uncut DNA. Migration distances of the molecular weight markers are shown. kb, kilobase.

stranded cDNA. Hybridization was detected with all but one of the restriction fragments known to contain *V* gene segments (S. Crews, personal communication). Furthermore, this probe hybridized to the GAT B cell cDNA colony which also annealed with the J_H probe (Fig. 5B). (3) Synthetic oligonucleotide probe: The amino acids Tyr-Tyr-Cys-Ala are highly conserved and found approximately at codons 95–97 at the 3′ end of murine V_H gene segments. The nucleotide sequences available also indicate little variation in this region. Using these sequences one of us (S.J.H.) has chemically synthesized the two undecamers shown in Fig. 8. The oligonucleotides were synthesized on a polymer support using the phosphite coupling procedure (Matteucci and Caruthers, 1980a,b) and were purified by high performance liquid chromatography. The sequences were verified by the method of Maxam and Gilbert (1980).

A computer search of 29 mouse V_H gene sequences has shown that seventeen have perfect homology to one of the two synthetic probes, ten have 10 of 11 homology to at least one of the probes, and two have less than 10 nucleotides homology to the two probes. Using a plasmid containing the S107 V_H gene sequence we have determined hybridization conditions in which perfect homology or 91% (10/11) homology is required to give a strong signal with minimal background.

As expected, a mixture of the two synthetic oligonucleotides hybridized with the putative GAT B cell V_H cDNA clone (data not shown). The clone which hybridized with our three probes was grown in quantity and mapped with restriction enzymes. It contains about 420 base pairs of mouse DNA inserted into the plasmid. Although the nucleotide sequence of the cDNA is not yet complete, the clone contains a V_H gene segment as well as the J_{H4} gene segment (data not shown). We will test GAT-responsive T cell clones for the presence of messenger RNA homologous to our probe.

2. *Can Universal V Region Probes Be Used to Screen T Cell cDNA Libraries?*

T cells may express V_H genes, but use the V_H repertoire differently from B cells. To test this hypothesis, we will make cDNA libraries from T cells (Fig. 4) and screen the resulting clones with both the synthetic oligonucleotide and J_H-primed spleen cDNA. As described in the previous section, both these probes

Protein Sequence:	Tyr Tyr Cys Ala	Tyr Tyr Cys Ala
Conserved DNA Sequences:	5′ TAT TAC TGT GC 3′	5′ TAC TAC TGT CG 3′
Synthesized Complementary Oligonucleotides:	3′ ATA ATG ACA CG 5′	3′ ATG ATG ACA CG 5′

Fig. 8. Synthetic oligonucleotide probes. The conserved oligonucleotide sequences found in immunoglobulin *V* gene segments, the amino acids these sequences encode, and the complementary undecamers we synthesized are shown.

will hybridize to many genes, and if a T cell cDNA clone hybridizes to both probes, it probably contains a V_H gene segment.

Although we have provided evidence on the diversity of V_H genes which do hybridize with these probes, it is clear these probes can not detect every V gene. Therefore, it is necessary to examine several different T cell lines. Currently, we are constructing cDNA libraries from three T cell hybridomas provided by the laboratory of J. Kappler and P. Marrack. These lines are antigen specific, responding either to ovalbumin, KLH, or human γ globulin (Kappler *et al.*, 1981). An analysis of these three distinct T cell lines with the DNA probes described above should constitute an important test of the proposition that the T cell receptor employs B cell V_H gene segments.

F. Summary

The early studies investigating immunoglobulin gene expression in T cells were plagued both by the impurity of the cells and the impurity of the nucleic acid probes utilized. With the availability of continuously growing T cell clones, experiments could be performed on cells which (in some cases) are absolutely free of B cell contaminants and which are known to respond specifically to antigen. Using cloned immunoglobulin probes, it has been determined that the heavy and light chain J and C genes are not part of the T cell antigen-binding receptor. Although rearrangement of J_H and transcription of C_μ sequences has been observed in a number of cloned T cells, these events are not required for receptor biosynthesis.

While some preliminary reports have been discouraging (reviewed by Robertson, 1981), the hypothesis that T cells express V_H gene segments remains a very attractive one. Using cloned idiotype positive T cells, efforts underway in this laboratory and a number of others should put this hypothesis to a critical test in the coming months. The presence of V_H idiotypic determinants on T cells and the activation of the heavy chain rearrangement mechanism in these cells support a role for V_H gene products in T cell antigen recognition. In addition, we have developed strategies for detecting V_H cDNA sequences which do not depend upon the assumption that B and T lymphocytes use the V gene repertoire in the same manner.

II. CLONING NONIMMUNOGLOBULIN GENES FROM T CELLS

If antigen-binding molecules from T cells do not contain immunoglobulin variable regions, it will be possible to characterize these molecules and even clone the genes which encode them. However, any approach will depend upon having a reliable assay for the T cell antigen receptor and/or secreted factor.

While in theory serological reactivities, antigen binding, or direct biological tests can be used to identify the relevant molecule, each of these assays presents some experimental difficulties. For example, a number of antisera are known to react with the surface of T cells and have an effect on antigen-induced T cell functions. These include antibodies to the Thy-1 antigen (McGrath *et al.*, 1980), Lyt-1 (Hollander *et al.*, 1981), and Lyt-2,3 antigens (Nakayama *et al.*, 1979; Hollander *et al.*, 1981). Some of these effects may be due to steric interference with antigen binding, rather than direct reactivity to the receptor molecule. Furthermore, the T cell receptor may have low avidity for antigen or could perhaps bind antigen only in the presence of histocompatibility determinants. Finally, direct biological assays can be cumbersome and often generate variable results. In practice, it appears that some of these difficulties may be circumvented by purifying soluble antigen-binding molecules from the supernatants of cloned T cells (Fresno *et al.*, 1981a,b).

Once the antigen-binding molecule has been identified, two strategies are available for cloning its gene and determining the primary structure of the corresponding protein. One method involves synthesizing cDNA libraries which are then screened by selecting homologous RNA, translating it *in vitro,* and then assaying the synthesized polypeptide. A second approach depends upon having partial amino acid sequence information which can be used to synthesize an oligonucleotide which can in turn be used to select a cDNA clone. In addition, we discuss a new technique in which DNA sequence information in conjunction with chemical peptide synthesis can be used to identify previously uncharacterized gene products.

A. Selection of a cDNA Clone through Assay of Its Corresponding RNA and Protein Product

1. *Methodology*

As summarized in Fig. 9, filter-bound DNA can be hybridized with cellular messenger RNA, such that the homologous RNA molecules can be purified. The hybridized RNA can be eluted from the DNA and translated *in vitro* to generate a protein which can be assayed as described above (serological reactions, antigen binding, bioassay on lymphocytes). This protocol was used in the isolation of the gene encoding β_2-microglobulin (Parnes *et al.*, 1981).

The number of clones which must be screened by these procedures can be greatly reduced by making the initial cDNA clones from a limited portion of the total RNA population. mRNA enrichment can be accomplished by (1) separating the RNA by molecular weight and choosing only that molecular weight fraction which can be translated into the protein of interest, and (2) selecting the RNA population used to make cDNA through specific hybridization. For example,

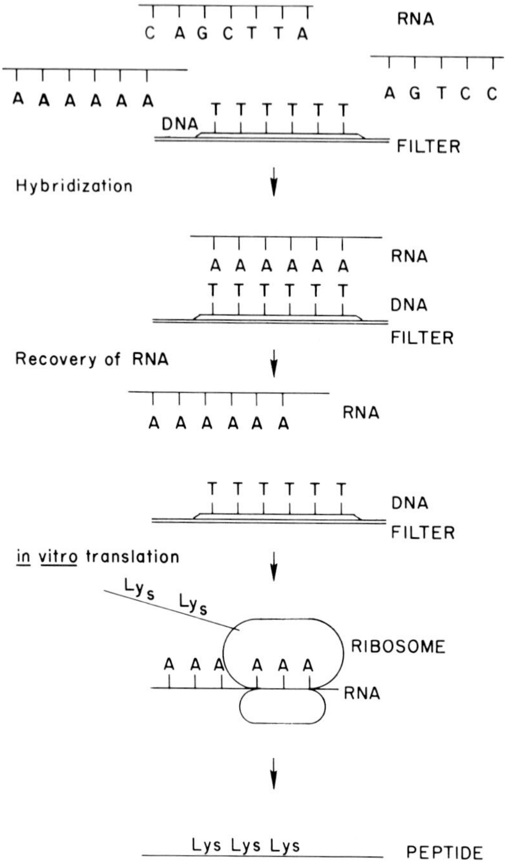

Fig. 9. Selection of a cDNA clone through assay of its corresponding RNA and protein product.

RNA from a Lyt-2-positive T cell can be hybridized to single-stranded cDNA from a Lyt-1-positive T cell and the unhybridized RNA can be selected by chromatography. This RNA population should contain Lyt-2 coding sequences and (probably) a relatively small number of other sequences. While this selection can be very powerful, only very small amounts of RNA may be available for synthesizing cDNA.

More rapid selection can be facilitated by inserting cDNA clones into bacterial expression vectors (Goeddel *et al.*, 1979). These vectors generally contain bacterial promoter sequences, which can be induced to give a high rate of transcription, and bacterial ribosome binding sites near the location of the cDNA insertion. Thus, the eukaryotic DNA sequence can be transcribed and translated, eliminating the need for separate RNA hybridization-selection and translation systems. Expression vectors have been used to clone interferon cDNA from leukocytes (Goeddel *et al.*, 1980).

2. *Potential Difficulties*

Given a collection of cDNA clones, selection can be complicated by the fact that the desired protein can only bind antigen or react with antisera after undergoing the proper posttranslational modifications (glycosylation, leader peptide cleavage, etc.) which will not occur in bacteria or standard *in vitro* translation systems. This difficulty can be circumvented by adding a microsomal fraction from pancreas (Dobberstein *et al.*, 1979) to the *in vitro* translation reaction or by injecting the selected RNA into *Xenopus* oocytes (Lane *et al.*, 1980). In both cases, the posttranslational processing system is effectively supplied. Another potential problem arises if the presence of an antigenic determinant or biological activity depends upon the presence of more than one polypeptide chain. This appears to be true for many anti-H-2 alloantisera which require the presence of β_2-microglobulin in order to recognize a protein product (Ploegh *et al.*, 1979). In this case, it is necessary to have an antigenic determinant or bioassay which depends upon one polypeptide chain only.

B. Selection of a Clone Using Partial Amino Acid Sequence and Oligonucleotide Synthesis

1. *Methodology*

Although nucleotide sequence analysis is in most cases more rapid than amino acid sequencing for obtaining the complete primary structure of polypeptides, partial amino acid sequence data can play an important role in obtaining clones coding for molecules produced in small quantities by T cells. With recent advances in amino acid sequence technology, it is possible to obtain sequence information from microgram quantities of unlabeled protein purified from polyacrylamide gels (Hunkapiller and Hood, 1980; Hewick *et al.*, 1981). The amino acid sequence can be translated into nucleotide sequence using the genetic code dictionary (Fig. 10). Part of the resulting nucleotide sequence can be synthesized to generate an oligonucleotide probe specific for a given gene. This probe can be used in three ways. First, the oligonucleotide can be radioactively labeled and used as a specific hybridization probe to select a clone from a cDNA library. Second, the oligonucleotide can be lengthened *in vitro* by hybridizing it to messenger RNA and extending the primer with reverse transcriptase. The resulting single-stranded cDNA should be long enough to allow stable hybridization to cDNA clones. Third, the oligonucleotide can be used as a specific primer to initiate the complete synthesis of cDNA clones as outlined in Fig. 4. A significant fraction of either the specifically primed cDNA clones or clones from

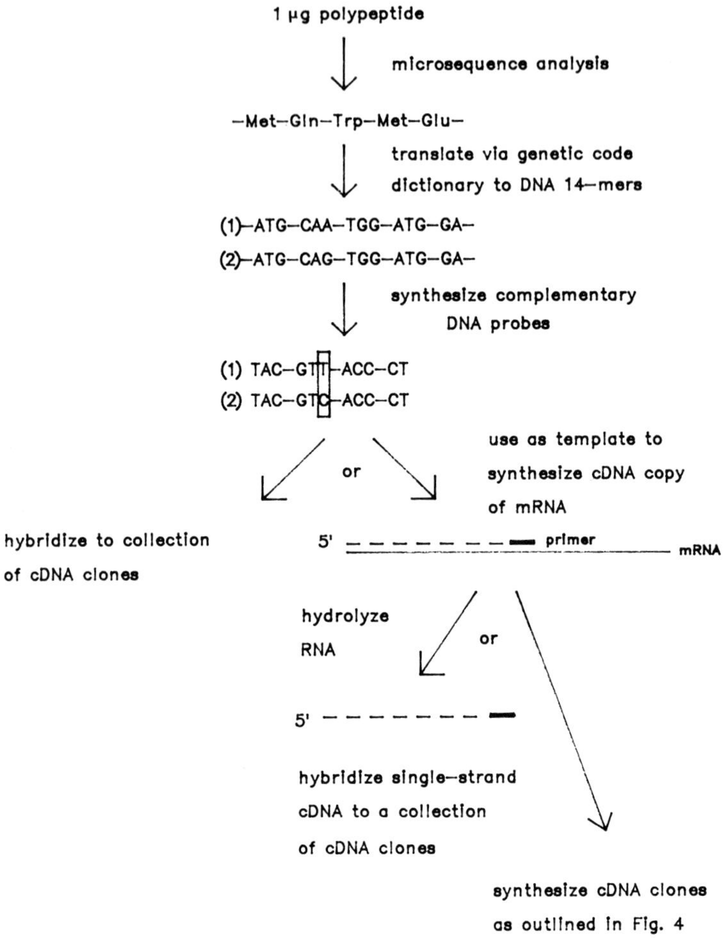

Fig. 10. Selection of a clone using partial amino acid sequence and oligonucleotide synthesis. Translation of a glutamine residue into nucleotide sequence generates two possibilities.

a cDNA library hybridizing with the oligonucleotide should contain the desired cDNA. This can be verified by nucleotide sequence analysis which should correlate with the known amino acid sequence. This type of strategy has been used to obtain a cDNA clone coding for an HLA antigen (Sood *et al.*, 1981).

2. *Potential Problems*

The major difficulty encountered in using an oligonucleotide as a specific gene probe is the detection of irrelevant sequences. To select a given sequence from the RNA (or cDNA) population of a typical eukaryotic cell, an oligonucleotide 14–15 bases in length is required (Szostak *et al.*, 1979). Shorter oligonucleotide probes will probably hybridize with a number of sequences in addition to the sequence of interest. In translating the protein sequence into DNA sequence, there may be ambiguities in the nucleotide sequence because most amino acids are specified by more than one codon. In fact, it is unlikely that a probe 14 or 15 nucleotides in length could be synthesized without ambigious residues given only the partial amino acid sequence of a polypeptide. With the automation of oligonucleotide synthesis, it is now possible to generate rapidly a mixture of probes which contain all possible residues at the ambiguous sites. The related probes do not interfere with hybridization of the perfectly matched sequences (Wallace *et al.*, 1981). Yet as the number of ambiguous residues and hence required probes increases, the specificity of the selection decreases. In practice therefore, the clones selected with an oligonucleotide may have to be further screened using a second assay.

C. Characterization of a Protein Encoded by a Cloned DNA Sequence

The strategies described in Sections II,A and II,B pertain to the situation in which a gene product has been characterized by antisera or other means and describe methods for then obtaining the gene. A cloned gene sequence may be used to identify closely homologous genes in the genomic DNA. Multigene families identified in this way may be larger than expected from biological studies, so a DNA sequence encoding a member of this family could be available before we have any information on the expression and function of the protein it encodes. Such a situation has occurred in our studies of the MHC; probes for the H-2K and H-2D molecules hybridize with 20–30 different DNA sequences, where only 3–5 homologous genes would have been expected (Steinmetz *et al.*, 1981). Recently, a new method has been developed which in many cases will allow unequivocal assignment of a protein product to a DNA sequence (see Fig. 11). Using the genetic code dictionary, an amino acid sequence can be obtained from a given nucleotide sequence. A peptide corresponding to a portion of the amino acid sequence can be synthesized (Marglin and Merrifield, 1970), covalently coupled to a carrier molecule, and subsequently used as an immunogen (Sutcliffe *et al.*, 1980). This method is usually successful providing the synthesized peptide is at least 7 amino acids in length and is derived from a hydrophilic portion of the protein (Lerner *et al.*, 1981). Antibodies raised against the peptide are suitable for answering a number of biological questions, such as the cell types expressing the protein, the developmental timing of its expression, the cellular location of the polypeptide, and whether there are cross-reactions with other antisera of known specificity.

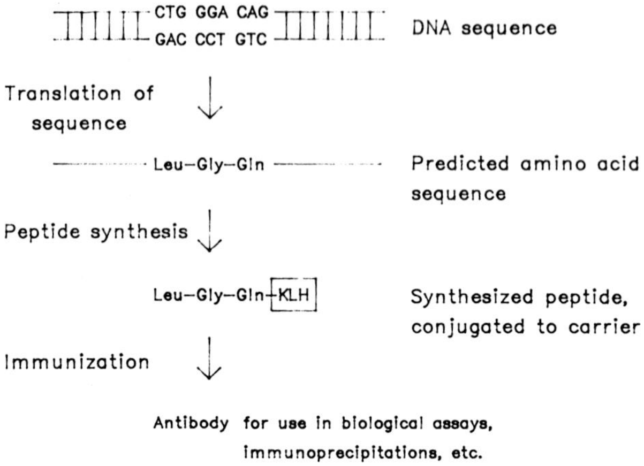

Fig. 11. Characterization of a protein encoded by a cloned DNA sequence.

The ability to go from protein to gene to related proteins greatly increases the number of biological questions which can be addressed using recombinant DNA technology. Moreover, it allows the rapid analysis of individual members of a multigene family.

III. CONCLUSIONS

A number of technical advances have greatly simplified the task of cloning cDNAs from rare messenger RNA molecules. Thus, whether or not V_H gene segments are involved in the T cell antigen binding receptor, the relevant genes can be isolated. Once receptor molecules have been identified a variety of cloned cell lines will be necessary to analyze the structure–function relationships of cell surface and secreted antigen-binding molecules produced by T cells. This analysis will certainly require extensive collaboration between molecular biologists and cellular immunologists in the years ahead. The techniques we have described are mostly concerned with the isolation and characterization of cloned sequences. In the future, we will be able to introduce genes into cloned T cells. We can then directly ask functional questions about individual gene sequences and therefore begin to analyze the molecular basis of cellular function and interaction in the immune system.

ACKNOWLEDGMENTS

We wish to thank the laboratories of Ron Germain, Philippa Marrack, and John Kappler, Ron Schwartz, and James Watson for the cell lines used in the studies reported. Thanks also to Steve Crews and Donna Livant for providing cloned DNA and unpublished sequence data, Phil Early and

John Frelinger for helpful discussions, and Gerald Siu and Martha Zuniga for careful reading of the manuscript. We are also grateful to Tim Hunkapiller for his patient instruction on the use of the computer and to Stephanie Canada for preparation of the manuscript. This work was supported by NIH research grants AI 17565, AI 16913 (S.J.H.) and AI 16590 (M.K.). E.K. is a postdoctoral fellow of the Cancer Research Institute.

REFERENCES

Altenburger, W., Steinmetz, M., and Zachau, H. G. (1980). Functional and non-functional joining in immunoglobulin light chain genes of a mouse myeloma. *Nature* (*London*) **287,** 603.

Alwine, J. C., Kemp, D. J., and Stark, G. R. (1977). Method for detection of specific RNAs in agarose gels by transfer to diazobenzyloxymethyl-paper and hybridization with DNA probes. *Proc. Natl. Acad. Sci. U.S.A.* **74,** 5350.

Bernard, O., Hozumi, N., and Tonegawa, S. (1978). Sequences of mouse immunoglobulin light chain genes before and after somatic changes. *Cell* **15,** 1133.

Binz, H., and Wigzell, H. (1975). Shared idiotypic determinants on B and T lymphocytes reactive against the same antigenic determinants. I. Demonstration of similar or identical idiotypes on IgG molecules and T cell receptors with specificity for the same alloantigens. *J. Exp. Med.* **142,** 197.

Binz, H., and Wigzell, H. (1977). Antigen-binding, idiotypic T lymphocyte receptors. *Contemp. Top. Immunobiol.* **7,** 113.

Cayre, Y., Palladino, M. A., Marcu, K. B., and Stavnezer, J. (1981). Expression of an antigen receptor on T cells does not require recombination at the immunoglobulin J_H–C_μ locus. *Proc. Natl. Acad. Sci. U.S.A.* **78,** 3814.

Coleclough, C., Perry, R. P., Karjalainen, K., and Weigert, M. (1981). Aberrant rearrangements contribute significantly to the allelic exclusion of immunoglobulin gene expression. *Nature* (*London*) **290,** 372.

Cory, S., Adams, J. M., and Kemp, D. J. (1980). Somatic rearrangements forming active immunoglobulin μ genes in B and T lymphoid cell lines. *Proc. Natl. Acad. Sci. U.S.A.* **77,** 4943.

Cosenza, H., Julius, M. H., and Augustin, A. A. (1977). Idiotypes as variable region markers: Analogies between receptors on phosphorylcholine-specific T and B lymphocytes. *Immunol. Rev.* **34,** 3.

Davis, M. M., Calame, K., Early, P. W., Livant, D. L., Joho, R., Weissman, I. L., and Hood, L. (1980a). An immunoglobulin heavy-chain gene is formed by at least two recombinational events. *Nature* (*London*) **283,** 733.

Davis, M. M., Kim, S. K., and Hood, L. (1980b). DNA sequences mediating class switching in α immunoglobulins. *Science* **209,** 1360.

Dobberstein, B., Garoff, H., and Warren, G. (1979). Cell-free synthesis and membrane insertion of mouse H-2D^d histocompatibility antigen and β_2-microglobulin. *Cell* **17,** 759.

Early, P., and Hood, L. (1981). Allelic exclusion and nonproductive immunoglobulin gene rearrangements. *Cell* **24,** 1.

Early, P. W., Davis, M. M., Kaback, D. B., Davidson, N., and Hood, L. (1979). Immunoglobulin heavy chain gene organization in mice: Analysis of a myeloma genomic clone containing variable and α constant regions. *Proc. Natl. Acad. Sci. U.S.A.* **76,** 857.

Early, P., Huang, H., Davis, M., Calame, K., and Hood, L. (1980a). An immunoglobulin chain variable region gene is generated from three segments of DNA: V_H, *D*, and J_H. *Cell* **19,** 981.

Early, P., Rogers, J., Davis, M., Calame, K., Bond, M., Wall, R., and Hood, L. (1980b). Two mRNAs can be produced from a single immunoglobulin μ gene by alternative RNA processing pathways. *Cell* **20,** 313.

Efstratiadis, A., Kafatos, F. C., Maxam, A. M., and Maniatis, T. (1976). Enzymic *in vitro* synthesis of globulin genes. *Cell* **7,** 279.

Eichmann, K. (1978). Expression and function of idiotypes on lymphocytes. *Adv. Immunol.* **26,** 195.

Eichmann, K., and Rajewsky, K. (1975). Induction of T and B cell immunity by anti-idiotypic antibody. *Eur. J. Immunol.* **5,** 661.

Forster, A., Hobart, M., Hengartner, H., and Rabbitts, T. H. (1980). An immunoglobulin heavy-chain gene is altered in two T cell clones. *Nature (London)* **286,** 897.

Fresno, M., Nabel, G., McVay-Boudreau, L., Furthmayer, H., and Cantor, H. (1981a). Antigen-specific lymphocyte clones. I. Characterization of T lymphocyte clone expressing antigen-specific suppressive activity. *J. Exp. Med.* **153,** 1246.

Fresno, M., McVay-Boudreau, L., Nabel, G., and Cantor, H. (1981b). Antigen-specific T lymphocyte clones. II. Purification and biological characterization of an antigen-specific suppressive protein synthesized by cloned T cells. *J. Exp. Med.* **153,** 1260.

Gearhart, P. J., Johnson, N. D., Douglas, R., and Hood, L. (1981). IgG antibodies to phosphorylcholine exhibit more diversity than their IgM counterparts. *Nature (London)* **291,** 29.

Germain, R. N., and Benacerraf, B. (1980). Helper and suppressor T-cell factors. *Springer Semin. Immunopathol.* **3,** 93.

Germain, R. N., Ju, S.-T., Kipps, T. J., Benacerraf, B., and Dorf, M. E. (1979). Shared idiotypic determinants on antibodies and T-cell-derived suppressor factor specific for the random terpolymer L-glutamic acid^{60}-L-alanine^{30}-L-tyrosine^{10}. *J. Exp. Med.* **149,** 613.

Gilmore-Hebert, M., and Wall, R. (1978). Immunoglobulin light chain mRNA is processed from large nuclear RNA. *Proc. Natl. Acad. Sci. U.S.A.* **75,** 342.

Gilmore-Hebert, M., Hercules, K., Komaromy, M., and Wall, R. (1978). Variable and constant regions are separated in the 10-Kbase transcription unit coding for immunoglobulin κ light chains. *Proc. Natl. Acad. Sci. U.S.A.* **75,** 6044.

Goeddel, D. V., Heyneker, H. L., Hozumi, T., Arentzen, R., Itakura, K., Vansura, D. G., Ross, M. J., Miozzari, G., Crea, R., and Seeburg, P. H. (1979). Direct expression in *Escherichia coli* of a DNA sequence coding for human growth hormones. *Nature (London)* **281,** 544.

Goeddel, D. V., Velverton, E., Ullrich, A., Heyneker, H. L., Miozzari, G., Holmes, W., Seeburg, P. H., Dull, T., May, L., Stebbing, N., Crea, R., Maeda, S., McCandliss, R., Sloma, A., Tabor, J. M., Gross, M., Familletti, P. C., and Pestka, S. (1980). Human leukocyte interferon produced by *E. coli* is biologically active. *Nature (London)* **287,** 411.

Harvey, M. A., Adorini, L., Miller, A., and Sercarz, E. E. (1979). Lysozyme-induced T-suppressor cells and antibodies have a predominant idiotype. *Nature (London)* **281,** 594.

Herzenberg, L. A., Black, S. J., and Herzenberg, L. A. (1980). Regulatory circuits and antibody responses. *Eur. J. Immunol.* **10,** 1.

Hewick, R. M., Hunkapiller, M. W., Hood, L. E., and Dreyer, W. J. (1981). A gas-liquid solid phase peptide and protein sequenator. *J. Biol. Chem.* **256,** 7990.

Hollander, N., Pillemer, E., and Weissman, I. L. (1981). Effects of Lyt antibodies on T-cell functions: Augmentation by anti-Lyt-1 as opposed to inhibition by anti-Lyt-2. *Proc. Natl. Acad. Sci. U.S.A.* **78,** 1148.

Hood, L., Davis, M., Early, P., Calame, K., Kim, S., Crews, S., and Huang, H. (1981). Two types of DNA rearrangements in immunoglobulin genes. *Cold Spring Harbor Symp. Quant. Biol.* **45,** 887.

Hunkapiller, M. W., and Hood, L. E. (1980). New protein sequenator with increased sensitivity. *Science* **207,** 523.

Jerne, N. K. (1974). Towards a network theory of the immune system. *Ann. Immunol. (Paris)* **125C,** 373.

Kapp, J. A., Araneo, B. A., and Clevinger, B. L. (1980). Suppression of antibody and T cell proliferative responses to L-glutamic acid^{60}-L-alanine^{30}-L-tyrosine^{10} by a specific monoclonal T cell factor. *J. Exp. Med.* **152,** 235.

Kappler, J. W., Skidmore, B., White, J., and Marrack, P. (1981). Antigen-inducible, H-2 restricted, interleukin-2-producing T cell hybridomas. *J. Exp. Med.* **153,** 1198.

Kemp, D. J., Harris, A. W., Cory, S., and Adams, J. M. (1980a). Expression of the immunoglobulin C_μ gene in mouse T and B lymphoid and myeloid cell lines. *Proc. Natl. Acad. Sci. U.S.A.* **77,** 2876.

Kemp, D. J., Wilson, A., Harris, A. W., and Shortman, K. (1980b). The immunoglobulin μ constant region gene is expressed in mouse thymocytes. *Nature (London)* **286,** 168.

Kemp, D. J., Harris, A. W., and Adams, J. M. (1980c). Transcripts of the immunoglobulin C_μ gene vary in structure and splicing during lymphoid development. *Proc. Natl. Acad. Sci. U.S.A.* **77,** 7400.

Kronenberg, M., Davis, M. M., Early, P. W., Hood, L. E., and Watson, J. D. (1980). Helper and killer T cells do not express B cell immunoglobulin joining and constant region gene segments. *J. Exp. Med.* **152,** 1745.

Kurosawa, Y., von Boehmer, H., Haas, W., Sakano, H., Trauneker, A., and Tonegawa, S. (1981). Identification of D segments of immunoglobulin heavy-chain genes and their rearrangement in T lymphocytes. *Nature (London)* **290,** 566.

Lahat, N., Moroz, C., and Ashkenazi, I. (1978). Immunoglobulin biosynthesis in mouse thymus cells. The expression of α and μ chains in BALB/c, C57B1 and intercrossed hybrid mice. *Immunochemistry* **15,** 883.

Lane, C. D., Colman, A., Mohun, T., Morser, J., Champion, J., Kourides, I., Craig, R., Higgins, S., James, T. C., Applebaum, S. W., Ohlsson, R. I., Paucha, E., Houghton, M., Matthews, J., and Miflin, B. J. (1980). The *Xenopus* oocyte as a surrogate secretory system. The specificity of protein export. *Eur. J. Biochem.* **111,** 225.

Lee, W., Cosenza, H., and Kohler, H. (1974). Clonal restriction of the immune response to phosphorylcholine. *Nature (London)* **247,** 55.

Lerner, R. A., Sutcliffe, J. G., and Shinnick, T. M. (1981). Antibodies to chemically synthesized peptides predicted from DNA sequences as probes of gene expression. *Cell* **23,** 309.

Loor, F. (1977). Structure and dynamics of the lymphocyte surface in relation to differentiation, recognition, and activation. *Prog. Allergy* **23,** 1.

McGrath, M. S., Pillemer, E., and Weissman, I. L. (1980). Murine leukaemogenesis: Monoclonal antibodies to T-cell determinants arrest T-lymphoma cell proliferation. *Nature (London)* **285,** 259.

Marchalonis, J. J. (1975). Lymphocyte surface immunoglobulins. *Science* **190,** 20.

Marglin, A., and Merrifield, R. B. (1970). *Annu. Rev. Biochem.* **39,** 841.

Matteucci, M. D., and Caruthers, M. H. (1980a). The synthesis of oligodeoxypyrimidines on a polymer support. *Tetrahedron Lett.* **21,** 719.

Matteucci, M. D., and Caruthers, M. H. (1980b). The use of zinc bromide for removal of dimethoxytrityl ethers from deoxynucleosides. *Tetrahedron Lett.* **21,** 3243.

Max, E. E., Seidman, J. G., and Leder, P. (1979). Sequences of five potential recombination sites encoded close to an immunoglobulin κ constant region gene. *Proc. Natl. Acad. Sci. U.S.A.* **76,** 3450.

Max, E. E., Seidman, J. G., Miller, H., and Leder, P. (1980). Variation in the crossover point of kappa immunoglobulin gene *V-J* recombination: Evidence from a cryptic gene. *Cell* **21,** 793.

Maxam, A. M., and Gilbert, W. (1980). Sequencing end-labeled DNA with base-specific chemical cleavages. *In* "Methods in Enzymology" (L. Grossman, and K. Muldave, eds.), Vol. 65, p. 499.

Nakayama, E., Shiku, H., Stockert, E., Oettgen, H. F., and Old, L. J. (1979). Cytotoxic T cells: Lyt phenotype and blocking of killing activity by Lyt antisera. *Proc. Natl. Acad. Sci. U.S.A.* **76,** 1977.

Nottenburg, C., and Weissman, I. L. (1981). C_μ gene rearrangement of mouse immunoglobulin genes in normal B cells occurs on both the expressed and nonexpressed chromosome. *Proc. Natl. Acad. Sci. U.S.A.* **78,** 484.

Parnes, J. R., Velan, B., Felsenfeld, A., Ramanathan, L., Ferrini, U., Appella, E., and Seidman, J. G. (1981). Mouse β_2-microglobulin cDNA clones: A screening procedure for cDNA clones corresponding to rare mRNAs. *Proc. Natl. Acad. Sci. U.S.A.* **78,** 2253.

Ploegh, H. L., Cannon, E. L., and Strominger, J. L. (1979). Cell-free translation of the mRNAs for the heavy and light chains of HLA-A and HLA-B antigens. *Proc. Natl. Acad. Sci. U.S.A.* **76,** 2273.

Rajewsky, K., and Eichmann, K. (1977). Antigen receptors on T helper cells. *Contemp. Top. Immunobiol.* **7,** 69.

Robertson, M. (1981). Genes of lymphocytes II: T-cell receptors, idiotypes and the MHC. *Nature (London)* **291,** 187.

Rogers, J., Early, P., Carter, C., Calame, K., Bond, M., Hood, L., and Wall, R. (1980). Two mRNAs with different 3′ ends encode membrane and secreted forms of immunoglobulin μ chain. *Cell* **20,** 303.

Sakamo, H., Huppi, K., Heinrich, G., and Tonegawa, S. (1979). Sequences at the somatic recombination sites of immunoglobulin light-chain genes. *Nature (London)* **280,** 288.

Sakano, H., Maki, R., Kurosawa, Y., Roeder, W., and Tonegawa, S. (1980). Two types of somatic recombination are necessary for the generation of complete immunoglobulin heavy chain genes. *Nature (London)* **286,** 676.

Sakano, H., Kurosawa, Y., Weigert, M., and Tonegawa, S. (1981). Identification and nucleotide sequence of a diversity DNA segment (D) of immunoglobulin heavy-chain genes. *Nature (London)* **290,** 562.

Sood, A. K., Pereira, D., and Weissman, S. M. (1981). Isolation and partial nucleotide sequence of a cDNA clone for human histocompatibility antigen HLA-B by use of an oligodeoxynucleotide primer. *Proc. Natl. Acad. Sci. U.S.A.* **78,** 616.

Southern, E. M. (1975). Detection of specific sequences among DNA fragments separated by gel electrophoresis. *J. Mol. Biol.* **98,** 503.

Sredni, B., Tse, H. Y., and Schwartz, R. H. (1980). Direct cloning and extended culture of antigen-specific MHC-restricted proliferating T lymphocytes. *Nature (London)* **283,** 581.

Steinmetz, M., Frelinger, J. G., Fisher, D., Hunkapiller, T., Pereira, D., Weissman, S. M., Uehara, H., Nathenson, S., and Hood, L. (1981). Three cDNA clones encoding mouse transplantation antigens: Homology to immunoglobulin genes. *Cell* **24,** 125.

Storb, U. (1978). Direct demonstration of immunoglobulin κ chain RNA in thymus T cells by *in situ* hybridization. *Proc. Natl. Acad. Sci. U.S.A.* **75,** 2905.

Sutcliffe, J. G., Shinnick, T. M., Green, N., Liu, F.-T., Niman, H. L., and Lerner, R. A. (1980). Chemical synthesis of a polypeptide predicted from nucleotide sequence allows detection of a new retroviral gene product. *Nature (London)* **287,** 801.

Szostak, J. W., Stiles, J. I., Tye, B.-K., Chiu, P., Sherman, F., and Wu, R. (1979). Hybridization with synthetic oligonucleotides. *In* "Methods in Enzymology" (R. Wu, ed.), Vol. 68, p. 419. Academic Press, New York.

Taylor, J. M., Illmensee, R., and Summers, J. (1976). Efficient transcription of RNA into DNA by avian sarcoma virus polymerase. *Biochim Biophys. Acta* **442,** 324.

Tonelle, C., Pierres, M., Ju, S.-T., Moinier, D., Fougereau, M. (1981). NH_2-terminal amino acid sequences of poly (Glu^{60}, Ala^{30}, Tyr^{10}) (GAT) and poly (Glu^{60}, Ala^{40}) (GA) monoclonal antibody heavy chains. *Molec. Immunol.* **18,** 979.

Villa-Komaroff, L., Efstratiadis, A., Bloome, S., Lomedico, P., Tizard, R., Naber, S. P., Chick, W. L., and Gilbert, W. (1978). A bacterial clone synthesizing proinsulin. *Proc. Natl. Acad. Sci. U.S.A.* **75,** 3727.

Walker, I. D., and Harris, A. W. (1980). Immunoglobulin C_μ RNA in T lymphoma cells is not translated. *Nature (London)* **288,** 290.

Wallace, R. B., Johnson, M. J., Hirose, T., Miyake, T., Kawashima, E. H., and Itakura, K. (1981). The use of synthetic oligonucleotides as hybridization probes. II. Hybridization of oligonucleotides of mixed sequence to rabbit β-globin DNA. *Nucleic Acids Res.* **9,** 879.

Zuniga, M. C., D'Eustachio, P., and Ruddle, N. H. (1982). Immunoglobulin heavy chain gene rearrangement and transcription in murine T cell hybrids and T lymphomas. *Proc. Natl. Acad. Sci. U.S.A.* (in press).

IX

Appendix

This Appendix is intended to serve as a source of methods as well as references to allow readers of this book to be able to isolate and quantify the lymphokines which allow T cell growth and to isolate and clone T cells. For each major section of the book, there will be a methodology section and reference list. The first series of methods will deal with the isolation and characterization of interleukin-1 (IL-1) and interleukin-2 (IL-2). In addition to these methodologies, there is a table listing the sources of available cell lines which either produce or are used for assaying the various lymphokines. There is a listing of methods available for the characterization of a variety of lymphokines which have been identified as being products of cloned murine T lymphocyte lines. Rather than go into detail with each of these methods, we have simply referenced the appropriate articles. The techniques used for T cell fusion have been reported in the literature and are basically simple derivatives of the elegant technology first described by Köhler and Millstein for the isolation of fusion products between a drug-marked myeloma and immune B cells. The description of Poisson statistics and clonal dilution analysis will provide readers with the necessary methodology for doing limiting dilution and clonal analyses. The generation of primary and secondary mixed lymphocyte reactions in bulk cultures as well as the isolation of murine T lymphocyte alloreactive clones follow methodologies which are used in the laboratories indicated. Methods for isolation of murine CTL clones also have been described. Murine T cell clones reactive with soluble antigens fall into two separate categories. The technology reported by Kimoto and Fathman has allowed the isolation of T cell helper clones. The somewhat different methodology used by Schwartz and his collaborators apparently selects for T lymphocytes at a separate point of differentiation probably due to the isolation of the T cell

ISBN 0-12-249920-4

clones soon after they have been taken from the immune mouse. Also included are methods which will allow the readers to generate and isolate clones of human alloreactive T cells. The generation of human antigen-reactive T cell clones has been described by Sredni and his associates. This Appendix has not outlined all of the techniques available for questions one might address with T cell clones. Rather, it includes the most pertinent methodologies and references which will allow the readers the opportunity of isolating T cell clones on their own.

I. FACTORS WHICH INFLUENCE THE GROWTH OF T LYMPHOCYTE CLONES

There is a large body of literature concerning isolation and assay of various lymphokines which support the growth of T cells. (Aarden *et al.*, 1979; Gillis *et al.*, 1978, 1980; Gillis and Mizel, 1981; Oppenheim *et al.*, 1979; Möller, 1980). The following several sections provide detailed methods for the assay of IL-1 activity (Oppenheim *et al.*, 1979; Gillis and Mizel, 1981) and the preparation of active supernatants containing TCGF (Gillis *et al.*, 1978, 1980) as well as methods for assaying I1-2 activities (Gillis *et al.*, 1978). Additional methods detail the biochemical purification of I1-2 and are presented by Gillis *et al.* (Appendix, Section IG).

REFERENCES

Aarden, L. A. (1979). Revised nomenclature for antigen non-specific T-cell proliferation and helper factors. *J. Immunol.* **123,** 2928.

Gillis, S., and Mizel, S. B. (1981). T cell lymphoma model for the analysis of interleukin-1 mediated T-cell activation. *Proc. Natl. Acad. Sci. U.S.A.* **78,** 1133.

Gillis, S., Ferm, M. M., Lu, W., and Smith, K. A. (1978). T cell growth factor: Parameters of production and quantitative microassay for activity. *J. Immunol.* **120,** 2027.

Gillis, S., Smith, K. A., and Watson, J. D. (1980). Biochemical and biological characterization of lymphocyte regulatory molecules. II. Purification of a class of rat and human lymphokines. *J. Immunol.* **124,** 1954.

Möller, G., ed. (1980). T cell stimulating growth factors. *Immunol Rev.* **5,** 1.

Oppenheim, J. A., Mizel, S. B., and Meltzer, M. S. (1979). Biological effects of lymphocyte and macrophage derived mitogenic "amplification" factors. *In* "The Biology of the Lymphokines" (S. Cohen, E. Pick, and J. J. Openheim, eds.), p. 291. Academic Press, New York.

A. Assay for Interleukin-1 (IL-1)

Igal Gery

Medium. The medium routinely used in this laboratory is RPMI-1640, with penicillin (100 U/ml) and streptomycin (100 μg/ml). When used for cell cultures, the medium is supplemented with fetal calf serum (FCS), at the concentration of 5%. Some authors add 2-mercaptoethanol to the culture medium (at 5×10^{-5} *M*), but we have found this unnecessary.

Tested Preparations. IL-1 is relatively stable, and samples may be stored at −20°C for weeks without a significant loss in activity. Tested samples are serially diluted in the medium with FCS, and aliquots of 100 μl are added in

ISOLATION, CHARACTERIZATION, AND UTILIZATION OF T LYMPHOCYTE CLONES

ISBN 0-12-249920-4

triplicate to 96-well flat bottom microplates (Falcon, Oxnard, California, or Linbro, Hamden, Connecticut). The dilution range routinely used in this laboratory is 1 : 5 to 1 : 320, which gives the final dilutions of 1 : 10 to 1 : 640.

Thymocytes. Mice of various inbred strains can be used. Strain C3H/HeJ has been used in many studies, particularly in order to avoid the effect of LPS on the thymocyte cultures, but thymocytes of strain CBA/N were found in this laboratory to be more sensitive to IL-1. The mice are usually used at the age range of 6–10 weeks, with the younger animals (6–7 weeks) yielding more cells per thymus, but often with lower mitotic responsiveness. The thymus is removed aseptically and teased, and the cells are spun down and washed once in the medium. Tissue aggregates are removed by gravitation, and the homogeneous thymocyte suspension is diluted to give a concentration of 15×10^6/ml. Before being added to the tested samples, the thymocytes are mixed with phytohemagglutinin (PHA-P, Difco, Detroit, Michigan), which has been diluted to 1 : 1000, to give a final concentration in the cultures of 0.05%. The thymocyte suspension is added in aliquots of 100 μl, and the cultures are incubated for 72 hr at 37°C with 5% CO_2 in air. Six hours before harvesting, the cultures are pulsed with [^{3}H]thymidine (Amersham, Arlington Heights, Illinois, 2 Ci/mmole, 0.5 μCi/10 μl/well). Harvesting is carried out by a MASH II harvester (M. A. Bioproducts, Walkersville, Maryland). The radioactivity retained on the filter discs is measured by scintillation counting.

Expression of Results. IL-1 activity may be recorded as the amount of [^{3}H]thymidine (in mean cpm ± SEM) incorporated by the thymocytes stimulated with a certain dilution of the tested sample. When high levels of IL-1 activity are present, the dose response may give a plateau. Recording the IL-1 activity of such samples may be more informative, therefore, when the results of two dilutions are included. Recently, an IL-1 unit system has been introduced. The advantages of this system are (a) the simplicity of data recording; (b) the standardization of data from different experiments and various laboratories; and (c) that this system takes into account the IL-1 activity at all dilutions of the tested sample. The unit value is assessed by dilution analysis of the tested sample and a standard preparation with a known unit value (Mizel, 1980). Standard samples used in this laboratory are calibrated routinely against those used in the laboratory of Dr. J. J. Openheim (NIDR, NIH, Bethesda, Maryland).

REFERENCES

Mizel, S. B. (1980). Studies on the purification and structure-function relationship of murine lymphocyte activating factor (IL-1). *Mol. Immunol.* **17,** 571.

B. T Cell Lymphoma Model for the Analysis of Interleukin-1 (IL-1)

S. Gillis and S. B. Mizel

The isolation and cloning of several murine tumor cell lines which produce IL-2 has led to elaboration of an interesting new assay for detection of IL-1 activity. Of the LBRM-33 clones assayed for IL-1 production following PHA stimulation (Gillis *et al.*, 1980), one nonproducing clone (1A5) was isolated. Since several investigators had shown recently that the macrophage requirement for IL-2 production by normal splenic T cells could be replaced by addition of IL-1 to mitogen-stimulated purified T cells, we questioned whether inclusion of IL-1 in cultures of 1A5 cell line cultures stimulated by phytohemagglutinin (PHA) might initiate IL-2 biosynthesis and secretion by a normally nonproducing cell line. Positive results from IL-1 addition experiments in fact led to the development of the sensitive assay for IL-1 activity. In the absence of the monokine, PHA-stimulated 1A5 cell failed to produce IL-1 (as assayed by the capacity of the resultant supernate to trigger proliferation of a T cell line), whereas in the presence of IL-1, PHA-stimulated 1A5 cells produced copious quantities of IL-2. The quantity of IL-2 produced by IL-1-stimulated 1A5 cells is equivalent in magnitude to that generated by mitogen-stimulated LBRM-33 IL-2-producing clones.

The observation that concentrations of IL-1 below levels detectable in the standard thymocyte mitogenesis assays (Mizell *et al.*, 1978) promoted IL-2 production by the mitogen-stimulated 1A5 cell line indicated that an assay using this cloned lymphoma cell line assay might be a more sensitive means of detecting concentrations of IL-1. In fact, simultaneous dose response experiments conducted in both systems revealed that the assay using the 1A5 cell line was approximately 10-fold more sensitive than the thymocyte mitogenesis technique (Gillis and Mizell, 1981).

Assays using the 1A5 cell line to measure levels of IL-1 are conducted by culturing 1A5 cells (10^6 cell/ml in RPMI 1640 medium, 10% fetal calf serum (FCS) with antibiotics and 2.5×10^{-5} *M* 2-mercaptoethanol) in triplicate in the presence of a $\log_2$ dilution series of samples suspected of containing IL-1 activity. Microplate wells also contain 1% PHA by volume (Gibco, PHA-M). The final volume is 200 μl. Twenty-four hours after initiation of PHA stimulation, 100 μl aliquots from each of the triplicate microwells for each concentration of IL-1 sample are pooled and assayed for the presence of IL-2 activity (see Appendix, Section I,G). Addition of as little as 1 unit/ml IL-1 has led to a maximal IL-2 production by 1A5 cells (between 50 and 200 U/ml IL-2 activity). Generally speaking, IL-1 activity at a concentration of 0.2–0.5 units/ml resulted in IL-2

ISBN 0-12-249920-4

production at half-maximal levels by PHA-stimulated 1A5 cells. Assay of a solution containing less than 1 U/ml IL-1 activity in standard thymocyte mitogenesis assays would show little if any capacity to augment PHA-triggered thymocyte replication. As is the case with mathematical interpretation of IL-2 units, IL-1 activity is quantified by a conventional dose response assay in which unknown samples are compared with an arbitrary standard solution (for example, 72-hr lipopolysaccharide-activated p388D_1 tumor cell supernate, Mizel *et al.*, 1978) and interpolation of resulting data by probit analysis (Gillis and Mizel, 1981).

REFERENCES

Gillis, S., and Mizel, S. (1981). T cell lymphoma model for the analysis of Interleukin-1 mediated T cell activation. *Proc. Natl. Acad. Sci. U.S.A.* **78,** 1133.

Gillis, S., Scheid, M., and Watson, J. (1980). The biochemical and biological characterization of lymphocyte regulatory molecules. III. The isolation and phenotypic characterization of interleukin 2 producing T cell lymphomas. *J. Immunol.* **125,** 2570.

Mizel, S. B., Oppenheim, J. J., and Rosenstreich, D. L. (1978). Characterization of lymphocyte activating factor (LAF) produced by the macrophage line p388D_1. I. Enhancement of LAF production by activated T lymphocytes. *J. Immunol.* **120,** 1497.

C. Preparation of TCGF from Rat Spleen Cells

Klaus Eichmann

The spleens of 10–40 Sprague-Dawley rats are removed, and single-cell suspensions are cultured for 24 hr at 5 × 10^6/ml in 70-ml portions of Iscove's modified Dulbecco's medium (IMDM) supplemented with 10% fetal calf serum (FSC), 10^{-5} *M* 2-mercaptoethanol (2-ME), 1% pencillin-streptomycin, 0.025 *M* HEPES, and 5 μg/ml concanavalin A (Con-A) in a 5% CO_2 atmosphere. The supernate that contained TCGF is collected by centrifugation, aliquoted, and stored at −70°C. The efficiency of each TCGF preparation is determined by its support of the proliferation of various T cell lines *in vitro*. The cell line HT2 is available as an indicator T cell line from C. G. Fathman. Samples of 1 × 10^4 of such T cells are cultured overnight in 200 μl of various dilutions of TCGF in IMDM in round-bottom Linbro microtiter plates (Linbro Chemical Co., Hamden, Connecticut), labeled with [^{3}H]thymidine for 4–6 hr, and ^{3}H incorporation is then determined. Optimal support of TCGF is at dilutions from 1:20 to 1:5. Most of the experiments described in Chapter 19 in the treatise were performed with a single TCGF preparation, which gave optimal results at a dilution of 1 : 20.

ISOLATION, CHARACTERIZATION, AND
UTILIZATION OF T LYMPHOCYTE CLONES

ISBN 0-12-249920-4

D. Preparation of TCGF from a T Cell Tumor (EL-4)

Chuan Chen and Ronald H. Schwartz

EL-4 cells (Farrar *et al.*, 1980) are grown to a density of 10^6/ml in RPMI-1640 medium with 5% fetal calf serum (FCS) and 50 μg/ml gentamicin. Stimulate each 10^6 cells/ml with 10 ng of phorbol myristate acetate (PMA). Our usual conditions are 100 ml of medium containing 10^8 cells in a 150 ml tissue culture flask plus 1 μg of PMA. The cells are incubated with the PMA for 48 hr at 37°C in a 5% CO_2 incubator. At the end of the incubation, the supernatant, which contains the T cell growth factor (TCGF), is collected by centrifugation (1200 *g* for 10 min), and the PMA is removed by adsorption with charcoal. Activated charcoal (2.0 g), Dextran T10 (0.5 g), and 165 ml RPMI-1640 supplemented with 5% FCS and 50 μg/ml gentamicin are mixed and centrifuged at 9000 *g* in a 200 ml plastic centrifuge tube in a Sorval centrifuge at room temperature for 5 min. The supernatant is decanted and the charcoal pellet washed again only with supplemented RPMI-1640. After decanting the second wash, the charcoal pellet is mixed with 165 ml of crude tumor factor containing the PMA and quickly centrifuged again at the same speed. At the end of the 5-min spin, collect the supernatant as soon as possible. This preparation is referred to as the crude tumor factor without PMA.

Purification of the TCGF can be achieved by concentrating the crude tumor factor without PMA about 20-fold with an Amicon membrane unit (YM 10) and passing the concentrate over a Sephadex G-100 column. Both the concentration and the column separation should be done in the cold. The active fractions are identified by their ability to support the growth of a TCGF-dependent T cell line. The active fractions are then pooled and filtered through a 0.45 μm Millipore filter unit (Sterifil D-HA) to sterilize the factor. The filtered material, which we refer to as purified tumor factor, is aliquoted and stored at −20°C until ready for use.

REFERENCES

Farrar, J. J., Fuller-Farrar, J., Simon, P. L., Hilfiker, M. L., Stadler, B. M., and Farrar, W. L. (1980). Thymoma production of T cell growth factor (interleukin 2). *J. Immunol.* **125,** 2555.

E. Production of Human TCGF

Elizabeth A. Grimm and Steven A. Rosenberg

Media. Culture media for IL-2 production is prepared by supplementing RPMI 1640 (Gibco, Grand Island, New York) with glutamine (2%) and if de-

ISBN 0-12-249920-4

sired antibiotics (penicillin, 100 U/ml and streptomycin 100 μg/ml, NIH Media Unit). Human AB serum is added to achieve a final 2% concentration of IL-2 production from peripheral blood lymphocytes (PBL) and thoracic duct lymphocytes (TDL); however, 10% AB serum has been found to be optimal for production of IL-2 from spleen cells. Freshly hydrated PHA-P (Difco, Detroit, Michigan) is added to a final concentration of 0.2% in the medium.

Cells. PBL are prepared from heparinized whole blood by Ficoll-Hypaque gradient separation and collection of the buffy interphase. PBL are washed twice in a buffered salt solution (BSS) and counted, then added to the culture medium at a final concentration of 5×10^6/ml.

Spleen cells are prepared by mincing human spleen tissue with scissors or scalpel to free the lymphoid cells. The spleen cells are washed in BSS and the red blood cells are lysed in a buffered ammonium chloride solution. The resulting cells are counted and adjusted to a final concentration of 5×10^6/ml in the culture medium. (The culture medium should be supplemented with 10% human AB serum for IL-2 production from human spleen.) TDL are prepared for IL-2 production from heparinized thoracic duct drainage are washed and prepared using the same procedure described for spleen.

Cells from the above tissues may be used from individual donors, or may be pooled, since no differences in IL-2 production have been found.

Culture and Incubation. Cells and medium can be cultured in a variety of vessels. Since we routinely prepare large quantities, we use the Falcon 3045 flask (Becton Dickinson Labware, Oxnard, California) to culture 150 to 200 ml. Flasks are incubated horizontally in a 37°C, 5% CO_2 humidified incubator for 48 hr. Cultures are harvested by centrifugation of the culture contents at 1500 rpm for 10 min. The supernatant is then collected and immediately frozen, or centrifuged at a higher speed (7000 rpm) to pellet subcellular debris and then frozen. Aliquots of the supernatant are saved for testing in the assays for IL-2, performed as described in Appendix IG.

F. Preparation of TCGF from Human Spleen Cells

Fritz Bach

The basic method used for deriving TCGF-containing medium from spleen cells is quite simple. Spleens are obtained at routine splenectomy from potential kidney transplant recipients prior to transplantation; all such individuals have received five 125 ml aliquots of blood. It is not known whether the immunization which may occur secondary to blood transfusion has any effect on the results we have obtained utilizing TCGF from these cells. Spleen cells, irradiated with 1000 R, are suspended at 1×10^6/ml in a total of 100 ml RPMI-1640 supplemented

ISBN 0-12-249920-4

with 3% human serum and 1% PHA-M, in 150-ml flasks (Corning) (100×10^6 cells/flask).

We have compared cultured supernatants for their TCGF activity (i) that have been incubated for 24 hr; (ii) that have been incubated for 48 hr; or (iii) that have been incubated for 24 hr following which the cells are resuspended to fresh medium plus 1% phytohemagglutinin (PHA) and recultured in the original flasks for an additional 24 hr, i.e., evaluating the supernatant present from 24 to 48 hr after initiation of culture. The TCGF activity, as assayed for its ability to stimulate day 10 reversion primary mixed lymphocyte culture (MLC) cells, is similar in the different preparations. Each of the preparations was somewhat inhibitory at a dilution of 1 : 2, i.e., 50% TCGF-containing medium, and showed peak activity at a dilution of 1 : 4, i.e., 25% TCGF-containing medium. Since the supernatant harvested following the first 24 hr of culture and the supernatant present from 24 hr to 48 hr of culture both showed approximately equal levels of activity, a double yield of conditioned medium can be obtained from a single batch of cells.

The supernatant factor derived from spleen cells is, in our hands, of consistent high activity and more potent than that derived from peripheral blood lymphocytes by a factor of approximately 2-fold.

G. IL-2 Microassay

Steven Gillis

The IL-2 assay is based on the dependence of cultured T cell lines on IL-2. T cells harvested from IL-2 dependent culture, washed, and placed back in culture in the absence of IL-2 invariably die within 24 hr. By using tritiated thymidine incorporation (^{3}H-TdR) as an index of cultured T cell replication, the IL-2 microassay provides a highly reproducible and quantitative indication of the amount of IL-2 activity present in a given sample of crude or biochemically manipulated conditioned medium (CM). To assay a CM or column fraction for IL-2 activity, serial ($\log_2$) dilutions of the sample are plated (100 μl volume) in replicate microculture wells (96 well flat bottom microtiter plate, No. 3596, Costar Inc., Cambridge, Massachusetts). Dilutions of the sample are made using RPMI 1640 medium supplemented with 2% heat-inactivated (56°C for 30 min) fetal calf serum, (FCS), 2.5×10^{-5} *M* 2-mercaptoethanol, 50 U/ml penicillin, 50 μg/ml streptomycin, and 300 μg/ml fresh L-glutamine. Sample concentration should range from 0.5 to 50%. Any IL-2-dependent T cell line can serve as an indicator cell for IL-2 microassay. Three thousand T cells harvested from long-term culture are then added in 100 μl of medium to each microplate well. After overnight culture at 37°C in an atmosphere of 5% CO_2 in air, each microwell culture is pulsed for an additional 4 hr with 0.5 μCi of ^{3}H-TdR (20 Ci/mm specific activity). Cultures are harvested onto glass fiber filter strips and ^{3}H-TdR

ISOLATION, CHARACTERIZATION, AND
UTILIZATION OF T LYMPHOCYTE CLONES

ISBN 0-12-249920-4

TABLE I

Cell Lines Capable of IL-2 Production

Cell line (Reference)	Species	Type	IL-2 production characteristics
FS6[a]	Mouse	T cell hybridoma	Mitogen inducible
123[b]	Mouse	T cell hybridoma	Mitogen inducible
1A8C3C10[c]	Mouse	T cell hybridoma	Constitutive
EL-4[d]	Mouse	Lymphoma	Phorbol ester inducible
LBRM-33[e]	Mouse	Lymphoma	Mitogen inducible
WEHI-7[f]	Mouse	Lymphoma	Mitogen plus IL-1 inducible
1A5[g]	Mouse	Lymphoma	Mitogen and IL-1 inducible
A4A[h]	Mouse	Initiated by conditioned medium from WEHI-3-initiated bone marrow cell lines	Phorbol ester inducible
MLA144[i]	Gibbon ape	Leukemia	Constitutive
Jurkat[j]	Human	Leukemia	Mitogen inducible
YK7[k]	Human	T cell hybridoma	Constitutive

[a] Harwell, L., Skidmore, B., Marrack, P., and Kappler, J. W. (1980). Concanavalin A-inducible interleukin-2-producing T cell hybridomas. *J. Exp. Med.* **152,** 893.

[b] Schrader, J., Arnold, B., and Clark-Lewis, I. (1980). A Con A-stimulated T-cell hybridoma releases factors affecting colony-forming cells and B-cell antibody responses. *Nature (London)* **283,** 197.

[c] Stull, D., and Gillis, S. (1981). Constitutive production of interleukin 2 activity by a T cell hybridoma. *J. Immunol.* **126,** 1680.

[d] Farrar, J. J., Fuller-Farrar, J., Simon, P. L., Hilfiker, M. L., Stadler, B. M., and Farrar, W. L. (1980). Thymoma production of T cell growth factor (interleukin 2). *J. Immunol.* **125,** 2555.

[e] Gillis, S., Scheid, M., and Watson, J. (1980). The biochemical and biological characterization of lymphocyte regulatory molecules. III. The isolation and phenotypic characterization of interleukin 2 producing T cell lymphomas. *J. Immunol.* **125,** 2570.

[f] Smith, K. A., Gilbride, K. J., and Favata, M. F. (1980). Lymphocyte activating factor promotes T-cell growth factor production by cloned murine lymphoma cells. *Nature (London)* **287,** 853.

[g] Gillis, S., and Mizel, S. (1981). T cell lymphoma model for the analysis of interleukin-1 mediated T cell activation. *Proc. Natl. Acad. Sci. U.S.A.* **78,** 1133.

[h] Lee, J. C., Enjuanes, L., Cicurel, L., and Ihle, J. (1981). T cell recognition of Moloney sarcoma virus proteins. II. Phenotypes of the different lymphocyte subpopulations producing and responding to blastogenic factors and their relative frequencies during tumor regression. *J. Immunol.* **127,** 78.

[i] Rabin, H., Hopkins, R. F., III, Ruscetti, F. W., Neubauer, R. H., Brown, R. L., and Kawakami, T. G. (1981). Spontaneous release of a factor with properties of T cell growth factor from a continuous line of primate tumor T cells. *J. Immunol.* **127,** 1852.

[j] Gillis, S., and Watson, J. (1980). Biochemical and biological characterization of lymphocyte regulatory molecules. V. Identification of an interleukin 2 producer human leukemia T cell line. *J. Exp. Med.* **152,** 1709.

[k] Okada, M., Yoshimura, N., Kaieda, T., Yamamura, Y., and Kishimoto, T. (1982). Establishment and characterization of human T hybrid cell secreting immunoregulatory molecules. *Proc. Natl. Acad. Sci., U.S.A.* (in press).

incorporation measured as an index of cellular proliferation. Using these procedures, IL-2-dependent indicator T cells will incorporate approximately 10,000 cpm of ^{3}H-Tdr in the presence of a saturating concentration of IL-2 (Gillis *et al.*, 1978). In the absence of IL-2, incorporated cpm of ^{3}H-TdR will be only marginally above background levels (approximately 100 cpm), consistent with the observation that independent T cells deprived of IL-2 for as little as 24 hr are greater than 95% dead. Units per milliliter of IL-2 activity is standardized and quantified by probit analysis of raw ^{3}H-TdR incorporation data (Gillis *et al.*, 1978). Roughly speaking, a 1 U/ml IL-2 sample will induce 50% of the maximum proliferation observed where IL-2 is saturating (50% of 10,000 cpm or approximately 5000 cpm) at a dilution of 1 : 4. Therefore, a 10 U/ml sample would induce 5000 cpm of T cell ^{3}H-TdR incorporation at a sample dilution of 1 : 40. Cell lines available for IL-2 production are listed in Table I.

REFERENCES

Gillis, S., Ferm, M. M., Lu, W., and Smith K. A. (1978). T cell growth factor: Parameters of production and quantitative microassay for activity. *J. Immunol.* **120,** 2027.

H. Purification and Characterization of IL-2

Steven Gillis, James Watson, and Diane Mochizuki

Preparative Purification of IL-2 from Human and Murine Mitogen CM

Twenty-four hour serum-free supernates harvested from cultures of either 1% PHA stimulated human peripheral blood lymphocytes (10^7 cells/ml) or concanavalin A (Con-A) (2.5 μg/ml) stimulated murine spleen cells (5×10^6 cells/ml) were concentrated by ammonium sulfate precipitation. Crude IL-2 supernates were brought to 80% saturation with $(NH_4)_2SO_4$ by gentle stirring at 4°C until dissolved. The resultant slurry was maintained at 4°C for a minimum of 12 hr prior to clarification by centrifugation at 10,000 *g* for 20 min. The precipitate was then resuspended in as little sterile 0.9% NaCl–25 m*M* HEPES, pH 7.2 (0.9% NaC1-HEPES) as possible prior to passage over gel exclusion columns.

AcA 54 Gel Filtration Chromatography

Precipitated material was fractionated on a 2 × 90 cm gel filtration column previously equilibrated in 0.9% NaC1–HEPES. The IL-2 preparate (5–20% of the bed volume) was applied to the column and eluted with 0.9% NaC1–HEPES into 7-ml fractions. The protein content of the column fractions collected was monitored with an LKB Uvicord 11 calibrated for absorbance at 280 nm. The

ISBN 0-12-249920-4

column was calibrated with the following molecular weight standards: bovine serum albumin (68,000), ovalbumin (43,000), soybean trypsin inhibitor (21,000), and cytochrome *c* (13,000). Under these conditions, assay of all fractions for IL-2 activity revealed a reproducible difference in size in size between human and murine IL-2. IL-2 activity fractionated from murine splenocyte CM chromatographed over a wide range of fractions and with a mean size of approximately 30,000 daltons (Watson *et al.*, 1979) whereas human IL-2 was detected in fractions which corresponded to mobility of molecules with a mean size range of 15,000 daltons. After detection of activity, fractions with appreciable IL-2 titer were pooled and dialyzed against 1000 volumes of 50 m*M* NaC1–HEPES prior to further separation over an ion exchange resin.

Ion Exchange Chromatography

Pretreatment of DEAE-Sephacel (Pharmacia Fine Chemicals, Piscataway, New Jersey) was conducted to minimize nonspecific sticking of IL-2 activity to the resin. After washing in 0.9% NaC1–HEPES, the matrix was then incubated for 4 hr in 0.9% NaC1–HEPES containing 2% FCS. Nonspecifically-bound proteins was removed by repetitive washing with 0.9% NaCl-HEPES. Finally, DEAE-Sephacel was washed with 0.1% Triton-X100 to prevent hydrophobic interaction, and 0.2 *M* sodium citrate to remove heavy metals. Following this series of treatments, DEAE-Sephacel columns (2 × 20 cm) were equilibrated in 50 m*M* NaCl-HEPES. Thirty-five to 75 ml of the AcA-54 passaged IL-2 solution was applied to the column. IL-2 activity was eluted by application of a salt gradient (2 column volumes) ranging from 50 to 500 m*M* NaC1–HEPES. The ionic strength of the eluted 5-ml fractions was determined using a conductivity meter. Assay of ion exchange column fractions revealed a fundamental difference in charge characteristic of human and murine IL-2 activity. Although human IL-2 activity did not bind to DEAE-Sephacel and could be recovered from the column run-through (Gillis *et al.*, 1980), murine IL-2 activity bound to the ion exchange resin and could be eluted with 185 m*M* salt. Human IL-2 activity, after run-through passage over DEAE-Sephacel (and therefore still in a solution of 50 m*M* NaCl–HEPES), was applied to a 1 × 10 cm column of carboxymethyl-Sepharose (Sigma Chemical Co., St. Louis, Missouri) equilibrated in 50 m*M* NaCl–HEPES, pH 6. Elution with two column volumns of 50 m*M* NaCl–HEPES resulted in recovery of no human IL-2 activity in the run-through solution, indicating that IL-2 applied to the column had adhered to the negatively charged resin. A control column, to which an equivalent amount of murine IL-2 was applied, bound less than 5% of the biological activity, a result expected on the demonstrated ability of murine IL-2 to bind to a positively charged ion-exchange resin. Salt gradient elution (50–1000 m*M* NaC1–HEPES) of carboxymethyl-Sepharose demonstrated that human IL-2 activity could be recovered from the negatively charged resin by competition with 225 m*M* NaC1-HEPES.

Preparative Isoelectric Focusing (IEF)

Following either one-step (DEAE for murine) or two-phase (DEAE carboxymethyl-Sepharose for human) ion exchange chromatography, active IL-2 fractions were pooled and dialyzed against 1% glycine, and 0.1% aspartate. Preparative flatbed IEF of IL-2 preparations was performed in horizontal layers of Sephadex using an LKB Multiphor apparatus. After dialysis, 2% ampholytes (pH 3–10) were added to the IL-2, the sample was then added to 4 g of Ultradex (specially treated Sephadex G-75), and the gel suspension spread in a gel tray. The slurry was dried to the appropriate crack point of the gel using a heat lamp and air blower. The tray was then transferred to a cooling plate (4°C) and electrophoresed for 24 hr under a constant current of 7 mA. During electrophoresis the voltage increased from 110–1000 V. After the gel reached electrophoretic equilibrium at 1000 V, it was sectioned into 30 portions and each section transferred in a steady manner onto a 1 × cm 5 column. The protein in each column was eluted with 5 ml of sterile distilled water. After pH determination, each eluted fraction was dialyzed sequentially against water and Hank's buffered salt solution (HBSS) containing 1 μg/ml polyethylene glycol (PEG) 6000. The extensive dialysis was to ensure adequate removal of ampholyte which inhibited IL-2 biological assays. Since little protein (less than 50 μg) was consistently associated with active IL-2 fractions, PEG was used in the dialysate to guard against loss of activity due to nonspecific adherence of IL-2 to either plastic tubes or dialysis membranes. Upon completion of dialysis procedures, IEF fractions were tested for IL-2 activity in a standard microassay.

Differences in basic physical characteristics between human and murine IL-2 continued to be evident upon analysis of IEF data. Human IL-2 migrated upon isoelectric focussing with a predominant p*I* value of 6.8, and with a minor peak of activity of p*I* 7.1 (Gillis *et al.*, 1980). Murine IL-2, however, appeared to be more acidic in nature and migrated as two distinct peaks of activity at p*I* 4.3–4.5 and 4.9–5.1.

Sample Preparation for SDS-Page

IL-2 purified by IEF was dialyzed against 50 m*M* ammonium bicarbonate, aliquoted into appropriate volumes, and lyophilized. Freeze-dried IL-2 was maintained at −70°C. Lyophilized fractions were rehydrated with sample buffer (10m*M* mono-Tris, 10% glycerol, 0.005% bromophenol blue, 0.01–1% SDS, 0–1% 2-mercaptoethanol) and heated to 70°C for 10 min immediately prior to electrophoresis.

Gel Systems

Depending on the amount of protein to be electrophoresed, either 10 × 0.6 cm tube gels or 12 × 12 cm slab gels were used. Tube gels were 13.5% acrylamide with a 9 cm, 10% acrylamide separation gel and a 2 cm, 5% acrylamide stacking gel. One to 2 cm slab gels were 13–15% acrylamide and were electrophoresed using a 13% acrylamide, 10 cm separation gel and a 5% acrylamide, 2 cm stacking gel. Stock acrylamide solution was 30% by weight acrylamide and 0.8% by weight N,N^1-bismethylene acrylamide (bis). Separation gels were 0.112 *M* mono-Tris, 0.029 *M* HC1, 0.05% TEMED, and 0.13% ammonium persulfate. Stacking gels were 0.0526 *M* mono-Tris, 0.052 *M* HC1, 0.1% TEMED, and 0.5% ammonium persulfate. Electrode buffer used was 50 m*M* bicine, 0.03% SDS. Tube gels were generally electrophoresed for 3–4 hr at a constant current of 2–3 mA/gel. During this time voltage normally increased from 65–230 V. Slab gels were routinely run overnight at a constant current of 25–30 mA. Voltage routinely increased in this time period from 65–230 V.

Recovery of Biological Activity from SDS-PAGE

Tube Gel. Following electrophoresis, tube gels were removed from container glass tubes and were immediately frozen at −70°C. The frozen gels were cut into 1-mm slices, and each gel slice was placed into a well of microtiter plate. The gel slices were washed twice with 200 μl complete media to allow diffusion of SDS and mono-Tris buffers from the gel slice. After the second wash, the media was aspirated, and the gel slices were minced. Two hundred microliters of complete media was added to each well containing a minced gel slice. IL-2 was allowed to diffuse from the gel pieces into media overnight at 37°C. Following incubation, the microtiter place was placed at 4°C for 1 hr to precipitate any residual SDS. The plate was then centrifuged at 2000 *g* for 15 min. The supernatant was removed and the IL-2 activity was determined in a standard microassay.

Slab Gel. Following electrophoresis, the gel was fixed and stained with 0.25% Coomassie Blue R (Sigma, St. Louis, Missouri) in 50% methanol, 7.5% acetic (prefiltered through Whatman no. 1). The gels were stained at room temperature while rocking for 15–30 min. The gels were destained in a solution of 20% ethanol, 7.5% acetic acid with multiple changes of the destaining solution over 2–3 hr. The individual protein bands (visualized with a light box) were cut out of the gel using a scalpel. The protein bands were then washed at room temperature (while rocking 15 min) with 5 ml of 50 m*M* Tris-acetate, pH 7.8, 0.1% SDS prior to electrophoretic elution.

Coomassie blue staining proteins were eluted from gel slices by electrophoresis using an apparatus obtained from CBS Scientific (Del Mar, California). The gel slices were first equilibrated in the electrode buffer (50 mM Tris-acetate, pH 2.8, 0.1% SDS) and then placed in the sample unit. The sample unit consisted of two vertical chambers with bore diameters of 0.1 and 0.25 cm, connected by a horizontal channel to allow buffer flow between the two chambers. A piece of dialysis membrane was held in place on the end of each chamber with rubber washers and screw caps. The gel slices were placed in the large bore chamber (anode). The two chambers were then connected with buffer. The sample was electrophoresed at constant voltage with 60–70 V (less than or equal to 0.25 W) for 15–20 hr with a buffer change every 7–10 hr. The proteins were eluted from the gel into the smaller bore buffer (cathode) chamber. At the end of the elution procedure it was possible to see the Coomassie stain adjacent to the dialysis membrane in the smaller bore chamber. Most of the buffer was then removed from the smaller elution chamber and the protein was resuspended in a small volume (100–200) of buffer by gentle pipetting. The protein sample was then assayed immediately in IL-2 microassay.

REFERENCES

Gillis, S., Smith, K. A., and Watson, J. D. (1980). Biochemical and biological characterization of lymphocyte regulatory molecules. II. Purification of a class of rat and human lymphokines. *J. Immunol.* **124,** 1954.

Mochizuki, D., Watson, J., and Gillis, S. (1980). Chemical separation of interleukin-2. *J. Immunol. Methods* **39,** 185.

Watson, J., Gillis, S., Marbrook, J., Mochizuki, D., and Smith, L. (1979). Biochemical and biological characterization of lymphocyte regulatory molecules. I. Purification of a class of murine lymphokines. *J. Exp. Med.* **150,** 849.

II. CELL FUSION AS A TECHNIQUE FOR GENERATION OF T CELL CLONES

T cell fusions have developed from simple modifications of the methodology used to fuse B cells and drug marked myeloma lines. The section by Marrack outlines how this T cell fusion is performed.

REFERENCES

Goldsby, R. A., Osborne, B. A., Simpson, E., and Herzenberg, L. A. (1977). Hybrid cell lines with T cell characteristics. *Nature (London)* **267,** 707.

Harwell, L., Skidmore, B., Marrack, P., and Kappler, J. W. (1980). Concanavalin A inducible interleukin-2 producing T-cell hybridoma. *J. Exp. Med.* **152,** 893.

Kishimoto, T., Suemura, M., Sugimura, K., Okada, M., Nakanishi, K., and Yamamura, Y. (1981).

Characterization of T cell derived immunoregulatory molecules from murine or human T cell hybridomas. *In* "Lymphokine Reports: A Forum for Nonantibody Lymphocyte Products" (M. Feldman, ed.), Vol. 4. Academic Press, New York.

Kontiainen, S., Simpson, E., Beverley, P. C. L., Herzenberg, L. A., Fitzpatrick, W. C., Vogt, T., Torano, A., Mackenzie, I. F. C., and Feldman, M. (1978). T cell lines producing antigen specific suppressor factors. *Nature (London)* **274,** 477.

Taniguchi, M., and Miller, J. F. A. P. (1978). Specific suppressive factors produced by hybridomas derived from the fusion of enriched suppressor T-cells and a T lymphoma cell line. *J. Exp. Med.* **148,** 373.

A. Production of Antigen-Specific, *H-2* Restricted T Cell Hybridomas

Philippa Marrack

Mice are primed in the base of the tail with between 20 and 100 μg of antigen in complete Freund's adjuvant (Corradin *et al.,* 1977). Seven days later, cell suspensions are prepared from the inguinal and periaortic lymph nodes. Cells are resuspended at 4×10^6/ml in modified Click's medium containing 1% normal mouse serum and about 100 μg/ml antigen. These are incubated for 4 days in 2% CO_2, 98% air. At this point dead cells are removed by centrifugation on Ficoll–Hypaque gradients. Live cells, which are enriched for antigen reactivity, are then resuspended at 10^5/ml in modified Mishell–Dutton medium containing 10% fetal calf serum, mouse interleukin-2 (IL-2) but no antigen. The exact concentration of IL-2-containing medium to be added varies with the batch, but is usually 20% of a concanavalin A (Con-A)-induced supernatant of AOFS 21.10.9, or 50% normal mouse spleen or FS6–14.13 Con-A-induced supernatant (Harwell *et al.,* 1980). This mixture is incubated for 3 more days in 10% CO_2, 90% air before harvesting and removal of dead cells on a Ficoll–Hypaque gradient. Cell yields vary with the antigen used but should be between 20 and 50% of starting cell number after 4 days incubation with antigen and removal of dead cells. This yield will increase between 2- and 4-fold during 3 days incubation in IL-2 (Schrier *et al.,* 1979).

These cells are fused to BW5147.G.1.4 Oua^r.1 or FS6-14.13.AG2 (Kappler *et al.,* 1981) as follows. About 2×10^7 tumor cells and 10^8 antigen-specific T cell blasts are thoroughly washed with balanced salt solution (BSS). They are then mixed in a 50-ml conical tube and cosedimented. The supernatant is removed, and the tub[illegible] .rifuged for a short time to spin any liquid adhering to the sides of the tube to the bottom. This is removed by suction. The cell pellet is then broken up over the cone of the tube by gentle tapping. The tube is placed in a 37°C water bath and 1 ml of a 1 : 1 mixture of polyethylene glycol 1540 (average molecular weight 1300–1600, Baker Chemical Co.) and serum-free medium (gassed with 10% CO_2, 90% air) at 37°C is added dropwise over the course of 45

ISBN 0-12-249920-4

sec. The mixture is left to stand at 37°C for a further 45 sec before slow dilution with 50 ml of medium at 37°C, again containing no serum. Dilution is achieved by dripping in 1 ml of medium in the first 30 sec, 2 ml medium in the next 30 sec, 3 ml medium in the next 30 sec, and 4 ml in the next 30 sec, before gentle addition of the remaining 40 ml of medium. During this period the polyethylene glycol, cells, and medium are only mixed by very gentle jostling of the tube.

After dilution, the mixture is left to stand for a further 5 min at 37°C. The cells are then centrifuged, washed once with BSS without vigorous resuspension of the pellent, and then gently resuspended in 40 ml modified Mishell–Dutton medium, 10% fetal calf serum, using a 10-ml pipette. The mixture is dispensed in 0.1 ml aliquots into 96-well tissue culture dishes applying as little shearing force as possible. The plates are incubated at 37°C in gassed boxes. One day later, 0.5 ml of 3× concentrated HAT in medium is added to each well. Medium is changed every 5 days. The presence of HAT is maintained in the medium for at least 3 weeks. The first hybrids from such a fusion must be harvested from these plates 9 or 10 days after fusion, though hybrids will continue to appear for about one month.

After removal from microcultures, hybrids are grown in 15-ml conical tissue culture tubes until they reach a concentration of about 2×10^5/ml in 2 ml. At this point 2×10^5 cells are removed and assayed for antigen specificity by IL-2 production in response to antigen stimulation (usually at about 1 mg/ml) and antigen-presenting cells (5×10^6/ml, 4000 R irradiated, spleen cells of appropriate *H-2* haplotype) (Kappler *et al.*, 1981). The remaining hybridoma cells are maintained in conical tubes during the 2-day assay period. Hybrids of interest are then grown up, cloned, and frozen. Plating efficiencies vary tremendously, ranging from less than 10% to nearly 100%, but are greatly improved by adding to the cloning medium either 10^5/ml HAT-sensitive L10A.2J B lymphoma cells, 10^6/ml irradiated thymocytes, or a 30% concentration of spent medium from a B cell lymphoma, L10A.2J.

Hybrids between BW5147 and normal T cells may be prepared by the same methods without prior selection for antigen reactivity. Con-A-inducible IL-2-secreting hybridomas, AOFS 21.10.9 and FS6-14.13, are available from our laboratory.

REFERENCES

Corradin, G., Etlinger, H. M., and Chiller, J. M. (1977). Lymphocyte specificity to protein antigens. I. Characterization of the antigen-induced *in vitro* T cell-dependent proliferative response with lymph node cells from primed mice. *J. Immunol.* **119,** 1048.

Harwell, L., Skidmore, B., Marrack, P., and Kappler, J. W. (1980). Concanavalin A-inducible, interleukin-2-producing T cell hybridoma. *J. Exp. Med.* **152,** 893.

Kappler, J. W., Skidmore, B., White, J., and Marrack, P. (1981). Antigen-inducible, *H-2* restricted, interleukin-2-producing T cell hybridomas. Lack of independent antigen and H-2 recognition. *J. Exp. Med.* **153,** 1198.

Schrier, R. P., Skidmore, B. J., Kurnick, J. T., Goldstine, S. N., and Chiller, J. M. (1979). Propagation of antigen-specific T cell helper function *in vitro*. *J. Immunol.* **123,** 2525.

III. CLONAL ANALYSIS BY LIMITING DILUTION

Techniques for analysis of precursor frequency have been developed from the original paper by Porter and Berry (1963). These methods have been applied by a variety of investigators to limiting dilution analysis (Eichmann *et al.*, 1980; Fischer-Lindahl and Wilson, 1977; Taswell, 1981), and several are presented in following chapters along with techniques for assaying functional activity of T cells obtained through limiting dilution techniques.

REFERENCES

Eichmann, K., Falk, I., Melchers, I., and Simon, M. M. (1980). Quantitative study on T cell diversity. I. Determination of the precursor frequencies for two types of Streptococcus A specific helper cells in non-immune polyclonally activated splenic T cells. *J. Exp. Med.* **152,** 477.

Fischer Lindahl, K., and Wilson, D. B. (1977). Histocompatibility antigen activated cytotoxic T lymphocytes. II. Estimates of the frequency and specificity of precursors. *J. Exp. Med.* **145,** 503.

Porter, E. H., and Berry, R. J. (1963). The efficient design of transplantable tumor assays. *Br. J. Cancer* **17,** 583.

Taswell, C. (1981). Limiting dilution assays for the determination of immunocompetent cell frequencies. I. Data analysis. *J. Immunol.* **126,** 1614.

A. Measurement and Calculation of CTL-P Frequencies

Helen Derry and R. G. Miller

The following is a sensitive yet simple method to measure CTL-P frequency in an MLR. The cultures and assay are done in the same wells—one merely removes some of the culture supernatant at the time of assay and replaces it with radiolabeled target cells. At the end of the assay, the supernatant is transferred to a gamma counting tube. Cultures are then scored as responding or nonresponding, and a computer program is used to calculate the CTL-P frequency.

Cultures are set up in 96 well V bottom tissue culture microtiter trays. Culture medium is Alpha MEM supplemented with 10% fetal calf serum (FCS) (heat inactivated at 56°C for 45 min), 10 m*M* HEPES buffer, 5×10^{-5} *M* 2-mercaptoethanol. Not all FCS will support a mixed leukocyte culture (MLC);

ISBN 0-12-249920-4

several batches should be tested for optimum response. Since culture volumes are small (0.2 ml), evaporation can result in erroneous results, particularly in wells at the periphery of the microtiter plate. Incubator floors should be filled with water to maximum depth possible.

Spleen cells or cells from axillary, brachial, and inguinal lymph nodes (LN) may be used as the responding population. Mesenteric lymph nodes can give different results. With spleen cells, the cell number should be increased about threefold, since the frequency of CTL-P in spleen is lower than in LN. For generation of MLC in microtiter trays, 3×10^4 LN cells and 3×10^5 irradiated spleen cells are sufficient to provide all the cells necessary. At lower than this number of LN cells, an accessory cell or factor must be provided to allow the expansion of an activated CTL-P. This is achieved in this culture system by the addition of nu/nu spleen cells to small numbers of LN cells. The nude spleen cells do not make CTL in response to the alloantigen but provide the means for the CTL-P to expand into detectable clones of CTL. Spleen cells thoroughly depleted of T cells by treatment with anti-Thy-1 and complement also can be used as accessory cells (Lutz *et al.*, 1981).

Prepare cell suspensions in 6 ml of culture medium and add to a 17 × 100 mm tube (Falcon No. 2057). Underlay the cell suspension with 3 ml of 6% BSA in phosphate buffered saline (or 100% FCS). Spin in a clinical centrifuge at 1000 rpm (160 *g*) for 5 min. The pellet will contain cells free of debris, enriched for live cells, and relatively depleted of RBC. Resuspend the pellet in 2–3 ml of culture medium. Stimulating spleen cells are irradiated (1500 rads).

A typical limiting dilution experiment to measure frequency of CTL-P is given in the tabulation below.

Group	Responder B6 nu/+ LN	Added cells B6 nu/nu S	Stimulator BALB/c nu/+ S 1500 rads	No. of culture replicates
1	0	0	3×10^5	12
2	0	10^5	3×10^5	12
3	100	10^5	3×10^5	24
4	300	10^5	3×10^5	24
5	1000	10^5	3×10^5	12
6	3000	10^5	3×10^5	12

The above six groups exactly fill one 96-well tray. If more replicates are wanted, the whole tray should be duplicated. Cultures without responder LN cells or nude spleen cells (group 1) are used to determine the spontaneous release (SR) for the target cells. This is used to score positive wells in the remaining groups and to find the lysis values for these groups. Where an experiment overlaps on two or more plates, group 1 must be repeated on each plate, since there is variation between plates depending on the plates themselves, position in the incubator, etc.

Cultures containing only accessory cells and stimulating cells (group 2) are included to ensure that no CTL-P are derived from these populations. In the event that there are CTL in these wells (i.e., positive cultures), the experiment should be discarded. This occasionally happens when nude mice older than 11 weeks are used as spleen cell donors or when depletion of T cells from normal spleen cells is incomplete. Cultures containing lower numbers of responding cells are prepared in replicates of 24 or more since the number of responding wells at these cell numbers is usually low.

In order to achieve the best replication within a group, all of the cells are first mixed together in a 12 × 75 mm tube (Falcon no. 2058) and then dispensed with a 200-μl Eppendorf pipette. Tape plate closed to minimize evaporation and place in incubator for 5–7 days depending on FCS used.

For a sensitive assay, the objective is to have as large and stable a target cell as possible. Large cells take up more radiolabel, and this allows smaller numbers of CTL to be detected. Stable cells will give a low spontaneous release (SR) with a small deviation. This will allow the detection of small amounts of released radiolabel over background. Target cells are labeled with ^{51}Cr (Miller and Dunkley, 1974). Two types of target cells are generally used.

1. Con-A blast target cells: These should be prepared 2 or 3 days before use. Under these conditions, the cells will label well and are most stable. Prepare spleen suspension as above using same strain as stimulator (or H-2 identical strain). To tissue culture flasks (Falcon no. 3013), add 10^7 viable cells and 20 μg Con A in 10 ml of culture medium. Place caps on almost tight and incubate 2 or 3 days.

2. Tumor targets. The most commonly used is the mastocytoma, P815 (*H-*2^d). We find that these cells are best as targets if kept *in vivo* and removed just prior to use by a needle puncture in the peritoneum. Cells for passage from mouse to mouse are suspended in saline without serum to prevent possible acquisition of new antigens. Other cell lines can be used as targets but should first be tested to ensure that they label well and have acceptable SR.

To prepare plates for assay, remove 0.1 ml of culture supernatant from each well with an Eppendorf pipette. Place pipette tip along wall of well almost to the top of cone part of the V to avoid disturbing the cell pellet. When target cells are ready, replace this volume with 100 μl of labeled target cells (equal to 3000 target cells). Try to add this to center of the well in order to disturb the pellet and allow better mixing of effector and target cells.

Include 12 control wells to determine quality of targets

4 × (100 μl assay media + 100 μl target cells) = total incorporated counts (T)
4 × (100 μl 1% glacial acetic acid in water + 100 μl target cells) = total releasable counts in cytoplasm (TR)
4 × (100 μl assay media + 100 μl target cells) = spontaneously released counts (SR)

Incubate 4 hr at 37°C. We find that it is not necessary to centrifuge the plates before this incubation. At end of 4 hr, remove 100 μl of supernatant from each culture well and transfer to gamma counting tube. It is not necessary to resuspend and centrifuge the cultures before this sampling.

For T, resuspend 4–5 times and remove 100 μl to counting tube. For TR, take 100 μl supernatant. For SR, take 100 μl supernatant. TR/T should be 80% or more. SR/TR should be 10% or less for tumor targets and approximately 20% for Con-A blasts. Results are unreliable if SR/TR is greater than 35%. The SR should be the same as group 1 in the experiment. If the SR with media alone is much higher than group 1 this indicates unstable targets.

To calculate CTL-P frequencies, first determine the number of cultures in each group mounting a detectable response. To do this, the ^{51}Cr release from each culture is compared with the (mean plus 2 standard deviations) release from a group of cultures from which responding cells were omitted (group 1). If greater, the culture is scored as responding. If the culture system is working well, the fraction of responding cultures in a group should not be substantially decreased if the response threshold is increased to 3 or even 4 standard deviations above the control mean. The numbers from all groups are then combined to make an estimate of the CTL-P frequency.

The steps involved in writing a computer program for the Porter and Berry (1963) fitting procedure are listed below. The notation has been left the same as in their study to facilitate comparison with their more detailed description.

1. For each group, enter N (number of cells/culture), n (number of cultures) and r (number of responding cultures).

2. Enter an estimate of the CTL-P frequency. Call this fe. A simple method to obtain this estimate is the graphical method outlined in Fig. 1 of Chapter 18 of this treatise.

3. For each group, calculate and store

(a) $Y = \log (feN)$

and (b) $q = r/n$

4. For each group, calculate and store

(a) $w = [10^{2Y} (\log_e 10)^2]/[\exp(10^Y) - 1]$

and

(b) $$\phi = \begin{cases} \phi_0 + qA & (q < 1) \\ \phi_1 & (q = 1) \end{cases}$$

where

$$\phi_0 = [1 - \exp(10^Y)]/(10^Y \cdot \log_e 10)$$
$$A = \exp(10^Y)/[10^Y \cdot \log_e 10]$$
$$\phi_1 = (10^Y, \log_e 10)^{-1}$$

5. Calculate

$$\bar{\phi} = (\Sigma nw\phi)/(\Sigma nw)$$

where the summation is over all groups.

6. Is $\bar{\phi} < 0.04$? If yes, go to (8). If no, go to (7).

The better the initial estimate *fe*, the smaller $\bar{\phi}$ will be. If $\bar{\phi}$ is too large, it is used to make an improved estimate of *fe* (or the associated *Y* values) which in turn are used to calculate a new value of $\bar{\phi}$. The process is continued until $\bar{\phi}$ is smaller than some arbitrary value which our experience has led us to take as 0.04.

7. Replace each *Y* value with $Y + \bar{\phi}$ and return to step (4).
8. Calculate $f_{\text{CTL-P}}$ and the range specified by the 95% confidence limits.

$$\text{(a)}\ f_{\text{CTL-P}} = 10^{(Y + \bar{\phi})}/N$$

The *Y* and *N* values for any of the groups may be used; all give the same result for $f_{\text{CTL-P}}$. We normally express the frequency as responding cells per 10^6 tested, i.e., the frequency calculated here is multiplied by 10^6.

$$\text{(b) Range} = f_{\text{CTL-P}} \cdot 10^{\pm 1.96(1/\Sigma nw)^{\frac{1}{2}}}$$

9. Calculate χ^2

$$\chi^2 = \Sigma nw^2 - (\Sigma nw\phi)^2/(\Sigma nw)$$

The value obtained here should be compared with the relevant entry of a χ^2 table ($p = 0.05$, degrees of freedom = one less than the number of groups; 5.99, 7.82, and 9.49 for group numbers of 3, 4, and 5, respectively). The experimental data could produce a χ^2 value as large or larger than the appropriate table entry only 1 time in 20 and still be sampled from a response which is actually determined by one-hit limiting dilution kinetics.

As an example, consider the data of Fig. 2, Chapter 18 of this treatise from which the data tabulated below are taken.

Group No.	*N*	*n*	*r*
1	200	48	14
2	500	48	31
3	800	48	39

From the figure, the CTL-P frequency is approximately 1 in 500 or 0.002 or 2000 per 10^6. Putting this estimate and the above data into a program based on the steps outline above, the program stops after 1 iteration ($\bar{\phi} = 0.001$) and yields frequency, range and χ^2 values of 2005, 1598–2516, and 0.414, respectively. If an initial frequency estimate of 1500 per 10^6 is made, the program stops after 2 iterations ($\bar{\phi} = 0.0002$) and yields identical frequency, range and χ^2 values.

To calculate cytotoxic activity per clone, first, calculate *p,* the mean specific fractional ^{51}Cr release for each group defined as

(Observed release - spontaneous release)/(total releasable - spontaneous release).

Include all cultures in the group, irrespective of whether they responded. The *p* values are a measurement of the mean number of target cells destroyed per culture of the group. What one actually wants is a measurement of the mean number of CTL per culture. No one has yet devised a simple procedure for doing this. However, Miller and Dunkley (1974) have shown that the quantity $\log_e(1-p)$ is roughly proportional to the number of CTL. We routinely calculate the quantity $-100 \log_e (1-p)$ which we call "cytotoxic activity." A value of 10 corresponds to 10% specific ^{51}Cr release, a value of 100 to 63% specific ^{51}Cr release. The mean cytotoxic activity per clone for any group is then $100 \log_e(1-p)/(f_{\text{CTL-P}} \cdot N)$ where N is the number of responding cells per culture.

REFERENCES

Lutz, C. T., Glasebrook, A. L., and Fitch, F. W. (1981). Enumeration of alloreactive helper T lymphocytes which cooperate with cytolytic T lymphocytes. *Eur. J. Immunol.* **11,** 726.

Miller, R. G., and Dunkley, M. (1974). Quantitative analysis of the ^{51}Cr release cytotoxicity assay for cytotoxic lymphocytes. *Cell. Immunol.* **14,** 284.

Porter, E. H., and Berry, R. J. (1963). The efficient design of transplantable tumour assays. *Br. J. Cancer* **17,** 583.

B. Limit Dilution Analysis of Functional T Cell Precursors

Klaus Eichmann

T cells are prepared by double nylon-wool passage of spleen cells which are then cultured at a density of 3×10^6/ml for 2 days with 5 μg/ml concanavalin A (Con-A) in RPMI-1640 (Grand Island Biological Co., Grand Island, New York) supplemented with 10% fetal calf serum (FCS), $10^{-5} M$ 2-mercaptoethanol, 0.025 M Hepes, 1% penicillin–streptomycin, and 0.2 mM glutamine. Thereafter, Con-A-activated T cells are purified by centrifugation over Ficoll (Pharmacia Fine Chemicals, Div. of Pharmacia, Inc., Piscataway, New Jersey).

ISBN 0-12-249920-4

Dilutions of such T cells are then placed in Linbro flat-bottom microtiter wells (7600305; Linbro Chemical Co.) that had received 1×10^4 3000-rad irradiated (^{60}Co) syngeneic peritoneal exudate cells/well as fillers, 2 days before. The dilutions of T cells should range from 2/well to 8×10^4/well and are cultured in 200 μl of appropriately diluted TCGF in Iscove's modified Dulbecco's medium IMDM with 10% FCS, supplemented with, 10^{-5} *M* 2-mercaptoethanol, 1% pencillin–streptomycin, and 0.025 *M* Hg. The medium is changed every 3 days by centrifugation of the plates followed by the removal and replacement of the medium with Titertek pipettes (Flow Laboratories, Inc., Rockville, Maryland). Routinely, 24 wells are set up for each cell concentration.

The frequency of cultures with growing cells is determined after 1 week of culture by visual examination with an inverted microscope. Filler cells are present mainly as fragments at that time and, therefore, do not interfere with the assessment of cell growth. Helper activity in each culture is determined on day 7 or 8 by adding the cells of each culture, after transfer into Click's medium, to a fresh Linbro flat-bottom microwell that contains antigen and 5×10^5 splenic B cells, purified by treatment with anti-Thy-1.2 and rabbit complement.

As antigens, we have used either 3×10^5 SRBC/well or 1×10^7 TNP-Strep A/well. Click's medium is used in these cultures in a 2% CO_2 atmosphere. After 4 days, responses are assessed by assay for direct plaque-forming cells (PFC) for TNP or SRBC. Positive PFC responses are determined by comparison with PFC responses of cultures that contain only B cells and antigen. Further processing of data is done by Poisson distribution.

Microcultures are assayed for cytolytic activity in a 4-hr ^{51}Cr release assay on the appropriate target cells. For this purpose, aliquots of the individual cultures are transferred to round-bottomed microtiter plates (Linbro IS-MRC 96; Linbro Chemical Co.), washed once with medium, and thereafter mixed with 2×10^3 ^{51}Cr-labeled P815 tumor target cells in a final volume of 0.2 ml. Spontaneous release is determined by transferring aliquots from control microcultures containing only target cells. An aliquot of the target cells is frozen and thawed four times for determination of maximum ^{51}Cr release.

C. Limit Dilution Analysis of T Cells Releasing Lymphokines

Peter Krammer

Culture of Con-A-Activated Spleen Cells at Limit Dilution

B6 spleen cells are treated with an isotonic phosphate-buffered ammonium chloride solution for 1 min to lyse erythrocytes. Cells are washed twice, and then cultured at a density of 5×10^6/ml for 2 days with 5 μg/ml Con-A in RPMI-1640 (Grand Island Biological Co., Grand Island, New York) supplemented with 10%

ISOLATION, CHARACTERIZATION, AND
UTILIZATION OF T LYMPHOCYTE CLONES

ISBN 0-12-249920-4

TABLE II

Test Systems for Lymphokines

Lymphokines	Test systems for analysis	Reference
Immune interferon (IFN-γ)	Virus plaque reduction assay	Campbell *et al.* (1975)
Macrophage activating factor (MAF)	Induction of cytotoxicity of purified bone marrow macrophages of P815 tumor cells	Lohmann-Matthes *et al.* (1979)
Colony stimulating factors (CSF)	Formation of colonies of hematopoietic cells in semi-solid agar cultures of bone marrow cells	Staber and Johnson (1980)
For neutrophilic granulocytes and macrophages (GM-CSF)		
For megakaryocytes (Meg/CSF)		
For eosinophilic granulocytes (Eo-CSF)		
For erythrocytes (E-CSF)		
Histamine-producing cell stimulating factor (HCSF)	Induction of an increase in histamine production by bone marrow cells	Dy *et al.* (1981)
T cell growth factor (TCGF)	Growth support of a TCGF-dependent T cell clone in long-term culture	See Appendix, Section I, C
T cell replacing factor (TRF)	Induction of anti-sheep red blood cell (SRBC) plaque forming cells in spleen cells from Nu/Nu mice immunized with SRBC	Schimpl and Wecker (1972)
B cell differentiation factors (BCDF)	Induction of IgM secretion and switch to IgG secretion by purified B cells	Isakson *et al.* (1981)

FCS, 10^{-5} *M* 2-mercaptoethanol, 0.02 *M* HEPES, 1% penicillin–streptomycin, and 0.2 m*M* L-glutamine. Thereafter, concanavalin A (Con-A)-activated cells are purified by centrifugation over Ficoll (1.077 g/cm^3) (Pharmacia Fine Chemical, Div. of Pharmacia, Inc., Piscataway, New Jersey). Different numbers of such cells ranging from 1 to 10^4/well are then plated in Linbro flat-bottom microtiter wells which had received 1 or 3 × 10^4 3300-rad irradiated (^{60}Co) AKR/J peritoneal exudate cells/well as fillers 2 days previously. The cells are cultured in 100 μl of appropriately diluted TCGF in RPMI-1640 with 10% fetal calf serum (FCS), supplemented as described above. Each well is fed with 100 μl of the above medium after 4 days of culture.

The frequency of cultures with growing cells analyzed according to Poisson distribution is determined after 7 to 12 days of culture by visual examination with an inverted phase microscope. Filler cells are largely present as fragments at that time and, therefore, do not interfere with the assessment of cell growth.

Preparation of Culture for Lymphokine Assays

To determine lymphokine secretion by cells in each individual well of the limiting dilution assay after 7 to 12 days of culture, cells in each culture well are washed twice in 200 μl fresh medium, resuspended in culture medium supplemented with 2% FCS or human serum (for HCSF) and 1% streptomycin, and stimulated with 10 μg/ml Con-A for 3 hr, then washed again and cultured in fresh medium, free of TCGF, for 24 hr. The supernatants from each well are then harvested and lymphokine activity is determined (Table II).

For frequency estimates analyzed according to Poisson distribution, supernatants from individual cultures from cells in limiting dilution are scored as positive when the lymphokine titer was equal to or higher than one or several (predetermined for each assay) standard deviations above the arithmetic mean of the controls. The controls are taken from culture wells of limiting dilution plates containing irradiated filler cells with no microscopically apparent growth of Con-A-activated cells. These wells are treated identically to the experimental group, i.e., washed twice in fresh medium, sham-induced with Con-A, washed again, and supernatants removed after 24 hr for the lymphokine assay.

REFERENCES

Campbell, J. B., Grunberger, T., Kochman, M. A., and White, S. L. (1975). Microplaque reduction assay for human and mouse interferon. *Can. J. Microbiol.* **3,** 1247.

Dy, M., Lebel, B., Kamoun, P., and Hamburger, J. (1981). Histamine production during the anti-allograft response. Demonstration of a new lymphokine enhancing histamine synthesis. *J. Exp. Med.* **153,** 293.

Isakson, P., Pure E., Witetta, E. S., and Krammer, P. H. (1982). T cell-derived B cell differentiation factor(s) (BCDF): Effect on the isotype switch of murine B cells. *J. Exp. Med.* **155,** 734.

Lohmann-Matthes, M.-L., Domzig, W., and Taskov, H. (1979). Antibody-dependent cellular cytotoxicity against tumor cells. I. Cultivated bone marrow-derived macrophages kill tumor target cells. *Eur. J. Immunol.* **9,** 261.
Schimpl, A., and Wecker, E. (1972). Replacement of T cell function by a T cell product. *Nature (London) New Biol.* **273,** 15.
Staber, F. G., and Johnson, G. R. (1980). The responses of hematopoietic precursor cells in mice to bacterial cell-wall components. *J. Cell. Physiol.* **105,** 143.

IV. MURINE T CELL CLONES REACTIVE WITH ALLOANTIGENS

The techniques for isolation of murine T cell clones reactive with alloantigens have been reported from several laboratories. Each technique has certain advantages and disadvantages. The "belt and suspenders" approach of Glasebrook and Fitch may well be the preferred approach for isolation of alloreactive T cell clones. One section describes an effective approach for induction and isolation of virus specific CTL.

REFERENCES

Glasebrook, A. L., and Fitch, F. W. (1980). Alloreactive cloned T cell lines. I. Interactions between cloned amplifier and cytolytic T cell lines. *J. Exp. Med.* **154,** 876.
Hengartner, H., and Fathman, C. G. (1980). Clones of alloreactive T cells. I. A Unique homozygous MLR stimulating determinant present on B6 stimulators. *Immunogenetics* **10,** 175.
Möller, G., ed. (1981). T cell clones. *Immunol. Rev.* **54,** 1.
Nabholz, M., Engers, H. D., Collavo, D., and North, M. (1977). Cloned T cell lines with specific cytolytic activity. *Curr. Top. Microbiol. Immunol.* **81,** 176.
Rosenberg, S. A., Schwartz, S., and Spiess, P. J. (1978). *In vitro* growth of murine T cells. II. Growth of *in vitro* sensitized cells cytotoxic for alloantigens. *J. Immunol.* **121,** 1951.
Sherman, L. A. (1980). Dissection of the B10.D2 anti-H-2K^b cytolytic T lymphocyte receptor repertoire. *J. Exp. Med.* **151,** 1386.
von Boehmer, H., Hengartner, H., Nabholz, M., Lernhardt, W., Schreier, M. H., and Haas, W. (1979). Fine specificity of a continuously growing killer cell clone specific for H-Y antigen. *Eur. J. Immunol.* **9,** 592.

A. Clones of Noncytolytic Alloreactive Murine T Cells

C. G. Fathman and Hans Hengartner

Primary MLR Sensitization. Lymph node responder cells (40×10^6) are cultured with 80×10^6 X-irradiated (3300 rad) stimulator spleen cells. Cells are cultured in plastic flasks (Falcon 3024) in 15 ml of MLR medium (this consists of RPMI 1640 containing 10% fetal calf serum 5×10^{-5} *M* 2-mercaptoethanol,

ISBN 0-12-249920-4

2 mM HEPES, 100 μg/ml of penicillin, and 100 U/ml of streptomycin; L-glutamine is added at the final concentration 2×10^{-3} M prior to use). The flasks are incubated in an upright position at 37°C in a water-saturated atmosphere of 5% CO_2 in air. These cells are harvested after 14 days, and viability is assayed with fluorescein diacetate (FDA). Briefly, FDA is added to an aliquot of cells to get a final concentrate of 5 μg/ml. After 1 min at room temperature, viable cells are brightly fluorescent when observed in the hemocytometer chamber on a Leitz Orthoplan microscope equipped with an Opak-fluor vertical illuminator by using appropriate excitation and barrier filters. Recovery of viable cells ranges from 10 to 50% of the initial responder cells. The recovered cells are referred to as primed responder cells (PRC).

Secondary MLR. PRC are recultured in 0.2 ml of fresh MLR medium in flat bottom microtiter plates (Falcon 3040), in the presence of 1×10^6 irradiated stimulator spleen cells (either syngeneic or allogeneic to the PRC). The number of PRC per well can be varied, but significant response can be seen with as few as 1×10^3 PRC/well. The PRC stimulator cell combinations are set up in triplicate. Such cultures are harvested either 2 or 3 days following initiation of culture. Proliferation is measured in terms of thymidine incorporation of an overnight pulse of 2 μCi of tritiated thymidine.

Cloning of Alloreactive T Cells. PRC obtained after several serial restimulations (restimulated more than four times) are restimulated with the priming stimulator cell at a cell density of 2×10^6 PRC and 5×10^7 X-irradiated stimulator spleen cells in 15 ml of MLR medium. Twenty-four hours after initiation of the mixed lymphocyte reaction, cells are centrifuged and 1×10^6, 3×10^5, 1×10^5, and 3×10^4 input primed responder cells resuspended in 1 ml of their supernatant. Each of these cell suspensions is mixed with 2 ml of 0.5% Bacto agar (Difco Laboratories) in MLR medium at 45°C and spread evenly on a 15 ml feeder layer of 0.5% Bacto agar in a 10 cm petri dish (Falcon 1001). Four to 7 days later, colonies can be observed in the soft agar layer, predominantly near the top of the soft agar. These colonies, which consist of 15–50 cells, are picked under an inverted microscope using a drawn-out Pateur pipette and transferred to 0.2 ml of fresh MLR medium containing 1×10^6 X-irradiated stimulated spleen cells in microtiter plates (Falcon 3040). These small colonies are cultured for 10 to 14 days in the microtiter plates before transfer and restimulation in Costar trays (Costar 3524) in 2 ml of MLR medium containing 1×10^7 X-irradiated stimulator cells. After transfer to Costar trays, the cells are allowed to grow for another 7 to 14 days at which time the expanded cells can be transferred into tissue culture flasks containing 5 ml of MLR medium and 4×10^7 fresh irradiated stimulator spleen cells. These mixtures are cultured upright in a water-saturated atmosphere of 5% CO_2 in air at 37°C. Following this expansion step, the cells can be assayed for reactivity as described above, expanded further, or after 24 hr of restimulation, frozen and stored as described below.

Subcloning of Alloreactive T Cell Colonies. Subcloning of colonies derived from soft agar cloning conditions described above are carried out in one of two ways. They can either be recloned in soft agar with the addition of 20% (v/v) of the supernatant from rat concanavalin A (Con-A)-activated spleen cells as a source of T cell growth factor in both the bottom and top layer of soft agar. Alternatively, they can be cloned by limiting dilution in the following manner. PRC are diluted to give a final concentration of 1 cell/ml. These cells are titrated into microtiter plates containing 100 μl of MLR medium and 1×10^6 irradiated allogeneic stimulator cells and 10% (v/v) volume rat Con-A supernatant. One hundred microliters of the cell suspension is put into each well, giving the average of 1 cell in every 10 wells. Such cells are cultured in the conditions described above at 37° until growth is observed by inspection using an inverted microscope. When growth is observed, the cells can be transferred to Costar wells in 2 ml of MLR medium in the presence of 10×10^6 irradiated allogeneic stimulator spleen cells. At this time it is possible to exclude the exogenous TCGF, although it can be added to ensure more prompt and reproducible growth of these cells (Hengartner and Fathman, 1980).

Storage of Alloreactive T Cell Clones. It is possible to freeze either long-term cultured alloreactive T cells or clones of T cells by restimulating these cells 10 to 14 days following the previous restimulation at a density of 2×10^5 cells/ml with 6×10^7 irradiated stimulator spleen cells in 15 ml of MLR medium. Twenty-four hours after initation of this culture, the cells are centrifuged, the supernatant is discarded, and the cells are resuspended in 1 ml of MLR medium containing 10% dimethyl sulfoxide (DMSO) at 4°C. The cells are frozen in storage vials by putting them in a Revco −70°C freezer overnight in a Styrofoam box. Freezing occurs at a rate of approximately 1°C/min. The following morning the cells can be transferred and stored in liquid nitrogen. Such cells are retrieved by thawing them in a 37°C water bath with shaking. At the moment the last ice crystal disappears, the cell suspension is diluted with 10 volumes of fresh MLR medium which is at 4°C. The cells are then centrifuged and resuspended in 15 ml of MLR medium and restimulated with 6×10^7 X-irradiated stimulator spleen cells in a 1-ml volume in culture flasks.

REFERENCES

Fathman, C. G., and Hengartner, H. (1978). Clones of alloreactive T-cells. *Nature (London)* **272,** 617.

Fathman, C. G., Collavo, D., Davies, S., and Nabholz, M. (1977). *In vitro* secondary MLR. I. Kinetics of proliferation and specificity of *in vitro* primed responder cells. *J. Immunol.* **118,** 1232.

Hengartner, H., and Fathman, C. G. (1980). Clones of alloreactive T cells. I. A unique homozygous MLR stimulating determinant present on B6 stimulator. *Immunogenetics* **10,** 175.

B. Cloning of Alloreactive Murine T Cells

A. L. Glasebrook and Frank W. Fitch

Cloning of both cytolytic and noncytolytic T cells is carried out, and the resulting cell lines are maintained in cultures prepared with both stimulating alloantigen and a source of IL-2 (Glasebrook and Fitch, 1980). Culture supernatant fluid (SF) from secondary mixed leukocyte cultures (MLC) is used for maintaining the cloned cells. Supernatants from concanavalin A (Con-A)-activated spleen cells (Con-A SF) may be used in the initial cloning culture; the yield of clones seems to be greater than when MLC SF is used initially. Although levels of IL-2 in MLC SF usually is lower than in Con-A SF, the phenotypic characteristics of cloned cells seem to be more stable when cells are maintained with MLC SF (and alloantigen) than when Con-A SF is used.

Culture medium consists of Dulbecco's modified Eagle's medium with additional folic acid and amino acids (Cerottini *et al.*, 1974), 5×10^{-5} *M* 2-mercaptoethanol, 10 m*M* morpholinopropanesulfonic acid, penicillin, streptomycin, and fetal calf serum (FCS) at concentrations indicated below. To prepare MLC SF, primary MLC are established by mixing 25×10^6 C57BL/6 responding spleen cells with an equal number of irradiated (1400 rads) DBA/2 stimulating spleen cells in 20 ml culture medium containing 2% FCS in plastic culture flasks (Falcon no. 3013). The flasks are incubated upright at 37°C in a humidified atmosphere. Fourteen days later, secondary MLC are established by mixing 3.5 to 5×10^6 viable primary MLC cells with 25×10^6 irradiated (1400 rads) DBA/2 stimulating spleen cells in 20 ml of culture medium containing 2% FCS. Culture supernatant is collected 48 hr later, centrifuged at 3000 *g* for 5 min, and stored at −20°C. The SF can be filtered, but there may be some loss of activity with some types of filters if small volumes of fluid are filtered.

Clones can be established from unstimulated spleen or lymph node cells, but the frequency of responding cells is much higher if the responding cells are stimulated with alloantigen *in vitro*. If unstimulated cells are used, several hundred cells must be added to each well. With secondary MLC cells obtained 48 hr after initiation of the secondary culture from MLC established as described above for preparing MLC SF, 0.1 to 1 cells are added to each well. The cells to be cloned are suspended in either MLC SF or Con-A SF, and a 100-μl aliquot is

ISBN 0-12-249920-4

added to each microwell of a tissue culture plate containing 10^6 irradiated (1400 rad) spleen cells in 0.1 ml of medium with 20% FCS. This cloning plate is then incubated at 37°C and is fed with 50 μl of additional medium with 11% FCS and 50 μl of SF after 4 days of incubation. Clusters of cells appear in the cloning wells at approximately 6 to 9 days of incubation. Screening for cytolytic activity using a sensitive micro ^{51}Cr release assay (Engers and Fitch, 1979) can be performed directly with an aliquot of cells from those wells which contain proliferating cells.

Cells of interest are expanded and maintained routinely by passage with irradiated alloantigen and MLC SF. From 1.6 to 3.2 × 10^4 cloned T cells in 100 μl of medium with 2% FCS are added to microwells (Linbro no. 76-033-05 or Costar no. 3524) which contain 0.5 ml of MLC SF and 6 × 10^6 irradiated (1400 rads) stimulating spleen cells in 1 ml of medium with 2% FCS. Cloned cells are passaged at 7 day intervals even though peak cell numbers usually are observed 5 days after transfer. Cells passaged at intervals shorter than 7 days have been found not to grow as well either in short- or long-term culture as cells passaged weekly.

Cell debris can be removed by centrifugation over a Ficoll-Hypaque gradient (Davidson and Parish, 1975). More than 95% of the cells remaining after culture for 7 days are the cloned T cells. Cloned T cells can be maintained for several passages using syngeneic spleen cells and either MLC SF or Con-A SF if it is necessary to avoid the presence of alloantigen. SF alone will support the short-term growth of T cell clones derived using the approach described above, but the yield of cells is much lower. T cells in the stimulating cell population can be depleted by treatment with anti-Thy-1 and complement if it is desirable for the cloned cells to be the only T cells present in the culture (Lutz *et al.*, 1981).

REFERENCES

Cerottini, J.-C., Engers, H. D., MacDonald, H. R., and Brunner, K. T. (1974). Generation of cytotoxic T lymphocytes *in vitro*. I. Response of normal and immune spleen cells in mixed leukocyte cultures. *J. Exp. Med.* **140,** 703.

Davidson, W. F., and Parish, C. R. (1975). A procedure for removing red cells and dead cells from lymphoid cell suspensions. *J. Immunol. Methods* **7,** 291.

Engers, H. D., and Fitch, F. W. (1979). An estimate of the minimal frequency of cytolytic T lymphocyte effector cells generated in allogeneic reactions. *J. Immunol. Methods* **25,** 13.

Glasebrook, A. L., and Fitch, F. W. (1980). Alloreactive cloned T cell lines. I. Interactions between cloned amplifier and cytolytic T cell lines. *J. Exp. Med.* **151,** 876.

Lutz, C. T., Glasebrook, A. L., and Fitch, F. W. (1981) Alloreactive cloned T cell lines. III. Accessory cell requirements for the growth of cloned cytolytic T lymphocytes. *J. Immunol.* **126,** 1404.

C. Isolation of Virus-Specific CTL Clones

T. J. Braciale and V. L. Braciale

Materials. Inbred mouse strains (The Jackson Laboratory, Bar Harbor, Maine), egg-grown influenza virus, Iscove's modified Dulbecco's medium (430–2200; Grand Island Biological Co., Grand Island, New York), fetal bovine serum (Sterile Systems Inc., Logan, Utah), 96-well flat bottom and 24-well tissue culture plates (Linbro Flow Labs, Hamden, Connecticut) and six-well cluster plates (Costar, Data Packaging, Cambridge, Massachusetts), crude rat concanavalin A (Con-A) supernatant, as source of TCGF, prepared according to the method of Lafferty and Woolnough (1977).

Methods. Mice are immunized intravenously at 7–12 weeks of age with 100–300 H.A.U. infectious egg-grown influenza virus and used as immune spleen donors 3 or more weeks after immunization (Braciale, 1977). Secondary cultures are prepared *in vitro* by coculturing 100 × 10^6 spleen cells from immunized mice with 20 × 10 influenza-infected syngeneic irradiated (2000 rads) spleen cells in 40 ml minimal essential medium (MEM) supplemented with 10% fetal bovine serum, antibiotics, and 5 × 10^{-5} *M* 2-mercapotethanol in a 75 cm^2 tissue culture flask (Braciale, 1977). Cultures are incubated at 37°C in a humid atmosphere of 7% CO_2 in air.

Spleen cells are obtained directly from immune mice or from secondary cultures *in vitro,* and viable cells are separated from erythrocytes and dead cells by centrifugation on Isopaque–Ficoll according to the method of Davidson and Parish (1975). Viable immune spleen cells are plated at limiting dilution in individual wells of 96-well microtiter plates with 1 × 10^6 syngeneic, influenza-infected, irradiated (2000 rads) stimulator spleen cells in 0.2 ml medium (Braciale *et al.,* 1981). The medium is Iscove's modified Dulbecco's medium supplemented with 5 × 10^{-5} *M* 2-mercaptoethanol 10% fetal bovine serum, and 10% (v/v) crude TCGF. Immune cells are plated in replicates of 48–96 wells at several concentrations ranging from 10^2 to 10^4 cells/well. Proliferating cell clusters in positive wells are visualized using an inverted microscope, and positive wells are selected for further expansion if the frequency of positive wells at that given responder cell dilution is 20%.

Clones are expanded by transferring the contents of positive wells to individual wells of 24-well tissue culture plates containing 5 × 10^6 irradiated, influenza-infected, syngeneic spleen stimulator cells in 2 ml of Iscove's medium supplemented as above. After 7 days, contents of individual wells are transferred to 6-well cluster tissue culture plates containing 20 × 10^6 irradiated stimulator cells in 5 ml of Iscove's supplemented medium. For routine passage, the cloned cell lines are reseeded at 5–7 day intervals at a concentration of 2–5 × 10^4

ISOLATION, CHARACTERIZATION, AND
UTILIZATION OF T LYMPHOCYTE CLONES

ISBN 0-12-249920-4

cells/ml in the presence or irradiated stimulator cells in fresh Iscove's supplemented medium containing 10% TCGF.

REFERENCES

Braciale, T. J. (1977). Immunologic recognition of influenza virus infected cells. *Cell. Immunol.* **33,** 423.

Braciale, T. J., Andrew, M. E., and Braciale, V. L. (1981). Heterogeneity and specificity of cloned lines of influenza virus-specific cytotoxic T lymphocytes. *J. Exp. Med.* **153,** 910.

Davidson, W. F., and Parish, C. R. (1975). A procedure for removing red cells and dead cells from lymphoid cell suspensions. *J. Immunol. Methods* **7,** 291.

Lafferty, K. J., and Woolnough, J. (1977). The origin and mechanism of the allograft reaction. *Immunol. Rev.* **35,** 231.

V. MURINE T CELL CLONES REACTIVE WITH SOLUBLE ANTIGENS

Several techniques have been described for isolation of T cell clones reactive with soluble antigens. T inducer (helper) cells can be obtained using the technique of Kimoto and Fathman (1980). Repertoire estimates can be approached using the technique described by Sredni *et al.* (1981) which isolates the T cell clones as soon as possible following induction of proliferation *in vitro*. Both of these latter techniques are described here.

REFERENCES

Kimoto, M., and Fathman, C. G. (1980). Antigen reactive T cell clones. I. Transcomplementing hybrid *I-A* region gene products function effectively in antigen presentation. *J. Exp. Med.* **152,** 759.

Schreier, M. H., and Tees, R. (1980). Clonal induction of helper T cells: Conversion of specific signals into non-specific signals. *Int. Arch. Allergy Appl. Immunol.* **61,** 227.

Sredni, B., Tse, H. Y., Chen, C., and Schwartz, R. H. (1981). Antigen specific clones of proliferating T lymphocytes. I. Methodology, specificity and MHC restriction. *J. Immunol.* **126,** 341.

A. Immunization and Long-Term Culture of Murine Immune Lymph Node Cells

M. Kimoto and C. G. Fathman

Mice of the haplotype selected for immunization (4–5 per group) are immunized with appropriate amounts of the soluble antigen selected, emulsified in complete Freund's adjuvant, subcutaneously at the base of the tail according to the method of Corradin *et al.* (1977). Seven days later, draining lymph nodes

ISBN 0-12-249920-4

(inguinal and paraaortic) are removed, and single cell suspensions are made and cultured in Costar trays No. 3524 with appropriate amounts of solbule antigen at a cell number of 5×10^6 cells/well in 1.5 ml of RPMI 1640 media supplemented with 10% horse serum, 3×10^{-5} *M* 2-mercaptoethynol 12 mM HEPES, 100 U/ml penicillin, and 100 μg/ml streptomycin; L-glutamine is added at a final concentration of 2×10^{-3} *M* before use. Four days later, the cells are harvested and blast cells are centrifuged on Ficoll-Hypaque at 2000 rpm for 20 min. Cells from the interface are collected, washed twice and recultured in Costar wells (No. 3524) with 5×10^6 irradiated (3300 rads) syngeneic spleen cells as filler cells, at a concentration of 1×10^5 primed T cells per milliliter in 2 ml of RPMI 1640 medium supplemented, with 10% fetal calf serum (FCS). After 7–14 days, cells are harvested and viable recovered cells are counted using the vital stain fluorescein diacetate (FDA). Briefly, FDA is added to an aliquot of cells to give a final concentration of 5 μg/ml. After 1–5 min at room temperature, viable cells are brightly fluorescent when observed in a hemocytometer using a fluorescent microscope. Viable recovered cells (2×10^5) are restimulated with appropriate amounts of soluble antigen in the presence of 5×10^6 syngeneic irradiated filler cells in 2 ml RPMI FCS media or assayed as described below. If recultured, after 4 days the cells are harvested, and blast cells are recultured with syngeneic irradiated filler cells in the absence of antigen at a concentration of 1×10^5 blast cells and 2.5×10^6 filler cells per milliliter in 2 ml RPMI FCS media for an additional 2–14 days. This period of rest in the absence of antigen is required only if the ultimate use of the cells is antigen-specific B cell help. If the cells are simply to be recultured and assayed for proliferation, the step of washing away excess antigen may be omitted and the cells simply may be left in the presence of residual antigen. Antigen-reactive T cells have been maintained by this cyclic restimulation for culture periods of greater than 2 years. In experiments where large numbers of cells are required, the cells can be restimulated and recultured in an upright position in tissue culture flasks (3024 Falcon Flasks) in a total volume of 15 ml of RPMI FCS media and the appropriate concentration of antigen-reactive T cells, antigen, and filler cells. These cells can be assayed for proliferative response 7–14 days after reculture. At this time, aliquots of viable recovered cells are assayed for their response following restimulation with appropriate amounts of the soluble antigen in the presence of 1×10^6 filler cells in 0.2 ml RPMI FCS media per well in microtiter plates for 48 or 72 hr. Two microcuries of tritiated thymidine are added 16 hr before harvest. Results are then expressed as the mean of triplicate cultures following standard scintillation counting.

REFERENCES

Corradin, G., Etlinger, H. M., and Chiller, J. M. (1977). Lymphocyte specificity to protein antigens. I. Characteriziation of the antigen-induced *in vitro* T cell-dependent proliferative response with lymph node cells from primed mice. *J. Immunol.* **119,** 1048.

B. Cloning of Soluble Antigen Reactive Murine T Inducer (T_h) Cells

M. Kimoto and C. G. Fathman

Antigen-reactive T cells are induced as described in the section on long-term culture of murine T cells (Appendix, Section V,A). After the fourth 2-week interval of culture, the cells can be restimulated with the appropriate amount of soluble antigen (usually 100 μg/ml) in the presence of syngeneic irradiated filler cells. Twenty-four hours later, the entire mixture of antigen-reactive T cells, filler cells, and antigen is mixed with 0.5% agar (1–2 volume/volume) and placed on a supporting layer of 0.5% agar for soft agar cloning as has been described previously (Fathman and Hengartner, 1978). The concentration of cells in soft agar should be varied from 0.25×10^5 to 5×10^5 antigen-reactive T cells in the presence of 50×10^6 filler cells. Within 7 days, colonies can be observed in soft agar using an inverted phase microscope. These colonies can be picked using a drawn out Pasteur pipette and replated in individual microtiter wells with 1×10^6 irradiated syngeneic filler cells in the presence of appropriate amounts of soluble antigen. For soft agar subcloning procedures, the same techniques are utilized, but with the addition of 10% concanavalin (Con-A)-activated spleen cell supernatant at each of the two initial steps (i.e., at the level of soft agar cloning and in the microtiter well). Approximately 7 days after antigen restimulation the cells can be transferred to Costar wells with fresh irradiated filler cells, (10×10^6/well) and fresh antigen. Subclones can but need not be removed from the influence of exogenous TCGF (Con-A supernatant) at this time. Seven days after this transfer, aliquots can be removed from Costar wells and assayed or expanded as described in the Appendix, Section V,A. An alternative method of cloning antigen reactive murine T cells is by limiting dilution cloning following four 2-week intervals of serial reculture as described above. For limiting dilutional cloning, 96-well microtiter flat-bottom plates are prepared by adding 1×10^6 irradiated syngeneic spleen filler cells per well in 100 μl of RPMI fetal calf serum (FCS) medium containing the optimal concentration of soluble antigen. To each well is added 100 μl of a cell suspension (of the long-term cultured antigen-reactive T cells which will be cloned) containing 1 cell/ml or approximately 1 cell in every 10 microtiter wells. Cloning at a frequency of 1 cell/10 wells generally results in the growth of clones derived from a single precursor cell. However, both soft agar cloning and limiting dilution cloning should be followed by subcloning to ensure clonality of the resultant populations. For limiting dilution cloning, the media is made 10% in rat Con-A supernatant as a source of T cell growth factor. The wells are observed under phase microscopy starting about 7 days after plating, and individual wells which are scored as positive for growth can be observed and the cells can be transferred into Costar wells in the presence of 2 ml RPMI FCS media, 10×10^6 irradiated

ISBN 0-12-249920-4

syngeneic filler cells, 10% rat Con-A supernatant as a source of T-cell growth factor, and the optimal concentration of soluble antigen. These cells are then simply expanded as above and can or cannot be maintained with exogenous T cell growth factor at 2-week feeding intervals.

REFERENCES

Fathman, C. G., and Hengartner, H. (1978). Clones of alloreactive T cells. *Nature* (*London*) **272,** 617.

C. Soft Agar Technique for Obtaining Antigen-Specific T Cell Clones

Chuan Chen and Ronald H. Schwartz

Mice are immunized with 20 to 100 μg of antigen per mouse. The antigen is emulsified in complete Freund's adjuvant and injected into each hind footpad and into the base of the tail. After 7 days, periaortic, inguinal, and popliteal lymph nodes are removed, and single cell suspensions are made from these lymph nodes and passed over nylon wool columns to separate T lymphocytes from B cells and macrophages. T lymphocytes (1×10^6) are cultured in complete EHAA (Click's) medium containing 10% fetal calf serum (FCS), 50 μM 2-mercaptoethenol, 0.6 mg/ml glutamine, 5 U/ml penicillin, and 50 μg/ml gentamicin and are stimulated with 100 μg/ml antigen in the presence of 1×10^6 irradiated (2000 rads) syngeneic spleen cells (Costar plates no. 3524). After 2–3 days of incubation of 37°C, the stimulated T lymphocytes are cloned in soft agar as described below.

One day before cloning, the agar suspension is prepared by suspending 3.3 g of Difco Noble agar in 100 ml of sterile distilled water in a sterile 250 ml Erlenmeyer flask that is covered with aluminum foil to prevent loss of water. This solution is boiled for at least 1 hr so that the agar will go completely into solution and the contents will become sterilized. Agar is prepared fresh for each cloning procedure. The stock solution is stored in a 45°C water bath until use.

To prepare the bottom layer of "hard agar," mix 5 ml of 1× EHAA, 1.5 ml of 2× EHAA, 2.0 ml of FCS, and 200 to 1000 μg of antigen (20 to 100 μg/ml), and place this solution in a 37°C incubator for 5 to 10 min to warm up the mixture prior to adding it to the agar. At the end of this 10 min incubation, add 1.5 ml of agar to this solution of antigen and media and distribute 2.5 ml of the mixture to each of 4 wells in a 6 well plate (Costar No. 3506). After the agar is solidified (5 to 10 min), store the plates in a humified incubator at 37°C in the presence of 5%

ISOLATION, CHARACTERIZATION, AND
UTILIZATION OF T LYMPHOCYTE CLONES

ISBN 0-12-249920-4

CO_2 for use the following day. The upper "soft agar layer" contains 1 to 2 $\times$ 10^6 stimulated T cells and 1 to 2 $\times$ 10^5 irradiated spleen cells. The procedure is the same as described for the hard agar layer except that 1.8 g of agar is suspended in 100 ml of sterile water for the soft agar layer. The T cells which are distributed in the upper layer come from liquid culture of cells which have been stimulated with antigen 2–3 days prior to harvest. The cells are mixed with agar to form a 0.33% agar solution and are added to the plates prepared the day before. These agar plates are than put back in the incubator and observed for cell growth using an inverted microscope.

After approximately 4 to 5 days, the colonies will be ready to pick. Colonies are removed from soft agar using Pasteur pipettes. Each colony is then transferred into one well of a 96-well U-bottom microtiter plate containing 1 $\times$ 10^4 irradiated spleen cells, 20 to 100 μg/ml antigen, and 5% TCGF supplemented medium in 100 μl. These microtiter plates are then incubated, and growth is observed using an inverted microscope. Growth can be seen as soon as 3–4 days following picking of the colonies. The cells are fed twice a week by removing 50% of the supernatant and adding back freshly prepared medium containing 5% TCGF supernatant. When cells grow to fill the bottom of the well completely, they are divided and distributed into two or more wells depending on how fast they are growing. After several weeks, the cells can be pooled into large Costar wells. Such cells can be recloned in an identical manner, except that only 50 to 100 cells from each colony are seeded into a 30-mm plate. Additionally, more irradiated spleen cells are put into the upper agar layer, usually 1 to 2 $\times$ 10^6 per plate. When the sublconed colonies are picked from soft agar they should be expanded in liquid culture using more irradiated spleen cells (1 $\times$ 10^6 per well for 96-well flat bottomed plates and 1 $\times$ 10^5 well for 96-well U-bottom plates).

VI. HUMAN T CELL CLONES REACTIVE WITH ALLOANTIGENS AND SOLUBLE ANTIGENS

Several laboratories have developed techniques for isolation of human T cell clones reactive with alloantigens (Möller, 1981; Kornbluth and Dupont, 1980; Bach *et al.*, 1979; Goulmy *et al.*, 1980). Two methods are described. Isolation of antigen-specific human T cell clones has recently been achieved (Sredni *et al.*, 1981), and this technique is described here.

REFERENCES

Bach, F. H., Inouye, H., Hank, J. A., and Alter, B. J. (1979). Human T lymphocyte clones reactive in primed lymphocyte typing in cytotoxicity. *Nature (London)* **281,** 307.

Goulmy, E., Blockland, E., van Rood, J. J., Charmot, D., Malissen, B., and Mawas, C. (1980). Production, expansion and clonal analysis of T cells with specific HLA restricted H-Y male lysis. *J. Exp. Med.* **152,** 182.

Möller, G. (1981). T cell clones. *Immunol. Rev.* **54,** 1.

Kornbluth, J., and Dupont, B. (1980). Cloning and functional characterization of primary alloreactive human T lymphocytes. *J. Exp. Med.* **152,** 164.

Sredni, B., Volkman, D., Schwartz, R. H., and Fauci, A. S. (1981). Antigen specific human T cell clones: Development of clones requiring HLA-DR compatible presenting cells for stimulation in the presence of antigen. *Proc. Natl. Acad. Sci. U.S.A.* **78,** 1858.

A. Cloning of Alloreactive Human T Cells

Fritz Bach

In our initial description of cloning PLT-reactive and cytotoxic T lymphocytes in man (Bach *et al.*, 1979), we utilized both seeding of cells in agarose and limiting dilution (LD) for PLT-reactive and CTL cells. At the present time, most of our experiments are performed utilizing the LD approach, since this allows ready quantification of the probability of clonality. TCGF-containing medium utilized for our human studies has for the most part been derived from PHA-activated peripheral blood lymphocytes (Inouye *et al.*, 1980b). The critical nature of TCGF production and the nature of the feeder cells are discussed separately in the Appendix, Section I,F.

Since we have published our techniques for generating PLT-reactive clones in some detail (Bach *et al.*, 1979, 1981; Inouye *et al.*, 1980a,b), we shall concentrate primarily on technical details relating to cloning of CTL.

Priming. Cells to be cloned are activated in primary MLC cultures in 25-ml Falcon flasks (No. 3013) using 5×10^6 responders and 5×10^6 irradiated (4000 R) stimulators in 10 ml of RPMI-1640 with 25 m*M* HEPES, supplemented with penicillin–streptomycin, L-glutamine, and 15% pooled human serum. The cells are cultured for 4 days at 37°C in a 5% CO_2-humidified atmosphere. In an attempt to avoid both recruitment by activated cells of other T lymphocytes that are not specific for the alloantigens used to induce the response, as well as to minimize the probability that we clone cells responding to phytohemagglutinin (PHA), the following approach has been used. Bulk mixed lymphocyte cultures (MLC) are prepared as described and on day 4, blasts are separated on a unit-gravity gradient (Miller and Phillips, 1969). Those fractions that contain only blasts and the first fraction which contains more than 66% blasts and no dead cells are pooled. This usually represents approximately 20% of the total cell recovery. Since no TCGF is added to those bulk cultures and since the blasts are recovered relatively early in the proliferative/cytotoxic response, we hope that a

ISBN 0-12-249920-4

majority of blasts present at that time are ones that are specifically alloantigen responsive. Cloning is performed from this pooled blast cell fraction.

Cloning. Blast cells are seeded in Terasaki wells (Cooke histoplate No. 236–72) at an average of 1 cell per 5 wells (probability of nonclonal growth in any well less than 0.1) in the presence of 1×10^4 irradiated feeder cells in 15 μl TCGF-containing medium. The plates are incubated at 37°C in a humidified 5% CO_2 atmosphere. Owing to the small volume of culture medium used in Terasaki wells, precaution against excessive evaporation and temperature change is particularly important.

Screening for Growth. Cell growth is determined by visual inspection using an inverted phase microscope and is scored as positive when more than one-third of the well is packed with cells. Growth is rarely seen during the first 6 days of culture, while the number of positive wells increases from day 7 to 10. Seldom is growth evident in hitherto negative wells after day 11.

Expansion of Clonal Populations. Cells in Terasaki wells are "picked" using a 20 μl microtiter pipette and sterile disposable tip. The contents of the Terasaki wells are transferred to U-bottom microtiter wells (Costar No. 3799) containing 200 μl of TCGF-containing medium and 5×10^4 irradiated feeder cells. On days 2 and 4 after transfer, the wells are replenished with TCGF medium, and, on day 6, they are fed with fresh feeders followed by further fresh changes of medium on subsequent alternate days. Cell expansion for the faster growing clones is usually evident as early as 4–5 days after transfer, while others may take as long as 2 weeks to expand to sufficient numbers for functional assays. At this stage of cell expansion, i.e, around 25–30 days after primary sensitization, the cells in positive wells can be screened for functional activity, i.e., PLT or CML.

Further expansion of cells is accomplished in 16 mm cluster wells (Costar No. 3524). The feeder layer consists of $5\ 10 \times 10^5$ irradiated peripheral blood lymphocytes (4000 R). The contents of the U-bottom microwell are transferred to the 16-mm well. Initially the culture is in 1 ml of TCGF-containing medium. Starting on day 2 after seeding in these wells, daily care of the clones appears to be required. Some clones grow exceedingly quickly and may require daily splitting into subcultures (without feeders added at those times).

Clones are usually harvested at weekly intervals, counted, and reseeded with new feeder cells. Although it appears that clones grow more successfully in the 16-mm wells (perhaps because conditions have been more nearly optimized for those wells), very rapidly dividing clones can be grown successfully in 25-ml flasks.

Alternate Cloning Procedures. In addition to the procedures described above, we have also cloned cells primed under various conditions such as from day 7 bulk MLC or from secondary bulk MLC culture. Although it is possible that different priming protocols may influence the types of lytic cells that are generated or can eventually be cloned (Widmer and Bach, 1982), the precise effect of different procedures is not known. We do know, however, that alloimmune CTL can be cloned from both primary and secondary MLC bulk cultures.

Cloning by limiting dilutions in 96-well microtiter plates has also been attempted using 1–2 $\times$ 10^4 feeders in 200 TCGF-containing medium. Similar plating efficiency (15–20%) from day 4 blast cells seeded at 1 cell per 5 wells is observed whether cells are cloned in Terasaki plates or in 96-well microtiter plates. Cloning of cytolytic cells in solid medium (agarose) has also been done as described in previous reports (Bach *et al.*, 1979; Wee *et al.*, 1981).

Testing of Different Feeder Cells. We have tested both X-irradiated LCL and X-irradiated peripheral blood lymphocytes as feeders for CTL clones. In addition, we have tested a "pool" of cells from several unrelated individuals as a feeder layer for the clone. Clonal growth can be observed with any one of these different feeders. It is our impression that the use of LCL as feeders leads to larger cell recoveries in each clone than do pooled feeders; however, more data are needed in this regard before any conclusion can be reached.

REFERENCES

Bach, F. H., Inouye, H., Hank, J. A., and Alter, B. J. (1979). Human T lymphocyte clones reactive in primed lymphocyte typing and cytotoxicity. *Nature* (*London*) **281,** 307.

Bach, F. H., Alter, B. J., Widmer, M. B., Segall, M. S., and Dunlap, B. (1981). Cloned cytotoxic and non-cytotoxic lymphocytes in mouse and man: Their reactivities and a large cell surface membrane protein (LMP) differentiation marker system. *Immunol. Rev.* **54,** 5.

Inouye, H. Hank, J. A., Chardonnens, X., Segall, M., Alter, B. J., and Bach, F. H. (1980a). Cloned PLT reagents in the dissection of HLA-D. *J. Exp. Med.* **152,** 143s.

Inouye, H., Hank, J. A., Alter, B. J., and Bach, F. H. (1980b). TCGF production for cloning and growth of functional human T lymphocytes. *Scand. J. Immunol.* **12,** 149.

Miller, R. G., and Phillips, R. A. (1969). Separation of cells by velocity sedimentation. *J. Cell. Physiol.* **73,** 191.

Wee, S. L., Wu, S., Alter, B. J., and Bach, F. H. (1981). Early detection and specificity analysis of human cytolytic T lymphocyte (CTL) colonies generated in soft agarose culture: A potential assay for definition of CTL defined (CD) determinants. *Hum. Immunol.* **3,** 45.

Widmer, M. B., and Bach, F. H. (1982). Submitted for publication.

B. Cloning and Expansion of Human Alloreactive T Lymphocytes

Bernard Mallisen and Claude Mawas

In order to derive a reliable technique for cloning cytotoxic T cells, we have taken advantage of our earlier work on the effect of various lectins on the induction of specific cytotoxicity in reverted primed lymphocytes (Malissen *et al.*, 1979). Phytohemagglutinin (PHA), concanavalin A (Con-A), pokeweed mitogen (PWM), and leucoagglutinin (Leucoa) were able to induce proliferation of primed cells, but only primed cells stimulated by PWM or Leucoa displayed specific cytotoxicity (for an interpretation of the differential effect of such lectins, cf. Malissen *et al.*, 1979). Furthermore, Leucoa or PHA allowed a strong expansion of primed cells when added simultaneously with irradiated peripheral bood lymphocytes autologous to the responder cells (Charmot *et al.*, 1980). The cloning protocol developed in our laboratory (Malissen *et al.*, 1981a,b) relies on these observations.

Culture Medium. All cultures are performed in RPMI 1640 (Gibco) supplemented with L-glutamine, sodium bicarbonate, antibiotics, and 10% (long-term cultures) or 20% (cloning step) human heparinized plasma from a random pool of 6 to 20 Australia antigen-negative donors, irrespective of ABO blood types. Batches of conditioned medium (CM) are prepared from tonsil cells activated for 48 hr by 1 μg/ml Leucoa (Pharmacia, Sweden).

Cloning Procedures. Cells to be cloned are carefully counted and diluted to the required concentration. A volume of 100 μl of the cell suspension are subsequently distributed into round-bottomed wells of microtiter plates (Greiner and Sohne) using a sterile multichannel pipette (Titertek, Flow Laboratories). At the same time, and in order to promote growth, each well also received in a volume of 100 μl, 5×10^4 irradiated (4000 R from a cobalt source, Gamma Cell, Atomic Energy of Canada) PBL from unselected blood donors plus Leucoa (1 μg/ml). For each experiment, microtiter plates containing only irradiated feeder cells plus Leucoa are set up as controls. Ten to 14 days later, growth is monitored in the original microplates using an inverted microscope. Growing cells are subsequently transferred to 24-well macroplates (Costar No. 3524) and to tissue culture flasks (Falcon No. 3013) for expansion. Functional screening of growing colonies is done as soon as enough cells are available.

Subsequent recloning is performed as the initial cloning step with the systematic addition of optimal doese of conditioned medium (CM) to the cloning

ISOLATION, CHARACTERIZATION, AND
UTILIZATION OF T LYMPHOCYTE CLONES

ISBN 0-12-249920-4

medium. Until now, this cloning strategy has permitted us to obtain (1) PLT and cell mediated lympholysis (CML) clones derived either from *in vitro* (Malissen *et al.*, 1981a) or *in vivo* (Malissen *et al.*, 1981b) alloactivated T cells, (2) anti-H-Y HLA-A2 restricted cytotoxic clones (Goulmy *et al.*, 1980), and (3) HLA-D restricted proliferative clones specific for soluble antigens like tuberculin (see Chapter 38 in this treatise).

Cloning efficiencies ranging from 10 to 100% were routinely obtained and Poisson distributions were always observed indicating that the obtained populations were derived from a single cell.

Expansion of Cloned Alloreactive T Cell Lines. Expansion of growing cells is obtained by using repeatedly two 4-days cycles of CM alone, followed by a 3–4 days passage on 4000 R irradiated PBL plus Leucoa (1 μg/ml). Using such a protocol, we have obtained from 10^9 to 10^{10} cells after 2 months of expansion.

Present Limitations. In order to be of use in immunogenetic investigations, cloned cytolytic T cell lines must demonstrate not only unlimited growth potential but also stability with regards to specificity and levels of cytotoxicity observed.

The availability of stable cytotoxic T lymphocyte hybridomas may only partially circumvent the absolute IL-2 requirement since some (Nabholz *et al.*, 1980) but not all (Kaufmann *et al.*, 1981) cytolytically active murine T cell hybrids reported until now need to be grown in the presence of IL-2 in order to show detectable cytolytic capacity.

Purification of IL-2 from PHA-stimulated lymphocyte CM (see, for instance, Gillis *et al.*, 1980; Mier and Gallo, 1980) will surely permit in the near future the isolation of the gene(s) coding for such product, opening the way for obtaining large amounts of pure human IL-2 by genetic engineering.

REFERENCES

Charmot, D., Malissen, B., Ghiotto, M., and Mawas, C. (1980). Expansion of human lymphocyte populations expressing specific immune reactivities. II. A comparison of immune reactivities in human T lymphocyte lines derived from allogeneically primed cultures and maintained with lectins or conditioned medium. *Tissue Antigens* **15,** 297.

Gillis, S., Smith, K. A., and Watson, J. (1980). Biochemical characterization of lymphocyte regulatory molecules. II. Purification of a class of rat and human lymphokines. *J. Immunol.* **124,** 1954.

Goulmy, E., Blokland, E., van Rood, J. J., Charmot, D., Malissen, B., and Mawas, C. (1980). Production, expansion and clonal analysis of T cells with specific HLA restricted male lysis. *J. Exp. Med.* **152,** 182s.

Kaufmann, Y., Berke, G., and Eshhar, Z. (1981). Cytotoxic T lymphocyte hybridomas that mediate specific tumor-cell lysis *in vitro*. *Proc. Natl. Acad. Sci. U.S.A.* **78,** 2502.

Malissen, B., Charmot, D., Liabeuf, A., and Mawas, C. (1979). Expansion of human lymphocyte populations expressing specific immune reactivities. I. Differential effects of various lectins on the expression of alloreactive cytotoxicity by primed cells. *J. Immunol.* **123,** 1787.

Malissen, B., Charmot, D., and Mawas, C. (1981a). Expansion of human lymphocyte populations expressing specific immune reactivities. III. Specific colonies, either cytotoxic or proliferative obtained from a population of responder cell primed *in vitro*. Preliminary immunogenetic analysis. *Hum. Immunol.* **2,** 1.

Malissen, B., Kristensen, T., Goridis, C., Madsen, M., and Mawas, C. (1981b). Clones of human cytotoxic T lymphocytes derived from an allosensitized individual. HLA specificity and cell surface markers. *Scand. J. Immunol.* **14,** 213.

Mier, J. W., and Gallo, R. C. (1980). Purification and some characteristics of human T-cell growth factor (TCGF) from PHA-stimulated lymphocyte conditioned media. *Proc. Natl. Acad. Sci. U.S.A.* **77,** 6134.

Nabholz, M., Cianfriglia, M., Acuto, O., Conzelmann, A., Haas, W., von Boehmer, H., McDonald, H. R., Pohlit, H., and Johnson, J. P. (1980). Cytolytically active murine T-cell hybrids. *Nature (London)* **287,** 437.

C. Establishment of Colonies of Antigen-Reactive Human T Cells

Benjamin Sredni

Peripheral blood mononuclear cells (PBMNC) from normal individuals who have been immunized are stimulated *in vitro* with the appropriate antigen for 5 days and are then seeded in soft agar (Sredni *et al.*, 1981). Four to 6 days after the soft agar seeding, these lymphocytes develop into recognizable colonies containing at least 50 cells each. (Figure 1 presents a schematic diagram of this procedure.)

Lymphocyte colonies develop only in the continuous presence of antigen which is essential both for the priming *in vitro* and in the subsequent cloning in soft agar. Colony development does not occur in control cultures without antigen. Following proliferation, the cells develop into two types of colonies which are morphologically distinguishable. Type I colonies are the larger of the two types, containing 50 to 500 cells. These develop within the upper agar layer 4 to 6 days after seeding and manifest a compact center with a diffuse periphery. Type II colonies appear about 2 days later and form on the exposed surface of the upper agar layer. These colonies contain 50–150 cells, are small and flat morphologically, and usually grow above the primary type I colonies. With regard to the kinetics of colony formation, the number of colonies increases with time after stimulation *in vitro*, reaching a maximum at days 4 and 5 for types I and II colonies, respectively (Fig. 2).

The concentration of antigen used in the lower layer of agar is a critical factor in optimal colony formation. For example, the optimal antigen concentrations for

ISBN 0-12-249920-4

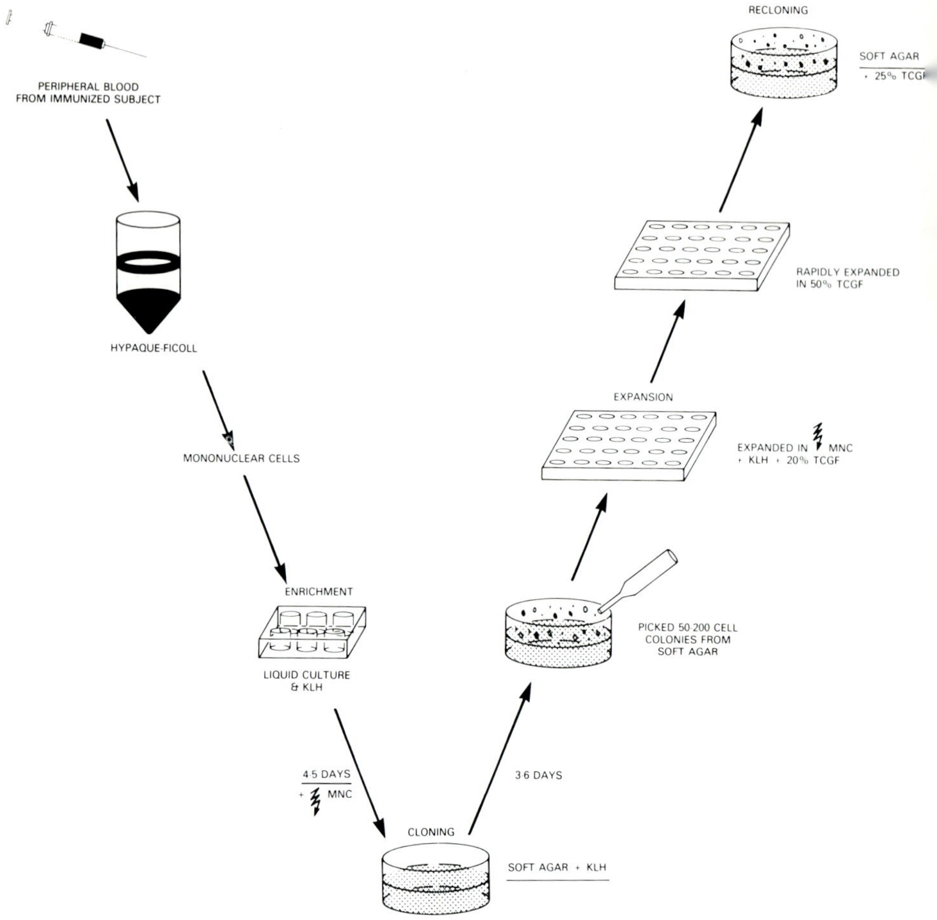

Fig. 1. A schematic diagram of the method for human T cell cloning.

type I and type II colonies are 25 and 50 μg of keyhole limpet hemocyanin (KLH) per milliliter, respectively. Too low a concentration of antigen yields fewer colonies for the same number of cells seeded. At concentrations greater than 50 μg/ml there is a plateau for both types of colonies (Fig. 3).

There is a direct proportion between the number of type I colonies formed and the number of cells seeded in the soft agar over the range 5×10^5 to 4×10^6 cells. The slope of the log–log plot of this line is 1, suggesting that each colony derived from one cell or functional unit (Tse *et al.*, 1980). This pattern is not seen with the type II colonies.

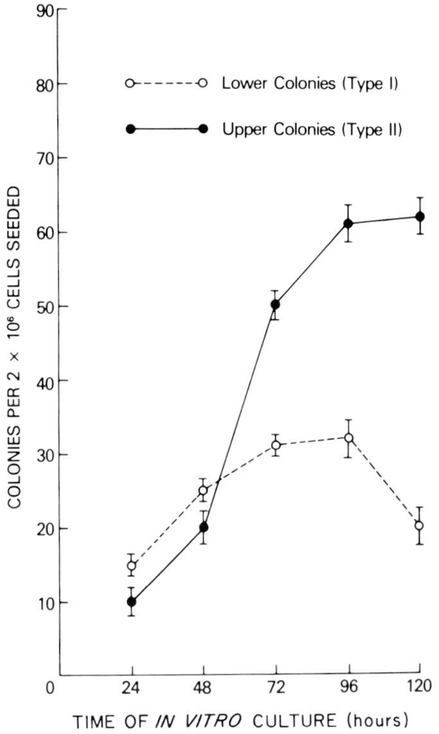

Fig. 2. Clonal frequency as a function of time after initial stimulation with antigen *in vitro*. The number of type I (○——○) and type II (●——●) colonies reached their maximum on days 4 and 5, respectively. Each point represents the mean ± SEM of three separate experiments.

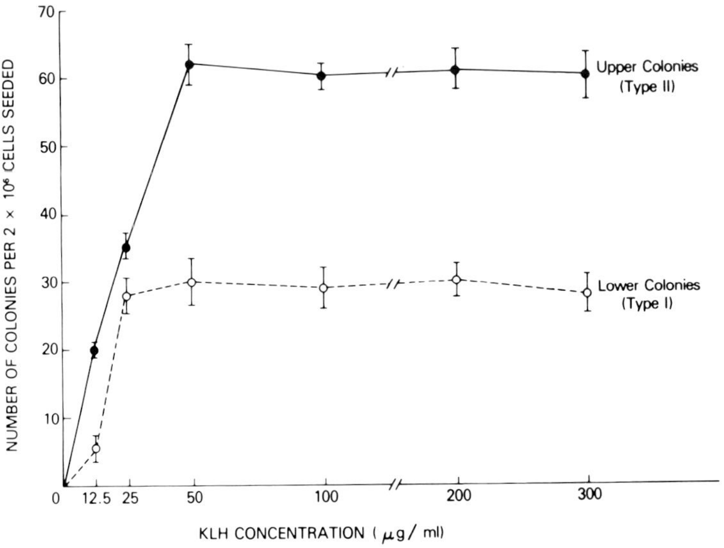

Fig. 3. Clonal frequency as a function of antigen concentration in the lower agar layer. After 5 days of growth in the agar, the number of colonies were counted. Each point represents the mean ± SEM of three separate experiments.

Recloning. The efficiency on recloning is about 85%. Representative clones derived from recloning of type I colonies possess identical specificity patterns in that they all respond only to the original stimulating antigen and not to other agents. Clonality of the T cell lines can be established by multiple reclonings at high plating efficiencies.

Surface Marker Characteristics of Antigen-Specific Clones. In a representative experiment, cells of a KLH antigen-specific clone, L.S.1.3, were identified at T cells by surface marker characteristics: 98% of the viable cells were erythrocyte-rosette positive and none were surface Ig positive or complement-receptor positive. In addition, 91% of cells bound the 3A1 monoclonal anti-T cell antibody and 98% bound a monoclonal anti-Ia antibody.

REFERENCES

Sredni, B. Volkman, D., Schwartz, R. H., and Fauci, A. S. (1981). Antigen-specific human T-cell clones: Development of clones requiring HLA-DR-compatible presenting cells for stimulation in presence of antigen. *Proc. Natl. Acad. Sci. U.S.A.* **78,** 1858.

Tse, H. Y., Schwartz, R. H., and Paul, W. E. (1980). Cell–cell interactions in the T cell proliferative response. I. Analysis of the cell types involved and evidence for nonspecific T cell recruitment. *J. Immunol.* **125,** 491.

Index

A

Accessory cell
  helper T cells' recognition of, 385–386, 388–389
  Moloney leukemia virus-specific cytolytic T cell clones, 298–299
  T lymphocyte interaction, 83–84, 86–87
Actinomycin D, interleukin-1 production, 46
Adherent cell, interleukin-2, 59–60, 62
Affinity chromatography
  PHA removal from culture supernatants, 67
  purification of GAT-TsF, 140–141
Agar cloning of T cells, 269, 377–378, 417–419, 439–442, 528–529
Alloantigens
  activation of T cells, 236
  murine T cell clones reactive with, 519–525
Alloreactive T lymphocyte, 245–251, 270–271, 274, 279, 358, 360
  antigen-specific T cells, 375–384
  anti-H-2 reactivity of Mls-specific clones, 331–339
  factors produced by, 276–278
  human T cells, cloning of, 530–535
  hybrid determinant recognition, 325–329
  influenza virus-specific CTL, 290, 293
  lymphokine production, 341–354
Allosensitized target-specific cytotoxic T lymphocyte, 74, 77
Allospecificity, 15
Allotypic determinants, T helper cells specific for, 397
Amino acid sequence, 483–485
Antibody
  effect of bursectomy on formation, 4
  interaction with suppressor factor, 132–134
  limiting dilution assays, 219–220
Antigen binding, 406, 481
  T cell hybridomas, 102–103, 110–115
Antigen-induced T lymphocyte, 83, 86–89, 270
  strategies for cloning, 266–269, 274
Antigen-presenting cell (APC)
  in analysis of antigen recognition by T cells, 368, 370–373
  human T cell culture, 440–441, 443–444
Antigen recognition, 112–115
Antigen-specific cytolytic T lymphocyte, 22
  receptor specificity analysis, 314–322
Antigen-specific, *H-2* restricted T cell hybridoma, 508–509
Antigen-specific T lymphocyte, 85, 95–96, 113, 359, 361–364, 368–369, 405
  alloreactivity, 375–384
  helper T cells, 22
  human T cells, establishment of colonies of, 535–538
  poly GAT-specific T helper cells, 397–404
  soft agar colonies of human T cells, 440–442
Antigen-specific T lymphocyte hybridoma, 96–99
  H-2 restricted, 119–126
Antigen-specific T lymphocyte suppressor factor (TsF), 97, 127–136
  antibody-suppressor factor interaction, 132–134
  B cells as targets, 129–130
  characterization, 137–148
  GAT-specific, 138–145
  genetic control of suppression, 130–132
  GT-specific, 139–145
  haplotype-specific suppressor factor, 149–155
Anti-PHA affinity column, 67–69

B

BCDF, *see* B lymphocyte differentiation factor
BCG-activated macrophage, interleukin-1 release, 47
BCHF, *see* B lymphocyte helper factor
BCSF, *see* B lymphocyte stimulating factor
B lymphocyte, 4, 16
 genetics, 468–479
 interleukin-1, 50
 limiting dilution assay, 220
 target for antigen-specific T hybrid suppressor factor, 129–130
 T cell activation of, 359–360, 385–395, 397–399
B lymphocyte differentiation factor (BCDF), test system for, 255, 257, 259–260
B lymphocyte helper factor (BCHF), 341, 347–349
B lymphocyte hybridoma, 173–174
B lymphocyte receptor, 285
B lymphocyte stimulating factor (BCSF), 341–346
Bone marrow cell, interleukin-1, 42
Bone marrow chimeras, antigen recognition, 376
Bone marrow-derived macrophage, 110–111
Bone marrow transplantation, 16
Bursectomy, effect on antibody formation, 4

C

Cancer immunotherapy, 451–466
Cell-mediated immune response, 4, 165, 265, 272
Cell-mediated lympholysis (CML), 425
Cell surface antigens, 143–144, 272
 human T lymphocyte clones, 421–422
Cell transfer assay, 219
Chicken gamma-globulin (CGG)
 specific hybridoma clone, 111–112
 T cell hybridomas, 123
Chicken red blood cells (CRBC), PHA removal from culture supernatants, 67–69
Chromosomal instability of T cell hybrids, 100
Cloning, 11–18, 357–358
 methods and strategies, 13–14, 266–269
  human T lymphocytes, 413–424, 530–538
  soft agar technique, 528–529
 uses of, 14–16
CM, *see* Conditioned medium
CML, *see* Cell mediated lympholysis
Colony stimulating factor (CSF), 5–6, 341–346, 349–350
 T cell clones, 278
 test system for, 255–257, 259–260
Concanavalin A (Con-A), 85
 activated suppressor T cells, 157, 160–161, 235
 antigen-specific *H-2* restricted T cell hybridomas, 120–121, 125
 clonal analysis of T cells, 234–237, 239–240
 ytolytic T lymphocytes, 167–168, 172
 ıterleukin-1, 49–50
 ınterleukin-2, 29, 60–61
 lymphokine production, 254–256, 346–348
 thymocyte response, 51–52
Conditioned medium (CM), 5–6, 22, 425
 cytotoxic T lymphocyte clones, 427
 interleukin-2 production, 26, 29
 noncytolytic T lymphocyte clones, 274
 sources, 268
Cortical thymocyte, interleukin-1, 49
CRBC, *see* Chicken red blood cells
Crisis period in lymphocyte growth, 69–70
Cross-reactivity
 of cytolytic T lymphocyte clones, 270–272, 279
 T cell lines with cross-reactive idiotype, 397–404
Crude T cell growth factor (TCGF), 58
CSA, *see* Cyclosporin A
CSF, *see* Colony stimulating factor
CTL, *see* Cytolytic T lymphocyte
Cutaneous T cell, interleukin-2, 60
Cyanogen bromide, T cells reactive to, 368–372
Cycloheximide
 interleukin-1, 46
 interleukin-2, 63
Cyclosporin A (CSA), interleukin-1, 50–52
Cytolytic (cytotoxic) T lymphocyte (CTL), 2, 6, 15–16, 58
 activation, 70
 alloreactive and *H-2*-restricted, 245–251
 antigen-specific, 22
 anti-HY-HLA specificity, 430–431
 clones, 233–244, 269–273, 279–280
 established lines, 166–169
 growth regulation, 193–203
 H-2 restricted influenza virus-specific, 285–295

human clones, 414, 417-423
interleukin-2, 69-76, 176-177
karyotype evolution, 183-191
kinetics of growth, 452
lymphokine production, 341-354
MHC specificity of alloreactive clones, 431-432
MLC-derived clones, 426-427
murine sarcoma virus-induced tumor antigens, recognition of, 297-311
mutants, 170-173
somatic cell genetic analysis of, 165-181
specificity, 177-178, 313-323
surface markers, 433-435
target interactions, 83-84
virus-specific clones, isolation of, 524-525
Cytolytic T lymphocyte-A (CTL-A) line, 167-169
antigen-loss variants, 172
karotype evolution, 188-190
and thymoma cell hybrids, 175
Cytolytic T lymphocyte-B (CTL-B) line, 167-169
karotype evolution, 183-190
mutants, 170-171
and thymoma cell hybrids, 175
Cytolytic T lymphocyte hybrid, growth factor dependence, lectin resistance, and cytolytic activity, 205-215
Cytolytic T lymphocyte precursor (CTL-P)
frequencies, 510-515
limiting dilution assays, 220-229
Moloney leukemia virus specificity, 297
receptor specificity analysis, 314-322
Cytomegalovirus-reactive clone, 16

D

Delayed-type hypersensitivity (DTH), 15, 83-84
Dinitrophenylated ovalbumin, *see* DNP-OVA
DNA, 467-486
activation of synthesis, 195-199
SIRS-mediated inhibition of synthesis, 159
DNP, 359
DNP-GAT, T helper cells for responses to, 397-404
DNP-OVA, T cells reactive to, 377-381
DTH, *see* Delayed-type hypersensitivity
Dual receptor theories, 122-123
Dual recognition-altered self controversy, 112-115

E

Effector T lymphocyte, 22
Epidermal growth factor (EGF), 194
Epstein-Barr virus-transformed, lymphoblastoid cell lines, 417-418
E-rosette-positive T lymphocyte, 59

F

FACS, *see* Fluorescence-activated cell sorting
FCS, *see* Fetal calf serum
Feeder cells, 266-269, 274
primed lymphocyte typing-reactive clones, 414
Fetal calf serum (FCS), 62, 85
Fibroblast growth factor (FGF), 194
Fluorescence-activated cell sorting (FACS), 97, 269
FLV, *see* Friend leukemia virus
FMR, *see* Friend, Moloney, Rausher leukemia virus group
Foreign antigen-specific T lymphocyte, 375-376
Frequency analysis
antigen-primed populations, 375
helper and cytolytic T cells, 233-244
Moloney leukemia virus-specific CTL precursors, 300-301
Friend leukemia virus (FLV), 271, 305-306
Friend, Moloney, Rausher (FMR) leukemia virus group, 305-306

G

GA, 363-364
T cells reactive to, 368
Galactose oxidase, interleukin-2, 61
GAT (L-glutamic acid^{60}-L-alanine^{30}-L-tyrosine^{10}), 138-145, 359, 361-364
poly GAT-specific T helper cells, 397-403
T cells reactive to, 368-369, 371-372, 474-478
GAT-TNP, 359, 361
Gaucher's disease, 46
Gel filtration chromatography, 503-504

Gene activations, T cell hybrids, 101
Genetically restricted, Ia-containing factor (GRF), 110
Genetics, 467–491
control of suppression in antigen-specific T hybrid line, 130–132
of repertoire, 313, 320–322
somatic cell genetic analysis, 165–181
Glucocerebroside (GL_1), interleukin-1 production, 46–47
L-Glutamic acid^{60}-L-alanine^{30}-L-tyrosine^{10}, *see* GAT
L-Glutamic acid^{50}-L-tyrosine^{50}, *see* GT
GRF, *see* Genetically restricted, Ia-containing factor
Growth factors
cytolytic activity, lectin resistance and, 205–215
mechanisms of action, 194–196
GT (L-glutamic acid^{50}-L-tyrosine^{50}), 138–145

H

Haplotype-specific suppressor factor (TsF-H), 149–155
HCSF, *see* Histamine-producing cell-stimulating factor
Helper T lymphocyte, 6, 15–16, 342, 359–362
antigen recognition, 369–370
B cell activation, 385–395, 397
cloned, 233–244, 279
genetics, 470
idiotype-positive, 397–404
interleukin-2, 59
Helper T lymphocyte hybridoma, 98–99
altered self–dual recognition problem, 112–115
characterization of hybridoma clones, 111–112
helper factor isolation, 116
H-2 restricted, 109–117
Ia antigens, 103
Ia-associated antigen complex, 109–111
Helper T lymphocyte precursor frequencies, 237–242
HGG, *see* Human gamma-globulin
High performance liquid chromatography (HPLC), purification of GAT-TsF, 141
Histamine-producing cell-stimulating factor (HCSF), test system for, 255, 259–260
HLA antigens, 15, 60, 417, 422, 427–428, 430–434, 442–445
HPLC, *see* High performance liquid chromatography
H-2 restriction
altered self–dual recognition problem, 112–115
antigen-specific T cell hybridomas, 119–126
cytotoxic T lymphocyte clones, 245–251
helper factor isolation, 116
helper hybridoma clones, 109–117
Ia-associated antigen complex, 109–111
influenza virus-specific cytolytic T lymphocytes, 285–295
Mls-specific T cell clones, 331–339
Moloney leukemia virus-specific CTL clones, 307
production of antigen-specific, *H-2* restricted T cell hybridoma, 508–509
responses to GAT and GT, 138–140, 142, 144
T cell recognition of B cells, 385–389
^{3}H-TdR assay
interleukin-2, 63–66, 69
phytohemagglutinin, 69
Human blood monocyte, interleukin-1, 48–49
Human gamma-globulin (HGG), T cell hybrids, 97
Human interleukin-2, 57–82
cellular sources, 27–30
culture conditions, 58–63
cytotoxic T lymphocytes, growth in, 69–76
cytolytic lymphocyte activation, 77–79
PHA removal from culture supernatants, 66–69
polyacrylamide gel electrophoresis, 33–35
production, 499–501
purification, 24–26
temperature, chemical, and enzymatic treatments, 26–27
testing of culture supernatant, 63–66
Human T lymphocyte, 22
cloning and expansion of, 413–424, 530–538
function, specificity, and cell surface markers, 425–437
karyotype evolution, 189–190
reactive with soluble antigens, 439–447
Humoral immune response, 4
Hybridoma, 95; *see also* B lymphocyte hybridoma; Helper T lymphocyte hybridoma; T lymphocyte hybridoma
H-Y HLA restriction, 430–431

I

Ia antigens, 327–328
  recognition by alloreactive T cell clones, 327–328
  restriction, 371–373
  role in antigen presentation, 370–371
  T cell hybrids, 103–105, 360
Ia-associated antigen complex (IAC), 109–111
Idiotype, 15, 362
  DNA probes from idiotype-positive B lymphocytes, 473
  T cell hybridomas, 102–103
  T cell lines and clones with cross-reactive idiotype, 397–404
IEF, *see* Isoelectric focusing
IFN, *see* Interferon
IL-1, *see* Interleukin-1
IL-2, *see* Interleukin-2
IL-3, *see* Interleukin-3
Immune response
  antibody-suppressor factor interaction, 132–134
  regulation by products of T cell clones, 405–409
Immune system, comparison with nervous system, 11–13
Immunoglobulins, 357
  degradation with proteolytic enzymes, 406–408
  genetics, 467–480
  in study of T cell lines bearing cross-reactive idiotype, 397–404
Immunological diseases, 12
Immunological memory, 3
Immunotherapy, 451–466
Inducer T lymphocyte, 405–406
Influenza virus, type A, 271–272
  cytolytic T lymphocyte specificity, 285–295
Interferon (IFN), 16, 341, 347–351
  activated suppressor T cells, 161
  T cell clones, 278
  T cell hybridoma, 120–121
  test system for, 254–257, 259–260
Interleukin-1 (lymphocyte activating factor), 22–23, 41–56, 84, 196, 341
  antigen binding, 110–111
  assay, 49–52, 495–498
  interleukin-2, 60
  mode of action, 51–52
  production, 42–49
    and release, 43–44
  T cell stimulation, 86–88
Interleukin-2 (T cell growth factor), 5–6, 16, 21–40, 84, 86, 88, 278, 341–353
  analysis of lymphokine release, 254–255, 258, 260–261
  antigen-specific *H-2* restricted T cell hybridomas, 119–122, 125
  cellular sources, 26–30, 502
  cloned T lymphocyte *in vivo,* 280
  Con-A activated T cells, 234–235
  culture conditions, 58–63
    human T cells, 440
  cytolytic lymphocyte activation, 77–79
  cytolytic T lymphocytes, growth in, 69–76, 168–170, 176–177, 193–203
    Moloney leukemia virus-specific clones, 298–299
  cytolytic T lymphocyte–thymoma cell hybrids, 175
  derivation of T cell clones, 266–269, 273–274
  future molecular prospects, 36–38
  H-2 restricted influenza virus-specific CTL, 288–289, 293
  human, 57–82
  immunotherapeutic effects of cells isolated and expanded in, 453–465
  interleukin-1 stimulation of production of, 50–51
  kinetics of T cell growth in, 452
  microassay, 24, 501–503
  noncytolytic T lymphocyte clones, 274
  PHA removal from culture supernatants, 66–69
  polyacrylamide gel electrophoresis, 30–35
  preparation, 498–501
  purification and characterization, 24–26, 503–507
  temperature, chemical, and enzymatic treatments, 26–27
  testing for, 63–66, 255, 257, 259
Interleukin-2-dependent cells, 63–65
  cytotoxic cell lines, 72–74
Interleukin-2 producer T cell, 22–23
Interleukin-2 responder T cell, 23
Interleukin-3, 274, 341
In vitro sensitization (IVS) cultures, cytotoxic T lymphocytes, 70–72, 77–79
Ion exchange chromatography, 504

I region, 96
restriction, 360–362
T cell hybridoma, 103–105
Ir gene control mechanisms, 138, 371–373
Isoelectric focusing (IEF), 505
Isotypic determinants, T helper cells specific for, 397, 402–403
IVS cultures, *see In vitro* sensitization cultures

J

Jurkat-FHCRC, 28–29, 60

K

Karyotype evolution, cytolytic T cells, 183–191
Keyhole limpet hemagglutinin, 440–441, 443–444
Keyhole limpet hemocyanin (KLH)
T cell hybridomas, 97–99, 122–124
T cells reactive to, 368, 372–373
T helper cells specific for activation of B cells, 386–395
Keyhole limpet hemocyanin-TNP, 359
Killer T lymphocyte, genetics, 470–473
KLH, *see* Keyhole limpet hemocyanin

L

LAF (lymphocyte activating factor), *see* Interleukin-1
Latex, interleukin-1 production, 43–44
LBL, *see* Lymphoblastoid cell line
LDCC, *see* Lectin-dependent cellular cytotoxicity
Lectin
cytolytic activity of CTL clones, 273–274
cytolytic T cell dependence, and lymphokine production, 350–351
Lectin-dependent cellular cytotoxicity (LDCC), 74
Lectin resistance, cytolytic T cell hybrids, 205–215
Leucine aminopeptidase, effect on interleukin-2, 26–27
Leukemia cells, limiting dilution assay, 219
Leukoagglutinin, interleukin-2 production, 60
Limiting dilution, 219–231, 234
cytotoxic T lymphocyte clones, 417–419
derivation of T cell clones, 268–269
isolation of tumor-reactive cells, 459
lymphokine release, 254–257, 261
specificity of CTL clones, 246
technique, 510–519
Lipopolysaccharide (LPS), interleukin-1 production, 43–45, 47–48, 50
Long-term cultures
cloned T cells derived from, 266–267
lymphokine production, analysis of, 258–261
LPS, *see* Lipopolysaccharide
Lyb-5$^+$ B cell, activation, 390–391, 393–395
Lyb-5$^-$ B cell, activation, 385, 390, 393–395
Lymph node cell, immunization and long-term culture of, 525–526
Lymphoblastoid cell (LBL)
antigen presentation studies, 370–371
interleukin-2, 62–63, 65–66
primed lymphocyte typing-reactive clones, 414, 417–418, 421
Lymphocyte, 1; *see also* specific types of lymphocytes
clones, 11
differentiation, 12
interleukin-1 stimulation, 50–51
long-term growth, 69–76
nonthymic, 4
Lymphocyte activating factor, *see* Interleukin-1
Lymphoid cells
human, culture of, 425
interleukin-2, 58–61
use in immunotherapy of cancer, 451–466
Lymphokine, 157, 161; *see also* specific lymphokines
antigen-specific *H-2* restricted T cell hybridomas, 119–122
production, 16
cytolytic and noncytolytic T cell clones, 341
murine T cells, 253–262
source, 16
Lymphoma treatment, 458–459
Lysosomal enzyme release, 47
Lyt antigens, 4, 481–482
binding, 110
cytolytic T lymphocytes, 172–173
cytolytic activity of CTL clones, 273
growth and kinetics of T cells, 235, 239–242

Moloney leukemia virus-specific CTL clones, 309
T cell expression of, and lymphokine production, 350–351
T cell hybrids, 101

M

Macrophage, 16
antigen binding, 110
effect on IL-2 producer T cells, 22–23
interleukin-1, 42–45
damaging agents, 46–47
production and release, 46–48
lymphocyte responses in culture, 41
T cell activation, 84, 88
Macrophage activating factor (MAF), 120, 341, 347–351
T cell clones, 278
test system for, 254–257, 259–260
Macrophage-derived suppressor factor (Mϕ-SF), 157–161
Macrophage Ia recruiting factor (MIRF), 120–121, 341
Major histocompatibility complex (MHC), 15, 143–145
cytolytic T lymphocyte clones, 270–272, 430–432
genetic control of suppression, 132
influence on receptor repertoire, 313, 320–322
noncytolytic T lymphocyte clones, 274–276
recognition and response to, 375–376, 379–382
restricted T cells, cross-reactivity, 279
restriction by GT-TsF, 143
restriction of human T cells, 442–445
T cell activation, 83–84, 87
T cell hybrids, 97
T helper cell recognition of B cells, 391–395
Mb, *see* Myoglobin
MBSA, *see* Methylated bovine serum albumin
Medullary thymocyte, interleukin-1 49
Methylated bovine serum albumin (MBSA)
GAT complexed to, 138
GT complexed to, 139, 142
MHC, *see* Major histocompatibility complex
Micromanipulation
derivation of T cell clones, 269
Moloney leukemia virus-specific CTL clones, 303–305
Migration inhibitory factor (MIF), 341
MIRF, *see* Macrophage Ia recruiting factor
Mitogen, growth factor acting as, 194
Mitogen-induced interleukin-2 production, 27, 60–61, 346
Mitogen-stimulated mononuclear leukocyte, 22
Mitosis, 195–196
Mixed leukocyte culture (MLC), 5, 425
Con-A-activated T cells, 235–236
cytolytic T lymphocytes, 166–169
factors produced by alloreactive T cell clones, 276–277
generation of cytolytic activity, 269–270, 273
interleukin-2, 61
murine T cell clones, 265
response of T cells to *Mls* locus antigens, 274
T cell clones derived from, 426–429
Mixed leukocyte–tumor cell culture (MLTC)
cytolytic activity, 271
murine T cell clones, 265
Mixed lymphocyte reaction (MLR), cytotoxic T lymphocyte precursor frequency, 220–229
MLC, *see* Mixed leukocyte culture
Mls locus, recognition by cloned *H-2* restricted CTL, 291–294
Mls locus determinants, T cells reactive to, 274–276, 279
Mls-specific T lymphocyte, anti-*H-2* reactivity, 331–339
MLTC, *see* Mixed leukocyte-tumor cell culture
Moloney murine leukemia virus (MoLv), 271
cytolytic T lymphocyte specificity, 297–311
Monoclonal antibodies (mAB), 433–435
Monocyte
interleukin-1, 48–49
interleukin-2, 59–60, 62
Mononuclear cells, interleukin-2, 58, 61
Mϕ-SF, *see* Macrophage-derived suppressor factor
Murine cytotoxic T lymphocyte
alloreactive and *H-2*-restricted, 245–251
established lines, 166–169
karyotype evolution, 183–191
Murine fibroblast interferon, 161
Murine interleukin-2
cellular sources, 27–30

Murine interleukin-2 (*cont.*)
polyacrylamide gel electrophoresis, 30-33
purification, 24-26
temperature, chemical, and enzymatic treatments, 26-27
Murine lymphocyte, human interleukin-2 stimulation of, 64
Murine macrophage, interleukin-1, 43-45
Murine sarcoma virus-induced tumor antigens, recognition by CTL clones, 297-311
Murine splenocyte, *in vivo* immunologic effects of cells expanded in TCGF, 453-456, 458, 463
Murine thymocyte
cyclosporin A, 51-52
interleukin-1, 41, 49-50, 496
Murine T lymphocyte
antigen recognition, 368
antigen-specific, 85
clones reactive with alloantigens, 519-525
clones reactive with soluble antigens, 525-529
derivation and analysis of, 265-284
lines, 22
lymphokine production, 253-262
reactivity with soluble antigens, 358-364
Mycobacteria, interleukin-1 release, 47
Myoglobin (Mb), T cells reactive to, 368-373

N

Natural killer (NK) cell, 23
Neoplastic T lymphocyte lines, 405
Nervous system, comparison with immune system, 11-13
Neuraminidase
interleukin-2, 61
treatment of T cell hybrids, 101
NK cell, *see* Natural killer cell
Noncytolytic T lymphocyte clones, 273-276, 278
Nucleotide sequence, 483-485
Nylon wool-purified T lymphocytes, 234-235

O

Oligonucleotide probe, 479-480, 483-485

P

PAGE, *see* Polyacrylamide gel electrophoresis
Papain, degradation of immunoglobulins, 406-408
Partially purified T cell growth factor (PP-TCGF), 77-79
PBL, *see* Peripheral blood mononuclear leukocyte
Peanut agglutinin (PNA)
binding of TsF-H, 153
thymocyte separation, 49-50
Peripheral blood lymphoid cell, *in vivo* immunologic effects of cells expanded in TCGF, 453-456, 463
Peripheral blood mononuclear leukocyte (PBL)
interleukin-2 58-61, 63-66
lytic activities, 72-73
MLC-derived T cell clones, 426-427, 429
PHA assay, 69
PFC, *see* Plaque forming cell
PHA, *see* Phytohemagglutinin
Phorbol ester, interleukin-2 production, 27
Phorbol myristate acetate (PMA)
interleukin-1, 43, 46
interleukin-2, 60
Phosphorylcholine (PC), T cell response to, 474
Phytohemagglutinin (PHA), 2, 5-6, 425
cytolytic T lymphocytes, 167
interleukin-1, 49-50
interleukin-2, 27, 29, 58-62, 64-66
removal from interleukin-2-containing culture supernants, 66-69
Plaque forming cell (PFC), 121
response to GAT, 138-139, 142
SIRS-mediated suppression, 159
suppression by TsF-H, 149-153
Plating efficiencies, 269
Moloney leukemia virus-specific CTL clones, 305
under limited dilution conditions, 418-419
PLT, *see* Primed lymphocyte typing
PMA, *see* Phorbal myristate acetate
PNA, *see* Peanut agglutinin
Pokeweed, interleukin-2, 61
Polyacrylamide gel electrophoresis (PAGE)
helpers, 116
interleukin-2, 30-35
Polyethylene glycol, somatic cell hybrids, 173

Porcine thyroglobulin, PHA removal, 67
PP-TCGF, *see* Partially purified T cell growth factor
Primed lymphocyte typing (PLT), human T cell clones, 413–417, 419, 422, 427–430
Prostaglandin, interleukin-2 production, 62
Puromycin, interleukin-2, 63

R

Rabbit reticulocyte interleukin-2, 36
Rat spleen cell, preparation of TCGF from, 498
Rausher leukemia virus (RLV), 305–306
Receptor repertoire, 11, 272, 313–323
Regulatory lymphocyte, 12–13
RLV, *see* Rausher leukemia virus
RNA, 36–37, 468–476, 481–486

S

Saturated ammonium sulfate (SAS), PHA removal from culture supernatants, 67–69
SDS-PAGE, *see* Sodium dodecyl sulfate-polyacrylamide gel electrophoresis
Sendai virus, somatic cell hybrids, 173
Serology, 16
Serum proteins, interleukin-2 production, 62
Sezary cell, interleukin-2, 60
Sezary syndrome, 59
Sheep red blood cells (SRBC)
  antigen-specific suppressor hybridoma, 99
  precursor cells reactive to, 237–238
  suppressor factor specific for, 127–136
  T suppressor clone specific for, 406
Short-term cultures, cloned T cells derived from, 266–268
Silica, interleukin-1 production, 44–48
SIRS, *see* Soluble immune response suppressor
Skin allograft rejection, 456–457
Sodium butyrate, interleukin-1 production, 46
Sodium dodecyl sulfate-polyacrylamide gel electrophoresis (SDS-PAGE), 116, 505–507
Soft agar technology, *see* Agar cloning of T cells
Soluble antigens
  human T cell clones reactive with, 429–430, 439–447
  murine T cell clones reactive with, 525–529
Soluble immune response suppressor (SIRS), 157–162
Somatic cell genetic analysis
  cell hybrids, 173–176
  cytolytic T lymphocyte functions, 165–181
Somatomedin, 194
Sperm whale myoglobin, T cells reactive to, 368–373
Spleen cell
  antigen-specific T hybrid line, 128, 130–131
  Con-A activated, 158, 205–214
  derivation of T cell clones, 267
  interleukin-2, 58, 60–61, 65–66, 498
  in vivo immunologic effects of cells expanded in TCGF, 453–456, 458, 463
  Moloney leukemia virus-specific cytolytic T cell clones, 298–299
  response to GAT and GT, 139, 142
  stimulation of T cells, 378–380
SRBC, *see* Sheep red blood cells
Suppressor factor
  antigen-specific, from T cell hybrids, 127–136
    antibody-suppressor factor interaction, 132–134
    B cells as targets, 129–130
    characterization, 137–148
    genetic control of suppression, 130–132
  composition, 362
Suppressor T lymphocyte, 84, 157, 362, 405–408
  identification of cells and their products, 138–140
Suppressor T lymphocyte hybridoma, 97–99
  Ia antigens, 103

T

T cell growth factor (TCGF), *see* Interleukin-2
TDL, *see* Thoracic duct lymphocyte
TGAL, 359, 361, 363–364
  T cells reactive to, 368–369, 371, 373
Th cell, *see* Helper T lymphocyte

Thoracic duct lymphocyte (TDL)
antigen-specific T hybrid line, 128–129
interleukin-2, 58–61
Thy antigens, 4, 481
cytolytic T lymphocytes, 172
T cell hybrids, 101
Thymectomy, 3–4
Thymocyte
cyclosporin A, 51–52
interleukin-1, 41, 49–50, 496
Thymoma cell, and cytolytic T cell hybrids, 174–179, 206–214
Thymus, 375–376
Tissue culture techniques, 5
Tissue rejection, 456–457
T lymphocyte, *see also* Cytolytic T lymphocyte; Helper T lymphocyte; Suppressor T lymphocyte
activation, 83–91
alloreactivity, 358, 375–384, 519–525
antigen recognition, 367–374
antigen-restricted recognition, 96
antigen-specific, 85, 361–362
anti-*H-2* reactivity of *Mls*-specific clones, 331–339
clones, 1–2, 5–7
cross-reactive idiotype, 397–404
derivation and analysis of, 265–284
function, specificity, and cell surface markers of human clones, 425–437
factors produced by, 276–278
growth factors, 495–507
immune response regulation by products of, 405–409
in vitro sensitization, 426–430
in vivo immunization, 430–432
cloning, 13–14, 357–358, 530–538
human T lymphocytes, 413–424
cross-reactivity, 241–242
effector functions, 15–16
fusions, 405–406, 507–510
historic overview, 1–9
hybrid determinant recognition, 325–329
interleukin-1, 50–52
interleukin-2 in proliferation of, 22
interleukin-2 production, 60
lymphokines
limiting dilution analysis, 516–518
production, 253–262, 341–345
reactivity with soluble antigens, 358–364, 439–447, 525–529
regulatory function, 16
specificity and heterogenity, 285–295
uses
immunotherapy of cancer, 451–466
in molecular genetics, 467–491
T lymphocyte hybridoma, 95–107; *see also* Helper T lymphocyte hybridoma
antigen-binding structures, 102–103
antigen-specific *H-2* restricted, 119–126
factor production, 120–122
karyotypic analysis, 124–126
receptor theories, 122–123
unexpected *H-2* specificities, 123–124
antigen-specific suppressor factor, 127–148
antibody-suppressor factor interaction, 132–134
B cells as target, 129–130
derivation and specificity, 128–129
genetic control of suppression, 130–132
catalog, 97–99
characterization, 111–112
dual recognition–altered self problem, 112–115
genetics, 470–471
haplotype-specific suppressor factor, 149–155
H-2 restricted hybrids, 109–126
interleukin-2 production, 29
I region, 103–105
isolation, 111
problems, 99–101
production, 508–509
soluble immune response suppressor, 157–162
T lymphocyte precursor
clonal analysis, 236–242
limiting dilution analysis, 515–516
T lymphocyte receptor, 14–15, 95–96, 113, 122–123, 137, 177, 270, 272, 285, 313–323, 357, 362–364, 367
genetics, 468, 481, 486
two-receptor controversy, 338
T lymphocyte replacing factor (TRF), test system for, 255, 257, 259–260
T lymphoma
genetics, 470–473
interleukin-1 analysis, 497–498
TNP-KLH, 360

TNP-specific cytotoxic T lymphocyte, *see* Trinitrophenyl-specific cytotoxic T lymphocyte
Tonsils
  interleukin-2, 58, 60
  PHA removal, 67
TRF, *see* T lymphocyte replacing factor
Trinitrophenylated *Streptococcus* A, precursor cells reactive to, 237–238, 241
Trinitrophenyl-specific cytotoxic T lymphocyte, 248–250
TsF, *see* Antigen-specific T lymphocyte suppressor factor
TsF-H, *see* Haplotype-specific suppressor factor
Type A influenza virus, *see* Influenza virus, type A

U

Ultraviolet radiation, T cell proliferation, 86–88

V

Vaccines, 16
Vicia villosa resistance, 171
  cytolytic T cell hybrids, 206–214
Viral products on T cell hybrids, 100
Virus-specific cytolytic T lymphocyte clones, 285–295
  isolation of, 524–525
VV resistance, *see Vicia villosa* resistance